AVIAN
MEDICINE:

PRINCIPLES AND APPLICATION

ABRIDGED EDITION

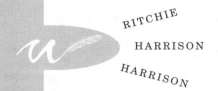

RITCHIE

HARRISON

HARRISON

ABRIDGED BY
DONALD W. ZANTOP

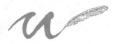

WINGERS PUBLISHING, INC.

Post Office Box 6863 Lake Worth, Florida 33466-6863

AVIAN MEDICINE: PRINCIPLES AND APPLICATION
Unabridged Edition, edited by
 Branson W. Ritchie, DVM, PhD
 Greg J. Harrison, DVM, Dipl. ABVP-Avian
 Linda R. Harrison

Library of Congress Card Catalog Number: 96-61840
ISBN: 0-9636996-5-2

Project Coordinator: Roy A. Faircloth
Editorial Director: Linda R. Harrison
Art Director: Kari W. McCormick
Production Assistant: Richard Larson
Medical Illustration: Leslie E. Sealing

AVIAN MEDICINE: PRINCIPLES AND APPLICATION
ABRIDGED EDITION

Abridged by
 Donald W. Zantop, DVM, Dipl. ABVP-Avian

©1997 Wingers Publishing, Inc.

FROM THE PUBLISHER

This abridged edition of *Avian Medicine: Principles and Application*, is designed to be used in conjunction with the original text, which remains an unparalleled classic. Our intention is to make the details included in the 9-pound, 1384-page comprehensive book and CD-ROM more accessible on a daily, quick reference basis.

We feel privileged that Dr. Donald Zantop was willing to take on the enormous task of abridging the work, for he is a model of the small animal practitioner for whom the book was originally written. Not only did he spend innumerable hours selecting the most pertinent clinical material to include in the condensed version, he added practical comments, as indicated, in the few areas where new information has become available. The Formulary, a continually evolving tool for the avian clinician, contains some additional data in this version.

We welcome your comments and appreciate your commitment to the practice of quality avian medicine and surgery.

WINGERS PUBLISHING, INC.

PREFACE

In 1976, I came to avian practice armed only with copies of Petrak's Diseases of Cage and Aviary Birds and Sturkie's Avian Physiology. A colleague, William Brunn, DVM, gave me a set of index cards on common diseases and treatments that became my first serious reference on avian medicine.

Today, a thorough understanding of avian medicine requires attention to many texts and journals, and this handbook does not replace the scholarly text that it abridges. Rather, it serves as a complement to that accumulated know-ledge, giving the avian practitioner readily available answers to problems encountered daily, "index cards" to refresh the mind.

My patients and I are indebted to these authors and to practitioners who, like Dr. Brunn, continue to share their knowledge with me. I encourage you to follow their example and share your knowledge with your colleagues.

DONALD W. ZANTOP, DVM

Diplomate, ABVP - Avian Practice
Fallston Veterinary Hospital
Fallston, Maryland

TABLE OF CONTENTS

THE AVIAN PATIENT

Ross A. Perry

In a single day, an avian practitioner may be presented with patients that belong to five different orders. Each of these orders is unique, having evolved specific anatomic, physiologic and behavioral characteristics that allow effective competition in a specific ecological niche. Which of the numerous avian genera will serve as an appropriate comparative model (ie, generic bird patient)? The avian clinician can be most effective by disposing of the philosophical handicap of basing medical decisions on a generic companion bird. For now avian veterinarians will continue to be required to diagnose and treat many medical problems subjectively until results from avian research efforts begin to satisfy the demand for information.

In developing a health plan, clients and veterinarians must strive to view the world from the bird's perspective, and, in so doing, caretakers will have greater empathy for the emotional as well as the medical needs of the bird. If the complete needs of a bird are not met (nutritional, environmental and psychologic), disease will inevitably follow. The veterinarian must prescribe health, not drugs. By being familiar with the behavioral attributes and species-specific medical problems that may occur, a veterinarian is more likely to recognize early signs of disease in an individual bird of a given species.

Selection of Companion Birds

In providing exceptional care and management advice, the veterinarian can become a model for responsible companion bird ownership. Unfortunately, many individuals obtain a bird for the wrong reasons (Table 1.1), instead of for the purpose of adding an intelligent, sensitive being to the family. Some clients rarely handle their birds, even if they do not bite. To highly social birds, this forced isolation must be a fate worse than death. Most clients are very appreciative of some supervised training from their veterinarian on how to handle their bird, but may be reluctant to ask for guidance (see Chapter 4).

Table 1.1   Misguided Reasons for Choosing Birds as Pets
• Entertainment
• Amusement
• Admiration
• Material acquisitions
• Self-admiration ("He says my name!")
• Toys for adults
• Toys for children
• Didn't want to see it suffer in the pet shop.

Bird Attributes

Individual clients are likely to differ as to which attributes of companion birds are desirable and which are undesirable. Avian veterinarians and aviculturists should also strive to match the correct personality of a bird with the personality of an owner. Bird clients who understand the "uniqueness" of avian species are usually happy with their birds' qualities.

Wild-trapped and Imported Birds

It is the belief of the author and editors that to be effective messengers for conservation and responsible stewardship, every avian veterinarian and aviculturist must strive to understand the damage induced by the harvesting of wild-caught birds, and to take every perceivable opportunity to stop these activities.

Captive-bred, Hand-raised Birds

Captive-bred, properly hand-raised birds make better pets than their wild-trapped conspecifics; however, malnutrition, candidiasis, stunting and various leg, toe, nail and beak deformities can occur in captive-raised birds. Bonding and breeding behavior in captive-bred and hand-raised birds (eg, masturbation, bizarre courting and behavioral rituals, excessive feather plucking and self-mutilation) can occur in improperly socialized birds as they reach sexual maturity. Male birds rubbing their backside and leaving "water" on their owner's hand is a common and notable example. Some clients will not accept that the bird is masturbating and needs behavioral modification support (see Chapter 4).

Some species such as Rose-breasted Cockatoos, large macaws, conures, Monk Parakeets and Sulphur-crested Cockatoos are particularly prone to excessive bonding and self-mutilation secondary to separation anxiety. The "mini" macaws, smaller Amazon parrots, Pionus parrots, *Poicephalus* species and Umbrella Cockatoos are less likely to develop these traits. These problems can be prevented in most birds by an effective socialization program when the bird is young. Repeated generations of captive birds become increasingly docile and more adaptive to captivity.

Taming Companion Birds

Young, hand-raised Psittaciformes adapt readily to new surroundings and handling procedures. They should be exposed early in life to novel situations (eg, car travel, hospital visits, multiple visitors in the household, other household pets) so that they are well adjusted to these events. Older birds, especially wild-

Table 1.3   Profiles of Common Companion Birds (Some characteristics are rated on a scale from 1 to 10, with 10 being the highest value)

African Grey Parrots (Africa)
Excellent talkers, individual variability (9)
Extremely intelligent - high-strung
Prolific breeders once initiated
Require attention (10)
Relatively playful (8)
Tend to form individual bonds

Amazon parrots (Mexico to South America)
Few enjoy "petting"
Excellent talkers (9), species-dependent
Extroverted personalities
Aggressive during breeding season
Tend to form individual bonds
Require attention (9)

Budgerigars (Australia)
Gregarious - easily tamed (10)
Good talkers but require work (7)
Quiet and nondestructive
Wild-type are most disease-resistant
Relatively gentle (8)

Canaries (Australia and Africa)
Color mutations are genetically weak
Breed prolifically in captivity
Males are vocal singers
Tidy and easy to care for
Do not like to be handled

Cockatiels (Australia)
Excellent companion birds (10)
Easily tamed and gentle (9)
Quiet and nondestructive (8)
Good whistlers - limited talkers
Mutations - weak

Cockatoos (Australia, New Zealand, South Pacific Islands)
Require attention (10)
Scream if neglected
Crave physical contact (10)
Hand-raised Umbrella Cockatoos are extremely gentle (9)
Intelligent, easily house-trained
Produce abundant powder (10)
Can be noisy; destructive; must be socialized
Mate aggression is common, particularly in Sulphur-crested

Conures (Mexico to South America)
Species variability
Smaller species are gregarious & playful
Enjoy and seek attention (9)
Noisy and destructive (7)
Generally poor talkers

Eclectus Parrots (Australia and South Pacific Islands)
Generally lethargic and unplayful
Dimorphic (males=green, females=red)
Males are more gentle than females
Tend to form individual pair bonds

Finches (Australia and Africa)
Melodious songs
Short-lived

Lories, lorikeets (Australia, South Pacific Islands)
Colorful, playful, active
Noisy and limited talking ability
High-carbohydrate liquid diet; messy
Frequently bathe

Lovebirds (Africa)
Relatively nondestructive, quiet
Hand-raised birds are calm
Parent-raised birds are hard to tame

Macaws (Mexico to South America)
Extremely intelligent
Require attention (10)
Can be destructive
Require large living space
Tend to be noisy (10)
Aggressive during breeding season
Blue and Gold most family-oriented
Hyacinth - least noisy, most mellow

Mynahs (India)
Prefer not to be handled
Good talkers (7)
Loose, messy droppings
Nondestructive

Pionus parrots (Mexico to South America)
Small and quiet
May hyperventilate when disturbed
Highly stressed
High altitude species cannot tolerate heat and humidity

Toucans (South America)
Quiet and antic
Prefer some live food (rodents)
Highly territorial
Messy, loose droppings

caught adults, are usually very difficult to tame. Patience, self-discipline, a sense of ritual, food bribery and reward are necessary to tame some adult birds (see Chapter 4). Even then, they are rarely trustworthy and may bite without provocation.

Genetic Factors

Determining the physical and behavioral attributes of related birds, especially the parents and siblings, can be of value in selecting a companion bird. It should be noted that large Psittaciformes have the capacity to live as long as humans, and adding a large psittacine bird to the family should be undertaken as a life-long commitment. Knowing the genetic background and characteristics of the relatives of a bird is particularly critical when choosing a pair of breeding birds.

Color Mutations

It should be noted that mutations in color are generally the result of continued inbreeding. In selecting for particular color mutations (eg, lutino cockatiels), scant priority is placed on other important attributes, so that decreased disease resistance, disorders, reduced longevity and birth defects often result.

Conformation and Size

Currently, show budgerigars are approximately twice the mass of their free-ranging conspecifics. Attempts to produce larger birds has also led to numerous undesirable characteristics including feathering that impairs flight, interferes with normal ambulation, accumulates excrement pericloacally and protrudes across and sometimes into the cornea.

Longevity

Some highly bred strains of birds may have life expectancies one-third to one-tenth the duration of "wild-type" or less highly inbred individuals of the same species. For example, it is believed that inbreeding has contributed to the reduction in the life expectancy of cockatiels from a record of 32 years to the present-day average of four to six years. When seeking a healthy companion bird that has the greatest potential of reaching its full life expectancy, clients should avoid highly inbred birds in favor of the wild-type characteristics.

Selected Species Recommendations

The Grey-cheeked Parakeet, Dusky and Maroon-bellied Conures and Monk Parakeets are reputed to be relatively resistant to common diseases and are longer-lived than most cockatiels, budgerigars and lovebirds. Grey-cheeked Parakeets have been described as quiet but playful; the conures are not as quiet, yet they can be tame and affectionate; and the Monk Parakeet is considered docile, quiet and relatively nondestructive. Other bird species that are considered relatively quiet include the Ring-necked Parakeet, Pionus species, Hawk-headed Parrot, Caique, Dusky-crowned Conure, Senegal Parrot, Jardines Parrot, Cape Parrot, Meyer's Parrot, Red-bellied Parrot and Brown-headed Parrot.

Choosing a Healthy Bird

Parameters that may increase the likelihood of adding a healthy, mentally stable companion bird to the family are:

- Obtaining the bird from a reputable breeder who specializes in the particular species or genus of bird that is desired and has a closed flock.
- Obtaining the bird from a reputable source who works in close liaison with an avian veterinarian.

Table 1.4 Suggested Longevity of Selected Companion Species

Bird	Maximum	Average
Gouldian Finch	unknown	4
Zebra Finch	17	5
Canary	20	8
Mynah	17	3
Toucan	unknown	4
Budgerigar	18	6
Agapornis sp.	12	4
Neophema	10	5
Cockatiel	32	5
Rainbow Lorikeet	15	3
Rosella	15	3
Eclectus Parrot	20	8
Galah	20	5
Bare-eyed Cockatoo	40	15
Sulphur-crested Cockatoo	40	15
African Grey Parrot	50	15
Pionus parrot	23	5
Amazon parrot	80	15
Macaw	50	15
Conure	25	10
Grey-cheeked Parakeet	15	8
Superb Parrot	36	6
Domestic pigeon	26	15

- Obtaining a young, recently fledged, parent- or hand-raised bird.
- Obtaining a well adapted companion bird from an individual who is no longer able to provide for the pet (due to age, moving, finances).
- Obtaining a bird that has normal-appearing feathers and droppings, a good appetite, appears to be bright, alert and responsive to its environment, and has not been exposed to birds from other sources.

Parameters that increase the likelihood of adding a diseased, unhappy bird to the family are:
- Obtaining a wild-trapped bird.
- Obtaining a recently imported bird.
- Obtaining a bird suspected of being smuggled.
- Obtaining a bird with an asymmetrical beak, excessively scaly legs, twisted digits, missing toes, a blocked nostril, slight swelling around the eyes, deformed eyelids, stained feathers above the nostrils, stained feathers around the vent, tail bobbing, fluffed appearance, soiled vent, poor feather quality, diarrhea, yellow urates, increased urine production, pectoral muscle atrophy, abdominal distention, fault lines and depigmented feathers (eg, black or yellow where normally green plumage occurs).

Identifying an overtly ill bird in a retail outlet should caution the consumer to purchase a bird from another source. Birds that are unusually inexpensive for the species may have a sordid past that can include specific diseases or exposure to pathogens that may cause problems when the birds are introduced to a home or aviary. Wild-caught birds, particularly those that are likely to be illegal imports (smuggled), should always be avoided.

Health Checks

A veterinarian is well advised to seek legal advice in developing a form to be used as a certificate of examination. The term "health certificate" should be avoided because it is impossible to certify "health." It is possible only to certify that no abnormalities were detected using a particular battery of tests. The expectations of a dealer or client regarding a veterinary examination may be quite different, and requirements and liabilities are likely to vary among countries and states.

Clients should always be offered state-of-the-art diagnostic, medical and surgical services that are available on a national level. It is then the client's choice to determine what level of care they desire for their pet. It is important to note in a patient's medical record what services were offered to a client and which of those services were chosen, in order to prevent accusations of negligence. A state-of-the-art health examination for birds can include a physical examination, CBC, biochemistries, radiographs, endoscopy, Gram's stain of the feces and rostral choanal slit, *Chlamydia* sp. screening and (where available) DNA probing for psittacine beak and feather disease (PBFD) virus and polyomavirus.

When all the data on a patient is collected and evaluated, the practitioner can state only that in his opinion, there were no detectable abnormalities at the time of testing. Table 1.5 lists some disease conditions that are frequently diagnosed in popular companion bird species.

Transporting the Bird

Clinicians will need to evaluate a bird's excrement for the day or two before an examination. If the bird's enclosure is too large to move (in most situations it should be), then clean butcher's wrap or any nonabsorbent paper should be placed on the bottom of the bird's enclosure for 12-24 hours before an appointment. The paper should then be brought with the bird to the veterinarian.

The Home Environment

Quarantine

If a client already has companion birds, any new additions to the household should be isolated (quarantined) for six to eight weeks. It should be noted that many avian infectious diseases involve a carrier state (eg, PBFD virus, polyomavirus, Pacheco's disease virus) and that quarantine alone is insufficient to ensure that one of these diseases is not introduced to a home.

Enclosures

Enclosures for companion birds should be as spacious as possible, with emphasis on length more than depth or height. The minimum size would allow a bird to spread its wings without touching the

Table 1.5 Common Diseases in Companion Birds by Species*

African Grey and Timneh Grey Parrots
Feather picking
Rhinoliths (bacterial, fungal, secondary to malnutrition)
Oral abscesses
Hypocalcemia syndrome
Hypovitaminosis A
Resistant bacterial infections - Klebsiella, Pseudomonas, E. coli, Staphylococcus, Aspergillus
Neoplasms (apparent higher incidence than other species)
Tapeworm infestation (imported birds)
Blood parasites (occasionally imported birds)
Reovirus
PBFD virus
Hematuria syndrome in infants
Non-regenerative anemia (neonates)
Neuropathic gastric dilatation

Amazon parrots
Bumblefoot
Hematuria with metal poisoning (Zn, Hg, Pb)
Egg-binding
Chronic sinusitis, pharyngitis, tracheitis
Hypovitaminosis A
Chlamydiosis - rhinitis, sinusitis, enteritis
Polyomavirus
Malcolored feathers (hepatopathy or malnutrition)
Oral abscesses
Lymphocytosis
Poxvirus infection (primarily imports)
Mutilation syndromes
Cloacal papillomatosis
Epilepsy in Red-lored Amazons (idiopathic)
Neoplasia (especially liver adenocarcinomas)
Herpesvirus-induced tracheitis
Coagulopathies

Budgerigars
Neoplasm (lipoma, testes, ovary, liver, kidney)
Goiter
Hypothyroidism (not documented)
Polyomavirus
Unilateral leg paralysis - renal or gonadal neoplasia
Knemidokoptes sp. mite infections
Feather mites and lice in Australian budgies
Retained feather sheaths
Overgrowth of beak and nails (malnutrition or hepatopathy)
Egg-binding
Pododermatitis
Gout
Trichomoniasis
Obesity
Diabetes mellitus
Hyperglycemia secondary to neoplasms
French Moult (acute PBFD or polyomavirus)
Polyfolliculosis
Chlamydiosis (usually chronic low grade)
Giardiasis
Megabacteria
Mycoplasmosis
Salpingitis
Ovarian cysts
Stroke (older budgerigars)
Coccidiosis
Splay leg in juveniles
Cere abscesses
Hepatopathy
Pancreatic insufficiency

Canaries
Feather cysts
Obesity - lipoma
Alopecia syndrome
Straw feather syndrome
Knemidokoptes sp. mite infection
Air sac and tracheal mites
Canary pox
Dry gangrene of extremities
Myeloproliferative disease
Egg binding, egg-related peritonitis
Dyspnea (acute, inhaled seeds)
Yolk emboli
Lymphocytosis
Eosinophilia with inflammation
Cataracts
Plasmodium sp. and toxoplasmosis

Cockatiels
Giardiasis (in USA)
Ascaridiasis in Australia
Mycoplasmosis
Spirochetosis
Obesity
Idiopathic neurologic dysfunctions
Diabetes mellitus
Egg-binding and egg-related peritonitis
Dyspnea (acute, inhaled seed)
Yolk emboli
Eosinophilia with inflammation
Sinusitis, conjunctivitis
Paralysis of lower eyelid, weak eye blink
Mouth and tongue paralysis (neonates)
Yellow feathers in lutinos (hepatopathies)
Pancreatitis
Liver failure - fatty liver, cirrhosis, neoplasia

Cockatoos
Self-mutilation (feathers, skin)
Psychotic behavior
Idiopathic liver cirrhosis
Tapeworm infestation (wild-caught)
Blood parasites (recently imported)
Proliferative foot lesions (herpesvirus)
Pododermatitis
Cere hypertrophy and occluded nares
Oral abscesses
Trematode infestation (imported birds)
Obesity
Lipomas (Rose-breasted and Sulphur-crested)
Cloacal prolapse (idiopathic)
Microhepatia

Corella, Short-billed and Long-billed
Acute and chronic PBFD virus
Malnutrition
Upper respiratory tract infections
Bumblefoot and leg calluses
Anti-social behavior
Jealousy and aggression (breeding season)

Table 1.5   Common Diseases in Companion Birds by Species* *(continued)*

Gang Gang Cockatoos
Malnutrition
Metabolic bone disease (juveniles)
Feather picking, barbering and self-mutilation
PBFD virus

Major Mitchell's Cockatoos
PBFD virus
Aspergillosis
Sinusitis
Metabolic bone disease in juveniles
Pododermatitis and leg calluses
Feather picking and barbering

Rosellas
PBFD virus
Feather picking
Aggression toward people & other birds
Flightiness
Pododermatitis (often severe)
Motile protozoa (fatal intestinal disease)

Conures
Black splotches in feathers (malnutrition, hepatopathy)
Pacheco's disease virus carriers (probably no more so than other South American species)
Polyomavirus
Bleeding syndrome
Screaming
Feather picking (severe)
Cannibalism
PBFD virus
Megabacteria
Heat stress
Neuropathic gastric dilatation
Hypocalcemia

Eclectus Parrots
Lead poisoning, biliverdinuria
Female aggressiveness
Annular toe deformities
Feather picking
Cataracts
PBFD virus
Polyomavirus
Hypovitaminosis A

Finches
Air sac mites - Gouldians
Tapeworms
Trichomoniasis
Bacterial infections (very susceptible)
Egg binding
Lymphocytosis
Foreign body constrictive toe necrosis
Dry gangrene of extremities

Frogmouths, Tawny (Australian captive)
Erysipelas
Subcutaneous white worms
Nutritional deficiencies (vitamin B complex-responsive neurologic signs)
Fatal pandemic convulsive syndrome
Obesity

Grey-cheeked Parakeets (*Brotogeris* sp.)
Sarcoptiform mange (*Metamicrolichus nudus*)
Chronic active hepatitis (*E. coli*)

Normally high AST values
Mycobacteriosis
Chlamydiosis
Feather picking refractory to therapy
Resistance to disease and stress
Screaming
Nail trimming lameness

Kakariki
Knemidokoptes sp. (new species in feathers)
PBFD virus

Kookaburra
Obesity and fatty liver syndrome (excess fat)
Vitamin B complex-responsive neurologic disorders
Gapeworm

King Parrots (Australia)
Acute PBFD virus (juveniles)
Chlamydiosis

Lorikeets
Hepatopathy
PBFD virus
Fungal infections
Coccidiosis
Ascaridiasis
Cestodes
Bacterial infections
Injuries
Necrotic enteritis (possibly clostridial)

Lovebirds (*Agapornis* spp.)
Aggression
Cannibalism
PBFD virus
Polyfolliculitis
Megabacteria
Heat stress
Lovebird pox
Epilepsy (idiopathic)
Viral infections
Obstetrical problems (egg binding)
Bilateral clenched foot syndrome
Capillariasis
Self-mutilation "stress dermatitis" axillae, patagium and base of tail

Macaws
Avian viral serositis
Neuropathic gastric dilatation
Sensitive to doxycycline, trimethoprim, gas anesthetics
Behavioral problems
Capillaria and ascarid infestation (imported birds)
Feather cysts in Blue and Golds
Oral and cloacal papillomatosis
Feather picking and mutilation
Herpesvirus feet lesions
Sunken eye sinusitis
Annular toe deformities in juveniles
Pancreatic dysfunctions
Cataracts
Polycythemia in Blue and Golds
Sensitive to vitamin D_3
Uric acid gout in young Blue and Golds
Upper respiratory tract infection and sneezing

Table 1.5	Common Diseases in Companion Birds by Species* (continued)
Malcolored feathers (turn black in Blue and Golds and miniature macaws) Polyomavirus Microhepatia Coagulopathies **Magpies, Australian** Soft pliable beaks and bones in juveniles (parathyroid gland dysfunction) Spiruroid throat worms Scaly leg mite (*Knemidokoptes*-like) **Mynahs** Hepatopathies Iron storage disease Cirrhosis of liver Chronic active hepatitis Combination hepatopathy Heart disease	Eye diseases (corneal scratches, keratitis, chronic keratoconjunctivitis) Epilepsy (idiopathic) **Pionus Parrots** Obesity Malnutrition Respiratory infections Poxvirus infection **Toucans** Hepatopathies Bacterial infections Giardiasis Coccidiosis Beak injuries Diabetes mellitus (Toco Toucans) Iron storage disease

This list is a guide to the most commonly reported clinical problems. All species discussed are susceptible to malnutrition, bacterial infections, fungal infections and toxicities. All Psittaciformes are susceptible to Chlamydia sp. to varying degrees. Unless a species has a particular propensity or a characteristic presentation, these problems are not mentioned. Diseases mentioned may be common in some localities or bird populations, whereas the same diseases are rarely encountered in other localities or populations.

sides of the enclosure. The enclosure should be clean and easy to service and should be constructed of a durable, nontoxic material. Newspaper, paper towels or paper bags appear to be the best substances for the bottom of the enclosure. They are inexpensive, easy to clean and do not promote the growth of pathogens as do wood chips or ground corncob. Cedar, redwood and pressure-treated wood chips should not be used for substrate or nesting material with birds.

Position of Enclosure

A bird's enclosure should be positioned so that at least some of the perches allow the bird to be at or above eye level of standing family members. Birds are generally more secure at this level than lower and are less likely to develop dominant or aggressive tendencies than if they are placed at higher levels. The enclosure should be positioned so that it partially receives direct sunlight on a daily basis and offers a shaded area. The need to avoid drafts is exaggerated. Covering birds is discouraged because fresh air is more important than being exposed to home lights. A bird is best kept in the dark for sleeping.

It is ideal for a companion bird to have a large outdoor enclosure in which it can be placed on a regular basis for exercise and exposure to fresh air and sunlight. An outdoor enclosure for a companion bird should be protected from extremes in weather as well as from predators and rodents.

Perches

Perches should be made from selected branches of clean, nontoxic hardwood trees and shrubs that have never been sprayed with pesticides or chemicals and are free from mold and wood rot. Variably sized perches should be provided; those with small diameters allow the toes to almost touch when wrapped around the perch and those with large diameters cause the feet to be flattened. The use of concrete perches in combination with wood perches is becoming increasingly popular and appears to be safe as long as the diet is balanced and natural perching is also available. Sandpaper perches should never be used in a bird's enclosure. They have no effect on nail length and may predispose a bird to foot problems.

Toys

Any toys available to a bird must be free of toxic metals, hooks, sharp objects or small, easily consumed components. Various gadgetry can be placed in a psittacine's enclosure to stimulate activity and satisfy its natural tendency to chew. There is no quality control for the avian toy market, and the client must be acutely aware of potentially dangerous toys. Toys designed for small birds should not be used with larger birds. There are some common toy components that are more dangerous than others. These include snap-type clasps, open chain links and bell clappers that can be removed and swallowed. Safer toys have a screw-type clasp with closed chain links. Most toys with a thin rope or substantial length of chain should be provided to a bird only while it is under direct supervision. If left in an enclosure, a bird can become easily entangled in these toys and die from asphyxiation. The most suitable toys for unsupervised birds include natural foods such as grass runners (eg, kikuyu, buffalo grass), various seed pods (eg, melaleuca, hakea, eucalyptus, callistemon and especially banksia for larger cockatoos), liquid amber, pine cones, vegetables, apple cores, clumps or tufts of grass freshly sprayed with water and short lengths of soft wood with bark attached (especially if live beetle larvae or borers are present).

Mirrors

Some mirrors contain mercury, which is toxic if consumed. Some properly made and designed glass and plastic mirrors are suitable for small birds but can be readily demolished and consumed by large Psittaciformes. Polished stainless steel mirrors are more suitable for large birds. Windows and large mirrors in rooms where birds are allowed to exercise should be covered to prevent inexperienced or startled birds from flying into these fixed objects causing severe head and neck trauma.

Hygiene and Sanitation

With a companion bird, it is better to be fanatical with cleanliness rather than to rely on disinfectants to prevent disease transmission in a dirty, contaminated environment. Water and food containers should be physically scrubbed or placed in the dishwasher on a daily basis to prevent the accumulation of slime and algae.

When disinfectants are necessary, chlorine or glutaraldehyde preparations are effective for most avian pathogens (see Chapter 2). Many disinfectants emit toxic fumes and should be used only with adequate ventilation and never near a bird. Disinfectants should be thoroughly rinsed from an enclosure to prevent the bird from contacting residual compounds.

Feeding and Watering Techniques

Healthy birds should always have a supply of clean, fresh, uncontaminated water. There is frequent discussion concerning the use of chlorhexidine in the water to reduce bacterial growth; however, in addition to reducing bacteria in water, this agent also alters the normal microbial population of the gastrointestinal tract (see Chapter 5). The routine addition of any disinfectant to a bird's water should be discouraged. Water that has been "sitting" in plastic or copper pipes can accumulate toxic levels of some chemicals, and pipes should be flushed for several minutes before collecting drinking water. Some city municipalities add disinfectants and algae inhibitors to the water that can be toxic to birds and fish. Many companion birds will readily adapt to a water bottle, which is easier to clean and keep free of contaminating food and excrement than a water bowl.

Birds should be provided fresh food in clean bowls on a daily basis. A combination of formulated diets (85%) supplemented with some fresh fruits and vegetables (15%) appears to keep a bird in the best health (see Chapter 31).

Grit

Whether or not to provide soluble shell grit and insoluble coarse sand grit to a bird is controversial. This practice is viewed with disfavor in the United States, especially if given free choice, which may lead to over-consumption and obstructive gastritis. In Australia, grit is frequently offered to companion birds with few ill effects; however, birds fed formulated diets are unlikely to need either insoluble or soluble grit. As a compromise, a cockatiel-sized bird can be offered five grains of grit biannually; a cockatoo-sized bird can be offered a half-teaspoon of grit biannually.

Preventive Care

Wing Clipping

The clinician should determine the client's expectations of the appearance and the reduced flight capacity of the bird prior to performing a wing clip. The client should authorize the trimming or removal of any feather that will alter the appearance or function of the bird, particularly with respect to show or racing birds. It is important to identify and avoid any pin feathers (blood feathers, blood quills), as a developing feather that is cut below the pulp cap will bleed profusely.

The goal of clipping the wings is to prevent the bird from developing rapid and sustained flight, *not* to make a bird incapable of flight. Excessive wing trims can result in fractures of the legs, wings or lacerations of the keel.

Nail Clipping

A short length (usually about 2 mm) of the nail can be removed by trimming or grinding without causing pain or bleeding. Short-blade podiatric nail clippers can be used to trim the tip of the nail with minimal risk of accidentally cutting adjacent toes.

Alternately, a motor driven hobby grinder (preferably with a rheostat foot switch) with a cone-shaped stone may be used for filing and shaping nails and beaks. Any bleeding that does occur is best controlled with a bipolar radiosurgical unit (beak), silver nitrate stick (nails) or Monsel's solution (both). It is best not to use a silver nitrate stick around the beak.

Bathing

Many birds enjoy a bath or shower and should be given the opportunity to determine the degree and duration of exposure to moisture. Frequent misting encourages normal grooming activity, which is critical to proper feather maintenance.

Identification Methods

Leg Band Removal

Open leg bands should always be removed from companion birds. Some closed leg bands aid in the identification of a bird and may suggest that the bird was captive-bred; however, they can constitute a health hazard.

It is generally recommended to anesthetize a bird with isoflurane to ensure that a band is safely removed. Small closed bands made of plastic or aluminum can be easily transected with Heath-type stitch removing scissors. Two diagonally opposing cuts are made and the band falls off in two halves. Large split bands are easiest to remove by using two pairs of locking pliers to apply opposing force at the site of the opening. Bands that are associated with constrictive accumulations of keratin (in-grown bands) can best be removed by using a variable speed hobby tool and a fine tip cutting bit.

Tattoos

Specific information placed in the skin of a bird by tattoo rarely remains legible. In practice, tattoos are generally restricted to indicating the gender of a bird following endoscopic evaluation of the gonads. By convention, tattoo ink injected into the left patagial membrane indicates a female and in the right patagial membrane indicates a male. The tattoo ink used should be sterilized to prevent the ink from serving as a nidus for bacterial granulomas

Microchips

Microchips are small electronic devices that are injected into the musculature (usually, the pectoral muscle of birds) to provide permanent identification. Unfortunately, there is no industry standard, and a single reader model cannot identify all available microchips. Microchips can be injected into the pectoral muscle of most birds without sedation or anesthesia, although given the option, the author prefers to perform the procedure in an anesthetized bird.

DNA Fingerprinting

DNA fingerprinting offers a technique for accurately identifying an individual bird and, with proper samples, identifying the bird's immediate relatives.

THE AVIAN FLOCK

Susan L. Clubb
Keven Flammer

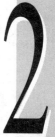

Avicultural medicine differs from clinical care of individual companion birds in several very important ways. In general, the health of the flock is of primary concern, and establishing a diagnosis or preventing exposure of the flock to an infectious agent is usually more important than providing supportive care for the individual ill bird.

The economics of the companion bird industry are changing. As production increases, sale prices for individual captive-bred birds decline. The commercial producer often operates on a slim margin of profit. Understanding the economics of the companion bird industry is vital for a successful avicultural practice.

Flock Preventive Medicine

The Veterinarian/Aviculturist Relationship

Table 2.1 lists routine veterinary services that are beneficial to aviculturists.

Veterinary/client confidentiality is of utmost importance for the avicultural client. Inappropriate discussions concerning disease problems in an avicultural facility can permanently and irreparably damage a facility's reputation. Clinical staff must be counseled in strict professional behavior to ensure they also maintain client/doctor confidentiality.

Table 2.1	Veterinary Services of Benefit to Aviculture

- Perform new bird examinations
- Perform resident bird examination
- Assist in establishing & maintaining records
- Establish a preventive medicine program
- Offer husbandry advice
- Provide emergency care for aviary birds
- Take appropriate action for disease outbreaks
- Evaluate reproductive failure
- Assist with incubation and pediatric problems

Flock Monitoring Team

The veterinarian should work closely with the aviculturist to establish an effective preventive medicine program. Quarantine procedures, parasite control techniques, pest control, identification systems, first aid procedures and subclinical disease testing (chlamydia, PBFD virus, polyomavirus) should be discussed. A healthy, pre-existing aviculturist/veterinarian relationship ensures fast action if a disease outbreak occurs.

Aviary Visits

Veterinarians and their staff should be aware of potential biosecurity hazards to avoid being mechanical vectors for disease transmission between individual patients or avicultural facilities. The veterinarian should visit only one avicultural facility a day, preferably in the morning prior to entering the hospital. If this is not feasible, it is best to have each facility maintain coveralls, scrubs and shoes that can be worn while evaluating that facility. These clothes then remain at the facility for laundering.

Selling Birds

Pre-sale testing for selected infectious diseases such as polyomavirus, PBFD virus or chlamydiosis, may help assure the buyer of good health. Pet retailers and breeders often require a veterinary examination within a certain period of time in order to activate a guarantee.

A suggested guarantee may last for 14-30 days post-purchase as long as the buyer has the bird examined within seven days. An immediate refund should be considered if the buyer's veterinarian determines that a bird has a health problem.

The New Bird

Acquisition

The purchase of captive-bred birds for breeding stock is logical for many species. Many psittacine and passerine species have adapted well to captivity and breed prolifically in properly designed aviaries. In some cases, hand-fed neonates are not thought to produce well in captivity, while in other cases these birds reach sexual maturity at a much younger age than expected and readily reproduce.

Although the purchase of culled breeders from another aviculturist should be viewed with suspicion, moving a pair of healthy, unproductive birds to a new environment frequently initiates breeding activity. The buyer should attempt to obtain as much information as possible about the seller and the birds before purchase. The first question to ask the potential seller would be, "Why is this bird or pair being sold?"

Evaluating a Prospective Purchase

The addition of new birds to an established aviary increases the potential for introducing an infectious disease. Additionally, new birds that are misrepresented (inaccurately sexed or sold, due to previous reproductive failure) represent a loss to the aviculturist by occupying space and requiring care that could be used for productive pairs. Examination of a breeding bird being considered for addition to the aviary should be more than a health exam. The bird's gender and the visual health of the reproductive tract should be confirmed by laparoscopy. Diagnostic testing should be based on the client's needs, species of birds, source of the birds and any questionable abnormalities detected on physical examination.

Quarantine

The type of examinations performed, length of the quarantine period and preventive techniques vary according to the resources of the aviculturist, the species and source of the birds being added and the type of collection. If a bird leaves a facility for any reason and is exposed to any other birds, it should be considered contaminated and must be placed in quarantine before being returned to its normal enclosure. Neonates that leave the nursery and come into contact with other birds should not re-enter the nursery.

Quarantine Facilities

Ideally, birds in quarantine should be housed separately from the remainder of the collection for a minimum of sixty days. Birds that are maintained in any enclosure (home or building) with the same air space should not be considered to be in quarantine.

New Bird Examination

Birds should be examined at the beginning of quarantine to establish any pre-existing problems and again at the end of quarantine to detect any clinical changes that may have occurred (see Chapter 8). It is critical for the aviculturist to understand that quarantine is only a "safety valve" in the prevention of infectious disease and does not ensure that a new bird is not an asymptomatic carrier of parasitic, bacterial or viral pathogens.

Suggested screening techniques would include a thorough physical examination, Gram's stain of feces and evaluation of a blood smear. Complete blood count, blood chemistry profile and cultures are useful to detect birds that require more extensive evaluation. By performing a complete CBC, biochemical profile and radiographs on each new bird in a facility, the veterinarian is able to establish a "normal value" for a particular test in a particular bird. Specific diagnostic screening tests that should be considered include ELISA tests for chlamydia and DNA probes for polyomavirus and psittacine beak and feather disease virus (see Chapter 32). Direct and flotation examination of feces for internal parasites should also be considered in birds that were recently imported or that are in flights with access to the ground (see Chapter 36). Any thin birds, especially species susceptible to neuropathic gastric dilatation (proventricular dilatation disease) should be examined radiographically.

Identification

Implantable transponders provide the least alterable identification with minimal risk to the bird. Closed bands can be used as an adjunct to or replacement for transponders but are not ideal. Properly fitting closed bands are an indication (not proof) that a bird was bred in captivity.

Closed bands are currently required for export of captive-bred birds of CITES-listed species. Unfortunately, the numbers often wear off closed bands and large birds may collapse them, resulting in leg or foot injuries. In addition, bands can catch on loose enclosure wires. These disadvantages should not dissuade the serious aviculturist from closed banding nor should they encourage the veterinarian to remove those bands.

Open bands are the least desirable but are none the less an effective means of identification. Metal bands must be removed from the legs of birds exposed to sub-freezing temperatures, as they contribute to frostbite.

The veterinarian can help the aviculturist establish a record system that is best for a particular facility, assist in developing and implementing effective identification systems and evaluate production records. Records that include all available medical information should be established at the time the bird enters the aviary.

Acclimation

New birds should be weighed upon arrival and observed closely for weight loss. Gavage feeding should be used only if the weight loss is dramatic (15% of initial weight) in order to avoid unnecessary stress. A bird that is reluctant to eat can be maintained on the diet to which it is accustomed and slowly changed to the diet used by the aviculturist. Changes in the quality of water may cause temporary intestinal upset. A species that will be housed outdoors must be slowly acclimated to its new climatic conditions. Tropical birds can tolerate northern temperate climates if acclimated for several months before being exposed to winter temperatures. Exposure to direct sunlight can cause burns on the unfeathered portions of the face. Biting insects may cause dermatologic reactions that can become quite severe in a new arrival.

Preventive Husbandry Practices

Fecal samples should be evaluated on an annual basis and can be grouped (no more than three to five pairs/sample) to facilitate testing for parasites in a large aviary. Infected groups can then be screened on an individual basis and treated as needed.

Annual prophylactic treatment for chlamydiosis is often advocated even in the absence of a diagnosis of chlamydiosis. This may be beneficial in birds housed outdoors and exposed to free-ranging birds, especially pigeons. In most cases, the indiscriminate use of antibiotics is not recommended. Egg production will typically decrease during treatment, and chicks that hatch from eggs laid during treatment may have developmental abnormalities.

Commercially available oil emulsion adjuvant vaccines for Pacheco's virus disease, pox and salmonella can be beneficial in populations at risk. In an avicultural collection, the benefits of vaccination must be weighed against any potential for adverse reactions (bruises, temporary skin nodules, handling stress).

Feeding Aviary Birds

Diets should be complete and balanced for optimal health and reproduction. In general, breeding birds should receive a formulated diet, a variety of fresh fruits and vegetables and some seeds and nuts. In-the-shell peanuts should be avoided because of their potential for exposing a bird to aflatoxins.

The seasonal provision of extra soft foods prior to the onset of the breeding season may stimulate reproduction.

Birds that are housed outdoors are exposed to natural sunlight and should not require supplemental Vitamin D_3. Macaws are especially susceptible to Vitamin D toxicity, which could be potentiated by unnecessary supplementation.

Facility Design

An aviary should be designed to be easy to maintain while providing safety, security and sanitary conditions for its inhabitants. It must also meet the psychological needs of the birds. A part of making a bird feel secure is to provide it with a defendable space. Additional factors in providing a secure environment include having visual barriers to separate the nesting areas of secretive birds, and keeping louder, more boisterous birds (eg, macaws) widely separated from quieter, more timid birds (eg, African Grey Parrots). Indoor/outdoor facilities provide the most natural conditions for the birds.

Indoor Facilities: Indoor housing has several advantages over outdoor facilities including improved pest control, the ability to manipulate lighting, temperature and humidity, and protection from inclement weather and theft.

Indoor aviaries also have disadvantages. They are generally more crowded than outdoor aviaries, the increased proximity of birds to each other potentiates the spread of infectious agents, and the lack of seasonal cycling of light and other unknown climatic factors may alter or prevent normal breeding behavior. Indoor areas require more frequent cleaning to prevent the accumulation of feces, food wastes and dust, all of which reduce the air quality and increase the likelihood of a disease outbreak.

The most important considerations when planning an indoor aviary are to avoid overcrowding and to ensure ease of cleaning and frequent air exchange. Walls and floors should be designed to allow pressure cleaning, and floor drains should be of sufficient size to prevent blockage by debris or feed.

The air in an indoor facility should be completely changed or filtered every two minutes. Tropical species may need additional humidity during dry winters.

Outdoor Facilities: Considerations include location of aviaries in relation to support buildings, flow of traffic through the aviaries, source of water and electric power, the effects of noise on neighbors and potential disturbances from people, free-ranging animals and traffic. The primary direction of wind and rain should be considered in the design of roofs in order to maximize protection of nest boxes and food bowls from rain.

Disadvantages to an outdoor breeding facility include the inability to control inclement weather, increased difficulty in pest control, the potential of noise irritation to neighbors and increased risk of theft. Some birds may be bothered by biting insects or aerosolized allergens.

Combination Indoor and Outdoor Facilities: Heated indoor facilities that are attached to outdoor flights are ideal for breeding birds in areas where the birds cannot remain outdoors year round.

Enclosures

The two primary styles of enclosures used in breeding aviaries are suspended wire enclosures and flights. Suspended enclosures are easy to construct, clean, modify or move, and are relatively inexpensive and secure. Birds have reduced exposure to their feces and accumulated food, simplifying disease and parasite control. These enclosures should be placed so that the perches are above eye level of aviary personnel to contribute to the security and contentment of the birds housed within.

Most enclosures for Psittaciformes are constructed from appropriate gauge welded wire (10 ga for larger macaws, 14-16 ga for cockatoos and Amazon parrots). Wire that is galvanized after welding is superior in strength to wire that is galvanized before welding. The galvanized coating that is used on welded wire does contain heavy metals. This wire should be thoroughly scrubbed with acetic acid using a wire brush and rinsed immediately to remove loose galvanizing material. "Weathering" the wire (ie, the practice of leaving rolls of wire in the open for six months to a year before use) does not reliably remove heavy metals (see Chapter 37).

Flight enclosures extend to the floor or ground. These enclosures are difficult to clean and to maintain pest- or parasite-free. Additionally, aviary personnel walking from one enclosure to the next can serve as mechanical vectors for the transmission of infectious agents.

Containers to hold the food bowls should be designed to reduce dumping, to prevent or reduce perching on the bowls and to keep the food dry. Food bowls should be positioned away from perches to reduce excrement contamination of the food and water containers.

Table 2.2   Suggested Minimum Sizes for Suspended Enclosures and for Nest Boxes

	Enclosures	Nest Box
Large macaws	6'x6'x12'	48"x16"x16"
Large cockatoos, medium macaws, obese Amazons	4'x4'x8'	36"x12"x12"
Amazons, African Grey Parrots	2'x2'x6'	24"x12"x12"
Pionus, mini-macaws	2'x3'x8'	24"x12"x12"
Conures, caiques	2'x2'x6'	18"x12"x12"
Small conures, cockatiels	2'x2'x3'	16"x10"x10"
Lovebirds, parrotlets, budgerigars	2'x2'x2'	8"x8"x24"

* Enclosure and box dimensions are height x width x depth

Some aviculturists are finding that the use of bottles serves as an effective method of maintaining a constant supply of clean, fresh water at all times. However, birds in a dry climate that are incubating eggs must have access to a bowl of water in which to bathe to help control egg humidity.

Perches must be secure and nonmovable in order to provide an optimal site for successful copulation. Wood perches that vary in diameter and surface texture provide the most natural standing surface. More permanent perches can be constructed of PVC, steel pipe or some synthetic materials. These should be used only in combination with some type of natural wood perch. Having wooden perches in an enclosure provides psychological stimulation (chewing) and will help maintain beak health. Some foot and leg problems may be associated with continuous perching on hard surfaces, especially in cold climates where chilling of the feet or frostbite may occur.

Nest Boxes

Nest boxes should be placed in or on the enclosure in such a way as to allow easy and frequent examination. Placing nest boxes on the same end as the feeding and watering station allows simultaneous feeding and nest box examination. Nest boxes must be waterproofed or placed so they do not get wet during heavy rains. The nest boxes should also be shielded from direct sunlight, which may cause overheating of the occupants.

Nest boxes may be constructed of many materials, with plywood being the most common. Lining the nest box with wire will decrease chewing damage; however, chewed wires can produce dangerous projections that can cause injuries to the chicks or adults. Nesting materials can contribute to disease problems. The use of potting soil, corn cob bedding, eucalyptus leaves or hay may contribute to fungal growth. There is a high incidence of cancer in laboratory rodents that are maintained on pine or cedar shavings. It is best to use large hardwood or aspen chips in the nest box.

Health Maintenance Program

The health maintenance program should be designed to address problems common in a species as well as endemic problems for a particular aviary. For example, Old World Psittaciformes housed in outdoor aviaries in southern coastal states must be protected from opossums to prevent an inevitable outbreak of sarcocystosis (see Chapter 36). Mosquito populations are high in the same geographic regions, and susceptible species of birds should be protected from poxvirus by vaccination.

Frequent disinfection of enclosures is not necessary if birds are healthy, organic debris is not allowed to build up in the enclosure and the food and water bowls are changed daily. Exceptional food hygiene is vital to prevent the spread of food-borne pathogens or the spoilage of moist foods within an enclosure. Hygiene is especially important when dealing with soft or fresh foods in which spoilage is rapid.

Vitamins should not be added to the drinking water; they oxidize rapidly and provide a growth media for bacteria and fungus. Water should be collected directly from a tap that is run for 30-45 seconds before filling a container. *Pseudomonas* sp. can frequently be cultured from garden hoses and from PVC pipe systems. Automatic watering systems reduce labor, ensure that birds have a clean fresh supply of water at all times and prevent food or fecal contamination of the water supply. Water should be flushed through the lines daily as part of the maintenance routine. Weekly flushing of water lines with hypochlorite or iodophores is necessary to keep the lines free of bacteria and algae. Automatic watering systems should be checked daily to ensure that they are working properly.

Food and water bowls should be made of stainless steel, hard plastic or crockery and should be washed daily. Bowls can be washed in soap and water and returned to the same enclosure. If cleaned as a group, the bowls should be disinfected (with Clorox) before reuse (Table 2.3).

Nest boxes should, at a minimum, be thoroughly cleaned on an annual basis, and nest material should be changed after each clutch if chicks were allowed to hatch in the nest.

Disinfectants: Organic debris must be removed from a surface before disinfecting. The constant use of powerful disinfectants in the absence of a disease threat is not beneficial, and continuous contact with these chemicals can be detrimental to the birds and aviary personnel. Chlorine bleach should be used only in well ventilated areas, and a 5% solution is effective for most uses.

Table 2.3   Commonly Used Disinfectants in an Aviary and the Organisms They Affect

Sodium hypochlorite (Clorox bleach)	Most bacteria
Quaternary ammonium (Roccal)	Most bacteria, recommended for *Chlamydia*
Phenol (One-Stroke)	Most bacteria, effective against *Mycobacterium* and *Candida*
Chlorhexidine (Nolvasan)	Most bacteria except *Pseudomonas* sp., less effective against *Candida*
Stabilized chlorine dioxide (Dent-A-Gene)	Most bacteria, fungi, viruses, protozoa, inactivates avian polyomavirus

Pest Control

Insects: Cockroaches that eat contaminated opossum feces can transmit *Sarcocystis falcatula* by defecating in a bird's food or by being eaten by a bird. Biological control of roaches is preferable to insecticides. Clean, sealed facilities reduce hiding places for roaches. Insectivorous animals (gecko lizards or chickens) can be used to consume the insects.

Ants can transmit some parasites such as the proventricular worm *Dyspharynx*. Ants may reduce food consumption by swarming food bowls or may build nests in the nest boxes. The incidence of mites and lice is low in captive psittacine birds but they may be introduced into an aviary by free-ranging birds. The red mite (*Dermanysis gallinae*) can be troublesome in some avicultural situations. This mite is nocturnal and hides in crevices in the aviary and nest boxes during the day. These mites are blood feeders and can kill chicks by exsanguination. For the control of mites inhabiting nest boxes, five per-cent carbaryl powder has been used successfully without apparent harm to chicks or adults. Mosquitoes can also be a problem for chicks in the nest box.

Rodents: Enclosures suspended on poles can be fitted with rat guards, or the poles can be greased to prevent climbing. Bait boxes should be used as needed and with caution. Snap traps baited with small quantities of ground meat are particularly effective.

Snakes: Snakes will occasionally enter enclosures and consume small birds, but will rarely attack larger Psittaciformes.

Evaluating and Treating Flock Problems

Emergency Care

The client should be well schooled in providing first aid and recognizing signs of illness that require veterinary intervention. The veterinarian should assist the aviculturist in preparing a first aid kit, in being prepared to provide post-examination nursing care and in having the necessary supplies to safely and effectively transport a sick bird (Table 2.4). The aviculturist should visually evaluate each bird every day during routine feeding procedures.

Table 2.4   Avicultural First Aid Considerations

- Quiet, isolated area with appropriate enclosure
- Enclosure that will provide heat, humidity and preferably oxygen
- Balanced electrolyte solutions
- Feeding tubes and syringes
- Syringes and needles
- Emergency medications (to be prescribed by the veterinarian)
- Bandage materials - nonstick elastic bandage material, adhesive tape, nonstick wound pads, antibiotic ointment, hydrogen peroxide or iodine solutions
- Scissors and forceps
- Coagulants for bleeding nails
- Disinfected container for transporting sick or injured birds

Managing Disease Outbreaks

In an avicultural setting, maintaining flock health must be the priority, and containing an infectious agent, determining its source and implementing control procedures are mandatory. Sick birds should be immediately removed from the collection and a thorough diagnostic evaluation performed. If the bird dies, a complete necropsy with collection of representative tissues from all organ systems is critical.

An easily and completely cleanable isolation area for new and sick birds should be available, and protocols should be established for managing this area.

Evaluating Reproductive Failures

Resident Bird Examination

Annual examinations of all birds in a collection can be used to detect flock problems, establish and confirm the accuracy of identification systems and collect data that may lead to the removal of unproductive individuals. The efficacy of husbandry practices and the plane of nutrition can be determined by assessing the physical condition of the birds.

The veterinarian working in unison with the aviculturist may be able to determine correctable physical, hormonal, nutritional, behavioral and psychological causes of reproductive failure.

Table 2.5 Evaluation of Reproduction Failure

- Obtain detailed histories
- Review health and production records
- Perform complete physical examination including cloacal mucosa
- Perform diagnostic tests as dictated by the findings
- Use laparoscopy to verify gender and visually evaluate the reproductive system and other organs
- Evaluate husbandry practices
  - Is diet appropriate, balanced, accepted?
  - Are enclosures appropriate in design and size?
  - Are nest boxes secure, dry, clean, free of pests and placed properly in the enclosure?
  - Are secure perches available for copulation?
  - Is the pair protected from environmental extremes?
  - Are aviary disturbances (visitors, pests) minimized?

Culling

Culling is a vital technique to improve the quality of captive breeding stock. Maintaining breeding birds that are not vigorous, that fail to adapt to captivity or that are of poor genetic lineage is a detriment to the future of aviculture and to the species.

Dealing with birds that are to be removed from a collection can challenge the ethics of the veterinarian. It is never advisable for the same veterinarian to represent both the buyer and the seller in a bird transaction.

Incubation and Pediatrics

Veterinarians should be involved in evaluation of incubation failures and management of the psittacine nursery. Ideally, all fertile eggs that fail to hatch should be examined in an attempt to detect patterns of mortality, which may be helpful in identifying problems associated with incubation (see Chapter 29).

A veterinarian who is experienced in nursery management can provide advice and management recommendations that could prevent the occurrence of clinical disease related to husbandry or nutritional problems of neonates (see Chapter 30).

NUTRITION

Randal N. Brue

A s aviculture has advanced over the past decade, sound feeding practices that are based on the eating habits of long-lived birds or on sustained reproductive successes have begun to emerge. Although most of this information is still anecdotal, there appear to be valid principles to support many of these practices. The majority of companion and aviary birds are considered opportunistic omnivores; that is, they will eat a large number of the foods that are available to them at any specific time. Even a relatively accurate analysis of 90% of a bird's intake may not be truly reflective of the total nutrient profile of the diet, because items consumed in trace amounts are difficult to quantitate and can have a significant impact on the bird's overall nutritional status. Additionally, most free-ranging birds do not live to their full genetic potential. This is due not only to predation and disease, but also to the frequency of malnutrition caused by seasonally insufficient supplies of nutrient-adequate foods.

Poultry Adaptations

Current nutrient recommendations for companion birds are derived from an extrapolation of the nutritional requirements for commercial poultry, the application of general nutritional principles that are fairly constant among all vertebrates, an evaluation of ornithological information (eating habits in free-ranging birds, the role of ecological niches, any known anatomic or physiologic differences) and information that has been generated through the years of trial and error feeding, which has resulted in certain species-specific or family-specific feeding practices. The culmination of this multifaceted approach has resulted in a general estimation of the nutrient needs for companion birds. It does not, however, determine the specific requirement of an individual nutrient or necessarily produce a diet that is totally optimized. It is doubtful that the nutritional needs of either the Psittaciformes or Passeriformes will ever be fully known.

Role of Nutrition in Bird Health

Without good, sound management techniques (see Chapter 2), an otherwise genetically strong and nutritionally sound bird will not maintain its good health. A properly balanced diet and a professionally administered health care program must be provided to ensure the long-term health of a bird.

Water

The quality of water provided to companion birds should be of utmost concern. Contamination in the water container, in addition to the aqueous medium and compatible environmental temperatures, provide all the requirements for microorganisms to thrive. Likewise, high-moisture foods such as egg foods, nestling foods, cooked foods, sprouts, fruits and vegetables provide excellent growth media for microorganisms. At warm environmental temperatures, these types of foods can become contaminated in as little as four hours.

Processed diets tend to increase the bird's water intake over that typical for a seed diet because they generally are dry, lower in fat and tend to have overall higher nutrient levels. Slightly moister feces are often observed in birds on a formulated diet.

Nutrient Interrelationships

There exists a vast array of interrelationships between the different nutrients. Ideally, these must all be evaluated to protect against nutrient imbalances and interferences, and to ensure that the proper amounts of nutrients are being both consumed and absorbed by the bird. It is critical to go beyond this quantitative approach and evaluate both the quality of the nutrient and the animal's actual intake of the nutrient. By evaluating the intake level and the quality (bioavailability), the total body uptake can be determined.

The Effective Energy Content of Food

It is important that the individual nutrient levels be balanced with respect to the energy content of the food, because the food intake by the animal is largely dependent on the total caloric density of that food. In the case of very low caloric density foods, the gastrointestinal tract capacity can become a limiting factor for adequate caloric intake. Conversely, if the dietary caloric density is extremely high, the appropriate feedback systems that regulate satiety may not have time to respond before the caloric needs are exceeded.

As the fat content of a diet increases, the rate of passage is slowed. This not only has an effect on the bird by prolonging satiety, but also improves digestibility of most nutrients in the food by increasing the length of exposure to digestive enzymes and the time for absorption. An example of this relationship is given in Table 3.1. Although there is a substantial difference in the metabolizable energy values of these two diets, the daily intake of protein and calcium is identical with respect to the energy content of the diet. This example illustrates how some seemingly dramatic differences in nutrient levels can actually give very similar results in the animal.

Table 3.1   The Effect of Dietary Energy Level on Intake and Proper Nutrient Density

	Diet A approx. 4% fat	Diet B approx. 22% fat
Energy content, kcal/kg	3015.0	4020.0
Intake, grams	30.0	22.5
Energy intake, kcal	90.5	90.5
Protein content, %	15.0	20.0
Protein intake, g	4.5	4.5
Calcium content, %	0.5	0.7
Calcium intake, g	0.15	0.15

Mineral Interrelationships

The most critical in companion bird nutrition, and in most species, is the relation between calcium and phosphorous. For proper growth, bone maintenance and health, a ratio of calcium to available phosphorous should be 1.5:1 to 2:1. The widest tolerable range of calcium to phosphorous ratio should be considered to be 0.8:1 to a maximum of 3.0:1 (3.3:1 produces rickets and leg abnormalities) Additionally, excess levels of calcium can precipitate deficiencies of magnesium, iron, iodine, zinc and manganese.

Vitamin Interrelationships

The most obvious example of vitamin interrelationship is the effect of the absorption of fat-soluble vitamins, in which an excess of one would decrease the absorption of the others due to competition for binding sites in the intestinal mucosa. There is also an interrelationship in the metabolism of folic acid and choline (and the amino acid, methionine) as they relate to the metabolism of single carbon units (ie, methyl groups).

Vitamin and Mineral Interactions

The most significant is the relationship of calcium, phosphorus and vitamin D_3. It is obligatory for adequate vitamin D_3 to be available for the proper absorption of both of these minerals to take place.

The other critical vitamin/mineral interaction is that between vitamin E and selenium, in which their biologic functions are essentially the same, but occur in different parts of the cell (lipid-based and aqueous, respectively).

Another example of a mineral and vitamin interrelationship is the increased absorption of iron in the presence of ascorbic acid.

Amino Acid/Vitamin Interactions

The most notable interrelationship between a vitamin and an amino acid is the relationship of niacin and tryptophan. In fact, a significant portion of the niacin requirement can be spared by an excess of tryptophan in the diet. Choline is an example of a vitamin that can directly spare the requirement of an amino acid, namely methionine.

Nutrient Antagonists (Anti-nutritional Factors)

Enzyme Inhibitors

Enzyme inhibitors are present in a large variety of foods, and most can be largely inactivated by thorough cooking. The largest group of enzyme inhibitors are the protease inhibitors, which inhibit the digestive enzymes trypsin and chymotrypsin and others. Ingestion of a diet high in active inhibitors results in poor protein digestion and pancreatic hypertrophy, stimulated by the direct inactivation of digestive enzymes or the effect of limited bioavailability of methionine. Protease inhibitors are present to some degree in all plants, with significant levels found in all of the legumes, barley, beets, buckwheat, corn, lettuce, oats, peas, peanuts, potatoes, rice, rye, sweet potatoes, turnips and wheat.

Tannins, found in a variety of plant sources, can bind protein, inhibit digestive enzymes and reduce the bioavailability of iron and vitamin B_{12}. At high levels, they can cause liver and epithelium damage. Tannins are found at high levels in acorns, carrots, rape seed, milo, grape seeds, tea, coffee, chocolate, bananas, grapes and raisins, lettuce, spinach, rhubarb and onions.

Some of the other enzyme inhibitors include amylase inhibitor in beans, wheat, rye and sorghum; plasmin inhibitor (inhibiting blood clotting) in some beans; kallikrein inhibitor in potato (decreases antibody formation); and cholinesterase inhibitors in asparagus, broccoli, carrots, cabbage, celery, radishes, pumpkin, raspberries, oranges, peppers, strawberries, tomatoes, turnips, apples, eggplant and especially potatoes.

Mineral Antagonists

Oxalate (oxalic acid) is an organic acid that efficiently binds calcium and other trace minerals. The highest levels of oxalate is found in tea, spinach and rhubarb, with lower levels found in peas, beets and beet greens, lettuce, turnips, carrots and berries. Potentially toxic levels are found in the leaves of rhubarb and the common house plant, diffenbachia. High levels of oxalates can cause vomiting, diarrhea, poor blood clotting and convulsions. Lower levels can result in decreased growth, poor bone mineralization and kidney stones.

Phytate or phytic acid is very effective at chelating minerals such as zinc, iron and calcium, resulting in an unavailable complex. Phytates are most commonly found in nuts, legumes, cereal grains (germ and bran) and, in lesser quantities, in green beans, carrots, broccoli, potatoes, sweet potatoes and berries.

Vitamin Antagonists

Thiaminase is a naturally occurring enzyme that destroys thiamine and is most often associated with raw fish, but it can also be found beets, Brussels sprouts, red cabbage and berries, some organ meats and as a product of certain microorganisms that can inhabit the gastrointestinal tract.

A compound found in flax seed (and therefore linseed meal) acts as an antagonist to pyridoxine (vitamin B_6).

Natural Plant Toxins

Lectins or phytohemagglutinins can cause kidney, liver and heart damage, destruction of gastrointestinal epithelium, red blood cell agglutination and cell mitosis interference. These compounds occur in legumes, especially the castor bean and black bean, and in lower levels in other plant seeds.

When saponins are consumed in high amounts, diarrhea and vomiting can occur. They are found in soybeans, alfalfa, spinach, asparagus, broccoli, potatoes, apples and eggplant.

Goitrogens are contained in soybeans, peanuts, pine nuts and the entire brassica family (turnips, rutabaga, broccoli, Brussels sprouts, cabbage, cauliflower, kale, kohlrabi and mustard). They are also found to a lesser degree in carrots, peaches, pears, radishes, strawberries and millet. Low-protein diets increase the effects of goitrogens.

Mycotoxins

Mycotoxins are compounds that are produced under certain conditions as metabolic by-products of molds. The difficulty with mycotoxins is that they are totally undetectable by sight, smell and taste.

Mycotoxins can have a broad range of effects on the body ranging from a toxic dose with mortality in two to three days to chronic exposure of moderate levels where decreased disease resistance is encountered along with lesions in the liver, kidneys, nervous system, reproductive system and integument. Carcinogenic, mutagenic or teratogenic effects may also be exhibited. Peanuts and corn are considered to be the human population's largest source of aflatoxin.

Table 3.2   Sources of Exposure and Pathology to Mycotoxin Ingestion

Mycotoxins	Common Feed Sources	Agent	Pathology
Aflatoxins	Corn, peanuts, cottonseed	*Aspergillus flavus,* *A. parasiticus*	Liver damage Hepatomegaly Immunosuppresion Kidney damage
Ochratoxin	Corn, barley, oats, wheat	*A. ochraceus* *Penicillum viridicatum*	Kidney and liver damage Hemorrhaging
Zearalenone	Corn, wheat	*Fusarium roseum* *F. graminearum*	Production of estrogen-like compounds
Trichothecenes (T_2 toxin)	Corn, wheat barley, oats, forages	*F. tricinctum* *F. roseum* *F. graminearum*	Oral inflammation & lesions Neural disturbances Immunosuppression Hemorrhaging
Vomatoxin (2-deoxynivalenol)	Corn, sorghum, wheat	*F. roseum* *F. graminearum*	Gastrointestinal inflammation Vomiting
Ergot	Rye, barley, wheat, oats	*Claviceps purpurea*	Tissue death Kidney and liver damage

Nutrient Needs During Different Life Stages

Embryonic

If a hen is fed a nutrient-deficient diet that will allow production, embryo development may progress, but will be abnormally affected. This most often is observed as early embryonic death, usually with the formation of a blood ring after approximately three days of development (vitamin A deficiency), losses immediately prior to hatch due to an embryo with insufficient strength to complete the hatching process (riboflavin, biotin, folic acid and vitamin B_{12} deficiencies) or embryonic malformation (zinc and manganese deficiencies).

Table 3.3   Recommended Nutrient Allowances for Companion Bird Diets

Nutrient	Anticipated Minimum Requirement	Recommended Allowance for Maintenance
Protein, %	10.00	12.00
Fat, %	—	4.00
Energy, kcal/kg	—	3000.00
VITAMINS		
Vitamin A, IU/kg of food	2500.00	5000.00
Vitamin D_3, IU/kg of food	500.00	1000.00
Vitamin E, IU/kg of food	15.00	20.00
Vitamin K, ppm	0.80	1.00
Thiamine, ppm	2.00	5.00
Riboflavin, ppm	4.00	10.00
Niacin, ppm	40.00	75.00
Pyridoxine, ppm	4.00	10.00
Pantothenic acid, ppm	12.00	15.00
Biotin, ppm	0.15	0.20
Folic acid, ppm	1.00	2.00
Vitamin B_{12}, ppm	5.00	10.00
Choline, ppm	750.00	1000.00
Vitamin C	No requirements demonstrated	
MINERALS		
Calcium, %	0.30	0.50
Phosphorus (available), %	0.15	0.25
Phosphorus (total) approx., %	0.30	0.40
Sodium, %	0.10	0.15
Chlorine, %	0.10	0.15
Potassium, %	0.30	0.40
Magnesium, ppm	500.00	600.00
Manganese, ppm	60.00	75.00
Iron, ppm	60.00	80.00
Zinc, ppm	40.00	50.00
Copper, ppm	6.00	8.00
Iodine, ppm	0.30	0.30
Selenium, ppm	0.10	0.10
AMINO ACIDS		
Lysine, %	0.45	0.60
Methionine, %	0.20	0.25
Tryptophan, %	0.10	0.12
Arginine, %	0.50	0.60
Threonine, %	0.35	0.40

Other essential amino acids are sufficient in common diets.

Growth

At hatch, the absorbed yolk sac serves as a temporary energy reservoir. This may be adequate to supply the chick with nutrients for the first one to three days, depending on the species. As the chick's digestive system becomes fully functional, the period of rapid growth begins. Due to the high metabolic rate and the rapid division and growth of cells, the amino acid, energy, linoleic acid, vitamin and mineral requirements are at the highest point of the animal's normal life.

Under normal situations, the absolute nutrient requirements decrease throughout the growth phase, since the level of growth proportional to body weight declines with age. If optimal nutrient levels are not present at an earlier growth phase, but are present in excess of requirement towards the end of the growing cycle, the bird will display compensatory growth. This is often observed when a baby is fed a nutritionally marginal diet (see Chapter 30).

Maintenance

Requirements for the maintenance of an adult bird are the lowest for the entire life cycle. Any increase in activity level, ambient temperature outside of the thermoneutral zone, molting and the exposure to any type of stress will alter the minimum nutrient levels required for maintenance.

Breeding

The increased requirements by the hen for breeding can be divided into two general categories: those required for egg production and those required for maximum hatchability of the embryo. On a dry matter basis, the egg (without the shell) consists of approximately 45% fat and 50% protein. Additionally, the shell, which comprises approximately 10% of the total egg weight, is approximately 94% calcium carbonate (38% calcium). These three constituents represent the largest increase in nutrient needs in order for the hen to produce eggs. The diet does require higher levels of protein, particularly of the sulfur amino acids (eg, methionine) and lysine. Calcium levels in the diet should be increased to minimize the decalcification of the bone and to prevent the formation of soft egg shells. To maximize hatchability of the embryo, increased levels of vitamin E, riboflavin, pantothenic acid, biotin, folic acid, pyridoxine, zinc, iron, copper and manganese are required over what is adequate for egg production.

Much of the reason for dramatically increasing the nutritional plane of a breeding bird's diet is to provide adequate dietary components for the chick to be fed.

Geriatric Nutrition

To date, there has been no research on the nutritional needs of geriatric psittacine birds. As the husbandry and veterinary care of these species continue to improve, proper geriatric nutrition will become a concern. Slight increases in vitamins A, E, B_{12}, thiamine, pyridoxine, zinc, linoleic acid and lysine may be helpful to overcome some of the metabolic and digestive changes accompanying old age.

Stress

Crowding, handling, exposure to unusual pathogens, unsanitary conditions and malnutrition may all be considered stress factors. Stresses tend to be cumulative, and a single stress often has very little clinical effect on the bird. However, when one or more additional stress is applied, the bird may be weakened to the point of clinical illness or death. Stress in young birds results in a decrease in weight gain and, if left uncorrected, weight loss and morbidity may occur.

The body's response to stress is the "flight or fight" syndrome, and the immediate response is to mobilize and produce glucose for the increased energy need. After carbohydrate stores are depleted (within approximately 24 hours), protein and fat stores are broken down, with the breakdown of skeletal muscle supplying amino acids for gluconeogenesis. Adequate diets should be provided to ensure the normal presence of sufficient body stores, which will also allow for satisfactory repletion of stress-depleted stores.

Table 3.4	Changes in Need for Nutrients During Periods of Debilitation
Vitamin C	The debilitated animal may not be able to adequately synthesize enough vitamin C, especially in the case of hepatic damage. Increased vitamin C in other species exposed to a number of different types of stresses has shown to improve production and health criteria.
Vitamin D	In diseases affecting the liver and kidneys, the enzymes required to produce the metabolically active form of vitamin D_3 will be impaired. In these situations, or in the case of a marginally deficient animal, it may be beneficial to provide vitamin D_3 therapy.
Vitamin K	For animals that have undergone extensive antibiotic therapy and are being maintained on an unsupplemented or marginally supplemented diet, it may be necessary to provide vitamin K because of its decreased synthesis by normal intestinal flora.
Vitamin B complex	In the case of an anorectic animal, it may be beneficial to supply additional B vitamins, especially thiamine. Other water-soluble vitamins such as riboflavin, pyridoxine and folic acid are particularly important in protein and energy metabolism; therefore, these vitamins have increased importance in the disease state.
Zinc	In a nutritionally compromised animal, zinc will improve healing and is an important component in protein synthesis; therefore, zinc is necessary for the maintenance of the immune system and phagocytic activity.

Disease

The most critical nutrient for the body to maintain during illness is water (see Chapter 15). Secondly, the necessary energy supplies to the body must be maintained. Because of the increased metabolic rate during illness, there is a higher energy need. Although much of this energy demand still falls within the normal maintenance requirement, it is critical to maintain or exceed the typical energy intake, which can be provided via carbohydrates, fats or protein.

Dietary protein is the third most critical component to be provided to the debilitated patient. With the increased metabolic rate, there is a subsequent increase in body protein turnover. There is also increased demand for amino acids because of the need for additional immune components and tissue repair. The exceptions to increasing the protein in the diet are during the acute phase of liver or renal disease.

Current Nutritional Knowledge

Protein Needs

Two of the best scientifically conducted studies that have been published investigated the total protein requirement and lysine requirement of the growing cockatiel. Chicks performed best and reached the weaning stage earliest on a 20% crude protein diet.

Lysine Needs

Cockatiel chicks showed the best growth responses when given diets in the range of 0.8-1.2% lysine. Unlike poultry species, which exhibit feather depigmentation (the formation of feathers lacking melanin pigment) during a lysine deficiency, all cockatiels, even those on the most severely deficient diet, had normal feather pigmentation. This suggests a metabolic difference between poultry and altricial birds (at least the cockatiel).

Energy

The approximate daily metabolizable energy (ME) needs for budgerigars appear to be between 12 and 16 kilocalories (kcal) per day in a normal maintenance situation. Canaries require approximately 12 kcal/day. A 350 g Amazon parrot would require an intake of 100 kcal/day, and a 1000 g macaw would require 220 kcal/day. Temperatures above or below 70°F would result in lower or higher needs, respectively.

Current Beliefs on Nutrient Requirements

Based on avicultural and clinical observations, there have been a number of hypotheses developed regarding species-specific differences in nutrient requirements.

Vitamin Differences

It has been suggested that several species may have increased needs for vitamin A over most other commonly kept species. Those most frequently seen to respond to "higher" levels are Eclectus Parrots, conures and certain Amazon parrots, most notably the Blue-fronted Amazon. The increased need for vitamin A in Amazon species is often linked to increased immunity against viral disease (poxvirus). Clinically, a level equivalent to 5000-10,000 IU per kg in the diet has proven successful in preventing deficiency symptoms.

Certain neonatal macaw species, especially the Blue and Gold Macaw and Hyacinth Macaw, seem more prone to the development of hypervitaminosis D_3 than other psittacine chicks. When a cross section of large psittacine babies was fed a moderately high level of vitamin D_3 (2500 International Chick Units [ICU]/kg dry mix; 1.0% Ca), Blue and Gold Macaws were the only species to develop mild signs of hypervitaminosis D_3, characterized by enlarged kidneys and mild, early calcification of the renal tubules. Similar findings have been reported on a hand-feeding diet containing between 1000 and 4000 ICU/kg, which resulted in crop

stasis, increased serum uric acid levels and the presence of articular gout and regurgitation after feeding. Radiographically, the
kidneys were found to be enlarged, with areas of calcification in
the kidneys and proventriculus. Subsequent necropsy showed
widespread soft tissue calcinosis. In both reports, other species fed
similarly on the same diets were not affected.

Minerals

Cockatiels have been noted to be particularly sensitive to high
calcium or high calcium and vitamin D_3 levels in the diet. Adult
diets containing over 1% calcium, particularly when accompanied
by generous levels of vitamin D_3 (over 2000 ICU/kg dry diet) have
been found to be excessive in long-term feeding studies. Normal
egg production criteria have been satisfied at dietary calcium levels as low as 0.3 and 0.35%.

Research in adult poultry has indicated that normal bone mineralization, plasma calcium and alkaline phosphatase levels can
be maintained at below 0.05% calcium in the diet. This is supported by a similar observation in cockatiels.

Energy

Large macaws, particularly the Hyacinth, appear to perform
better on a higher fat diet than other species. An increase of approximately 25% fats over that adequate for other species has
been found to be necessary to support maximum growth.

Rose-breasted Cockatoos and budgerigars are very prone to
obesity and are probably examples of birds with slightly lower energy requirements. Amazon parrots frequently become obese due
to their sedentary behaviors.

Differences in Nutrient Metabolism and Requirements Based on Evolutionary Diversion

There is no generic companion bird with respect to nutritional requirements. Based on the ecological diversity in which species have
evolved, differences can be expected. Budgerigars, cockatiels and a
number of the grass parakeets and finches range into the vast, arid
interior of Australia. These birds are expected to have developed biological adaptations allowing them to conserve both nutrients and
water for existence in this sparse habitat. Conversely, psittacines of
the neotropics tend to consume a wide variety of foodstuffs, including an abundance of fresh vegetative matter. Birds in this environment have not had the need to develop any nutrient-conserving
mechanisms, and may, therefore, have somewhat higher needs.

Nutritional Labeling of Commercial Products

All pet foods are required by law to list levels of crude protein,
crude fat, crude fiber and moisture. Protein and fat are listed as
minimums, because they are of specific nutritional value and are
among the most expensive components of food. In a processed
food, these levels are generally close to the guarantee because of
the significant added cost in oversupplying these nutrients.

The protein guarantee is determined from the amount of nitrogen in the product (usually calculated as % crude protein = % ni-

trogen x 6.25). It provides no estimation of protein quality (ie, the product's amino acid profile).

Fiber and moisture are required to be listed as maximum amounts in the product, because both are traditionally considered of little nutritional importance and can, at higher levels, create quality problems.

Other nutrient guarantees are optional, except when the product specifically states that it is supplemented with certain nutrients (or category of nutrients), in which case those nutrients must be guaranteed.

Ingredient Statement

Companies are required to list the ingredients contained in the food in their order of dominance. While still maintaining accuracy in labeling, manufacturers may opt for labeling techniques that become vague or "hide" ingredients that have poor consumer perception. Instead of listing each ingredient by its full, approved term, "collective" terms can be used to group similar products together under an umbrella term. The collective term "grain products," can be used to describe the product's total content of cereal grains (corn, wheat, oats, barley), regardless of its form (whole, ground, heat processed). Likewise, the term "animal protein products" can be used to reflect a wide variety of ingredients such as meat meal, blood meal, dried milk, hydrolyzed feathers or fish residue.

Antioxidants

Some form of protection against product oxidation is essential to maintain nutritional adequacy of the product, to ensure a high-level of palatability and to prevent the formation of oxidative by-products, some of which are carcinogenic.

Table 3.6   Control of Product Oxidation

1. **Environmental control** - Lowering the product temperature to decrease the rate of oxidation (refrigerating), or modifying the atmosphere to remove the available oxygen (packing in nitrogen), minimizes the amount of oxidation.

2. **Rapid product use** - Oxidation is minimized by using the product as quickly as possible after the ingredients are mixed and processed. This is particularly critical with a complete, processed food that does not contain antioxidants, because the presence of trace minerals acts as a catalyst for the oxidation process.

3. **The use of antioxidants** - Either natural or chemical antioxidants can be used. Natural antioxidants such as vitamin E (and other tocopherols) and vitamin C tend to have a limited antioxidant life and do not give the product the length of protection that is possible with chemical antioxidants. Chemical antioxidants (ethoxyquin, BHT, BHA) provide the longest period of protection. There are no scientific studies detailing the effects of any preservatives on the long-term health of companion birds.

Grit

Grit is not required in the normal, healthy psittacine or passerine bird. Grit, (generally granite or quartz) is required in birds that consume whole, intact seeds. Examples are pigeons, doves, free-ranging gallinaceous species and Struthioniformes. There have been numerous examples of birds not having grit for 15-20 years and still not showing any signs of decreased performance or poor digestion. There have also been numerous reports of birds, especially with health problems and depraved appetites, consuming copious quantities of grit and developing crop or gastrointestinal impactions. Considering the small chance of benefit and the potential risk, ad libitum feeding of grit should be avoided.

Food Selection

Psittacines, in particular, have individual preferences for foods based on previous experience (or habit), food placement (position in the cage), particle size, fat content, texture, shape, color and taste. These preferences can be strong, and most clients encourage them by providing what the bird is most likely to readily eat. Birds must be trained to eat new foods. This is best accomplished by providing limited portions, or meals, to encourage consumption of everything offered, as opposed to a virtual ad libitum feeding program where the bird can reach satiety by eating only one or two of its favorite ingredients. Providing a large variety of foods immediately pre- and post-weaning is a very effective way to develop good eating habits that will tend to persist throughout life.

Essential Nutrients and Their Biological Functions

Essential nutrients are those that are required to properly drive biochemical reactions within the body.

Energy

The total amount of energy, or the gross energy contained within the feed, is broken into several fragments as it is metabolized in the body. During the process of digestion, potential energy sources are lost through the feces, urine and urates. What remains is the metabolizable energy (ME). A portion of the ME is lost as heat (the heat increment). The remaining energy (net energy value of the food) is available for maintenance of the bird. Any energy that remains after satisfying the basic maintenance requirements is available for production activities such as growth of body mass and feathers, deposition of fat, production of eggs and for exercise.

The bird derives energy from proteins, fats and carbohydrates. Protein is the least efficient source of energy, because the body must deaminate the amino acid, excrete the nitrogen as uric acid and then use the remaining carbon skeleton for glucose or fat synthesis. The average gross energy of protein is 5.65 kilocalories/gram. After the losses through deamination and subsequent metabolic reactions, protein yields a net of 4.1 kcal/g.

Carbohydrates are the most important energy source for the body because they are the only energy form that the brain can use. Lactose, the disaccharide contained in milk, is a very poor energy source for avian species because of an inefficient supply of lactase. Carbohydrates are efficiently metabolized with an ME value of 4 kcal/g.

Carbohydrates also form the fiber fraction of the diet, broadly classified as indigestible carbohydrate. This fraction consists mainly of cellulose, which is essentially undigested because of the bird's lack of the enzyme cellulase. Fibrous agents generally minimize the absorptive space in the gastrointestinal tract. The hemicellulose, psyllium, is an exception, as it acts to increase absorption.

Dietary fat is not only an important source of energy but it is the primary storage form of energy in the body. The ME in fat is concentrated with a value of 9 kcal/g, 2.25 times greater than that of either carbohydrates or protein.

Essential Fatty Acids

Animals and birds have no requirement for fat per se, but they do have a requirement for the individual fatty acids that make up fat. The primary essential fatty acid for animals and birds is linoleic acid. This compound cannot be synthesized in the body. Arachidonic acid is sometimes considered to be an essential fatty acid; however, it can be synthesized from linoleic acid.

Common vegetable oils are generally high in linoleic acid (eg, corn oil, soybean oil, peanut oil = 50%; sunflower oil = 60%; safflower oil = 75%). Tropical oils, such as coconut oil, contain substantial amounts of medium chain fatty acids, and are therefore poorer sources of linoleic acid.

Generally, oleic and linoleic acids are the most efficiently absorbed by the bird. This occurs because of the ease with which these fatty acids form mixed micelles with the bile salts, thereby improving their digestion by pancreatic lipase.

The essential fatty acids are used as structural components in the cell with particular importance in the cell membranes. They are also precursors of prostaglandins.

Based on the general requirements for most other species, it can be safely predicted that the linoleic acid requirement for companion and aviary birds is 1.0-1.5% of the diet. In seed-based diets, this would rarely fall short, but in a processed, low-fat diet there could be a marginal deficiency.

Amino Acids and Protein

The essential amino acids are lysine, arginine, histidine (basic amino acids), methionine (sulfur-containing), tryptophan (heterocyclic), threonine, leucine, isoleucine, valine (aliphatic) and phenylalanine (aromatic).

The quality of a dietary protein is determined by two primary factors. The first is the balance of amino acids within that protein. To be optimally utilized, the protein should have an amino acid profile similar to that of the animal's body. If this occurs, each individual amino acid will be present in approximately the right proportion that the body needs with no major excesses or deficiencies of any one amino acid. This profile is achieved only in a few foods, most notably in eggs and in milk. It seems obvious that these two protein sources would fit the profile of the body, because they provide the only source of food during early periods of rapid growth. Very few ingredients have an amino acid profile that ap-

proaches ideal. With proper selection, the ingredients work together in a synergistic manner to enhance the overall performance of the mixed diet.

The second criteria that affects protein quality is the availability of the amino acids within the foodstuff. Certain ingredients have
structural characteristics or contain chemical compounds that will
decrease the bioavailability of an amino acid. An example would be
the trypsin and chymotrypsin inhibitors in unprocessed soybeans
that prevent normal proteolytic activity of these digestive enzymes,
thereby decreasing digestibility. The specific structure of an amino
acid chain can also render a protein indigestible. An example of this
is the extremely poor digestibility of keratin.

Vitamins

Vitamins are defined as natural food components that are present in minute quantities, are organic in nature and are essential
for normal metabolism. They will cause specific, characteristic deficiency symptoms when they are severely limited in the diet.
Vitamins are generally not synthesized by the body in amounts
sufficient to meet the physiologic requirement.

Vitamins are now subcategorized into two general groups
based on their solubility characteristics. The fat-soluble vitamins
are comprised of vitamins A, D, E and K. The water-soluble vitamins include thiamine (vitamin B_1), riboflavin (vitamin B_2),
niacin, pyridoxine (vitamin B_6), pantothenic acid, biotin (vitamin
H), folic acid (vitamin M), vitamin B_{12} (cyano-cobalamin), choline
and ascorbic acid (vitamin C).

Vitamin A

Vitamin A occurs in several forms: retinol (alcohol), retinal
(aldehyde) and retinoic acid. Plants do not contain active vitamin
A, but instead contain vitamin precursors. These exist in the form
of carotenoid plant pigments, with the carotenes being the most
important of the pro-vitamin A compounds.

The most critical action of vitamin A in avian medicine is its effect on the growth and differentiation of epithelial tissues. It is in
this function that vitamin A is obligatory for normal disease resistance because it is required for the maintenance of mucous
membranes and for the normal functioning of secretory tissues.

Vitamin A is also required for normal mucopolysaccharide formation and apparently affects the stability of cell membranes and
of the subcellular membranes (such as the mitochondria and lysosomes). Vitamin A also functions in the proper growth of bones
and in the maintenance of normal reproduction.

Vitamin A apparently acts by the increased production and differentiation of immune related cells, while the carotenoids possibly improve the activity of lymphocytes.

The liver will typically contain over 90% of the total body stores
of vitamin A with the preferential storage form being retinyl
palmitate.

Vitamin A is usually considered safe up to approximately ten
times the requirement in monogastrics (including poultry).

Experimentally, vitamin A toxicities have been achieved by feeding over 100 times the daily requirement for extended periods of time. Probably an excess of 1000 times requirement would be necessary to induce an acute intoxication. Carotenoids in the diet do not contribute to potential vitamin A toxicity. At excessive levels, they may result in a temporary yellow pigmentation of the skin and fat.

Vitamin D

There are two predominant forms of vitamin D: ergo-calciferous (vitamin D_2), a plant derivative, and cholecalciferol (vitamin D_3), produced exclusively in the bird's body. Vitamin D_3 is considered to be 30-40 times more potent than vitamin D_2. Vitamin D_3 levels are quantified in International Chick Units (ICU) as a way to differentiate it from vitamin D_2 or total vitamin D.

Unlike other vitamins, the active metabolite actually acts as a hormone in the body being transported to the intestines, bones and other target organs where it exerts its role in the metabolism of calcium and phosphorus (see Chapter 23).

The most important physiologic role of vitamin D is the homeostasis of calcium and phosphorus levels in the body.

Hypervitaminosis D_3

In a prolonged feeding study with cockatiels on a diet containing 1.0% Ca, 0.5% P and 4000 ICU vitamin D_3 (18% crude protein and 3150 kcal/kg), high egg production for approximately one year was followed by a rapid decline in reproductive performance, concurrent with the onset of polyuria in all birds. Most had signs of anorexia and lethargy, with some exhibiting signs of diarrhea or lameness. Radiographs indicated the presence of nephrocalcinosis. Several females were lost, with necropsies showing extensive soft tissue mineralization, especially of the kidneys.

Vitamin E

Vitamin E is a compound of plant origin with eight active forms derived from four tocopherols and four tocotrienols. The compound of the greatest biologic importance in the avian species is alpha-tocopherol. Vitamin E is essentially a biologic antioxidant that functions at the intercellular and intracellular level by preventing the oxidation of saturated lipid compounds in the cell, thereby maintaining membrane integrity.

Working in conjunction with vitamin E are several metaloenzymes, which block the initiation of peroxidation in the aqueous phase of the cell. These enzymes incorporate manganese, zinc, copper, iron and selenium as active components. Glutathione peroxidase (GSHp) is probably the most important of these metalloenzymes because of its integral relationship with vitamin E. This selenium-containing enzyme is very active in the destruction of peroxides before they cause membrane damage. Because of their similar activity, selenium and vitamin E tend to have a sparing effect on each other. Exudative diathesis, the condition observed in poultry, generally appears only when both selenium and vitamin E are limited in the diet.

There is considerable evidence in poultry that levels higher than those required for optimum growth can increase immunity.

Vitamin E is absorbed through passive diffusion and is dependent upon normal lipid digestion requiring proper micelle formation and the presence of bile salts and pancreatic juices. Any malabsorption syndrome will decrease uptake. Liver and plasma stores of vitamin E are the most readily accessible to the body in times of need. Vitamin E stores of the body tend to be relatively stable and may not be effective in preventing a vitamin E deficiency from occurring. It appears that lipolysis of fatty stores may be required for vitamin E to be released.

Vitamin E is abundant in plant materials (particularly those high in oil) and in plant leaves. In cereal grains, vitamin E is concentrated in the germ. Alfalfa leaves are a particularly high source of vitamin E.

Vitamin K

Vitamin K comes from three sources: 1) green plants (phyloquinones - K_1 series), 2) bacteria (menaquinones - K_2 series) and 3) synthetic forms (menadione - K_3). The microbial synthesis of vitamin K_2 is significant in most species.

Natural vitamin K compounds require the presence of dietary fats and bile salts for proper absorption from the gastrointestinal tract; therefore, altered micelle formation (eg, decreased pancreatic and biliary function) will impair the normal absorption of vitamin K. Generally, vitamin K is stored only briefly in the liver before it is released into the body and transported to all tissues via lipoproteins. It is believed that menadione is well absorbed but poorly retained, while phylloquinone is rather poorly absorbed but retained much longer in the body.

A number of plasma clotting factors (eg, prothrombin) are dependent on vitamin K for their synthesis. The bone also contains a vitamin K-dependent protein (osteocalcin), which acts in the regulation of calcium phosphate incorporation into bone.

Thiamine (Vitamin B_1)

Thiamine is fairly common in food sources, but generally at only low concentrations. Several compounds in nature possess antithiamine activity, many of which exhibit competitive inhibition with thiamine based on their structural similarities. An example of this is amprolium, which inhibits thiamine absorption from the intestine and prevents thiamine phosphorylation. Another well known compound is thiaminase, contained in some raw fish and produced by certain types of bacteria. Thiamine is not stored for any length of time in the body. It is excreted primarily through the urine and in lesser amounts through the feces.

The active form of thiamine is thiamine pyrophosphate and is an important cofactor in carbohydrate metabolism. Deficiency results in polyneuritis, weakness, anorexia and poor growth.

Riboflavin (Vitamin B_2)

Riboflavin contained in plant materials is generally less available than from animal sources because of decreased digestibility of the flavin complexes in plants. Very little riboflavin is stored in the body; the highest concentrations are found in the liver, kidney and heart. Riboflavin as part of the coenzymes flavin mononucleotide (FMN) or flavin adenine dinucleotide (FAD), which are flavoproteins, act in a large number of enzyme complexes that are responsible for essential reactions in the utilization of carbohydrates, fats and proteins.

Niacin

Niacin exists in two major forms, nicotinic acid and nicotinamide. Niacin is widely distributed in foods, but that found in plants has low bioavailability. Bioavailability in animal products tends to be very high. Niacin can also be synthesized from the essential amino acid tryptophan; however, the amino acid's preferential use is for protein synthesis, so only tryptophan in excess of the animal's needs will be available for bioconversion to niacin.

The greatest concentrations of niacin compounds are in the liver, but no true storage occurs.

The coenzymes NAD and NADP are important components in carbohydrate, fat and protein metabolism, being especially important in the energy-yielding reactions of the body. These functions are critical to the generation of energy for the body as well as for normal tissue integrity, especially of the skin, alimentary tract and the nervous system.

Pyridoxine (Vitamin B$_6$)

Vitamin B$_6$ refers to the group of three compounds: pyridoxal, pyridoxamine and pyridoxal phosphate. Pyridoxal is the form predominantly found in plants.

The various forms are then converted and phosphorylated to the predominate tissue form, pyridoxal phosphate, which requires both niacin (as NADP) and riboflavin (as FMN) for the enzyme systems. Minimal amounts of the vitamin are stored in the body.

The metabolically active form of vitamin B$_6$, pyridoxal phosphate, is involved in a number of enzyme systems as a coenzyme. It is required in essentially all major areas of amino acid utilization, the synthesis of niacin from tryptophan and in the formation of antibodies. It is required in the decarboxylation of glutamic acid to form gamma-aminobutyric acid (GABA), the lack of which has been shown to cause seizures. A deficiency of pyridoxine creates a deficiency of many other important metabolites and hormones such as serotonin and histamine. Evidence also suggests that it may play a role as a modulator of steroid hormone receptors.

Pantothenic Acid

Tissues convert pantothenic acid to coenzyme A (predominantly), with the greatest concentrations found in the liver, adrenals, kidneys and brain. The majority of the pantothenic acid in the blood is found as CoA in the erythrocytes. CoA is one of the most critical coenzymes in tissue metabolism, forming the compound acetyl CoA. Acetyl CoA acts as the entry point into the citric acid cycle for carbohydrate metabolism, a point of entry for amino acid degradation and as an essential component in fatty acid biosyn-

thesis and degradation, the synthesis of triglycerides and phospholipids, as well as in the formation of compounds such as acetylcholine, mucopolysaccharides, cholesterol, steroid hormones and
many more.

Biotin

Biotin is widely distributed in foods but generally at low concentrations. There is evidence that suggests that the synthesis of
biotin by intestinal microflora is important in an animal.
Microbial-derived biotin would be manufactured and absorbed in
the large intestine.

The largest concentrations of biotin in the body are found in the
liver; however, this storage site seems to be poorly mobilized during times of biotin deprivation.

Biotin is an active part of four different carboxylase enzymes in
the body, and is responsible for the fixation of carbon dioxide (car-
boxylation). These enzymes have important functions in the metabolism of energy, glucose, lipids and some of the amino acids.

Folic Acid (Folacin)

Folic acid is the compound pteroylmonoglutamic acid. At one
time, PABA was believed to be essential in the diets of vertebrates, but it has since been determined that if the requirement
for folic acid is met, PABA provides no additional benefit. Folates
are generally widely distributed in foods and are present as the
polyglutamic derivatives of folic acid.

Folic acid's primary metabolic role is in the transfer of single-
carbon moieties in a wide variety of reactions. This function is particularly important in amino acid metabolism, in the bioconversion of amino acids and in the biosynthesis of nucleotides. Because
of folic acid's requirement in the synthesis of three of the four nucleic acids, a deficiency results in impaired cellular division and
an alteration of protein synthesis. This is particularly noticeable
in the young growing animal. Additionally, due to impaired cell
mitosis in a deficient bird, females do not physiologically prepare
for breeding, as noted by a lack of oviduct hypertrophy in the presence of estrogen. Further, there is an effect on normal red blood
cell maturation, resulting in the characteristic macrocytic anemia. Similarly, deficiencies result in immune system impairment
due to the effects on cell replication and protein synthesis. Folic
acid is involved in the formation of uric acid, so there is an increased requirement when high-protein diets are provided. Folic
acid is required for the production of white blood cells and a severe deficiency can reduce immunologic response through decreased WBCs or reticuloendothelial cells.

In some species, a deficiency of zinc has been found to impair
the utilization of dietary sources of folic acid. Sulfa drugs (eg, sul-
fanilamide) may increase the requirement of folic acid since they
will compete with structurally similar PABA in the bacterial synthesis of folic acid. Vitamin C and iron may improve the bioavailability of folates in food.

Vitamin B$_{12}$

Vitamin B$_{12}$ or cyanocobalamin is a product of bacterial biosynthesis and therefore must be obtained by consuming a bacterial source or animal tissues that accumulate the vitamin. The only exceptions are a few plants, such as peas, beans, spirulina and kelp, that may be able to synthesize minute amounts of this vitamin.

Most of the vitamin B$_{12}$ in the body is found in the liver with secondary stores in the muscle. Vitamin B$_{12}$ is stored efficiently, with a long biological half-life (approximately one year in humans).

Vitamin B$_{12}$ is a critical component of a large number of metabolic pathways. Similar to folic acid, most of the metabolic reactions of vitamin B$_{12}$ involve single carbon units and are very important in the synthesis of nucleic acids and protein as well as carbohydrates and fats.

Like folic acid deficiencies, vitamin B$_{12}$ deficiencies result in an impairment of protein synthesis causing failure or delay of normal cell division. This affects growth rate and feed intake, may result in nervous disorders and poor feathering, perosis, anemia, ventricular erosion and fat accumulation in the heart, liver and kidneys. Deficiency of vitamin B$_{12}$ can also create a folic acid deficiency.

Some research indicates that vitamin B$_{12}$ absorption is decreased in the presence of protein, iron or vitamin B$_6$ deficiencies or by dietary tannic acids.

Choline

Natural sources of choline are widely distributed and occur primarily in the form of phosphatidylcholine (lecithin). Choline can be synthesized in the body but in the avian species tested to date, it cannot be synthesized at high enough levels to meet the needs of the young bird.

Choline has four general metabolic functions: 1) As a component of phospholipids, choline is an essential part of the cell membrane and is required for maintaining cell integrity; 2) Choline is required for maturation of the cartilage matrix of bone; 3) Choline is involved in fat metabolism of the liver by promoting fatty acid transport and utilization, and is therefore necessary to prevent hepatic lipidosis in the normal bird; 4) Choline is acetylated to form the neurotransmitter acetylcholine.

Because of their interrelated functions, the requirement for choline is dependent upon the levels of folic acid and vitamin B$_{12}$ available to the animal. Excess protein increases the choline requirement, as do diets high in fat. Dietary levels of choline chloride (the normal supplemental form) should not exceed twice the requirement.

Vitamin C (Ascorbic Acid)

Vitamin C has not been demonstrated to be a required nutrient for any of the avian species, except for a few highly evolved, largely frugivorous species (Willow Ptarmigan and Red-vented Bulbul). Vitamin C is easily manufactured in birds with the enzyme L-gulonolactone oxidase. This process occurs in the liver in most passerine species, and in the kidneys of psittacines and other older phylogenetic orders of birds. Biosynthesis of ascorbic acid can be inhibited by deficiencies of vitamin A, E and biotin.

The metabolic functions of vitamin C are related to its ability to act in oxidation and reduction reactions. Its best understood role is in the synthesis of collagen, where it is involved in the hydroxylation of procollagen residues.

Vitamin C is also an excellent antioxidant, acting to neutralize free radicals that are produced in the body. Ascorbic acid can also regenerate vitamin E (the active lipid antioxidant).

Stressful conditions that have been shown to improve with supplemental vitamin C are: 1) dietary deficiencies of energy, protein, vitamin E, selenium or iron; 2) high production or high growth rates (the newly hatched chick has a slower rate of ascorbic acid synthesis); 3) management stresses, eg, handling, insecure environment, transportation, crowding; 4) extreme temperature variations from normal; 5) health stresses: fever and infection reduce blood ascorbic acid and diseases with liver involvement decrease synthesis while increasing overall requirement for ascorbic acid.

Minerals

Minerals are essentially classified in one of two groups: macro minerals and trace or micro minerals. The required trace minerals are magnesium, manganese, zinc, iron, copper, iodine, selenium and, in certain situations, cobalt and molybdenum.

Calcium

Calcium is the predominant mineral in the body (approximately 1.5% of body weight) with primarily skeletal system containment. Calcium is also contained in the body fluids, where it plays an essential role in blood coagulation and membrane permeability, and maintains normal excitability of the heart, muscles and nerves. Several enzyme systems are also activated by calcium. Low Ca^{++} concentrations result in a decrease in electrical resistance and an increase in membrane permeability (to sodium and potassium) of nerve tissue, which causes hyperexcitability of neural and muscle tissue and can result in spontaneous fiber discharge.

Calcium absorption occurs predominantly in the upper small intestine by an active transport system involving a calcium-binding protein. This is regulated by the active metabolite of vitamin D_3 in response to low plasma calcium levels. Compounds such as phytate (in cereal grains), oxalates (in spinach, rhubarb and related vegetation) and phosphates will decrease absorption of calcium due to the formation of complexes. Regulation of calcium metabolism involves parathyroid hormone, calcitonin and vitamin D_3 (see Chapter 23).

For maintenance of proper bone tissue, the calcium to available phosphorus ratio should be approximately 2 to 1. A range of 0.5:1 to 2.5:1 can be tolerated. During growth of most species, ratios of approximately 1:1 are required to support adequate growth. High egg-producing hens (poultry) may be provided with dietary ratios in excess of 10:1 in order to support daily shell production. This must not be confused with the significantly lower needs of a hen (most companion birds) that produces a periodic clutch of eggs.

Levels of over 1.0% calcium in the diet have been observed to decrease the utilization of proteins, fats, vitamins, phosphorous, magnesium, iron, iodine, zinc and manganese.

Phosphorus

In addition to being an important bone constituent, phosphorus is also a component of proteins, carbohydrates and lipid complexes that perform vital functions in the body. Phosphorus has a wider range of biological functions than probably any other element.

Like calcium, circulating levels are regulated by parathyroid hormone and calcitonin, with plasma levels being inversely related to plasma calcium levels. Excretion of excess amounts of phosphorus takes place primarily through the kidneys.

In plant sources, phosphorus is often complexed with phytin, making it unavailable to all monogastric animals because of their lack of the enzyme phytase. As a general rule, phosphorus from animal products or inorganic supplements is almost completely available, while that from plant sources is generally considered to be approximately 30% available.

When kept within the range of acceptable calcium: phosphorus ratios, moderately higher phosphorus does not create a significant problem. Amounts of phosphorus outside these acceptable ratios, however, will cause decreased performance and will interfere with the absorption of calcium from the gastrointestinal tract. Additionally, high serum phosphorus levels can induce nutritional secondary hyperparathyroidism by suppressing serum calcium, resulting in stimulation of the parathyroid. In some species, increased excretion results in the development of urolithiasis. It is estimated that the level of available phosphorus, when balanced with calcium and vitamin D, can be supplied at approximately two times the requirement without adverse effects.

Magnesium

Most of the body's magnesium is present in the bone, complexed with calcium and phosphorus. In tissues, magnesium serves as an activator for many of the enzymes involved in phosphate transfer and metabolism. Levels of calcium and phosphorus in a diet affect the magnesium requirement, with high levels of either of the former tending to increase the requirement of the latter.

Potassium

Potassium is widely distributed in most foods, making deficiencies unlikely in adult animals. Unlike sodium, potassium is located primarily intracellularly, and is found at the highest levels in muscle, erythrocytes, brain and liver. Potassium is the primary intracellular cation, affecting acid-base balance and osmotic pressure. It is also involved in protein biosynthesis, cellular uptake of amino acids and as a cofactor in a number of enzyme systems.

Excess potassium is excreted through the kidneys under the influence of sodium and aldosterone levels. Severe stress can create hypokalemia because of an increase in renal potassium excretion caused by elevated plasma proteins. This hypokalemia can be extended during the adaptation to the stress as potassium stores are replenished in the muscle and liver.

Potassium toxicity is not likely due to the capacity of the unimpaired kidney to excrete large concentrations of the mineral. Excesses of three times the required amount have presented no problems in avian species.

Sodium

Sodium is the primary cation of the extracellular fluid, and is predominantly responsible for the regulation of the body's acid-base equilibrium by associating with either chloride or bicarbonate. Sodium is critical in the maintenance of the proper osmotic pressure in the body, protecting against excessive fluid losses. It is also involved in the transmission of nerve impulses, the permeability of cells and acts to inhibit mitochondrial enzyme systems that are otherwise activated by the intercellular ions, potassium (K+) or magnesium (Mg++).

Excess sodium, on the other hand, can be efficiently excreted through the kidneys by an increase in water consumption. Sodium retention is regulated by the adrenal hormone, aldosterone, which maintains proper plasma sodium levels and regulates sodium excretion.

The body has a specific mechanism for concentrating sodium in the extracellular fluid while concentrating potassium in the intracellular fluid. This high concentration gradient is maintained by the sodium-potassium/ ATPase pump system. This system transports Na+ out of the cell, while transporting K+ in. This is an energy-requiring process that uses intracellular ATP as an energy source. Intracellular sodium activates the enzyme system, which uses Mg++ as a cofactor.

Moderate increases in dietary sodium are relatively nontoxic providing adequate (low sodium) water is provided for renal excretion. Levels of five to ten times the requirement can be provided before there is a decrease in growth and loss of appetite in a young bird. Higher levels of sodium intake result in poor feathering, polydipsia, polyuria, nervousness, edema, dehydration and mortality.

Chlorine

Chlorine, metabolically active as the chloride ion, is closely associated to sodium in foods, in the body and in metabolic processes, and both will be excreted under the same conditions. Chloride is also essential in maintaining the body's acid-base balance, osmotic pressure and water balance.

It is critical to evaluate the overall dietary sodium, chlorine and potassium levels together. In the diet there must be a balance of the total sodium and potassium content with the total chloride and sulfate content in order to maintain the proper acid-base balance in the blood.

Essential Trace Minerals

Iron

The functions of iron in the body are almost entirely related to the cellular respiration processes. In the body, iron exists as heme iron (which is chelated with a porphyrin group) and non-heme iron (which is found bound to proteins).

Iron is unique in that body reserves are conserved and recycled very efficiently with negligible excretion. The primary method of iron depletion is through bleeding. Because the body has no normal pathway for the excretion of excess iron, intestinal absorption is carefully controlled to prevent accumulation. Under normal situations, the absorption of iron from the gastrointestinal tract is poor, however, if the body becomes marginally deficient, the absorption is improved until the situation is corrected.

Normally, heme iron (from animal sources) is considered to be approximately 20-25% available to the animal, while non-heme, vegetative sources are usually less than 5% available. Additionally, the non-heme iron present in most foods is in the ferric form (Fe +++), which is poorly absorbed. In order for proper absorption to take place, ferric iron must be reduced to the ferrous state (Fe ++). In the ferrous form, iron becomes more soluble and therefore absorption is improved. This can be accomplished by any reducing compound in the food, with ascorbic acid being one of the more efficient agents. Proteins also enhance absorption, probably by forming soluble amino acids chelated with the iron. Additionally, absorption may be improved by dietary organic acids (eg, citrate, lactate), fructose and vitamin E, as well as by diets low in phosphorus.

In the normal, healthy animal there should be no toxicity symptoms from moderate excesses of dietary iron because of the efficient controls the body has over iron absorption and metabolism. Chronically high iron intake can result in elevated blood levels, increased tissue concentrations (especially of the liver and spleen) and the eventual development of hemosiderosis and possibly hemochromatosis (skin pigment changes). Iron storage diseases have been predominantly seen in mynahs and toucans, possibly being caused by a combination of genetic and dietary factors.

Copper

Copper is a component of several proteins, enzymes and certain natural pigments. It is required for hemoglobin synthesis, proper collagen (bone), elastin and keratin formation and maintenance of the nervous system.

Zinc

Zinc is critical to the animal for growth, reproduction and normal longevity because of its involvement in tissue repair and wound healing. It functions in a number of reactions in protein and carbohydrate metabolism, cell division and mucopolysaccharide formation. It also functions in the mobilization of vitamin A from the liver. Zinc is required in a large variety of enzymes, either as an enzyme activator or as a component of certain metalloenzymes.

Zinc is widely distributed in foodstuffs, but generally is not present in adequate supply to fill the needs of the young or producing animal.

Manganese

Manganese is present in most plant sources at moderate to poor levels. Bile salts are important in the absorption, excretion and reabsorption of this mineral. Recycling appears to occur several times before the mineral is finally excreted in the feces.

Manganese has several functions in the body. It is essential for normal bone structure, being required for the formation of the organic bone matrix through involvement in the synthesis of chondroitin sulfate (at two separate points in its synthesis).

Iodine

Iodine's sole metabolic function is for the biosynthesis of the thyroid hormones. Thyroid hormone functions to control the rate of energy metabolism in cells. Moderate increases in dietary iodine do not present a problem because of the efficient excretion process in the body. Prolonged intake of high dietary levels of iodine causes reduced iodine uptake by the thyroid with antithyroidal or goitrogenic effects.

Selenium

To a greater degree than other trace minerals, selenium content in foods is largely dependent upon the soil selenium content in which they were grown. Other than the enzymatic form, there are no stores of selenium, making the selenium pool quite labile.

Selenium's metabolically active form is as a component of glutathione peroxidase. This enzyme is located in the aqueous phase of the cell and is responsible for oxidizing reduced glutathione, allowing it to act as a biological antioxidant. Reduced glutathione serves to protect membrane lipids and other cellular constituents by preventing oxidative damage by neutralizing any hydrogen peroxide and fatty acid hydroperoxides that are formed in the body.

Vitamin E and selenium are interdependent, each having the ability to spare the other. Selenium and vitamin E work together in the prevention of exudative diathesis. This disease is characterized by generalized edema (first appearing on the breast, wing and neck) due to abnormal capillary permeability, resulting in the leaking and accumulation of fluid. This is accompanied by decreased growth, leg weakness and mortality. Exudative diathesis has not been shown to occur except when both vitamin E and selenium are deficient.

The protection of lipid membranes from exposure to free radicals is not only important for the cell membrane, but also for the membranes of the mitochondria and microsomes. Because these act to both fuel and protect the cell, it is necessary for adequate vitamin E and selenium to be present for the cell to maintain its defense mechanisms.

PERSPECTIVE ON PARROT BEHAVIOR

Greg J. Harrison

Veterinarians who treat companion birds must be knowledgeable about not only avian medicine and husbandry, but also behavior. Every year many birds are euthanized, sent to zoos or breeding facilities, released, abused or ignored because a client is not able to tolerate or change a bird's abnormal behavior.

To understand the behavior of companion birds, it is necessary to remember that many captive-bred birds are only one generation removed from the wild and thus retain many of the characteristics of their free-ranging conspecifics. This, coupled with their relatively high level of intelligence, can make them challenging pets.

Some species of free-ranging parrots have been noted to spend all waking hours flying, eating, preening and vocalizing with their mates. For such intensely social birds, life in an enclosure with no companionship must be the ultimate "psychological torture." It has been suggested that large birds, especially macaws, should never be kept as a single bird unless the client can meet their extensive needs for social interaction.

Companion Bird Behavior

Birds have been shown to be capable of discrimination, tool use, numerical competency and problem solving involving simple labeling and intermodal associations. They have further been shown to be able to transfer learned information and thus are considered to have abstract thought.

A Blue and Gold Macaw learned to smack a stick of wood on the table, imitating the owner in an effort to discourage the house cat from coming near its enclosure. A Boat-tailed Grackle, after repeated unsuccessful attempts to kill a frog with its beak, was video-taped using a stick to impale and kill the frog.

Hand-raising

Birds raised by human foster parents will imprint as people, not birds. As they mature, their natural instincts to choose a mate may cause objectionable behaviors (eg, feather picking, screaming). An imprinted bird will spend all of its time attempting to drive unwanted individuals, other pets or objects out of its territory, while trying to find one chosen person with whom to mate.

Molding a companion bird's behavior should begin when it is a neonate. It should be raised in an area where there is lots of activity and opportunity for new experiences. It should be handled and fed by different people using a variety of feeding methods. Chicks that are exposed to different situations are more stable as adults. Chicks raised "en masse" in boxes without a variety of socializing experiences will be less tolerant and more fearful of new situations as adults. These birds rarely enjoy handling or close contact with people.

Weaning

Weaning is an important part of early training, and it is crucial that human foster parents understand that begging and whining are a natural part of the weaning process. Overindulgent clients can inadvertently teach the chicks that screaming, begging and throwing food get the results they are seeking (eg, food, attention).

The weaning area should be free of perches, toys and other distractions so that the new food will be the entertainment. A flat plate covered with the formulated diet and several kinds of soft vegetables and fruit can be placed on the bottom of the enclosure. When the bird begins to reject hand-feeding, the midday feeding should be eliminated. As it begins eating more on its own, the other feedings can be gradually decreased in volume, with the evening feeding being the last to be eliminated.

Varying the type of feeding utensil (eg, spoon, syringe), adding small chunks of whole food to the formula, or gradually moving the utensil from the bird to the feeding dish may help. It is a common practice by some aviculturists to offer foods from the hand or mouth; however, it should be noted that as a bird becomes older it is capable of seriously injuring the lips or face of the feeder.

Preventing Behavioral Abnormalities

In order for the bird to recognize that it is a bird, not a human, it must understand its boundaries. Clear, consistent communication through words and actions will make the bird feel secure and realize that it is the follower, not the leader.

Herd and flock animals are guided by natural desires to lead or to follow. If a bird is allowed to lead, it will determine who can and cannot enter its territory. It will also demand that certain foods or items be present in its territory. As it matures sexually, the demands increase and it becomes more and more frustrated, if allowed to lead.

Training

Model-Rival Training

Free-ranging parrots use other members of the flock as models for behavior. This natural learning process can be used by clients in a model-rival training program to teach birds what is and is not acceptable behavior. This program involves the use of one person as the trainer, while a second person acts as the bird's rival, and models both good and bad behavior.

For example, the goal of a training session for the African Grey Parrot, Alex, was to review and improve his pronunciation of the label "five." To accomplish this goal, two trainers, A and B, were used in a model-rival training program. The dialogue included:

- **A** (acting as trainer): "Bruce, what's this?"
- **B** (acting as model/rival): "Five wood."
- **A**: "That's right, five wood. Here you are... five wood." **A** hands five wooden popsicle sticks to **B**, who begins to break one of the popsicle sticks apart in a manner similar to that of Alex.
- Alex: "I wood."
- **B** (now acting as trainer, quickly replaces broken stick and presents them to Alex): "Better."
- Alex: "No!"
- (**B** turns from Alex to establish visual contact with **A**.)
- **A**: "What's this?" (presents sticks)
- Alex (now acting as model/rival): "I wood."
- **B**: "Better." (Turns, then resumes eye contact): "How many?"
- **A**: "FIVE wood." (Takes wooden sticks.) "Five wood." (Now acts as trainer, directs gaze to Alex and presents sticks to him.) "How many wood?"
- Alex: "Fife wood."
- **A**: "OK, Alex, close enough. Fivvvvve wood. Here's five wood." (**A** places one stick in his beak and the others within reach.)

Goals and Reinforcers

A list of goals for desirable behavioral attributes for a companion bird might include: be loving and gentle, be quiet, be clean, be willing to consume a balanced diet, come when called, stay where placed, allow wings and feet to be handled, get on a perch, be controllable and be house trained. Once the behavioral goals for a bird have been established, they can be taught by using positive reinforcers.

A primary positive reinforcer is any item or action that will stimulate a behavior to recur. Trainers have traditionally used highly desirable food items, praise or affection as primary reinforcers, but it has been suggested that the use of object rewards increases the speed of learning. The bird is allowed to play with a variety of items until it chooses a favorite. That object is then used as a reward for that day's lessons. Using the same reward every day causes boredom and slows learning. In talking lessons, it is best to use the item being taught as the reward. For example, to teach the word "strawberry," a strawberry should be the reward.

The intensity and amount of interaction with the reinforcer, or the most desirable item of the day, should be varied. The first positive response should elicit a large positive reinforcement, and each succeeding response would be a little less dramatic and much less time-consuming.

After choosing a highly desired item as a primary reinforcer, it is a good idea to also choose a secondary reinforcer. These are items or events that, through repetition, have become associated with the primary reinforcer. The advantage is that they can be interchanged with each other. For example, a sound such as a kiss, a bell, a whistle, or a clicker, can be given as a secondary reinforcer. Each time the primary reinforcer is offered, the bird develops a Pavlovian response to the secondary reinforcer. This is important because it is not always easy or appropriate to offer the primary reinforcer. The bird may be doing a series of actions and rather than stop to offer a primary reinforcer, the sound can be offered and the bird knows the desired action has occurred and is likely to repeat the performance.

Negative Reinforcement

A negative reinforcer is something that a bird is willing to work to avoid and can be used to diminish or extinguish unwanted behavior. Negative reinforcement should be used only as a last resort after the bird has successfully completed as much of the positive training program as it is able; it is the trainer's responsibility to make certain the tasks given the bird were not too difficult. Frequently, clients try negative reinforcement first, and the bird learns that negative actions get attention. Intelligent birds consider the negative reinforcers as a form of entertainment. Especially violent negative reinforcement may destroy the bird's will to learn and cause it to reach a permanent learning plateau. Birds that are frightened may behave, but they would not be expected to seek interactions with the client or enjoy learning.

As with positive reinforcement, negative reinforcement must be given at the exact time the negative event occurs. Immediately placing the bird in a small "time-out" enclosure on the ground is an effective negative reinforcement. Neither the traveling enclosure nor the regular enclosure should be used as a negative reinforcing area. A sturdy cardboard box works well. Other possible negative reinforcers include spraying the bird with water, leaving the room and scolding.

Verbal negative reinforcers should be presented fairly, using commanding, not violent, tones. Identifying certain shapes or colors the bird dislikes may be useful. Merely showing a disliked item from a nonthreatening distance at the moment a negative action is beginning may be a deterrent. Perhaps the use of a remote or voice-activated shocking perch would be effective for feather picking and screaming.

Initiating Training

When training a chick, a commitment of at least 15 minutes, three times a week, for three to six months is a minimum. Training sessions should be uninterrupted, and begin and end at the same time each day. They should be held in an unfamiliar place, away from the bird's play or living area. Training of juvenile birds should begin with simple, one-word commands given over and over to elicit a chosen response. The command must be the same each time, and the bird's response must be the same each time in order for the bird to receive reinforcement. Commands should be issued in a command tone that is sharp, louder than a normal talking voice and delivered with authority.

During the early part of training, the minimal effort on the bird's part must be rewarded, and every time the desired action is repeated it is reinforced. Timing of reinforcement is critically important. The reinforcing event must occur at the exact second that the positive action has been completed. This makes it easy for the bird to understand what is being reinforced and increases the possibility of a repeat performance.

After the desired behavior is established it is recommended to attempt two performances to get reinforcement, then three, four and so on until ten behaviors in a row are performed for one reinforcement. At that point, the reinforcement should be changed from a predictable schedule (ten behaviors = one reinforcer) to a random schedule. Thus, a reinforcer may require 10 behaviors one time and two the next. It takes a while to establish random scheduling, but once established it will produce the strongest performance.

Teaching Commands

In order to be good companions, birds should respond to a minimum of six or seven commands such as "come," "up," "stay," "wing," "foot," "hood" and "go potty."

Training should begin while the neonate is still being hand-fed and the pin feathers are just beginning to open. In order to teach the bird to come, a desired item should be presented to it while giving the command, "come." Beginning with a feeding utensil first thing in the morning often works well, especially if no food has been left in the enclosure overnight. The "stay" command should be taught second, while placing a hand in front of the bird in a stop-sign fashion.

With the bird already on a perch, the "stay" command should be given. While the trainer's hand remains in a stop-sign fashion, a second perch is presented to the bird. The "up" command is given and the bird is encouraged to step up onto the perch.

The "wing" command is accomplished by gently taking each wing from the folded to the open position. Repetition and reinforcement may be needed for ten to twelve weeks. By the time of the emergence of the first pin feathers, the bird should be able to lift its wing on command. Once fledging age is reached, the primary feather tips may be easily clipped one portion at a time by using the commands "stay" and "wing."

Likewise, "stay" and "foot" commands are taught for nail trimming. Over a period of weeks, the bird learns to present its foot and allow the nails to be filed.

For ease of mouth examination, "stay," and "tongue" commands are used. The bird can be taught to allow its tongue to be held for up to ten seconds.

By covering the head with a hood, most birds can be easily handled for nail and wing clips and even minor surgery. This has been shown to be an effective way of calming pionus parrots, cockatiels, conures, cockatoos, some Amazon parrots and macaws. A doll bonnet can be modified by stitching a length of cloth to the brim and inserting a draw string in the bottom edge, making a sort of bee keeper's bonnet. Towels and plastic trash liners have also been used successfully. The hood should be slowly introduced during play time, making sure it does not frighten the bird. Gradually, over several play sessions, the hood can be placed on the bird's head. Hooding time can be extended to accommodate long periods of time such as those that occur with travel. Hooding prior to anticipated times of stress (eg, visits to the veterinarian) is a good way to prevent fear reactions.

House Training

Many birds have a natural inclination to keep the nest clean. They will defecate over the edge or in an area away from the nest. Companion birds usually defecate when they are aroused first thing in the morning. Other common times are when first picked up and every few minutes thereafter on a fairly predictable schedule. With some patience, ingenuity and reinforcement, most birds can be house trained. Each time the bird is picked up, it should be held over the "toilet" area and the "go potty" command should be given. Signs of impending defecation such as legs apart, squatting and leaning back are cues for moving the bird to the "toilet" and issuing the command. Some larger psittacine birds can be trained in a week, but smaller species make less obvious preparation for defecation and are somewhat more difficult. Nervous birds can be expected to go more often and should be presented with the opportunity to do so.

Diet Changes

The first step in changing a bird's behavior is a thorough physical examination to detect any subclinical disorders. It is difficult to change behavior in a bird that is ill. Included should be a blood panel for biochemistries and CBC, Gram's stain, possibly radiographs and cultures. If the bird is on a seed diet, the injection of vitamins and minerals, and oral lactulose should precede the diet change by three weeks.

For many large birds, offering a highly palatable diet alone for 24 hours is sufficient. If they refuse to eat, mixing the new diet in the old seed diet or adding a treat such as popcorn, fruit juice, cheese or other sweet or fatty items may help. Table food may also be mixed with the new diet for several days, and then gradually decreased. Frequently, the biggest obstacle in correcting an improper diet is the client. Most birds will switch to the new diet within five days if they are placed in a different environment separate from the client.

Many birds are so accustomed to seeds and the familiar surroundings in their enclosure, that adding anything new is stressful. A bird may sit on the opposite side of its enclosure for weeks after a piece of carrot or a new toy has been added. For these birds, a diet change is often more successful if food is not the only change made. The bird is placed in a box, aquarium, bath tub or travel enclosure with no bowls, toys or perches. The food is sprinkled on the floor of its new enclosure, and after several hours of walking on the food, the fear is gone. The natural picking curiosity returns and the food is eaten. Placing food over a mirror on the floor may also help. Use of a bird already on the diet as a model is often rewarding.

A number of formulated diets are available today based on nutritional requirements of various companion bird species. Some are more readily accepted than others. As a general rule the extruded diets are more palatable than pelleted diets. Subtle shades of black, brown, yellow and green (naturally occurring colors of food) have been shown to be most acceptable. The use of dyed grains has been found to decrease the acceptance of food in several studies.

Birds are able to taste, which is supported by the presence of taste receptors. Preference testing experiments showed responses to sweet, bitter, acid and salt solutions. Sugar or fat can be added to a diet to facilitate its acceptance; however, the continued use of 10% sugar and 15% fat by weight in a formulated diet has been shown to be detrimental. Birds have been shown to avoid foods treated with pesticides if given a choice.

Behavioral Modification

Although it is ideal to train birds when they are young, adult birds with behavioral problems can also be trained. The quickest route to an obedient bird is to let the bird know it must depend on you for leadership.

A handheld perch and portable stand perches of several heights (all shorter than the handler's shoulders) are required for the training sessions. Plastic jugs or buckets can be cut to scabbard the arm, keeping the bird off the arm and shoulder and also preventing biting, while a hand cover may be cut from a sheet of dark plastic or a garbage can liner. A hood should also be available.

The bird's favorite color may be discovered by using children's beads or other toys that are similar in size and shape but of different colors. The color the bird chooses to play with is considered a favorite and should be used on perches, clothes and reinforcers. The training routine and the commands used must remain consistent. The same stands, perches and reinforcers should be used at each session, and the trainer should even wear the same uniform (eg, a favorite hat or shirt in the bird's favorite color).

DEFENSE MECHANISMS OF THE AVIAN HOST

Helga Gerlach

5

The defense mechanisms of avian species are generally comparable to those of mammals despite fundamental differences in the structure of the system. Detailed information is available only for the chicken, which serves as the model for studying the development of bursa- and thymus-derived lymphocytes.

Many captive birds have been inbred for color mutations. This inbreeding may weaken the immune system and cause these birds to be more susceptible to disease than their free-ranging relatives.

The purpose of the defense system is not only to protect the individual against invasive organisms, but also to eliminate abnormal body cells. The defense system also functions in the recognition of foreign cells, as is observed in graft rejection phenomena. For this system to function properly, it is mandatory that the body be able to distinguish between normal body cells (self antigens) and those antigens that are unlike self (foreign antigens). If the body becomes intolerant of its own cells, then an autoimmune disease occurs.

Epithelial Surfaces

The primary barriers to pathogen access to the body are the skin and the mucosal linings of the intestinal, respiratory, urinary and reproductive tracts. The native flora of the skin is specified and regulated by factors such as desquamation, desiccation and a relatively low pH. Changes in local environmental factors can damage the flora and allow invasion by other microorganisms.

Autochthonous Flora

The normal or autochthonous flora of the intestinal tract is developed in the newly-hatched chick during the first three to four weeks. This flora is species-specific. The acquired flora takes up the available space, occupies receptors and acts competitively against invaders by various mechanisms. Natural development of the immune system also depends on continuous antigenic stimulation by the autochthonous flora. Mucosa-associated lymphatic tissue forms the so-called lymphoepithelial system, which appears to function by capturing and processing antigens from the mucosal surface.

The mucosa of the respiratory, urinary and reproductive tracts of birds is similarly colonized by specific flora whose compositions are relatively unknown. The mucosal surfaces contain goblet cells that secrete a tenacious mucus. The mucus serves to cover cellular receptors for bacteria or viruses. This mucus also contains lysozyme (which has antibacterial and antiviral activities) and immunoglobulin (IgA).

Myeloid System

This system consists of three cell types that all originate from the bone marrow: polymorphonuclear granulocytes (the most important of which is the heterophil), thrombocytes and mononuclear cells, which differentiate into macrophages.

Leukocytes

Generally speaking, the nucleus of the avian heterophil is multilobulated when it leaves the bone marrow. Therefore, the left shift seen in mammals is difficult to ascertain. Heterophils are rather short-lived (a few hours or days), and their granules are packed with a variety of enzymes (peroxidases, proteases, hydrolases) and lactoferrin. Lactoferrin serves to bind free iron, which is a required growth factor for many bacteria. The main function of heterophils is to phagocytize and destroy "foreign" material or damaged cells without having to process them as antigens for presentation to the immune system.

The second way in which heterophils eliminate bacteria is by producing OCl-, hydroxyl radicals, and singlet oxygen. OCl- causes oxidation of bacterial capsular proteins, and the latter two substances are highly unstable and react with lipids to form toxic, bactericidal hydroperoxides.

The information on avian eosinophils is still rather poor. In contrast to mammals, birds are not generally thought to respond to parasitic invasion with an increase of eosinophils. It appears that avian eosinophils participate in hypersensitivity reactions. The degree of involvement is thought to be dependent on the species, inciting antigen and age of the individual.

Avian basophils are morphologically and functionally identical to tissue mast cells. Their granules contain vasoactive amines and proteins, prostaglandins and activators for the coagulating cascade, as well as anticoagulants such as heparin. These cells function to accelerate inflammation at the site of antigen deposition.

Thrombocytes

Unlike mammalian platelets, avian thrombocytes are capable of phagocytosis. It is currently undetermined if the phagocytic process is the same as that used by heterophils.

Macrophages

All macrophages are derived from the bone marrow and enter the peripheral blood as monocytes. The morphologies of the macrophages vary according to their location and functional state.

Table 5.1   Macrophage Morphology by Location

Morphology	Location
Monocyte	Peripheral blood
Histiocyte	Various tissues
Kupffer's stellate cell	Liver sinus
Multinucleated giant cell	Granulomatous tissue
Langhan's giant cell	Tuberculous granuloma
Epithelioid cell	Macrophages with intraplasmatic inclusion
Microglial cells	Brain

Cells corresponding to the alveolar macrophages of mammals have not been demonstrated in the avian lung. However, the entire epithelial surface in the parabronchi, atria and part of the infundibulum is capable of taking up particulate matter and transporting it into phagosomes, which are subsequently processed by interstitial macrophages.

Macrophages have a long life-span unless they are destroyed by the material they ingest. They are equipped with lysosomes containing various substances that can be set free according to their respective functions. These substances are involved in phagocytosis, promoting fever (much rarer in birds than in mammals), inducing inflammation, processing antigens to stimulate an immune response and tissue healing. Macrophages are activated by interferon released by T-lymphocytes. Activation causes macrophages to increase in size, mobility and metabolic activity.

Macrophages are active factors in the inflammatory process. They are chemotactically attracted to the site of microbial invasion where they help to eliminate the intruder.

Not all foreign material is totally ingested or destroyed in macrophages. Some antigen molecules remain on the cell surface for long periods of time. The surface of this macrophage subpopulation expresses special antigens (class II histocompatibility antigens: cell membrane antigens on macrophages, B-cells and activated T-cells) that regulate the interaction between the antigen-presenting macrophage and the antigen-recognizing cells (lymphocytes).

Macrophage-like cells (called dendritic cells) are characterized by long, filamentous cytoplasmic processes and are distributed throughout the spleen and lymph follicles in the parenchymal organs. The dendritic cells have poor phagocytic activity, but they have surface receptors for complement, antibodies and class II histocompatibility antigens. Antigens that are bound to dendritic cells are very powerful immunostimulants that may play a major role in anamnestic response to antigens.

Immune Modulators

Several immune modulators, including adjuvants and paramunity inducers, function principally at the macrophage level. Adjuvants function in various ways to enhance the immune response to antigens. Many of them, such as aluminum hydroxide or some oils, function only to inhibit the resorption of antigens.

Paramunity inducers, especially those consisting of inactivated components from various poxviridae, can stimulate phagocytosis by macrophages and granulocytes, natural killer (NK) cells and, depending on the strain of poxvirus used, the production of interferon and the prostaglandins E and A. The activation of NK cells seems to be an important factor in the nonspecific defense mechanism, especially against virus infections and virus-induced tumor cells.

Antibiotics, especially some tetracycline preparations, inhibit the immune system to varying degrees. An indirect effect is a transient increase in the serum corticosterone level, which depresses macrophage activity. Direct effects include interference with protein synthesis, phagocytosis and antigen processing.

Specific Defense

The specific defense mechanism relies mainly on antigen-sensitive cells, B- and T-lymphocytes, to recognize each antigenic epitope (antigenic determinant) and to produce organism-specific antibodies (humoral immune system), or to provoke cell-mediated reactions (cellular immune system). Depending on whether the host has been exposed to the particular antigen before or if it is an initial encounter, specific defense responses to an antigen may be delayed for two to three or even five to ten days, respectively.

For a substance to be immunogenic, it must be a structurally stable macromolecule and foreign to a host, and it must possess surface structures (epitopes) against which the immune response will be focused. Individual epitopes may induce antibody production, cell-mediated reactions, tolerance or immunosuppression. Since epitopes are specifically defined and occupy rather small areas on an antigen, an antibody produced against one antigenic site may react with an epitope on another totally unrelated antigen. This cross-reaction between totally different antigens can create diagnostic problems in some serologic tests

In addition to macromolecules, small molecules (called haptens) that are linked to a carrier may also provoke an immune response. Haptens of particular interest to the clinician are small, metabolized molecules of drugs, which may bind to serum (or other) proteins. These molecules are recognized as foreign and often induce hypersensitivity responses. Responses to hapten-carrier molecules indicate that production of antibodies to epitopes of the haptens is possibly independent of the carrier molecule itself. Nevertheless, cell-mediated response may be initiated against the hapten-carrier as such, and is therefore called "carrier-specific."

Humoral System

Immunoglobulins

The primary function of the humoral immune system is the production of antibodies directed mainly against extracellular phases of antigens. Antibodies are immunoglobulins, with the major part of the molecule containing ligands for membrane receptors, complement activation and isotype-specific (antigenically

unique) structures. Immunoglobins can be differentiated into isotypes (IgM, IgG, IgA and, in mammals, also IgD and IgE).

IgG: (synonym IgY because of its structural and weight difference from mammalian IgG) is the most common antibody in the
serum, and due to its small size, it can penetrate into tissue spaces
and across body surfaces. IgG can opsonize, agglutinate and precipitate antigen.

IgM: is the major isotype produced following the initial contact
with an antigen. Because of its size (19 S), IgM is normally confined to the peripheral bloodstream and is more active than IgG
in opsonization, agglutination, virus neutralization and complement activation.

IgA: exists in both monomeric and polymeric forms and when
coupled with a secretory component, is excreted onto the mucosal
surfaces of the respiratory, genitourinary and digestive tracts. In
the chicken, IgA also occurs in the bloodstream and in pigeons,
this immunoglobulin is found in high concentrations in the crop
milk. IgA does not activate the complement cascade, nor can it act
as an opsonin. It can agglutinate particulate antigens and neutralize viruses. Its major task is to prevent antigens from adher-
ing to the mucosal surfaces of the body.

Antibody Production

As a rule, birds with high antibody titers against a certain infection are better protected than those with a low titer. However,
there are many exceptions to this generality, particularly with respect to antibodies directed against bacteria. In many instances,
an effective response requires the interaction of antibodies and
components of the cell-mediated immune system. The fate of the
antibody-antigen complex is either phagocytosis or lysis with the
aid of the complement cascade.

Newly hatched chicks receive maternally derived antibodies
(IgG) transmitted via the yolk. The type and quantity of antibodies that the chick receives depend on the immunologic status of
the hen. Vaccination (plus a booster) of the breeder hens with the
appropriate antigens is carried out four to six weeks prior to the
beginning of egg production in order to ensure significant levels of
IgG in the yolk.

Maternal antibodies may present an obstacle to early vaccination programs by neutralizing the vaccinal antigen and, at the
same time, depleting the chick's natural protection. It is also
known that IgM and IgA secreted by the oviduct diffuse from the
albumen into the amniotic fluid where they are swallowed by the
embryo, thus coating the surface of the intestine with a protective
covering of these immunoglobulins.

Lymphocyte Activity

The cellular basis of humoral immunity is the B-lymphocyte,
which is the antigen-sensitive cell. Precursor cells colonize and
develop in the cloacal bursa during embryonic life.

Around hatching time, the mature B-lymphocytes migrate in
large numbers from the bursa into the secondary lymphatic or-

gans (spleen, cecal tonsils, Peyer's patches, Meckel's diverticulum, lymph follicles in the various organs, paraocular and paranasal lymphatic tissue) where they start to function. The Harderian gland is particularly important, and parts of the cloacal bursa, which act as a secondary lymphatic organ. There are some indications for the existence of extrabursal sites of B-cell differentiation (suggested to be gut-associated lymph tissue, Harderian gland, and bone marrow). Around hatching, the Harderian gland has already accumulated actively secreting plasma cells within the interstitial space prior to antigen exposure.

The binding of antigen to the membrane of a B-cell stimulates proliferation of the cellular clones and ends in the differentiation of two functional cell populations: plasma cells and memory cells. The proliferation of B-cells is rigorously controlled and occurs only if certain additional factors are present: 1) The antigen has to be presented fixed to the surface of certain cells, mainly macrophages (which secrete IL-1 and possess class II histocompatibility antigens); 2) T-helper cells must also respond to the same antigen and secrete soluble mediators.

The T-cell then secretes two proteins: the B-cell growth factor (IL-4) and IL-2. IL-2 binds to the IL-2 receptors (produced under the influence of IL-1) on the B-cell, where it stimulates DNA synthesis and division.

Plasma cells differentiate from B-cells to form a series of intermediates until they attain their typical morphology (eccentric wheel-like nucleus and copious cytoplasm). The specificity of the immunoglobulin is the same as in the B-parent cell. Plasma cells can produce up to 2,000 Ig molecules per second, and these antibodies are normally secreted by reverse pinocytosis. Plasma cells survive for only three to six days due to gradual catabolism of the immunoglobulins.

In order to maintain high serum immunoglobulin levels, it is necessary to expose a bird to a second dose of antigen to achieve a so-called booster effect. The memory cells, which survive for many months or even years (perhaps not strictly as individuals, but as clones), are stimulated by the proper antigen, inducing the production of more antigen-sensitive cells. The resulting immunoglobulin production is both faster and more vigorous than the initial response.

Function of the Cell-mediated System

The cell-mediated system is essential for protection against viruses, virus-infected cells, intracellular bacteria, foreign tissue grafts, parasites, fungi and some tumor cells. Thymus-derived lymphocytes (T-cells) also mediate the inflammatory response known as delayed hypersensitivity. T-cells form the basis of the cell-mediated system, but in contrast to the uniform B-cells, T-cells form many subgroups including:

- effector cells, which produce lymphokines provoking cytotoxicity
- helper cells, which produce lymphokines
- suppressor cells, which inhibit the responses of other B- or T-cells.

As in a B-cell response, three mutually interacting cells are necessary for a cell-mediated immune reaction to occur: the antigen-presenting macrophage, the effector cell and the CD4 helper cell. The epitope must be closely linked to the class I histocompatibility antigen in order for the effector cell to be able to recognize the antigen. Once an antigen is recognized, the helper cell secretes IL-2, causing T-cell proliferation and leading to the production of both effector and memory cells. The effector cells are capable of performing various functions. They can secrete several lymphokines, or they can cause direct toxic reactions on contact with foreign or modified cells.

In addition to the cells listed above, vascular endothelial cells, keratinocytes, and cutaneous Langerhans cells have also been found to be capable of presenting antigen. Langerhans cells play an especially important role in the development of skin allergies, delayed hypersensitivity reactions, and allergic contact dermatitis.

Immune Tolerance

Tolerance is defined as a host's failure to respond to produce reactions against a specific antigen. The most important example of tolerance is the absence of antibodies against normal body components. Tolerance to self-antigens is established during embryonal life. An embryo may develop tolerance to viruses or some bacteria that are egg-transmitted.

Disturbance of the Defense System

Both the nonspecific and the specific defense systems can be impaired at almost any site. Depending on whether a stimulatory or suppressing portion of the system is damaged, impairment can result in either deficiency or exaggeration of the system. In addition to the aforementioned immunosuppression caused by antibiotics, certain mycotoxins and many tumors, particularly the virus-induced tumors, can decrease the efficiency of the defense system. A variety of viruses (Newcastle disease virus, several herpesviruses, adenovirus and reovirus) are known to inhibit the immune system. Other viruses, such as PBFD virus and polyomavirus that frequently cause degeneration or necrosis in lymphatic organs are almost certainly also immunosuppressive.

Autoimmunity

Autoimmune antibodies are directed against self-antigens. At a very low level they can be considered as normal, but in higher concentrations they may cause disease. Autoimmune diseases have rarely been reported in birds. The obese strain chickens produce antibodies against thyroid cells, thus causing hypofunction and thyroiditis.

Hypersensitivity

An excessive immunologic reaction can cause a type of inflammation called hypersensitivity. Four different types of hypersensitivity reactions have been described in mammals. Type I occurs rarely in birds because birds do not have IgE, which is essential for the reaction in mammals. Nevertheless, birds have large numbers of mast cells in their lymphatic tissues, particularly in the thymus.

Type I = immediate hypersensitivity. IgE isotypes can attach to mast cells (= basophils) by their Fc fragment. If antigen is fixed to such a cell-bound antibody, the basophil releases vasoactive substances (including histamine), which cause a local inflammation within minutes.

Type II = cytotoxic hypersensitivity. The destruction of cells can be carried out either by antibodies activating complement or by cytotoxic cells. Heterophils, macrophages and some lymphocytes have receptors for Fc immunoglobulin fragments and may, therefore, lyse target cells that are coated with immune complexes.

Type III = immune complex hypersensitivity. Immune complexes are able to activate complement, even in tissues. The C5a component, which leads to vasoactive anaphylatoxins, is also a potent heterophil attractor. As these heterophils try to digest the immune complexes, they release proteolytic enzymes, thus causing tissue damage. The Arthus phenomenon and immunogenic glomerulonephritis are common examples.

Type IV = delayed hypersensitivity. This reaction is caused by cell-mediated immune responses occurring at least 24 hours after antigen contact with sensitized T-cells.

Immune Complex Reactions

Chronic lesions caused by immune complexes can occur in the form of amyloidosis. Although amyloids differ in their composition, the amyloid proteins share the common feature of having polypeptide chains arranged in ß-pleated sheets. This uniquely stable molecular configuration renders the fibers virtually insoluble and almost completely resistant to proteolysis.

FUTURE PREVENTIVE MEDICINE

Branson W. Ritchie

Traditional methods of detecting infectious disease agents have relied on recovering the inciting organisms from samples or indirect demonstration that an organism has been present in the body through the detection of a host immune response. All of these detection systems have inherent problems.

Nucleic acid amplification and detection technologies will continue to improve and will compensate for many of the problems associated with other diagnostic techniques. Nucleic acid probe technology is currently being used to detect microorganisms, determine gender and detect genetic abnormalities.

Overview of DNA and RNA

The ability to selectively amplify and detect nucleic acid from pathogens is based on the fact that unique sequences of DNA or RNA are present in all living organisms. As a review, DNA is a polymer made of four units (bases): adenine (A), guanine (G), cytosine (C) and thymidine (T). RNA is a polymer made of four bases: adenine, guanine, cytosine and uracil (U). In the cell, the replication of DNA or RNA is catalyzed by specific enzymes (polymerases). Specifically derived heat-stable polymerases can be used *in vitro* to reproduce nucleic acid.

When double-stranded DNA is heated, the individual strands will separate (melt) from each other. When the strands are allowed to cool, the individual strands will rebind (reanneal) to their complementary strand of DNA, so that adenine from one strand binds to thymidine on the other strand, and cytosine on one strand binds to guanine on the other strand.

If two strands of DNA, a synthetically produced DNA probe and a target sequence of pathogen DNA, bind together, the process is called hybridization. This hybridization process is the basis of using pathogen-specific DNA probes to detect the presence of an organism's nucleic acid.

DNA Probe Technology

Use of DNA Probes

The sensitivity and specificity of nucleic acid probe technology, the speed of obtaining results and the fact that the process can be used to detect organisms that will not replicate *in vitro*, may ultimately lead to nucleic acid probes replacing culture techniques as the gold standard in detecting pathogens.

The identification of subclinically infected animals requires that the reservoir site for the infectious agent be identified, and that samples be collected from the appropriate site at the correct stage of the infection. Depending on the organism and the host, these reservoir sites may be blood cells, hepatocytes, enterocytes, neurons or possibly any cell within the body.

Given the correct conditions, synthesized DNA probes will bind to specific, complementary target DNA (in a diagnostic test this is pathogen DNA), and the hybridization that occurs can be detected by using a number of visual indicator systems.

For a DNA probe to be specific, it must be developed from a known genomic sequence of the organism in question.

The key to a DNA probe detection system is to identify a pathogen-specific nucleic acid sequence and to synthesize nucleic acid probes to bind specifically to this sequence. The specific nature of the probe prevents cross-reactions with other pathogens, imparts specificity and reduces false-negative results.

Specificity of Nucleic Acid Probes

Nucleic acid probes can be designed to be so specific that they can differentiate between two related organisms that are antigenically similar (induce production of similar antibodies) but have differences in nucleic acid sequence that alter the pathogenicity of the organism.

From a diagnostic perspective, probes are extremely valuable because they can be developed for pathogens so that they are genera-, species- or strain-specific, depending on which portion of a nucleic acid sequence they are designed to detect. For example, a probe could be developed that would detect any *E. coli* or only an *E. coli* that had a unique biochemical function.

Once a probe has been developed, it can be used to detect nucleic acid that is extracted from a sample and attached to a membrane, or it can be used to detect pathogen-specific nucleic acid in a section of paraffin-embedded, formalin-fixed tissue that has been processed for histopathologic evaluation (*in situ* hybridization).

In situ hybridization using pathogen-specific nucleic acid probes is particularly effective when a pathogen is present in relatively small numbers or produces a lesion that histologically resembles that induced by other pathogens. For example, the intranuclear inclusion bodies caused by polyomavirus can appear morphologically similar to the intranuclear inclusion bodies caused by PBFD virus or adenovirus. *In situ* hybridization using viral-specific DNA probes can quickly and correctly determine which of these viruses induced the identified inclusion bodies. When compared to antibody staining techniques for the identification of pathogens in tissues, nucleic acid probes are more specific and more sensitive than other pathogen detection techniques.

In addition to confirming the presence of a pathogen in tissue, *in situ* hybridization can also be used to detect the type of cell infected and whether the pathogen's nucleic acid is present in the cytoplasm or nucleus of the host cell. This last finding is of particular importance in understanding the replication scheme of many viruses, which can be critical for understanding how infections can be treated or prevented.

Sensitivity of Nucleic Acid Probes

Detection of a pathogen in excretions or secretions where numbers of the organism may be small requires further processing. To increase the likelihood of finding an organism in a diagnostic specimen (increased sensitivity), a sample to be tested is often subjected to a group of reactions that will amplify the number of pathogen DNA molecules in the sample, thus improving the ability of the probe to detect the organism.

The most commonly employed technique for amplifying target nucleic acid is the polymerase chain reaction (PCR). When used in combination with pathogen-specific nucleic acid primers, PCR can use one copy of a nucleic acid sequence to produce 1,000,000 copies. The most important component of this process is the pathogen-specific oligonucleotide primer. It is these oligonucleotide primers that allow the process to preferentially increase the number of pathogen nucleic acid molecules without increasing the number of all other contaminating nucleic acid molecules that would be present in a sample.

For example, a fecal sample collected for polyomavirus testing might contain 10 polyomavirus particles, 300 *E. coli*, 10,000 *Staphylococcus* spp., 150 host-derived WBCs (nucleated and containing DNA) and 300 *Candida* spp. It would not be possible to detect only ten copies of the target (polyomavirus) DNA. By using PCR amplification, the 10 polyomavirus particles can be increased to 10,000,000, which can be easily detected.

A PCR cycle involves heating the target DNA (from the pathogen in a sample) to cause ds DNA to become ss DNA, thus exposing the target sequence on the pathogen's DNA to the oligonucleotide primers, where they can anneal to prime the generation of new sequence. The temperature of the reaction is then adjusted so that an enzyme (DNA polymerase) will synthesize a new strand of nucleic acid starting from one end (3') of the primer. At a specified time (determined for each pathogen-specific set of primers), the reaction is heated to stop the DNA polymerase and separate the created ds DNA into new target ss DNA.

This process is cyclic and is usually performed 40 times. The synthesized strands of ss DNA serve as new templates for the reaction, and each cycle results in an exponential increase in molecules.

Sample Collection

Minimal contamination of a diagnostic sample can be a problem with the amplification step that is used to increase the sensitivity of the test. If a clinician were testing a bird to determine the presence of PBFD virus in the blood, and the blood sample was collected from a toenail, a positive result may indicate the presence of PBFD virus either in the blood or on the bird's toenail. A blood sample properly collected into a sterile syringe by venipuncture would be less likely to result in a contaminated sample.

Vaccines

Conventional Vaccines

Modified live vaccines have inherent risks including possible reversion to a virulent form or an attenuation that alters the antigenicity of the vaccine strain to such a degree that it is not protective against a field strain of a virus. Modified live vaccines may be virulent in animals that are immunosuppressed, may be immunosuppressive themselves, may cause a low level of morbidity that affects reproduction and must be handled with care to prevent inactivation.

Killed vaccines require exposing the vaccinate to a large dose of antigen and frequently require the addition of harsh adjuvants that can cause unacceptable tissue reactions in the vaccinate.

Subunit Vaccines

To develop a subunit vaccine, the protein from a pathogen that induces a protective immunologic response in the host must be identified. The nucleic acid sequence (gene) that codes for this protein is then inserted (cloned) into a plasmid of an *E. coli* or other organism, which then produces the desired protein. The immunologic protein is then purified away from the producing organism and can be used as a vaccine. Subunit vaccines allow proteins that would protect an animal against different serotypes to be included in the same mixture.

In the development of subunit vaccines, it may be advantageous to combine several proteins from the same pathogen in order to stimulate both virus-neutralizing and T-cell immune responses. Subunit vaccines also create the possibility for incorporating several proteins from numerous pathogens into one vaccine.

Antimicrobial Therapy

Conventional antimicrobial therapy depends on using chemotherapeutic agents that selectively interfere with metabolic processes that are unique to bacteria, parasites or fungi, while having little or no effect on the metabolism of the host cell. While this is generally effective for bacteria, parasites and fungi, it is ineffective for most viruses and tumor cells, which use the host cell metabolic pathways for energy production and replication

Liposomes have been shown to be effective in transporting agents with immunologic activity against antigen-expressing tumors into the affected cells. For treating cancer, this type of immunotherapy would be far superior to chemotherapeutic methods currently used, because immunotherapy could be targeted specifically for the cancer-producing cells with no effects on normal cells within the affected host. Liposomes can also carry chemical compounds, which increase macrophage activity.

Monoclonal antibodies have been used as a therapeutic agent for some types of cancers with antigen presenting capabilities. By binding cytotoxic agents to the monoclonal antibodies, high concentrations of therapeutic agents are delivered directly to the affected cells to which the antibodies bind.

Antisense RNA Therapy

In the process of replicating DNA, the cell produces a complementary copy of the DNA in the form of a messenger RNA. This mRNA is then used as a copy to make new DNA molecules. In the 1960s, a concept was developed of inhibiting the replication of DNA by introducing a nucleic acid sequence that would bind to the mRNA and prevent its use as a template for replication. This was termed antisense RNA therapy.

When fully implemented, antisense RNA therapy will revolutionize the way that neoplastic and viral diseases are treated. By binding specifically to mRNA, the antisense RNA would inhibit the replication of cancer cells or viruses, while having no adverse affect on unaffected host cells.

To be clinically applicable in the treatment of viral and neoplastic diseases, antisense RNA technology must advance to the point where therapeutic nucleic acid sequences can be introduced to the body in such a way that they enter an affected cell, and subsequently interfere with replication of a virus or neoplastic cell.

PRACTICE DYNAMICS

Cathy A. Johnson-Delaney

For veterinarians with a strong interest in treating companion birds, the advantages of incorporating avian medicine into the small animal practice are numerous. With only minimal equipment additions and some intense continuing education with the desire to learn, the practitioner can increase patient diversity and practice volume and be introduced to the challenge of avian diagnostics and therapeutics.

Membership in the Association of Avian Veterinarians (AAV) and participation in conferences with carefully planned programs are necessary to keep abreast of the rapidly expanding information on the diseases and treatment of companion birds. *The Journal of the Association of Avian Veterinarians,* other journals, textbooks and bird magazines are essential reading for serious practitioners.

Veterinarians with limited experience in treating birds should be realistic about their expertise and be ready to refer complicated cases that require advanced diagnostic, surgical or therapeutic techniques.

Staff Responsibilities

Staff members play a major role in the success of any practice. They should be familiar with the clinic's general recommendations on diets, husbandry and preventive health care. It is critical that staff members' and clinic birds be screened for infectious diseases to prevent them from serving as a source of infection for clients' birds. Assistants should also be encouraged to attend continuing education seminars.

Communicating with the Client

When a client calls for an appointment, the receptionist must instruct the client on the proper way to transport the bird to the clinic so that an evaluation of enclosure management and diet can be made. The water dish should be emptied before transport, but enclosure substrates should not be changed so that droppings from the past several days can be evaluated. The client should also be instructed to collect several fresh fecal samples at home by placing plastic wrap under the perch. Samples should be folded in the plastic and refrigerated until transport to the clinic. A paper towel placed over the enclosure substrate will help identify fresh droppings produced during the trip to the hospital. The client should also bring previous medical records, samples of the normal diet and samples of any abnormal discharges.

If the bird is showing signs of illness, the client should be instructed to warm the enclosure interior to 85-90°F and to cover it in such a way that this temperature may be maintained on the way to the hospital.

Detailed information about the diet and home environment are crucial in evaluating the avian patient, as malnutrition and improper management are common causes of medical problems.

Hospitalization Protocol

A patient that is highly bonded to its family and becomes depressed when separated (beyond its illness) may greatly benefit from regular visitation. The client may also be able to entice a reluctant patient to eat. On the other hand, if the bird has a contagious disease or is recovering from a serious injury or surgical procedure, the excitement and activity associated with a visit may be contraindicated.

Before a bird is discharged from the hospital, the technician should instruct the client on how to administer medications and provide the recommended care, including provisions for keeping the bird warm on the way home.

Travel Considerations

Most airlines are now refusing to transport wild-caught birds, and many domestic carriers are refusing to ship companion birds on the grounds that it is difficult to differentiate between domestically raised and imported birds. Airlines that will ship companion birds within the United States will specify the type of carrier they will accept and the conditions of release from liability that must be authorized. According to aircraft manufacturers and airline engineers, temperature ranges in the cargo bins, which are designated for carriage of animals, vary from 40°F to approximately 70°F.

Carrier specifications for international shipment are set by the International Air Transport Association, and many airlines use these standards for domestic flights as well. It is advisable to be familiar with these carrier specifications and to contact the state veterinarian regarding what is considered a properly completed health certificate for a companion bird. Use of the term "health certificate" should be discouraged because it is impossible to determine from a physical examination if a bird is healthy. Use of a "Certificate of Veterinary Inspection" to accompany the state regulatory form may be appropriate.

Accommodating the Avian Patient

Housing

Appropriate enclosures for avian patients must also be considered. A separate avian housing area that can be maintained at 80-85°F is preferable, but not essential. Birds may be housed in aquariums with screened covers, intensive care units or converted small animal enclosures. Heating pads placed under or along one side of the aquarium can raise the interior ambient temperature to 85-90°F.

Commercial and custom-designed aquariums heated with warm water make excellent housing units for sick birds. Some hospitals use avian isolation units, complete with separate heat and ventilation.

Existing small animal kennels can be converted by installing a removable perch and lining the enclosure with brown wrapping paper or butcher paper. Heating pads or clamp-lamps provide supplemental heat, and towels, plastic wrap, acrylic or plexiglass sheets can be placed over the front of the enclosure to retain heat. Spraying a light coat of Pam cooking oil or silicone on the bars will facilitate the removal of excrement.

Preventing the Spread of Disease

Many avian pathogens can be spread through aerosol and feather particulates, and an efficient ventilation system of laminar flow design will minimize hospital contamination. As fresh air enters one side of the room, it passes across the examination area and is pulled outside by exhaust fans; vents are placed approximately two feet above floor level in the opposite wall from the fresh air vent. Air filtration systems (purifiers) designed to decrease particulates and pathogens to the 0.1-1.0 micron range are recommended for use in the reception, examination, treatment and housing areas. The maintenance requirements and volume of air exchanged vary with each system. These units reduce aerosolized hair, dander, feathers, dust and contagions that would otherwise accumulate in the environment. In initially designing a hospital, areas with separate air flow systems should be incorporated to allow for the separation of patients that require routine care from those that may have infectious diseases. Hospital suites for housing sick birds should be divided into small, easily cleaned areas that also have separate air flow systems.

All equipment used on avian patients should be thoroughly disinfected between patients. It should be stressed that all disinfectants are toxic and must be handled with care to prevent problems in hospital premises or patients. Quaternary ammonia solutions (quats) are satisfactory for use as table washes or in cold sterilization trays, and can be used to clean enclosures and soak capture nets, dishes, perches and grooming tools. Because these solutions may be nephrotoxic to birds, equipment must be thoroughly rinsed after being soaked in quaternary ammonia compounds. Quats are the disinfectants of choice against chlamydia and have a wide range of effectiveness against many other pathogenic bacteria and viruses. A phenol-type disinfectant is recommended by the United States Department of Agriculture (USDA) for use in quarantine stations and other avian facilities. It has activity against the Newcastle disease virus and many other pathogens. Phenols may be used for cleaning enclosures and other equipment, but because they are irritating to skin, rubber gloves should be worn, and enclosures and instruments must be thoroughly rinsed prior to direct contact with birds.

Chlorhexidine has the advantage of being gentle to tissues and equipment and is effective against viruses and candida, but it is not effective against chlamydia and many other pathogenic bacteria. It can be used in some cases in the drinking water or as a wound or sinus irrigation solution or in liquid diets and hand-feeding formulas. Other types of disinfectants useful in the avian practice are isopropyl alcohol for cleaning surfaces and instruments; iodophores such as povidone iodine solutions (hand soaps, scrubs and wound irrigations) and chlorine bleach for cleaning nonmetal surfaces, equipment and utensils. Good ventilation is important when using any disinfectant, and surfaces must be thoroughly rinsed and dried before coming in contact with birds.

The order in which hospitalized avian patients should be maintained follows the same pattern as that for working with other animals: clean, feed and treat beginning with the healthiest and ending with the most highly contagious and critically ill. Any bird within the hospital that is sick for an unconfirmed reason should be considered highly contagious until proven otherwise. When working with a patient with a highly infectious disease, it is advisable for the attendant to wear a mask and hospital gown that can be changed.

Equipment

The specialized equipment needed to practice avian medicine is minimal. Many small animal practices already have isoflurane anesthesia (mandatory for avian practice), ophthalmic-sized surgical instruments and suture materials, an endoscope, a radiosurgery unit and radiographic equipment. Additional equipment acquisitions should include a high quality gram scale, avian mouth speculums, gavage needles and a radiographic positioner. Bandaging and splinting supplies, protective collars and dental acrylics for orthopedics and beak repair are also necessary.

It is important that hospital perches be made of nonporous material such as heavy plastic or epoxy/resin composites. Perches of porous material (eg, wood) should be disposed of after use.

Diagnostic Equipment

Equipment necessary for basic in-house avian diagnostic tests includes a binocular microscope with oil immersion capability (1000x), hematocrit centrifuge, refractometer, hemacytometer, bacteriologic incubator, alcohol lamp or Bunsen burner, and basic laboratory supplies such as staining kits, coverslips, slides, hematocrit tubes, serum separators and culturettes.

Several serum chemistry testing systems are commercially available. Those currently used in avian practices are the Kodak DT60 Analyzer, the VetTest 8008, the Reflotron and the Seralyzer. Both the Kodak and the VetTest units can run a typical avian profile including AST, uric acid, glucose, calcium, total protein and albumin.

Although many clinics perform in-house diagnostic tests, most find it necessary to use the services of consultants from time to time. Board certified radiologists and histopathologists who have had experience diagnosing avian cases are especially helpful. Commercial clinical pathology laboratories that specialize in avian and exotic patients are indispensable for isolation and identification of avian pathogens that require specialization beyond the capacity of most veterinary hospitals.

Submitting Samples to an Outside Laboratory

Considerations for choosing an outside laboratory include experience in avian diagnostics, types of services and tests available, sensitivity and specificity of the tests offered, policies regarding laboratory supplies and transport media, mailers, billing and invoice policies, direct fees for tests, turnaround time for results being reported and method of reporting (telephone, fax, computer, mail). A laboratory that is reporting sensitive data by fax should require that the clinician sign a release form stating that the fax is secure to receive confidential information. There are potential legal ramifications of laboratories reporting sensitive information regarding infectious diseases by phone, and high quality laboratories will provide this information only by mail or to a secure fax machine. Submitted samples should always be clearly identified and accompanied by a written report indicating the tests requested, a brief history of clinical signs, differential or tentative diagnosis and any medications being used. Ideally, all samples submitted should meet the following criteria:

1. Baseline samples should be taken prior to administration of medication. Correct sample collection techniques should be used (free-flowing blood, not nail clip, for blood work).
2. Samples should be collected aseptically from anatomic sites likely to contain pathogens.
3. Samples should be taken during the acute phase of the disease rather than the chronic stage.
4. A relevant synopsis of the disease process or flock outbreak should be included.
5. Any pertinent background information and differential diagnoses should be provided.

Most samples for bacteriologic screening should be kept moist in an appropriate transport medium, refrigerated but not frozen and sent immediately with cold packs. Chlamydia isolation may be more successful if tissues are frozen and shipped with dry ice, rather than refrigerated immediately and then shipped on regular ice. Fecal samples or cloacal swabs in specific chlamydia transport medium may be submitted for antemortem diagnosis. Refrigerants must be sealed in leak-proof plastic bags, and dry ice should be packed to allow for the carbon dioxide to escape after sublimation, without contaminating the samples. Refrigerants should constitute about 50 percent of the weight of the contents of the package. Styrofoam-lined boxes with sturdy cardboard, wood or plastic exteriors are preferred for shipping refrigerated specimens. To comply with legal and medical responsibilities, specimens should be packed with sufficient material to absorb any leaking fluid as well as to protect the specimen from damage.

Pharmaceuticals

Very few pharmaceuticals are specifically licensed for use in avian species, but the Federal Drug Administration (FDA) has exercised discretion in enforcing extra-label drug use in companion animals to avoid the adverse impact on animal health that could result if the human drugs were unavailable for veterinary use. Avian practitioners should be aware that the promotion, distribution and use of human drugs in animals results in violation of the Federal Food, Drug and Cosmetic Act when:

1. A drug labeled for human use accompanied by labeling which prescribes, recommends, or suggests a use for animals, for which the product is not generally recognized as safe and effective, is an unsafe new drug under section 512(a) and is adulterated under section 501(a)(5) of the Act.
2. The use or intended use of a human drug in animals by a veterinarian causes such drug to be considered a misbranded drug under section 502(f)(1) of the Act.
3. A drug labeled for human use that is promoted, distributed or otherwise intended for animal use is misbranded under section 502(f)(1) of the Act if its labeling fails to bear adequate directions for animal use.
4. The use of a human drug in food-producing animals may cause adulteration of the food. If the residue is a human drug, the food is adulterated under section 402(a)(2)(A) of the Act.

Regulatory action has not ordinarily been considered concerning the distribution of human drugs for use in companion or non-food-producing animals provided all of the following conditions exist:

1. Intended animal use of the human drug is not established by labeling, advertising, promotional activity or in any other overt manner.
2. There is no approved veterinary drug version of the human drug available.
3. The human drug does not represent a significant risk to the animal when prescribed, dispensed or administered by a veterinarian.

Environmental Responsibility

Most leading professional, avicultural and conservation-oriented organizations are actively promoting domestically raised, not wild-caught, birds for pets. Throughout the world there are increased legislative efforts to stop or at least control importation of wild-caught birds. The avian practitioner should promote the purchase of domestically raised birds and keep clients informed of conservation efforts.

Imported birds that have passed through USDA quarantine stations are banded with a stainless steel band with a code of three letters followed by three numbers. The quarantine system is designed strictly to prevent diseases of importance to the poultry industry from entering the United States. Quarantine procedures for imported birds include a 30-day stay in an approved quarantine facility, screening for Newcastle disease, and a 30-day treatment with chlortetracycline for chlamydiosis. Information concerning the importation and quarantine process, USDA regulations, ports of entry and health certificates for shipment of birds out of the country is available from state veterinary offices or regional APHIS/REAC offices. Other regulatory agencies in the United States involved in bird trade are the US Department of the Interior, The Convention on International Trade in Endangered Species (CITES) and the US Department of Treasury — Customs Service, which watches for smuggled birds. The Fish and Wildlife Service is charged with restricting imports and exports of many species of birds which may require special permits if listed in CITES. Information about transporting listed species may be obtained through the US Fish and Wildlife Service, PO Box 3507, Arlington, VA 22203-3507; 703-358-2093.

If a bird is diagnosed with exotic Newcastle disease (VVND) virus and definite proof of proper importation cannot be produced, the bird along with any birds that have been in direct contact may be confiscated, tested and euthanized. Many states also require proof of hatching or legal importation before issuing a license to an aviary or breeding facility. The avian veterinarian should record a bird's band number, tattoo number, microchip number, or any pertinent physical information in the medical record. If the band is removed, the client should keep a copy of this record along with the removed band.

MAKING DISTINCTIONS IN THE PHYSICAL EXAMINATION

Greg J. Harrison
Branson W. Ritchie

The purpose of the relationship between an avian veterinarian and the client is to ensure a long, comfortable, disease-free life for the companion bird. Clinicians must thoughtfully combine information from the anamnesis, physical examination and minimum database to advise clients on how to prevent medical problems.

In the practice of avian medicine there is a decisive difference between the diagnosis and treatment of obvious problems and the ability to detect, identify and correct subtle abnormalities. By careful and systematic evaluation of the patient and its environment, subtle abnormalities become increasingly obvious. Avian species attempt to hide signs of disease.

Clients should be instructed to evaluate the movement, body posture, head position, behavior, appetite, attitude, ocular clarity and excrement of their birds on a daily basis. This will help identify abnormalities before a disease progresses to an irreversible point.

Clients that are taught to observe a bird's fecal output (not food consumption) can be instructed to seek immediate medical assistance when changes are noted.

To help identify management and disease-related problems early, it is advisable to perform a complete physical examination on a new patient twice in the first year, and annually thereafter.

Anamnesis

Early identification and correction of subtle abnormalities caused by environmental stresses (eg, exposure to cigarette smoke, kerosene heaters, chemical fumes, disinfectants), management flaws (poor hygiene) or nutritional inadequacies (eg, all-seed diet, excess vitamin supplementation) are clinically more rewarding than attempting to stabilize a chronically compromised patient with an acute, life-threatening metabolic crisis.

Developing the Anamnesis

When and where was the bird obtained? Birds obtained from traveling dealers are frequently exposed to infectious diseases and may be illegal imports that have not been through a USDA quarantine system.

Specific Questions for Developing the Anamnesis

- What is the duration of observed problems?
- Are there other pets?
- What exposure does the bird have to other birds?
- Are other pets or family members ill?
- Has the bird had other medical problems?
- Has the bird received any medications?
- When was the bird first introduced to the home?
- Where was the bird obtained?
- Did the bird come with a health guarantee?
- Where is the bird kept in the home?
- What substrate is used in the enclosure?
- Is the home heater electric or gas?
- What temperature is the home?
- What houseplants does the bird have access to?
- Is the bird frequently exposed to fresh air and sunlight?
- Is the photoperiod natural and regulated, or random and irregular?
- Are exterminators used?
- Is the bird exposed to cigarette smoke?
- What potential aerosols is the bird exposed to (household chemicals, disinfectants, hair sprays)?
- What disinfectants are used in the enclosure and how often?
- Have any changes recently occurred (new enclosure, different diet, painted house, new carpet, moved bird to new location or new residence, new pet or strangers in the house)?
- What types of foods are offered?
- What types of foods are consumed?
- What feeding schedule is used?
- Are any dietary supplements used?
- Is the appetite increased or decreased?
- Have droppings changed color, frequency, consistency or quantity?
- Has the water intake changed?
- Any coughing, sneezing, diarrhea or vomiting?
- Have noted changes remained the same or progressed?

How long has the bird been in the household? Recently obtained birds (within the last year) are more likely to be suffering from problems associated with infectious disease or stress, while long-term pets are more likely to have problems with malnutrition or chronic systemic diseases.

Have any new birds recently been added to the household or aviary? New birds can invariably be a source for previously unencountered pathogens.

Has there been a change in food or water consumption? Subtle increases or decreases in food or water consumption can be signs of disease.

Are other pets or family members ill? If other pets or family members are ill, the clinician should consider a common etiologic agent (infectious disease or exposure to an environmental toxin).

Is the bird restricted to an indoor environment? Frequent exposure to fresh air and sunlight is important for a bird's overall health. Drafts have no effect on healthy birds that are acclimated to normal temperature fluctuations.

Is the bird exposed to toxic compounds, particularly aerosols? Commonly encountered, but infrequently discussed, toxins that could have a dramatic effect on the health of a bird include cigarette smoke, fumes from disinfectants (eg, Clorox, ammonia, Lysol), furniture polish, floor wax, paint, hair spray, dry cleaning fluid and carpet and furniture cleaners (see Chapter 37).

Have any medications already been administered? Some breeders and pet retailers recommend the use of over-the-counter (OTC) medications (usually tetracyclines or erythromycin) for the treatment of sick birds. These OTC preparations usually have little or no therapeutic value and further complicate the disease picture by weakening the immune system and encouraging the proliferation of secondary bacterial or fungal pathogens.

Have there been changes in a bird's behavior? Excessive sleeping, resting fluffed, decreased talking, singing or playing? Personality changes, including increased aggression, screaming, scratching or increased preening?

What is the bird's reproductive status? Seeking seclusion, tearing up paper, a crouched copulatory stance and masturbatory actions are suggestive of breeding behavior.

Physical Examination

The physical examination can be viewed as a three-part process: observing a bird's response to its environment, examining the bird's environment and systematically examining the patient. By carefully performing the same thorough physical examination on each patient, the practitioner can develop an image for the average and a perspective of what should be considered clinically normal.

Evaluating the Bird in its Environment

Birds that are stressed will frequently alter their behavior in an attempt to hide signs of disease. This is particularly true while a patient is in the examination room, and it is a challenge for the clinician to distinguish between stress-related behavior, normal behavior and a disease process. A bird that the client describes as listless at home may appear bright, alert and responsive when subjected to the stress of the hospital environment.

The general appearance, attitude, posture and activity level of the bird should be determined while it remains securely within its enclosure. Some avian species (notably Amazon parrots and *Pionus* spp.) may pant when stressed. Excessive chest movement, excessive tail motion when breathing (tail-bobbing), open-mouthed breathing, neck-stretching, yawning, extending the wings away from the body, and forward movement of the head (bobbing) on inspiration or expiration are all indications of respiratory system compromise. Dyspnea associated with the upper respiratory tract or lungs is frequently accompanied by open-mouthed breathing. Lung and lower respiratory tract problems are usually associated with a rhythmic tail-bob.

Acute dyspnea in an apparently healthy bird usually results from exposure to aerosolized toxins, dislocation and movement of tracheal plaques (from malnutrition or infectious agents) or aspiration of foreign bodies (particularly seed husks or enclosure substrates).

Table 8.1 Normal Heart and Respiratory Rates of Birds (per min)*

Weight	Heart Rate (Rest)	Heart Rate (Restraint)	Resp. Rate (Rest)	Resp. Rate (Restraint)
25g	274	400-600	60-70	80-120
100g	206	500-600	40-52	60-80
200g	178	300-500	35-50	55-65
300g	163	250-400	30-45	50-60
400g	154	200-350	25-30	40-60
500g	147	160-300	20-30	30-50
1000g	127	150-350	15-20	25-40
1500g	117	120-200	20-32	25-30
2000g	110	110-175	19-28	20-30
5000g	91	105-160	18-25	20-30
10kg	79	100-150	17-25	20-30
100kg	49	90-120	15-20	15-30
150kg	45	60-80	6-10	15-35

*The resting or flying heart rate of any sized bird can be estimated with the formulas: Resting HR in beats/sec = $12 \times (4 \times Wg)^{-0.209}$. Flying HR beats/sec = $25 \times (1 \times Wg)^{-0.157}$. Multiply results of either by 60 for beats per minute.

Table 8.2 Effects of Aging in Macaws

- Muscle wasting > 40 years old
- Joint stiffness suggestive of arthritis
- Loss of skin tone and elasticity
- Neurologic disease
- Decreased feather production > 40 years old
- Twisting deformities of the carpi > 40 years old
- Pigment spots, polyps, wart-like blemishes, cysts, wrinkling facial skin
- Thinning of the skin on the face and feet > 40 years old
- Cataracts > 35 years

Excrement

The amount and character of feces is a more accurate reflection of a bird's condition than the owner's impression of the body weight and food consumed.

A normal budgerigar may produce from 25-50 stools per day, while a Blue and Gold Macaw may defecate 8-15 times a day. A reduced quantity of excrement can be an indication of decreased food intake, an increased gastrointestinal transit time or a blockage. Dry, scant droppings may indicate dysphagia or food and water deprivation.

The normal excrement should consist of a fecal component, urates and liquid urine. Normal feces may be green, light- to dark-brown and be slightly loose-to-firm in consistency. Normal urates should be white and the urine should be clear. The physical characteristics of feces can be influenced by the species and age of the bird, the time of day, type of diet consumed, quantity of food and water available, reproductive status, medication administered, renal disease, liver disease and the presence of parasitic, bacterial, chlamydial, fungal or viral pathogens.

It is common for a bird in the exam room to have a stress-induced polyuria or diarrhea. Over-consumption of fruits, vegetables or a recent change in the diet can alter the color and consistency of the feces. Birds that consume heavily pigmented foods (eg, blackberries, blueberries) can produce oddly colored feces.

Dark-colored feces (not caused by fruit consumption) is indicative of melena. This is a common finding in budgerigars on an all-seed diet, but may be abnormal considering that the melena stops when birds are placed on a formulated diet. Blood in the excrement can originate from the GI tract, oviduct, kidneys, testicles or cloaca. Frank blood in the excrement may be associated with coagulopathies, liver disease, cloacal pathology, pre- or post-oviposition, malnutrition or enteritis. Bright-green, loose feces and yellow, green or brown urates may indicate hemolysis or hepatitis and are common with malnutritional, toxic, chlamydial, bacterial or viral hepatitis. Clay-colored feces are indicative of maldigestion or malabsorption.

Birds consuming some formulated diets or large quantities of fruits and vegetables will produce a loose voluminous feces and more urine than birds on a principally seed diet. Neonates fed most standard formulas have soft, semiformed voluminous feces, as do hens in the pre- and post-ovulatory period. Voluminous droppings may also indicate malabsorption (eg, gastrointestinal disease, pancreatitis, peritonitis or parasites), diabetes or renal tumors. For some birds, especially house-trained birds, a voluminous feces is a normal morning dropping.

A granular or rough stool can indicate abnormal digestion. The presence of undigested food in the feces is not normal and must be differentiated from food that has fallen into the feces. Excreting poorly digested food can be an indication of maldigestion, malabsorption or hypermotility caused by parasites, pancreatitis, proventriculitis, ventriculitis or intestinal disease.

Diarrhea is rare in companion birds. Loose, watery feces are normal in lorikeets and birds that consume liquid or nectar diets. In psittacine birds, most cases of diarrhea reported by clients are actually polyuria. Finding bubbles (gas) in the feces is common in birds with true diarrhea. Diarrhea can occur with various parasitic, fungal, chlamydial, viral and bacterial infections, systemic diseases and following the administration of some medications.

Direct examination of the feces should include a Gram's stain (to detect fungi, bacteria and inflammatory cells), fecal flotation (for helminths), direct wet mount examination for protozoa and determination of pH. The normal pH of the cloaca is 6.5-7. A basic pH (>7.5) favors the growth of yeast and Enterobacteriaceae.

Urine and Urates

The stress of being transported to the clinic will cause most birds to be polyuric when they are examined by the attending clinician. The presence of hematuria in any form is abnormal. Blood that is in the urine may originate from the GI tract, oviduct, kidneys, testicles or cloaca.

Yellow-green urates are indicative of hemolysis or liver disease. Idiopathic, reddish-brown urates have been described in some hand-fed babies that seem to be otherwise healthy with normal growth patterns. This phenomenon is more common in birds that are receiving an animal protein-based diet, and some cases will resolve when a neonate is switched to a plant protein-based formula.

The avian urinalysis should include cytology and determination of the pH, glucose, sediment, color and specific gravity. Glucose should be completely absorbed and is not normally detected in the urine. The presence of ketones is abnormal and may suggest diabetes mellitus. The presence of casts is an indication of renal disease. Uric acid crystals can be dissolved by adding several drops of sodium hydroxide to a urine smear. This will facilitate the identification of casts, bacteria and cellular debris.

Urine may be excreted without urates when birds are nervous, polydipsic or consuming fruits and vegetables with a high-water content. Polyuria may be noted in birds that are egg laying, feeding chicks or holding their droppings overnight. It is also common in hand-fed babies and birds that are excited or housed in hot environments. Pathologic causes of polyuria include diabetes, renal disease, wasting disease, certain medications (eg, aminoglycosides, steroids, medroxyprogesterone) and exposure to various toxins.

Vomiting vs Regurgitation

The distinction between regurgitation and vomiting is not as easily made in birds as in mammals. The expulsion of ingesta from the crop is considered regurgitation. The pH of material regurgitated from the crop is generally neutral to slightly alkaline. Regurgitation can occur as part of the normal mating activity. If regurgitation is part of courtship activities, the patient will be of normal weight and will have no other clinical signs of disease.

Vomiting is considered the expulsion of ingesta from the proventriculus. Vomitus is usually acidic, may be bile-tinged and generally contains partially digested food. An acute onset of vomiting caused by a pathologic process is often accompanied by depression, severe dehydration and shock.

Odors

Normal fresh excrement from companion birds is basically odorless. Foul breath is rare in birds and, when present, indicates an abnormality that might include candidiasis, oral or upper gastrointestinal tract ulcerations, oral or upper GI abscesses or gastroenteritis. Unpleasant skin and feather odors are usually associated with necrotic tissue secondary to cysts, abscesses or neoplasias. Pasty droppings that adhere to the vent and produce a metallic, offensive odor are frequently noted in cockatoos. These birds generally have abnormally acidic feces of unknown etiology.

Birds consuming high animal fat diets may have a rancid oil odor that can persist for several weeks after a diet change.

Gram's Stain

Gram's stains of samples from the feces, cloaca, choanal slit and crop can be used to evaluate a bird's overall health by estimating microbial populations. Fresh feces appear to be the most useful sample to evaluate.

In general, the digestive tract of grain- and fruit-eating Psittaciformes contains a gram-positive bacterial flora with a few yeast. A normal fecal Gram's stain should contain 100-200 bacteria per high-power field with 60-80% gram-positive rods and 20-40% gram-positive cocci. A few yeast or gram-negative bacteria per high-power field could be considered normal but should alert the clinician to carefully evaluate the patient for subtle abnormalities.

Gram-negative bacteria are common in the oral cavity and in feces of clinically normal carnivorous or insectivorous Passeriformes, raptors, Galliformes and Anseriformes. The feces of canaries and finches normally have a reduced population of bacteria and often show various types of yeast one-fourth to one-half the size of *Candida*.

In most psittacine birds, an absence or decrease in the number of bacteria, the detection of WBCs, a shift from a gram-positive to a gram-negative bacterial population or the presence of a high number of yeast (> 5/HPF) in samples from the choana, cloaca or feces may indicate a primary microbial infection or that immunosuppression with colonization by secondary pathogens has occurred. Some formulated diets and most breads contain brewer's yeast, which can be passed in the feces and morphologically resembles *Candida* spp. In general, yeast of clinical concern will be budding, while brewer's yeast will not.

Properly interpreting a Gram's stain requires that the clinician determine if the organism detected is pathologically colonizing a mucosal surface. A clinically normal bird with an abnormal Gram's stain should be observed for changes that could indicate a problem. The management practices associated with the bird should be carefully evaluated to identify problems that could increase a bird's exposure to pathogenic bacteria or that could be weakening the immune system. A shift from an abnormal to a normal Gram's stain over a three- to six-week period is common in birds that are changed from an all-seed to a formulated diet.

An improperly evaluated Gram's stain can result in unnecessary antibiotic therapy that is detrimental to an individual bird or to an aviary as a whole. Damage to the normal flora caused by the indiscriminate use of antibiotics or contact with disinfectants precipitates the colonization of opportunistic pathogens.

Examination of the Patient

The initial consideration in performing a physical examination is in handling the patient in a safe and efficient manner. A client should be informed that handling a critically ill bird can destabilize the patient to a point where it can no longer compensate.

The examination room used for birds should be secluded, sealable, easily cleaned, contain minimal furniture, have dimmable lights and should not have ceiling fans or uncovered windows. With smaller, easily stressed species (eg, finches, canaries), performing the physical examination in a dimly lighted room will help calm the patient.

The clinician should wear ear protectors to prevent hearing loss when handling large screaming psittacine birds. The use of a magnifying loupe, operating microscope or slit lamp will help in discerning subtle changes associated with the skin, feathers, head, cloaca, oral cavity, eye and limbs. The ear canal of birds can be examined using a small otoscope cone. An otoscope may also be useful in evaluating the oral cavity, cloacal mucosa and pharyngeal area. With practice, a thorough examination can be performed on a critically ill patient in less than three minutes.

While a physical examination can be performed using different regional or anatomic approaches, the key to detecting subtle abnormalities is to consistently use the same approach (using a physical examination form may be helpful).

A paper or cloth towel can be used for removing larger patients from their enclosures. Paper towels are best for handling birds because they can be discarded after use. If cloth towels are used, they should be laundered and autoclaved between each bird to prevent nosocomial infections. With practice, the most refractory psittacine birds can be easily restrained using a towel. Gloves should never be used to restrain psittacine or passerine birds.

Small birds can be restrained with one hand by placing the bird's head between the second and third fingers. Larger birds can be initially removed from the enclosure with a towel or net and then restrained by placing the thumb and index finger on either side of the mandibles. A bird must be able to move the sternum in order to breathe, and excessive force on the chest can result in asphyxiation. The bird should be held upright or parallel to the floor. Holding a sick bird upside down can compromise respiratory effort.

The Dermis and its Unique Adaptations

The feather condition of a bird is an excellent indication of its overall health. The feathers and skin should be evenly colored, sleek, clean and dry. Feathers should be complete and intact throughout their length and width. Bent, malformed, broken or frayed feather edges are indications of a problem.

The normal feather brilliance or "sheen" is derived from a combination of physical color, structural reflection of light (structural color), the presence or absence of powder from the powder down feathers (if present) and oil from the preen gland (if present). A bird loses its sheen if abnormalities occur in any of the factors that contribute to the reflectivity of the feathers.

Malnutrition in general may cause these kinds of feather problems. Such birds appear sparsely feathered, not because the feathers are reduced in number but because the feathers that are present are abnormal.

The skin over most of a bird's body is thin, soft, dry and relatively translucent. Small portions of discarded feather sheaths are normally found on the skin and should not be confused with dry, flaky skin. Uric acid deposits may be noted under the skin in cases of gout. Examination of subcutaneous tissues can be enhanced by wetting the overlying feathers with warm water or alcohol.

Balding, thinning, swelling, peeling or ulcerations of the skin or scales of the feet and legs are indications of abnormalities. The skin and feathers of birds consuming an all-seed diet are rarely normal.

When a bird is relaxed, the feathers lie flat and follow the natural contour of the body. Feathers that are out of place may indicate abnormalities. Localized feather abnormalities should alert the clinician to carefully evaluate certain areas of the body. Wet, sticky or stained feathers around the nares are indications of rhinitis. Generalized feather abnormalities indicate systemic abnormalities that should be evaluated.

One of the many functions of feathers is to retain body heat. A bird that is diseased may be "fluffed" because it is chilled or because it is consuming insufficient energy to maintain a proper metabolic rate and compensate for normal heat loss. Birds may also fluff their feathers when they are content or when they wish to be preened or as a part of the mating ritual. A bird that is fluffing due to illness will show other signs of disease.

Feather problems should be divided into those that occur before, during or after development. Lesions occurring before development are caused by damage in the follicle, and the feathers do not emerge properly, if at all. Damage that occurs to a feather during development is characterized by an abnormal feather structure or color that is evident as the sheath is removed from the differentiated feather. Dark lines located transversely across several feathers (stress lines) indicate that an adrenocortical surge occurred while the affected feather was developing. Post-developmental feather problems are characterized by an abnormal rachis, barb or barbules but a normal follicle and calamus.

The molting process varies with the individual bird. Some birds (eg, canaries, raptors, pheasants) molt seasonally (typically after breeding season) while other birds molt continuously (budgerigars and cockatoos). The normal molt should be orderly and uneventful with an old feather being forced out by a newly developing feather (see Chapter 24). Birds should lose the feather sheath from the differentiated portion of a feather within days. Retention of the feather sheath is not normal, and may indicate malnutrition, pansystemic disease or an infectious agent. Birds will normally preen the head, neck and facial feathers of a companion.

Damaged pin feathers cut or broken off at the surface may be black and mistaken for mites. These damaged feathers may cause pruritus and excessive preening. Head feathers may appear abnormal in canaries that are malnourished, especially in reproductively active hens. The skin of the neck is frequently hyperkeratotic in these cases. The powder down feathers of the prolateral region should be examined for the presence of powder formation or feather deformities. Moist lacerations or ulcerations may be noted in the axillary region in some birds with dermatitis.

Birds that are fed a marginal diet, that are not exposed to fresh air and sunlight and that are not allowed to bathe regularly have feathers that appear worn and tattered. The feathers that are replaced may have retained sheaths that give the bird the appearance of having an excessive number of pin feathers. Birds that are provided an inadequate diet may enter a molt cycle when their nutritional requirements are satisfied. Following a diet change, these birds may go through a period when they seem to scratch and preen excessively.

Head

Scabs, scars or active pustules on the lid margins may be indicative of poxvirus (particularly in Amazon parrots).

Periophthalmic swelling, epiphora or conjunctivitis all indicate ocular or sinus abnormalities. Conjunctivitis is most common in cockatiels, lovebirds and Amazon parrots. In cockatiels and lovebirds, bacterial, mycoplasmal, chlamydial or viral conjunctivitis may damage the lids resulting in dry eye. A common problem in cockatiels is partial lid paralysis, with ectropion and conjunctivitis.

Cere

An immature budgerigar will have a flesh-colored cere that normally turns dark blue (male) or stays light blue or pink (female) as the bird matures. Some browning of the cere is normal in reproductively active budgerigar hens. An abnormal accumulation of keratinized tissue on the cere (brown hypertrophy of the cere) can occur in some budgerigars with endocrine abnormalities. Estrogen-producing tumors may cause a male budgerigar's cere to change from blue to brown. Hyperkeratotic swelling and hypertrophy of the cere that causes occlusion of the nares may be noted in some Umbrella and Moluccan Cockatoos. A crusty cere and beak may be indicative of *Knemidokoptes* spp. mites.

Nares

The nares and operculum (keratinized plate inside the nostril) should be smooth, relatively dry, symmetrical and evenly sized and colored. The feather configuration around the nares varies among species. Cockatoos have dense feathers that completely surround the nares. By comparison, Amazon parrots have sparse bristle-type feathers around the nares. In cockatiels, Amazon parrots and lories, the nares are round, while in cockatoos the opening forms a slit. Any degree of moisture around the nares should be considered abnormal.

Nasal discharges may be unilateral or bilateral and may appear clinically as dirty, malpositioned or moist feathers around the nares. Mild cases of rhinitis may be accompanied by severe cases of air sacculitis, sinusitis and caseous accumulations in the nares or sinuses. Periorbital swelling usually indicates a sinus infection. Signs of previous respiratory disorders may include grooves in the beak or loss of feathers associated with the nares.

Pathology in the sinus or nasal cavities may alter the normal flow of air, causing the skin over the infraorbital sinus to move in and out as a bird breathes. This abnormality may be subtle and the bird may otherwise appear normal. Mild blockages that are not corrected can progress and cause severe sinusitis and conjunctivitis (cockatiels) or atrophic rhinitis (African Grey Parrots) with structural damage to the rhinal cavity and surrounding bony structures (sunken sinus syndrome in macaws). In some species, transillumination of the sinus areas may help identify pockets of debris.

The ear canals can be evaluated for discharge or the abnormal accumulation of desquamated hyperkeratotic skin by parting the feathers on the side of the head. The glistening, translucent ear drum can be visualized and will move slightly with respiration.

The surface of the beak should be smooth, shiny and uniform regardless of the species. Dry, flaky layers on the beak and skin around the cere are abnormal and may signal poor management or systemic disease. Physical damage (bite wounds) to the epithelial growth centers of the beak can cause similar lesions. Proliferative growths associated with the beak are common with *Knemidokoptes* sp. infections.

Oral Cavity

Evaluation of the oral cavity can be augmented by using a speculum or gauze strips to open the mouth. A detailed examination of the oral or pharyngeal mucosa may require isoflurane anesthesia.

The tongue has a dry sheen while the choanal slit and pharyngeal and laryngeal mucosa are slightly moist. Choanal papilla are well formed in some species (Amazon parrots and macaws) and less distinct or absent in other species. Excessive moisture in the mouth may indicate inflammation in the oral cavity, choanal slit, sinuses or pharyngeal and laryngeal areas.

Accumulations of debris or food, abnormal coloration, erosions or ulcerations, sticky white mucus or perichoanal, pharyngeal or sublingual swellings are abnormal. White plaques that are easily removed and blunting or swelling of the choanal papillae are common with hypovitaminosis A. Shallow yellow or white plaques that are attached and difficult to remove are common with pox or bacterial ulcerations. White or brown cheesy lesions are suggestive of candidiasis or trichomoniasis. Accumulations of desquamated hyperkeratotic epithelium, recognized clinically as small white bumps on the dorsal surface of the tongue base are common in cockatiels. Birds with these lesions are frequently infected with *Candida* sp.

A decreased jaw tone may indicate a systemic weakness. Vitamin E or selenium deficiency and giardia have been suggested as causes of this problem in cockatiels. These birds may not be able to crack seeds and frequently have poor tongue control resulting in food accumulation in the oral cavity.

Respiratory Tract

A bird that is in severe respiratory distress may require oxygen before it can tolerate the stress of a physical examination. In a normal bird, the respiratory rate should return to its pre-exercise rate within two minutes of ceasing the exercise. A sustained tachypnea can indicate respiratory disease, cardiovascular disease or a mass that is blocking air flow in and out of the caudal air sacs.

Auscultation

A pediatric stethoscope is ideal for auscultating the avian lungs, heart and air sacs. The heart rate will vary from 45-600 beats per minute depending on the species and level of excitement.

Hearing a slight rush of air is normal. Detected cracks, pops, wheezes or whistling sounds are indications of severe respiratory tract abnormalities. Most abnormal respiratory sounds in birds are associated with rhinoliths, infraorbital sinusitis, tracheal stenosis or air sac disease.

Body Examination and Palpation

The submandibular and neck areas should be palpated, with particular attention to the esophagus and crop. The esophagus as it extends down the right side of the neck can be palpated for swellings. If distended with food, the crop can be quite large, and care should be exercised when handling the bird (particularly a neonate) to prevent regurgitation, which may lead to aspiration pneumonia. Peristalsis of the crop is easy to observe (one to three per minute), particularly in neonates.

The crop and esophagus can be visually examined by wetting the feathers around the thoracic inlet and placing a small, high-powered light (eg, endoscope light) on one side of the crop. Using this transillumination technique, the relative thickness of the crop mucosa and its vascularity can be determined. If empty, expanding the crop with air and holding it in place by digital pressure on the esophagus allows improved transillumination. Thickening or increased vascularization of the crop or esophagus is an indication of inflammation. The patient's general condition can be subjectively evaluated by palpating the pectoral muscles to determine the ratio of muscle mass to sternum.

A bird's weight in grams should be determined with each visit. A scale that has been fitted with a perch can be used for tame birds.

The feathers over the sternum and abdomen should be moistened with alcohol to visually determine the amount of subcutaneous fat deposits. The abdomen should be slightly concave or flat.

Abdominal organs are difficult to palpate in birds, particularly in small species; however, the ability to palpate unusual structures in the abdomen can provide important information. Normally, the abdomen should be flat, tight and slightly concave in the center. With liver enlargement, ascites, proventricular or ventricular distension or displacement, egg development, egg-related peritonitis or mass formation, the abdomen may appear distended, doughy and convex. The right liver lobe extends further caudally than the left and can be detected most easily if enlarged. Gentle palpation under the caudal edge of the sternum should not be painful, and if a bird responds to this procedure it could indicate hepatitis. Palpation on a bird with a swollen abdomen should be performed gently. If fluid is present in the peritoneal space and an air sac is ruptured by excessive digital pressure, fluid can rush into the lungs causing asphyxiation.

Extra-abdominal wall swellings caused by hernias or lipomas may be visualized and palpated.

In a well muscled, low-body-fat canary or finch the abdominal musculature is almost transparent, and portions of the gastrointestinal tract and liver (especially with hepatomegaly) can be visualized.

Cloacal Area

A pericloacal accumulation of excrement may indicate enteritis or polyuria or can be associated with cloacal dysfunction. The pericloacal feathers of a bird with chronic biliverdinuria are often stained greenish or greenish-yellow.

Inspection of the cloacal mucosa can be accomplished using a moistened cotton-tipped applicator. The applicator is gently inserted into the cloaca and slowly withdrawn while pushing the tip to one side.

The cloacal mucosa should be carefully checked for papillomatous growths. Five percent acetic acid (apple cider vinegar) will cause papillomatous tissue to turn white and can facilitate visualization of subtle lesions. The cloaca normally everts in reproductively active Vasa Parrots.

The openings of the urinary, gastrointestinal and genital tracts can be examined using an otoscope cone, vaginal speculum, human nasal speculum or endoscope. This procedure induces some level of discomfort and is best performed in an anesthetized bird. In sexually mature hens, the cervix may be observed in the left lateral wall of the urodeum.

The uropygial gland, located dorsal to the cloaca at the end of the pygostyle, is well developed in some species (canaries) and absent in other species (Amazon parrots). If present, the gland should be smooth, evenly colored and contain a small amount of yellow, creamy material. Infections and neoplasia are the two most common causes of abnormalities.

The internal temperature of a bird can vary from 107-112°F and temperatures often elevate rapidly during periods of stress.

Wings, Legs and Feet

Green discoloration (bruising) of subcutaneous tissues usually represents the breakdown of extravascular hemoglobin. In general, it takes about two days after a traumatic event for this green color to appear, providing the clinician with an indication of the chronicity of an injury.

Hemorrhagic, necrotic, dystrophic feather shafts are an indication of damage to the developing feather that can be caused by a number of infectious or metabolic problems. Mites may be observed moving on the underside of the wing or the nits may be attached to the feather vanes. Increased translucency, color alterations or structural changes in the flight feathers can be an indication of malnutrition or mismanagement. The ventral surface of the wing and prolateral region are common locations for feather picking in cockatiels, African Grey Parrots, cockatoos, Grey-cheeked Parakeets and Quaker Parrots.

Ulnar vein turgidity and skin consistency on the neck, abdomen and dorsal surface of the digits can be used to evaluate the hydration status of the bird. Flat veins that do not immediately refill when depressed may indicate hypoproteinemia, anemia, dehydration or shock.

The feet and legs should be uniform in texture and color. The feet should have prominent scale patterns on both the dorsal and plantar surfaces. Changes that result in smoothing of the plantar foot surface can instigate chronic and severe foot and leg problems. Common etiologies of foot abnormalities include hypovitaminosis A, a lack of sunlight, contact with nicotine sulfate (from the hands of cigarette smokers) and improper perches. Any ulcerative lesion or swelling of the feet should be addressed immediately. Ulcerative lesions can rapidly become infected (bumblefoot) and can be life-threatening if infectious agents invade associated tendon sheaths and bones. Bacteremia is common in many birds with ulcerative lesions on the feet. The accumulation of exfoliated, dried hyperkeratotic scales is common in malnourished Passeriformes. Proliferative lesions on the feet of canaries (tasselfoot) are common with *Knemidokoptes* infections.

The length of a bird's nails should be evaluated and the client should be instructed to carefully monitor the nail growth at home. Overgrown nails are common in birds with hepatopathies and can result in trauma to the foot pads (inducing bumblefoot) or entanglement in enclosures or toys. Hemorrhage in unpigmented nails is an indication of trauma or liver disease.

A weak grip can indicate systemic weakness or specific neuromuscular disease of the feet or legs (see Chapter 28). Leg paresis, ataxia and muscle atrophy may occur in birds with abdominal tumors. This lameness is typically the result of tumors that place pressure on the ischiatic nerve. Unilateral lameness is most common, but bilateral lameness may also occur. Bilateral lameness can also be a direct result of primary neural lesions (eg, aspergillosis, Marek's disease virus, lymphoid leukosis, spinal injuries, vitamin E or selenium deficiencies and B vitamin deficiencies).

Once the physical exam is completed, the minimum database can be collected. The decision of which test to perform is based on the condition of the patient. For the most accurate results, blood samples for CBC and biochemistries should be drawn when a bird is not stressed. Leaving a bird in a dark clinic overnight so that blood may be drawn the first thing in the morning may be the best solution.

Table 8.4 Suggested Ideal Examination Database for Medium and Large Psittacines	
• Physical examination	• Radiographs
• Body weight	• Fecal Gram's stain
• CBC	• Chlamydia testing
• Biochemistries - TP, Glucose, CA, AST, LDH, CPK, UA, Bile acids	• DNA probe testing for PBFD virus, polyomavirus

HEMATOLOGY

Terry W. Campbell

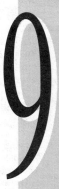

The techniques involved in the evaluation of the avian hemogram are easily performed by in-house veterinary laboratory personnel. Because avian blood does not store well (eg, during transport), hematologic results obtained soon after collection are preferred over those performed several hours later.

Blood volume in birds depends on the species and varies from 5 ml/100g in the Ring-necked Pheasant to 16.3 ml/100g in the racing pigeon. In general, birds are better able to tolerate severe blood loss than mammals, which is due to their greater capacity for extravascular fluid mobilization In healthy Mallard Ducks and racing pigeons, a blood volume equivalent of up to three percent of the body weight can be collected. In Passeriformes, pheasants and Psittaciformes, up to one percent of the body weight can be collected with few ill effects (0.9 ml from a 90 g cockatiel).

For best results, venous blood should be collected for hematologic studies. Blood collected from capillaries (eg, blood from clipped nails) often results in abnormal cell distributions and contains cellular artifacts such as macrophages. Blood to be used for hematology should be collected into a tube containing EDTA as the anticoagulant. Other anticoagulants, such as heparin, interfere with cell staining and create excessive cell clumping, resulting in erroneous cell counts and evaluations.

Blood Collection

Right jugular venipuncture is a procedure that can be used for collecting blood from most avian species. It is the method of choice for small birds that do not have other blood vessels large enough for venipuncture. Extending the neck encourages the highly movable jugular vein to fall into the jugular furrow. Lightly wetting the feathers with alcohol in this area will aid in the visualization of the vein. Improper attention to technique and hemostasis can cause a large hematoma to form during or following jugular venipuncture. However, jugular venipuncture becomes a skill perfected with practice, and complications are infrequent in skilled hands.

Venipuncture of the bascilica or wing vein is a common method for obtaining blood from medium to large birds. Hematoma formation, which can be severe, is common when the ulnar vein is used for blood collection. A needle with an extension tube, such as a butterfly catheter, aids in stabilization during sample collection to minimize tearing of the vein.

Venipuncture of the medial metatarsal (caudal tibial) vein, which lies on the medial side of the tibiotarsus at the tibiotarsal-tarsometatarsal joint, is another common method for blood collection in medium to large birds. The primary advantages of this method over other methods of blood collection are that the surrounding leg muscles protect the medial metatarsal vein from hematoma formation and, in some species, the leg is more easily restrained than the wing.

Laboratory Techniques

After the blood is collected, a blood film is made. The film can be made either from blood containing no anticoagulant (especially if blood parasites are suspected) or blood containing EDTA. EDTA will cause hemolysis of erythrocytes in some birds including Corvidae, currasows, Crowned Cranes, hornbills and Brush Turkeys. Prolonged exposure to EDTA may result in increased disruption of cells in the blood film in some species. When preparing a blood film, the standard two-slide wedge technique used in mammalian hematology usually works well with avian blood. It is advisable to use precleaned, bevel-edged microscope slides to minimize cell damage during preparation of blood films. Peripheral blood films can also be made using a two-coverglass technique. A drop of blood is placed in the center of one coverglass; a second coverglass is placed on top of the first, and the two are pulled apart as the blood begins to spread between the two surfaces.

A variety of hematologic stains can be used to evaluate the air-dried blood film. Romanowsky stains, such as Wright's, Giemsa, Wright-Giemsa, Wright-Leishman or May-Grunwald and their combination, are preferred.

After making a blood film, the remainder of the blood sample is used to obtain a packed cell volume (PCV), hemoglobin concentration and cell count. The hemoglobin concentration is measured spectrophotometrically by using the manual or automated cyanmethemoglobin method after centrifugation removal of free red cell nuclei and membrane debris.

The red blood cell (RBC) count is obtained either by automated or manual methods. The two manual methods that can be used are the erythrocyte Unopette system (standard method in mammalian hematology) or Natt and Herrick's method. The latter method requires the preparation of a methyl violet 2B diluent. A 1:200 dilution of the blood is made using this solution and a diluting pipette. After mixing, the diluted blood is discharged into a Neubauer-ruled hemacytometer and the cells are allowed to settle to the surface for five minutes before enumeration. The red blood cells are counted using the four corner squares and one central square of the central large primary square of the hemacytometer. The number of red cells counted is multiplied by 10,000 to obtain the RBC count per microliter of blood. Appropriate secondary squares are counted on each grid and the counts are averaged.

The mean corpuscular values can be calculated using the PCV, hemoglobin and RBC count values. The mean corpuscular volume (MCV) and mean corpus-corpuscular hemoglobin concentration (MCHC) are useful in the characterization of the erythrocytes, especially in the evaluation of anemia.

$$MCV = \frac{PCV \times 10}{RBC \ count}$$

$$MCH \ (pg) = \frac{Hemoglobin \times 10}{RBC}$$

$$MCHC = \frac{Hemoglobin \times 100}{PCV}$$

A reticulocyte count can be useful in the evaluation of the red cell regenerative response. The erythrocytes are stained with a vital stain, such as new methylene blue stain, and the reticulocytes are identified as red blood cells that contain distinct rings of aggregated reticulum encircling the cell nucleus.

The white blood cell (WBC, leukocyte) count of birds is obtained using manual techniques because the presence of nucleated erythrocytes and thrombocytes interferes with the counting of white blood cells using electronic cell counters. The current methods of choice for obtaining a total leukocyte count in birds are the indirect method using the eosinophil Unopette brand 5877 system or the direct leukocyte count using Natt and Herrick's method. Estimation of leukocyte numbers from a blood film should be reserved for those occasions when a quantitative count is unavailable or when there is suspicion of error in a value obtained from the other methods.

The indirect eosinophil Unopette brand method involves the filling of the 25 microliter pipette with blood, mixing the blood with the phloxine B diluent in the vial provided in the system and charging the hemacytometer chamber for cell counting. The blood-phloxine mixture should not be allowed to stand in the Unopette vial for longer than five minutes or erythrocytes may also be stained. The charged hemacytometer should stand undisturbed for at least five minutes to allow the cells to settle to the surface of the counting grid. It is advisable to keep the charged hemacytometer in a humid chamber to prevent dehydration of the sample if the chamber is going to sit for longer than five minutes. The granulocytes that stain distinctly red (heterophils and eosinophils) are counted in both sides of the hemacytometer (representing 18 large squares). A WBC count is obtained by determining a leukocyte differential from the peripheral blood film and using the formulas in Table 9.1.

A total thrombocyte count can be obtained using the Natt and Herrick's method; however, thrombocytes tend to clump, making an accurate count difficult to achieve. A subjective opinion as to the number of thrombocytes present can be made from the peripheral blood film. An average of one to two thrombocytes is present in monolayer oil immersion (100 x) fields in blood films of normal birds. An estimate of the thrombocyte count can be made from the peripheral blood film by obtaining the average number of thrombocytes in five monolayer oil immersion fields. This represents the average number of thrombocytes per 1000 erythrocytes in most species of birds.

A more accurate method would be to count the number of thrombocytes per 1000 erythrocytes in the blood film. The number of thrombocytes per 1000 erythrocytes is multiplied by the erythrocyte count and divided by 1000 to obtain an estimated thrombocyte count per ml of blood. If the actual erythrocyte count is not known, then 3,500,000 can be used to represent the average number of erythrocytes per ml of blood in most species of birds having an average PCV of 45%. If the PCV is below 40 or above 50, the estimated thrombocyte count (est T) can be corrected using the following formula:

$$\text{Corrected est T} = \frac{\text{est T X observed PCV}}{\text{normal PCV (averages 45\%)}}$$

Table 9.1 Formulas for Determining WBC Counts

The total heterophil and eosinophil count T(h+e) is obtained by using the formula given for the eosinophil Unopette brand system:

$$\text{T(h+e)/mm}^3 = \text{cells counted x 10 x 32 / 18}$$

The total leukocyte count (TWBC) is obtained using the leukocyte differential and the following formula:

$$\text{TWBC/mm}^3 = \text{(T(h+e) / \% heterophils+eosinophils x 100}$$

The TWBC can be calculated using the formula:

$$\text{TWBC/mm}^3 = \frac{\text{number of cells counted x 10 x 32 x 100}}{\text{(\% heterophils+eosinophils) x 18}}$$

This formula can be simplified by using the formula:

$$\text{TWBC/mm}^3 = \frac{\text{number of cells counted x 1.111 x 16 x 100}}{\text{\% heterophils+eosinophils}}$$

or

$$\text{TWBC/mm}^3 = \frac{\text{number of cells counted x 1778}}{\text{\% heterophils+eosinophils}}$$

The Natt and Herrick's method is a direct method for obtaining a TWBC and utilizes the same dilution and charged hemacytometer used to obtain a RBC count. The dark-staining leukocytes are counted in the nine large squares of the hemacytometer chamber. The TWBC is obtained using the following formula:

$$\text{TWBC/mm}^3 = \frac{\text{(total leukocytes in 9 squares) x 10 x 200}}{9}$$

or simplified to:

$$\text{TWBC/mm}^3 = \text{(total leukocytes in 9 squares + 10\%) x 200}$$

Cell Identification (Blood)

Erythrocyte Morphology

The normal mature avian erythrocyte is oval with a centrally positioned oval nucleus. The cytoplasm is abundant and stains a uniform orange-pink, resembling the cytoplasm of mammalian erythrocytes. The nucleus of the mature erythrocyte is condensed and stains dark purple. The nuclear chromatin is uniformly clumped. The red cell nuclei vary with age, becoming more condensed and darker staining as the cells age.

Avian erythrocytes frequently demonstrate diffuse polychromasia. Polychromatic erythrocytes demonstrate cytoplasmic basophilia and have nuclei that are less condensed compared to mature erythrocytes. Immature round erythrocytes (eg, rubricytes) may also be found in the peripheral blood of birds.

Leukocyte Morphology

The granulocytic leukocytes of birds are heterophils, eosinophils and basophils. The heterophil is a round cell with distinct eosinophilic cytoplasmic granules. These granules are oval to spindle-shaped and often contain a distinct refractile body in the center of the granule. The mature heterophil nucleus is lobed, usually containing fewer lobes than mammalian neutrophils. The nuclear chromatin contains heavy chromatin clumping. The cytoplasm of normal mature heterophils is colorless and nonvacuolated.

Avian eosinophils are round granulocytes and contain distinct round-to-oval cytoplasmic granules that lack the central refractile body seen in heterophil granules. The cytoplasmic granules of eosinophils typically stain brighter or differently from heterophil granules in the same blood film. The cytoplasm of avian eosinophils stains clear blue. The eosinophil nucleus is lobed and generally stains darker than the nuclei of heterophils.

The normal basophil is slightly smaller than the heterophil and has a colorless cytoplasm that contains strongly basophilic granules. These granules often dissolve or coalesce in alcohol-based stains, such as the Romanowsky stains. Avian basophils have round-to-oval, non-lobed nuclei that are often hidden by cytoplasmic granules.

The mononuclear leukocytes found in the peripheral blood of birds are lymphocytes and monocytes. The mature avian lymphocytes are round cells that frequently "mold" around adjacent cells in the blood film. These cells have high nucleus to cytoplasm (N:C) ratios. The nucleus is usually centrally positioned and round with a scant amount of homogeneous blue cytoplasm appearing as a small band surrounding the nucleus. Avian lymphocytes often vary in size, and the larger lymphocytes that have pale-staining nuclei may be confused with monocytes. The nuclear chromatin of mature lymphocytes is densely clumped. Occasionally, the cytoplasm of small mature lymphocytes may contain irregular projections.

Monocytes are the largest leukocytes found in the peripheral blood films. They vary in shape from round to ameboid. Monocytes have an abundant amount of cytoplasm compared to lymphocytes.

The cytoplasm generally stains darker than the cytoplasm of normal lymphocytes. The cytoplasm of monocytes has a finely granular, blue-gray appearance and often contains vacuoles. Often two distinct cytoplasmic zones can be seen in monocytes: a light-staining area adjacent to the nucleus and a darker staining area on the periphery. The cytoplasm of monocytes may occasionally contain fine, dust-like eosinophilic granules. The nucleus of monocytes generally contains less nuclear chromatin clumping as compared to mature lymphocytes. The shape of the monocyte nucleus is variable, ranging from round to bilobed.

On occasion, abnormal-appearing leukocytes are found in the peripheral blood films of birds. Immature heterophils are abnormal findings in avian blood films. In general, immature heterophils have increased cytoplasmic basophilia, nonsegmented nuclei and immature cytoplasmic granules compared to mature heterophils. Usually when immature heterophils are found on a blood film, mature heterophils can also be found.

Mature heterophils appear to show toxic changes in a manner similar to the toxic changes identified in mammalian neutrophils. Signs of toxicity include increased cytoplasmic basophilia, vacuolation, abnormal granules, degranulation, and degeneration of the nucleus. The degree of toxicity is reported subjectively on a scale of +1 to +4. A +1 toxic heterophil shows increased cytoplasmic basophilia. A +2 toxic heterophil has increased cytoplasmic basophilia, vacuolation and partial degranulation. A +3 toxicity shows a deeper cytoplasmic basophilia, vacuolation and abnormal granulation.

Abnormal granulation is indicated by the presence of granules that vary in appearance from the typical rod-shaped eosinophilic granules (eg, large, pale, round eosinophilic granules and small, deeply basophilic granules). A +4 toxic heterophil resembles a +3 toxic heterophil except the cell nucleus has undergone karyorrhexis or karyolysis. The number of toxic heterophils present is an indication of severity and suggestive of duration of an inflammatory response. A slight number (25% or less) of toxic heterophils may be present in the early stages of disorders responsible for their occurrence. As the disorder becomes increasingly severe, the number of toxic heterophils will increase. A marked number (greater than 25%) of toxic heterophils is common in birds showing this heterophil abnormality. It is common for birds with toxic heterophil changes to have all of their heterophils affected on the blood film. Clinically, these birds will be severely compromised.

Cytologic indications for reactivity in lymphocytes include increased cell size, increased cytoplasmic basophilia, the presence of azurophilic cytoplasmic granules and smooth nuclear chromatin. Blast-transformed lymphocytes have a deeply basophilic cytoplasm and smooth nuclear chromatin. Blast-transformed lymphocytes may also have nucleoli and distinct Golgi. Occasionally, plasma cells can be found in the peripheral blood of birds. These are relatively large lymphocytes with eccentric, mature-appearing nuclei; abundant, deeply basophilic cytoplasm; and prominent Golgi adjacent to the nucleus. Lymphocytes containing azurophilic granules (large purple cytoplasmic granules) are considered abnormal in birds.

An occasional monocyte having a few cytoplasmic vacuoles is normal, but the presence of large numbers of highly vacuolated monocytes is abnormal.

Cells that contain large granules that fill the cytoplasm are frequently found in blood films of birds. Often these granules fail to stain or may stain blue. These cells are common in blood films of some species of birds (eg, cockatoos) and suggest either staining artifact or represent variation owing to different cytochemical properties of these cells compared to other avian species. The differential for the type of cell involved includes eosinophils, basophils and rarely, Mott cell variant of plasma cells.

Careful examination of the blood film most often reveals normal staining basophils and no evidence of lymphoid reactivity (which may support the possibility of Mott cells being present), but there are no eosinophils present that stain normally. Based on these characteristics, the majority of these cells have been identified as eosinophils.

Thrombocyte Morphology

Birds have nucleated cells (thrombocytes) rather than cytoplasmic fragments as platelets that participate in blood coagulation. Mature thrombocytes are small oval cells that appear more rounded than the erythrocytes. The nucleus is pyknotic and the cytoplasm is colorless in mature cells. The cytoplasm may contain one or more red granules and small vacuoles or clear spaces. Thrombocytes, like mammalian platelets, tend to clump in blood films. Thrombocytes are differentiated from small, mature lymphocytes by having a colorless, nonhomogeneous cytoplasm; small, round, red cytoplasmic granules; and a smaller N:C ratio. Small mature lymphocytes have high N:C ratios with a scant amount of blue, homogenous cytoplasm.

Abnormal thrombocyte cytology includes the presence of reactive and immature thrombocytes. Reactive thrombocytes are usually found in aggregates, have a diffusely eosinophilic cytoplasm (suggesting release of chemicals from the granules) and irregular cytoplasmic margins. Reactive thrombocytes tend to be more spindle-shaped than nonreactive thrombocytes.

Interpretation of the Erythron

The normal PCV of birds ranges between 35 and 55 percent. A PCV less than 35 percent is indicative of anemia, and a PCV greater than 55 percent is suggestive of dehydration or polycythemia. An increase in red cell polychromasia is indicative of red blood cell regeneration. In normal birds, the number of polychromatic erythrocytes (or reticulocytes) found in the peripheral blood film ranges between one and five percent of the erythrocytes. An anemic bird with a five percent or less degree of polychromasia (or reticulocytosis) is responding poorly to the anemia or there has not been enough time for the bird to demonstrate a significant response. An anemic bird showing a ten percent or greater degree of polychromasia is exhibiting a significant regenerative response. The presence of immature erythrocytes (eg, rubricytes) in the peripheral blood along with an increase in poly-chromasia is indicative of a marked regenerative response.

Table 9.3 Causes of Anemia in Birds

Blood-loss Anemia (Appears regenerative except in the peracute stage)
1. Traumatic injury
2. Parasitism (ticks, *Dermanyssus* mites, coccidia)
3. Primary coagulopathy (rarely reported in birds)
4. Toxicity resulting in a coagulopathy (aflatoxicosis and coumarin poisoning)
5. Organic disease (ulcerated neoplasm, gastrointestinal ulcers, organ rupture)

Hemolytic Anemia (Regenerative)
1. Red blood cell parasites (*Plasmodium, Aegyptianella* and, rarely, *Haemoproteus* and *Leucocytozoon*)
2. Bacterial septicemia (salmonellosis and spirochetosis)
3. Toxicity (mustards and petroleum products)
4. Immune-mediated (rarely reported in birds)

Depression Anemia (Nonregenerative)
1. Chronic disease (tuberculosis, chlamydiosis, aspergillosis, neoplasia)
2. Hypothyroidism
3. Toxicity (lead poisoning and aflatoxicosis)
4. Nutritional deficiencies (iron and folic acid deficiencies)
5. Leukemia (lymphoidemia and erythroblastosis)

Hypochromasia can be associated with certain nutritional deficiencies in birds, especially iron deficiency. Hypochromasia has also been seen in lead toxicosis. Lead toxicosis may also create a dichotomous population of erythrocytes in the blood film of a non-anemic bird. In such cases, small senescent, mature erythrocytes with pyknotic nuclei and young erythrocytes (eg, rubricytes) are present in the blood film without the appearance of normal, mature erythrocytes. This condition resembles the inappropriate release of nucleated erythrocytes in the blood of non-anemic dogs suffering from lead poisoning. Basophilic stippling in the cytoplasm of erythrocytes is a rare finding with lead poisoning in birds. Basophilic stippling may be associated with erythrocyte regeneration and hypochromic anemia.

Polycythemia is rarely reported in birds. Increases in the PCV (relative polycythemia) are usually associated with dehydration in birds; however, absolute polycythemia can also occur. The conditions often associated with absolute polycythemia in mammals are expected to be the causes of this condition as well.

Interpretation of the Leukogram

There is wide variation in the normal leukograms among birds of the same species. Preparing normal reference values on healthy individual birds is the best method for evaluating blood parameters of a bird during illness.

In general, total leukocyte counts greater than 10,000/microliter are considered suggestive of leukocytosis in tame, adult psittacine birds. The total leukocyte count in the blood of normal psittacine birds not accustomed to handling may be high (greater than 10,000/microliter) owing to a physiologic leukocytosis.

Although avian heterophils lack the myeloperoxidase and alkaline phosphatase of mammalian neutrophils, studies of their ultrastructure, cytochemistry and function suggest they perform a similar function in the inflammatory response. Although avian heterophils do not produce hydrogen peroxide during phagocytosis, they do contain lysosomal enzymes and have a bactericidal function. A leukocytosis and heterophilia can be associated with infectious agents (eg, bacteria, fungi, chlamydia and parasites) and noninfectious etiologies (eg, traumatic injury and toxicities). A slight to moderate leukocytosis, heterophilia and lymphopenia can result from either an exogenous or endogenous excess of glucocorticosteroids (stress response). A marked leukocytosis and heterophilia are often associated with chlamydiosis, avian tuberculosis and aspergillosis.

Immature heterophils occur rarely in the peripheral blood of most species of birds. When present, they generally represent an overwhelming peripheral demand for heterophils and a depletion of the mature storage pool in the hematopoietic tissues.

The presence of toxic heterophils is also uncommon in the peripheral blood of birds. When present, they suggest the presence of a septicemia or toxemia (especially associated with bacterial toxins affecting the microenvironment of the hematopoietic tissue).

The general causes of leukopenias in birds are depletion of peripheral leukocytes and depression or degeneration of leukopoiesis. Leukopenias associated with heteropenias can be associated with certain viral diseases (eg, Pacheco's disease virus) and overwhelming bacterial infections. A degenerative response is indicated by the presence of a leukopenia, heteropenia, immature heterophils and toxic heterophils. Leukopenias associated with lymphopenias have been reported in early response to corticosteroids in some species of birds. A lymphopenia also may be expected with certain viral diseases; however, viral causes have not been well documented in birds.

A lymphocytosis may be expected with antigenic stimulation associated with certain infections. The presence of many reactive lymphocytes is also suggestive of antigenic stimulation. A marked lymphocytosis with or without the presence of immature lymphocytes can occur with lymphocytic leukemia. A marked lymphocytosis, with the majority of cells appearing as small mature lymphocytes with scalloped cytoplasmic margins, is suggestive of lymphoid neoplasia.

A monocytosis can be found with certain diseases that produce chemotactic agents for monocytes. These conditions include avian chlamydiosis, mycotic and bacterial granulomas and massive tissue necrosis. A monocytosis can also occur in birds on a zinc-deficient diet.

The function of the avian eosinophil is unclear. Although this avian granulocyte was given the name *eosinophil*, there is evidence that its function may differ from the mammalian eosinophil. Thus, conditions responsible for inducing avian eosinophilias most likely differ from those causing mammalian eosinophilias. Studies suggest that avian eosinophils may participate in delayed (Type IV) hypersensitivity reactions.

As with avian eosinophils, the exact function of basophils in birds is unknown. Avian basophils are similar to mammalian basophils in their ability to produce, store and release histamine. Basophils appear to participate in the initial phase of the acute inflammatory response in birds, but this is not always reflected as a basophilia in the leukogram.

Interpretation of Thrombocyte Changes

Avian thrombocytes play a primary role in hemostasis in a manner similar to mammalian platelets. They may also have a phagocytic function and participate in removing foreign material from the blood. A normal thrombocyte count ranging between 20,000 and 30,000/microliter of blood can be used as a general reference for most birds. Thrombocytopenias are usually indicative of excessive peripheral demand for thrombocytes, although a depression in thrombopoiesis should be considered. Thrombocytopenias are often seen with severe septicemias, where a combination of excessive peripheral demand for thrombocytes and depression of thrombocyte production may occur.

Identification of Common Blood Parasites

For a complete review of avian parasites see Chapter 36.

Haemoproteus Only the gametocyte stage of this organism appears in the peripheral blood, whereas schizogony occurs in the tissues (eg, lung, spleen and liver). The mature gametocyte contains yellow-to-brown, refractile pigment granules. The typical mature gametocyte occupies greater than 50 percent of the red cell cytoplasm, partially encircles the host cell nucleus forming the classic "halter-shape" and causes little displacement of the red cell nucleus. Macrogametocytes stain blue with Romanowsky stains and have pigment granules dispersed throughout the cytoplasm of the parasite. The smaller microgametocytes stain pale blue to pink with pigment granules appearing in spherical aggregates. If blood containing *Haemoproteus* organisms is allowed to stand at room temperature for a few hours prior to preparing a blood film, gametes may be released from the cells and found in the extracellular spaces of the blood film. When gametes are found, it should be considered as an artifact of blood film preparation because these structures normally leave the host red cell following ingestion by the intermediate insect host (hippoboscid flies).

Leucocytozoon is easily identified from blood films because it grossly distorts the host cell (usually immature erythrocytes) that it parasitizes. Like *Haemoproteus*, only the gametocyte stage of *Leucocytozoon* occurs in the peripheral blood of birds. The large, round-to-elongated gametocytes cause the host cell to enlarge and appear to have two nuclei: the host cell nucleus pushed to the margin of the cell and the parasite nucleus, a pale-pink nucleus within the parasite. The parasitized cell usually has tapered ends with the remnants of the cell membrane trailing away from the cell. The macrogametocyte stains dark blue with a condensed nucleus and occasional cytoplasmic vacuoles. The microgametocyte stains light blue with a diffuse, pale-pink nucleus. Gametocytes of *Leucocytozoon* lack the refractile pigment granules found in *Haemoproteus*.

The intraerythrocytic gametocytes of **Plasmodium** spp. are often confused with those of *Haemoproteus* spp. because they also contain refractile pigment granules. However, *Plasmodium* gametocytes usually occupy less than 50 percent of the host cell cytoplasm, and those of some species alter the position of the red cell nucleus. Two key features that aid in the detection of *Plasmodium* are the presence of schizogony in the peripheral blood and gametocytes or schizonts in blood cells other than erythrocytes. Schizonts appear as round-to-oval intracytoplasmic inclusions that contain dark-staining merozoites. The number of merozoites produced depends upon the species of *Plasmodium*. As with *Haemoproteus*, *Plasmodium* macrogametocytes stain darker than the microgametocytes. Both *Plasmodium* and *Haemoproteus* infections may reveal small, ring-like forms (trophozoites) in the cytoplasm of infected erythrocytes. In rare cases, only these forms may be seen, and it is impossible to identify the parasite involved. Mosquitoes (*Culex* and *Aedes* spp.) are the intermediate hosts for *Plasmodium*.

Microfilaria are frequently found in the peripheral blood of a variety of birds.

Atoxoplasma sp. is identified by its characteristic sporozoite within the cytoplasm of mononuclear leukocytes, especially lymphocytes. The sporozoites appear as pale-staining, round-to-oval intracytoplasmic inclusions that compress the host cell nucleus and create a characteristic crescent shape to the nucleus. This organism can be found in the peripheral blood films or imprints of tissues such as the lung, liver and spleen.

Aegyptianella can occur within the cytoplasm in one of three forms: 1) anaplasma-like initial bodies appearing as small (less than one micrometer in diameter), round, basophilic inclusions; 2) intermediate stages resembling *Babesia* and measuring between one and two micrometers in diameter; and 3) large, round-to-elliptical forms measuring between two and four micrometers in length. *Aegyptianella* spp. are considered to be pathogenic to many species of birds.

A bone marrow sample should be obtained for cytologic evaluation in avian patients with persistent nonregenerative anemia, thrombocytopenia, panleukopenia and heteropenia. Bone marrow evaluation is also indicated for suspected cases of leukemia or if unexplained abnormal cells are found in the peripheral blood. An evaluation of the hemogram should accompany any bone marrow evaluation to properly assess hematopoiesis.

Bone Marrow Collection

In general, the proximal tibiotarsus just below the femoral-tibiotarsal joint (knee) is the preferred site for bone marrow collection in most birds. After surgical preparation of the skin either on the cranial or medial aspect of the proximal tibiotarsus, a small stab incision through the skin is made using a scalpel blade. A bone marrow aspiration biopsy needle is pushed through the thin cortex and into the marrow space using clockwise-counterclockwise rotational movements. Once the needle has entered the marrow space, the stylet is removed from the needle and a syringe is attached to gently aspirate a small amount of marrow into the needle lumen. Excessive pressure during aspiration should be avoided to prevent peripheral blood contamination of the sample.

Bone marrow biopsy needles commonly used include pediatric Jamshidi bone marrow biopsy-aspiration needles and disposable Jamshidi Illinois-Sternal/Iliac aspiration needles. Disposable spinal needles can be used to sample small birds because they contain a stylet to facilitate passage of the needle through the cortex without occlusion of the needle lumen with bone.

10

CYTOLOGY

Terry W. Campbell

Cytology is designed to be a rapid, inexpensive "in-house" diagnostic procedure, and the use of cytodiagnosis should be easily within the realm of any veterinary clinician. The basic cytodiagnosis of inflammation, tissue hyperplasia, malignant neoplasia and normal cellularity are easily differentiated from each other. The goal is to achieve a quick presumptive or definitive diagnosis during the patient's initial visit to the veterinary clinic in an effort to provide an immediate and specific treatment plan. Cytology can then be used to monitor the success of therapy by evaluating changes in microbial and cell populations within or on the host. Cytology should be considered as a part of the minimum database in birds with discharges, masses or swellings. Cytologic evaluation of tissue imprints and fluids collected during a postmortem examination can be used to develop a presumptive diagnosis that can guide disease management decisions within the flock until a definitive diagnosis is provided by culture, DNA probe or histopathology.

Sample Collection by Aspiration

A hypodermic needle (eg, 22 ga, one-inch needle) attached to a syringe (12 ml or larger) is inserted into the tissue to be sampled. A full vacuum is applied to the syringe using the syringe plunger. The needle is moved at different angles in the tissue without releasing the vacuum. It is important to release the vacuum before withdrawing the needle from the tissue, because the aim of the procedure is to obtain a small amount of sample in the lumen of the needle only, not in the syringe itself. Once the needle has been withdrawn from the tissue, it is detached from the syringe and the syringe is filled with air. The needle is reattached to the syringe, and with the point of the needle lying against the slide surface, the air within the syringe is used to force the sample onto a glass microscope slide. A second glass microscope slide placed on top of the first allows the sample to spread between the two glass surfaces when the slides are pulled horizontally apart.

Abdominocentesis is an aspiration biopsy procedure used to collect cytologic samples from birds with abdominal fluid accumulation.

It begins with a surgical preparation of the site along the ventral midline just distal to the point of the keel. The needle (21-25 ga, one-inch) is attached to a syringe and is directed through the body wall at the midline, pointing caudally toward the right side of the abdomen to avoid the ventriculus, which lies to the left of the midline. The abdominal fluid is aspirated into the syringe and prepared for cytologic examination, either by making a direct smear as one would prepare a blood film or by using a concentration method.

Fluid samples having low cellularity require a concentration procedure for easier examination of the cells. A variety of techniques can be used to concentrate cells on microscope slides. A simple method is to marginate the cells on a smear made by the conventional wedge technique used for making blood films. Just prior to reaching the end of the smear, the spreader slide is quickly backed slightly into the advancing smear, just before lifting it from the surface of the slide containing the smear. This should produce a slide with the marginated cells concentrated at the end of the film.

Cells can be concentrated by centrifugation in a manner similar to that used in mammalian urinalysis procedures. Unlike urine sediments, cytologic sediments from poorly cellular fluids do not have a visible button or pellet at the bottom of a spun tube. Therefore, the concentrated cells are usually obtained by aspirating the fluid at the bottom of the tube into a pipette or syringe. The sample is then placed onto a microscope slide and a smear is made in the manner described for concentrating cells in a smear.

Cytologic evaluation of the ingluvies (crop) can be performed from samples obtained by aspiration. This is indicated in birds showing clinical signs of regurgitation, vomiting, delayed emptying of the crop or other crop disorders. A crop aspirate is obtained by inserting a sterile plastic, metal or rubber feeding tube through the mouth and esophagus into the ingluvies.

In cases where material cannot be aspirated for examination, a wash sample can be obtained by infusing a small amount of sterile isotonic saline into the crop and aspirating the fluid back into the tube and syringe.

Aspiration of the infraorbital sinus of birds suffering from sinusitis can provide diagnostic material for culture and cytologic examination. One technique of sinus aspiration in psittacine birds samples the large sinus between the eye and the external nares (Figure 10.4). With the head and body properly restrained, a needle (eg, 22 ga one-inch) is passed through the fleshy skin at the commissure of the mouth. The needle is directed toward a point midway between the eye and external nares, keeping parallel with the side of the head. The needle passes under the zygomatic bone, which lies between the lower corner of the rhinotheca (upper beak) and the ear. Often the passage of the needle is improved by keeping the bird's mouth open with an oral speculum.

It is important to note that in some species (eg, some passerine birds), the sinuses may not communicate with each other as they do in psittacine birds. Therefore, a bilateral sinusitis may require bilateral aspirations.

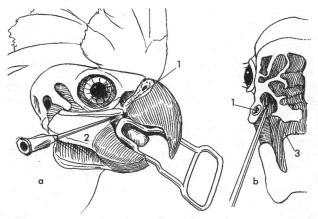

FIG 10.4 Aspiration of the infraorbital diverticulum of the infraorbital sinus in psittacine birds can be performed by **a)** passing a needle through the fleshy skin at the commissure of the mouth and directing it toward a point midway between the eye and external nares, **b)** keeping parallel with the side of the head and passing under the zygomatic arch. 1) zygomatic arch 2) mandible 3) oral cavity.

A second site of sinus aspiration is the small sinus immediately below the eye. This sinus usually yields a smaller sample volume than the previously described sinus. This sinus can be entered directly by inserting the aspiration needle at a perpendicular angle through the skin just below the eye (Figure 10.5). It can also be approached from a rostral direction by entering through the commissure of the mouth, directing the needle under the zygomatic bone and ending in the sinus cavity below the eye (Figure 10.6).

Wash samples are aspiration techniques in which a small amount of sterile isotonic saline is infused into an area and immediately reaspirated in an effort to collect a cytologic sample from locations that may be difficult to sample or that provide a poorly cellular field. Tracheal washes are commonly performed in birds suspected of having respiratory disease of the trachea, syrinx and bronchi. Depending on the patient, this procedure can be performed with or without general anesthesia. A soft, smooth-tipped, sterile plastic or rubber tube or catheter is inserted through the open glottis. The tube is passed to the level of the thoracic inlet near the syrinx. An oral speculum should be used in birds capable of biting off the tube. The animal is held parallel to the floor, and sterile saline (0.5-2 ml/kg body weight) is quickly infused into the trachea and immediately reaspirated to complete the wash sample. Similar wash techniques can be used to collect cytologic samples from the air sacs, ingluvies and infraorbital sinus.

Contact Smears

Cytologic samples can also be obtained by direct contact between the tissue being sampled and the microscope slide. Often referred to as contact or impression smears, these samples are used to evaluate postmortem tissues or antemortem tissue biopsies. Imprints of solid tissues should be made from freshly cut sur-

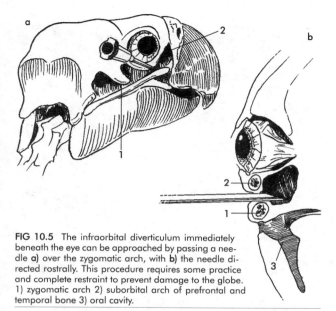

FIG 10.5 The infraorbital diverticulum immediately beneath the eye can be approached by passing a needle **a)** over the zygomatic arch, with **b)** the needle directed rostrally. This procedure requires some practice and complete restraint to prevent damage to the globe. 1) zygomatic arch 2) suborbital arch of prefrontal and temporal bone 3) oral cavity.

faces that have been blotted with a clean paper towel to remove the excess fluid and blood. It is best to lay the slide against the tissue surface using the weight of the slide to make the imprint. If the tissue is brought to the slide, too much force is used and the resulting specimen is too thick for evaluation.

Contact smears made from tissues that exfoliate poorly (eg, connective tissue) may require traumatic exfoliation to improve the cellularity. One method of improving cellular exfoliation is to scrape the tissue to be sampled with a scalpel blade and to make the contact smear from either the scraped surface or the material remaining on the scalpel blade.

Scrapings are commonly performed to collect cells from the palpebral conjunctiva, cornea, oral cavity or tissues that normally yield poorly cellular samples. A metal or plastic spatula is used to gently scrape these tissues, and the exfoliated cells are transferred to a microscope slide.

Cytologic samples can also be obtained using a sterile swab. Once the sample has been collected, the swab is gently rolled across the surface of a clean microscope slide, using light pressure in order to avoid cell damage. The swab should be rolled in one direction only and not rolled back and forth across the smear to prevent the creation of an excessively thick smear. Cytologic samples of internal tissues can be obtained using endoscopic equipment. Samples can be obtained either from the tip of the endoscope or by using brushes or biopsy forceps. The sample is applied directly to a microscope slide.

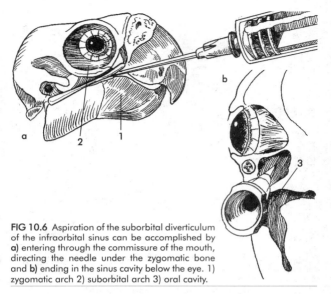

FIG 10.6 Aspiration of the suborbital diverticulum of the infraorbital sinus can be accomplished by **a)** entering through the commissure of the mouth, directing the needle under the zygomatic bone and **b)** ending in the sinus cavity below the eye. 1) zygomatic arch 2) suborbital arch 3) oral cavity.

Classification of Cells and Cellular Responses

The cells observed in the cytologic sample can be classified as either hemic, epithelial, mesenchymal or nervous tissue cells. Hemic cells are those cells found in the blood and the hematopoietic tissues (see Chapter 9). It is extremely important to recognize hemic cells because these cells can be either important features of the cellular response or common contaminants of the cytologic sample.

Epithelial cells typically exfoliate easily and are found in clusters or sheets. Epithelial cells vary in shape depending upon their origin. They can be oval, cuboidal, columnar or polygonal (eg, squamous epithelial cells). Epithelial cells typically have an abundant cytoplasm, small round-to-oval nuclei and distinct cytoplasmic margins. Cells from secretory epithelium may contain cytoplasmic granules or vacuoles.

Mesenchymal cells tend to exfoliate poorly and normally occur as single cells. These cells vary in shape and usually have indistinct cytoplasmic margins. The fibroblast is the most frequently encountered cell of this group. Fibroblasts are typically spindle-shaped with small nuclei that usually follow the shape of the cell.

Nervous tissue cells are rare in cytologic specimens. They may be seen as deeply basophilic, stellate cells with cytoplasmic projections.

During the cytologic examination, an assessment of the cells is made by identifying the majority of the cell types, the morphology of the cells and character of the non-cellular background. The goal of cytology is to identify the cellular message and classify the cell response into one of the basic cytodiagnostic groups. These groups include inflammation, tissue hyperplasia or benign neoplasia, malignant neoplasia and normal cellularity.

Inflammation

The inflammatory cells of birds are heterophils, lymphocytes, plasma cells and macrophages. It should be emphasized that heterophils found in tissues and fluids other than peripheral blood may not appear the same as those found in hemic tissue. Heterophils found in inflammatory lesions often degranulate and may resemble mammalian neutrophils. Plasma cells are large, oval lymphocytes with an abundant, deeply basophilic cytoplasm; an eccentric, mature nucleus; and a prominent perinuclear halo (Golgi). Macrophages are large cells with an abundant cytoplasm that may contain small granules, vacuoles or foreign material. Macrophages and their nuclei vary in shape and can coalesce into multinucleated giant cells.

Eosinophils may be included in the list of inflammatory cells; however, eosinophilic inflammation is either extremely rare in birds or difficult to detect based on routine cytologic methods.

The inflammatory response is classified as either heterophilic, mixed-cell or macrophagic inflammation. Heterophilic inflammation is represented by a predominance of heterophils (greater than 70 percent of the inflammatory cells) in the cellular response. Heterophilic inflammation indicates an acute inflammatory response in birds. It is important to examine the heterophils closely for signs of degeneration or phagocytized material.

Degenerate heterophils indicate a toxic microenvironment, usually caused by microbial toxins. Degenerative changes in heterophils include increased cytoplasmic basophilia, vacuolation, degranulation and nuclear karyolysis. If bacterial phagocytosis can be demonstrated, the cytodiagnosis of septic heterophilic inflammation can be made.

Because macrophages migrate quickly (within a few hours of onset) into inflammatory lesions, mixed-cell inflammation is the most commonly found inflammatory response in birds. Mixed-cell inflammation is represented by the presence of heterophils and mononuclear leukocytes. Heterophils represent at least 50 percent of the inflammatory cells in mixed-cell inflammatory responses. Mixed-cell inflammation usually represents an established, active inflammation. The heterophils in this type of inflammation are usually nondegenerate.

Macrophagic inflammation is indicated by the predominance of macrophages (greater than 50 percent) in the inflammatory response. This type of inflammation does not necessarily imply chronicity, but may be suggestive of a number of etiologies (eg, intracellular pathogens). Macrophagic inflammation is common to certain avian diseases. These include avian tuberculosis, chlamydiosis, foreign body reaction, mycotic infections and cutaneous xanthomatosis. Multinucleated giant cell formation is often associated with macrophagic inflammation. Giant cells can appear within hours of the onset of some inflammatory responses and, unlike in mammals, their presence does not imply chronic inflammation.

Tissue Hyperplasia or Benign Neoplasia

Cells from hyperplastic tissue appear mature and do not exhibit much pleomorphism. Proliferating cells may also exhibit an increase in mitotic figures; however, the nuclear features do not show immaturity.

Malignant Neoplasia

Cells obtained from malignant neoplasms show varying degrees of pleomorphism. The severity of the malignancy increases with the greater degree of pleomorphism. Increased nuclear size, which is reflected by an increased nucleus to cytoplasm ratio, is suggestive of an abnormal cell. Nuclear anisocytosis (variation in size) and nuclear pleomorphism (variable nuclear shapes) are features of malignant cells. Multinucleation can also be a feature of malignancy.

Coarse, hyperchromatic chromatin is suggestive of neoplasia. Other nuclear features of malignant cells include abnormal nucleoli (very large or multiple, such as greater than five), irregular nuclear margins, abnormal or increased mitotic figures and abnormal lobation, especially in cells that normally do not have lobed nuclei.

Cytoplasmic features of malignant cells include increased basophilia, abnormal vacuolation or inclusions, decreased volume, variation in cell margins and variability in the staining.

The four basic classifications of malignant neoplasms based upon cytologic features include carcinomas, sarcomas, discrete-cell neoplasia and poorly differentiated neoplasia. Carcinomas are malignancies of the epithelial cells; therefore, the abnormal cells in the sample have features of epithelial cells. Cytologic evidence of adenocarcinomas includes epithelial cells that tend to form giant cells, have cytoplasmic secretary vacuoles and tend to occur in aggregates (eg, balls, rosettes or loose groupings). Sarcomas are malignancies of mesenchymal cells and therefore tend to exfoliate cells poorly. Fibrosarcomas are the most frequently encountered sarcomas of birds. Cells from fibrosarcomas are abnormal-appearing fibroblasts, which are spindle-shaped cells that typically exfoliate as single cells.

A common discrete or round cell neoplasm of birds is lymphoid neoplasia. The abnormal lymphocytes found in this type of neoplasm exfoliate extremely well. Cellular features of malignant lymphocytic tissue include a marked increase in the number of lymphoblasts, nuclear and cellular pleomorphism, increase in cytoplasmic basophilia and mitotic figures, and abnormal or multiple nucleoli.

Poorly differentiated neoplasms produce cells having features of malignant neoplasia; however, the cells are difficult to classify as carcinomas or sarcomas.

Abdominal Fluids

Abdominal effusions can be classified based upon cellularity, types of cells present, protein content, specific gravity and gross appearance. Abdominal fluids are classified as transudates, modified transudates, exudates, hemorrhage and malignant effusion. Transudates are odorless, transparent fluids characterized by a low cellularity (total cell counts usually less than 1000/mm³), a specific gravity less than 1.020 and a total protein less than 3.0 g/dL. These poorly cellular fluids contain primarily macrophages and occasional mesothelial cells. Transudates occur as a result of oncotic pressure changes or other circulatory disturbances. These include hepatic cirrhosis, cardiac insufficiency and hypoproteinemia.

Modified transudates have an increased cellularity (total cell counts usually less than 5000/mm³ but greater than 1000/mm³). The mononuclear leukocytes predominate in this type of effusion with occasional mesothelial cells and rare heterophils. The mesothelial cells usually appear reactive. Reactive mesothelial cells tend to be round or oval with increased cytoplasmic basophilia. The cell margins often have a scalloped or villus-like appearance. The nuclei have coarse chromatin and prominent nucleoli. Multinucleation, cytoplasmic vacuolation and mitotic activity are often associated with reactive mesothelial cells. Care should be taken not to mistake these cells for malignant neoplasia. Modified transudates result from hydrostatic pressure changes or irritation of long-standing transudative effusions.

Exudative effusions are characterized by high cellularity (total cell counts usually greater than 5000/mm³), a specific gravity greater than 1.020 and a protein content greater than 3.0 g/dL. The majority of the cells found in exudative effusions are inflammatory cells. Acute exudative effusions demonstrate primarily a heterophilic inflammatory response; however, macrophages quickly move into the fluid, creating a mixed-cell inflammatory response within a few hours of onset. Lymphocytes and plasma cells are often seen in long-standing exudative effusions. Exudative effusions vary in color and turbidity. They are frequently viscous, have a foul odor and tend to clot. Abdominal lesions often associated with exudative effusions include septic peritonitis, egg-related peritonitis and abdominal malignancies.

Hemorrhagic effusions are identified by the presence of erythrocytic phagocytosis in the fluid sample. Thrombocytes disappear rapidly in hemorrhagic effusions. Proof of erythrophagocytosis is made by the detection of macrophages that have phagocytized erythrocytes (suggestive of recent hemorrhage), or that contain iron pigment or hemosiderin crystals resulting from erythrocyte degradation (implying a duration greater than 48 hours). Iron pigment appears as gray to blue-black pigment in the cytoplasm of macrophages using Wright's stain. Hemosiderin appears as diamond-shaped, golden crystals within the macrophage cytoplasm.

Malignant effusions have features of either exudative or hemorrhagic effusions, but contain cells compatible with malignant neoplasia.

Urate peritonitis is a rare effusion that can occur in the abdomen of birds when urinary fluids leak into the abdominal cavity. The cytology of the acute lesion is poorly cellular but contains a marked number of sodium and potassium urate crystals. These crystals are the same ones found in the urate portion of the bird's droppings. Urate crystals are spherical (2-8 mm) and have a spoke-wheel appearance.

Cytology of the Alimentary Tract

The differential diagnoses for common oral lesions include septic stomatitis, candidiasis, trichomoniasis and squamous cell hyperplasia.

Smears made from a bacterial abscess reveal either a heterophilic or mixed-cell inflammation with bacterial phagocytosis. Heterophils may appear degenerate if bacterial toxins are present.

Cytologic evidence for candidiasis is the presence of numerous narrowly based budding yeast. Candida yeast are typically oval and often stain deeply basophilic with the Romanowsky stains. Occasionally they stain poorly, however, and may appear as "ghosts" in the cytologic specimen. Because these organisms can be part of the normal flora of the upper alimentary tract of birds, low numbers of the yeast do not usually elicit an inflammatory response. However, an inflammatory response often occurs when the infection has involved the mucosa indicating the condition has become more serious. The presence of hyphae formation also indicates a potential lethal infection and suggests a systemic involvement by the yeast.

Trichomoniasis is best diagnosed by observing the movement of the piriform flagellate protozoa in a wet mount preparation. However, it is important to recognize these organisms in a stained cytologic sample if wet mount preparations are not part of the cytologic routine or trichomoniasis is not suspected. Trichomonads appear as basophilic, piriform cells with flagella on Wright's stained smears. The cell nucleus usually stains more eosinophilic than most cell nuclei. An eosinophilic axostyle can often be seen as a straight line running from the nucleus to the opposite pole of the cell. Eosinophilic flagella at the nuclear end and an undulating membrane on one side of the cell are usually present. An inflammatory response is usually found associated with trichomoniasis lesions.

The gross appearance of lesions caused by squamous hyperplasia and metaplasia from hypovitaminosis A can resemble lesions caused by bacteria, yeast and protozoa; however, the cytology has a very different appearance. Normally, squamous epithelial cells exfoliate as single cells or small groups following gentle scraping of the oral cavity. However, lesions resulting from squamous cell hyperplasia produce smears containing large numbers of cornified squamous epithelial cells that exfoliate in large sheets or aggregates. One does not see inflammatory cells (at least in acute lesions), yeast or protozoa. As this lesion becomes increasingly chronic, secondary bacterial infections often occur, creating a septic inflammatory response associated with the squamous cell hyperplasia on the cytologic sample.

Cytologic evaluation of the esophagus and ingluvies is indicated in birds with clinical signs of regurgitation, vomiting, delayed crop emptying or other suspected esophageal and crop disorders. The normal cytology reveals occasional squamous epithelial cells and a variable amount of background debris and extracellular bacteria (represented by a variety of morphologic types). A rare yeast is accepted as normal.

The same lesions and cytodiagnoses described for the oral cavity also apply to the normal cytologies of the esophagus and crop. Another cytologic indication of a disorder involving the esophagus and crop is the presence of many bacteria represented by one morphologic type, even though there is no apparent inflammatory response. This condition is typical of a peracute ingluvitis, and the disorder is often referred to as "sour crop." The pH is often greater than 7, whereas normal crop pH is 6.5-7. Capillaria ova may be detected in cytologic samples from the esophagus or crop of some birds with capillariasis.

Examination of the cloacal cytology is indicated whenever a disorder of the lower intestinal tract, reproductive tract, urinary tract or cloaca is suspected. Abnormal findings would include the presence of inflammatory cells, large numbers of yeast and a uniform population of bacteria. Special stains may be required for the detection of pathogens, such as *Mycobacterium* and *Giardia* spp.

Abnormal urinary fluid is watery and may contain cellular elements such as inflammatory cells and cellular casts.

Cytology of the Respiratory Tract

The normal cytology of the nasal cavity and infraorbital sinuses of birds reveals occasional non-cornified squamous epithelial cells and low numbers of extracellular bacteria with little background debris. The normal cytology of tracheal wash samples consists of a few ciliated respiratory epithelial cells and goblet cells. An occasional squamous epithelial cell may be found. Ciliated respiratory epithelial cells are columnar or prismatic in shape and have an eccentric nucleus at the small pole of the cell. Eosinophilic cilia are located at the opposite, larger pole of the cell. Goblet cells are columnar cells with eccentric nuclei. They lack cilia but contain eosinophilic cytoplasmic granules and vacuoles.

Cytologic evidence for periorbital sinusitis is provided by the presence of inflammatory cells in the aspirate. Lesions with a bacterial etiology are indicated by a septic, heterophilic or mixed-cell inflammation. Mycotic lesions often reveal either a mixed-cell or macrophagic inflammation with the presence of fungal elements, such as yeast, hyphae or spores. Sinus infections associated with chlamydia often reveal a mixed-cell or macrophagic inflammation. Chlamydial inclusions appear as small, blue-to-purple spherules, often in dense clusters, within the cytoplasm of macrophages when stained with Wright's stain. The chlamydial inclusions appear red, and the host cells appear blue-green with Gimenez stain. The chlamydial elementary bodies stain red, and the larger initial bodies stain blue with Macchiavello's stain.

A septic tracheobronchitis is identified from a tracheal wash sample by the presence of inflammatory cells showing bacterial phagocytosis. In severe cases, the ciliated respiratory epithelial cells appear degenerate. Degeneration and fragmentation of the ciliated respiratory epithelial cells in association with a macrophagic and lymphocytic inflammation are suggestive of a viral etiology. Inflammation of the trachea and bronchi usually results in an increase in goblet cells and mucin formation, which causes an increased thickness to the non-cellular background.

Aspergillosis is characterized by thick, septate hyphae that branch at 45° angles. Occasionally conidiophores can be seen. Other fungal lesions, such as phycomycosis, may reveal non-septate, branching hyphae. Mycotic lesions usually reveal a mixed-cell or macrophagic inflammation. Aspiration of foreign material also results in a macrophagic inflammation. A mixed-cell inflammation generally occurs when secondary bacterial pathogens become involved.

The cytologic evaluation of the lower respiratory tract (lungs and air sacs) is made from either biopsy samples, endoscopy impressions or imprints from necropsy specimens.

Normal air sac samples are poorly cellular with the presence of a few non-cornified epithelial cells. Bacterial infections show the typical septic inflammatory patterns. Chlamydial and mycotic lesions demonstrate mixed-cell or macrophagic inflammation with the presence of chlamydial inclusions or fungal elements, respectively.

Cytology of the Skin

Bacterial infections involving the skin are usually associated with a heterophilic or mixed-cell inflammation. Bacterial phagocytosis must be demonstrated to detect a septic inflammatory lesion.

Foreign bodies typically create a macrophagic inflammatory response with multinucleated giant cell formation. If a secondary bacterial infection has been established, lesions caused by foreign bodies may show a mixed-cell inflammatory response.

Cutaneous xanthomatosis is a unique condition of birds caused by an excessive accumulation of lipids in the skin. A macrophagic inflammatory response with multinucleated giant cells and cholesterol crystals is observed on the cytologic specimen. Cholesterol crystals appear as angular, translucent crystals that vary in size and shape.

Subcutaneous lipomas produce a cytologic specimen that appears "greasy" on the unstained slide. The cytology reveals numerous lipocytes, which vary in size.

Cutaneous and subcutaneous malignant neoplasms are rare in birds, but can be detected on cytologic examination. Lymphoid neoplasia produces a highly cellular sample of immature lymphocytes. These lymphoblasts and prolymphocytes are large, round cells that exfoliate as single cells. They have large nuclei with fine chromatin and multiple or large prominent nucleoli.

Cutaneous melanosarcomas have also been found in birds. Poorly differentiated melanosarcomas reveal mesenchymal cells that contain few cytoplasmic melanin granules. The gross appearance of the involved skin shows dark pigmentation. The malignant cells usually exfoliate as single cells, and the background may contain melanin granules from ruptured cells. The round melanin granules vary from black to dark brown to golden in color.

Avian poxvirus lesions reveal clusters of squamous epithelial cells that contain large cytoplasmic vacuoles. These cytoplasmic vacuoles often contain small, pale eosinophilic inclusions with oil immersion examination of Wright's stained smears.

Cytology of the Cornea and Conjunctiva

Normal conjunctival scrapings provide poorly cellular samples with little background material. The cells normally found are epithelial cells that may contain intracytoplasmic pigment granules. The normal cytology of the cornea is also poorly cellular and consists of occasional non-cornified squamous epithelial cells. Inflammatory lesions involving the cornea and conjunctiva reveal inflammatory cells and increased numbers of exfoliated epithelial cells. Chronic inflammatory lesions may show an increase in the number of epithelial cells that contain pigment granules. Chronic lesions may also reveal the presence of cornified squamous epithelial cells that are not normally found in the conjunctiva or cornea.

Cytology of Synovial Fluid

The amount of fluid in synovial joints of most birds is normally too small for sampling. Normal synovial fluid is poorly cellular. The cells are mononuclear cells, representing either synovial lining cells or mononuclear leukocytes. The background of normal synovial fluid cytology consists of a heavy, granular, eosinophilic substance representing the mucin in the fluid.

An increase in the inflammatory cells and change in the color, clarity, and viscosity of the fluid is indicative of inflammatory joint lesions. There may be a decrease in the granular eosinophilic background material, suggesting a decrease in mucin content. Erosion of the articular cartilage may result in the presence of multinucleated osteoclasts in the synovial fluid. Spindle-shaped fibroblasts suggest erosion into the fibrous layer of the articular capsule.

Articular gout produces a cream-to-yellow-colored deposit in affected joints. The cytology of this material reveals numerous, needle-shaped crystals (monosodium urate). These crystals are birefringent under polarized light. They occasionally stain eosinophilic with Wright's stain. Inflammatory cells are often present and the mucin content is often reduced.

Cytology of Internal Organs

Avian lymphoid tissue appears as lymphoid aggregates in the walls of the intestines, internal organs (especially the spleen and liver) and skin. The cloacal bursa of young birds is a sac-like lymphoid nodule found in the dorsal wall of the proctodeum of the cloaca. The cytology of normal lymphoid tissue shows a predominance of small mature lymphocytes (greater than 90 percent of the lymphoid cells). Reactive lymphoid tissue demonstrates an increase in the number of immature lymphocytes (prolymphocytes and lymphoblast) and plasma cells. Lymphoid hyperplasia causes an increase in the lymphoid tissue mass; however, the cytology appears normal with the exception of a slight increase in the number of prolymphocytes. Lymphoid neoplasia produces a marked increase in the number of immature lymphocytes, especially lymphoblasts. The neoplastic cells may show varying degrees of cellular features of malignant neoplasia.

Cytologic samples of the liver are usually highly cellular with a predominance of hepatocytes, erythrocytes and free nuclei. Hepatocytes are large epithelial cells that occur in sheets or clusters or as single cells. Normal hepatic cytology reveals uniform-appearing hepatocytes. These cells have an abundant, basophilic, finely granular cytoplasm and a round-to-oval, slightly eccentric nucleus. Binucleation is occasionally seen. Normal hematopoiesis is occasionally found because the liver is a common location for ectopic hematopoiesis. Also, macrophages containing iron pigment are occasionally seen.

Inflammatory lesions of the liver reveal numerous mature heterophils and an increase in the number of macrophages and plasma cells. It is important not to confuse normal ectopic granulopoiesis with heterophilic inflammation. If developing stages of the heterophils can be found, the cytology is representative of granulocytopoiesis. The hepatocytes may demonstrate degenerative changes in the presence of hepatic inflammation.

Avian tuberculosis produces a macrophagic inflammatory response in the liver. The cytology reveals numerous macrophages and multinucleated giant cells. When stained with Romanowsky stain, the background of the smear contains numerous large bacterial rods that do not stain. Likewise, macrophages may contain numerous bacterial rods that do not stain. An acid-fast stain is required to demonstrate the tubercle bacilli, which stain red.

Avian chlamydiosis often results in a mixed-cell or macrophagic inflammation in the spleen or liver with a marked increase in the number of plasma cells. Small, blue-to-purple, intracytoplasmic inclusions suggestive of chlamydial elementary and initial bodies may be seen in macrophages.

Hepatic lipidosis produces cytologic specimens that appear "greasy" on gross examination. The stained smears reveal enlarged hepatocytes that contain round, cytoplasmic vacuoles. The background material also contains these round vacuoles suggestive of lipid material.

Primary neoplasm of the liver reveals hepatocytes showing features of malignant neoplasia.

Occasionally, parasites may be found on hepatic imprints. Those commonly seen are schizogony of *Haemoproteus* and *Leukocytozoon*, sporozoites of *Atoxoplasma* and microfilaria.

Normally, cytology of the spleen shows a marked number of erythrocytes and lymphocytes, reflecting the cytology of a lymphoid tissue. Macrophages are also present and occasionally contain iron pigment from erythrophagocytosis of senescent red cells. Excessive splenic iron pigment is seen in birds with hemolytic anemia owing to increased red cell degradation by the spleen. Chlamydial infections often cause a marked increase in the number of splenic plasma cells. Macrophages often demonstrate intracytoplasmic chlamydial inclusions. Developmental stages of blood parasites may also be found in splenic samples. Systemic bacterial or fungal infections may result in an increase in the number of inflammatory cells, especially mature heterophils, in the spleen. Often, the etiologic agent can be found either within the leukocytes or in the non-cellular background.

The normal kidney produces a highly cellular sample that contains numerous epithelial cells with an abundant, slightly basophilic cytoplasm and slightly eccentric, round-to-oval nuclei. Abnormal cytology includes an increase in the number of inflammatory cells or the presence of cells having features of neoplasia. Epithelial cells from renal adenomas show increased cytoplasmic basophilia, slight pleomorphism and occasional mitotic figures. Renal adenocarcinomas produce epithelial cells having features of malignant neoplasia. Nephroblastomas (embryonal nephroma) produce poorly differentiated epithelial and mesenchymal cells. The cuboidal epithelial cells are associated with spindle-shaped cells of the fibrous stroma, and the background may contain a heavy, eosinophilic substance.

Table 10.3 Staining Procedures

Acid-fast Stain
1. Air dry then gently heat fix
2. Cover with carbol fuchsin
3. Steam over water bath (3-5 min.)
4. Rinse with tap water
5. Decolorize with acid alcohol until most red color is removed
6. Rinse twice in tap water
7. Cover with methylene blue stain (1 min.)
8. Gently rinse with tap water (air dry)

Gram's Stain
1. Air dry and gently heat fix slide
2. Cover with crystal violet (1 min.)
3. Gently rinse in tap water
4. Cover with Gram's iodine (1 min.)
5. Gently rinse in tap water
6. Decolorize with 95% ethyl alcohol (15-30 sec.)
7. Gently rinse in tap water
8. Cover with safranin (1 min.)
9. Gently rinse in tap water (air dry)

Macchiavello's Stain
1. Air dry then heat fix
2. Cover with basic fuchsin (5 min.)
3. Quickly rinse in tap water
4. Dip in citric acid 1-10 times (1-3 sec.)
5. Rinse in tap water
6. Cover with methylene blue (20-30 sec.)
7. Rinse in tap water (air dry)

Modified Gimenez Stain
1. Air dry then heat fix
2. Cover with carbol fuchsin (1-2 min.)
3. Rinse in tap water
4. Cover with malachite green (6-9 sec.)
5. Rinse in tap water
6. Recover with malachite green (6-9 sec.)
7. Rinse with tap water (air dry)

Sudan III Stain
1. Apply stain to wet or dry smear
2. Apply coverslip

New Methylene Blue Stain
1. Completely air dry or use as a wet mount
2. Apply small drop of stain
3. Add coverslip

Stamp Stain
1. Air dry smear then heat fix
2. Cover for 10 min. with carbolated fuchsin as used for Gram's stain diluted 1:4 with water
3. Rinse with tap water
4. Differentiate in 0.5% H_2SO_4 until the preparation looks gray; time according to thickness of the smear
5. Counterstain with 5% malachite green or methylene blue (15 sec.)
6. Rinse with tap water (air dry)

Wright's Stain
1. Air dry slide
2. Flood with Wright's stain (stand 1-3 min.)
3. Add equal amount of Wright's buffer
4. Gently mix by blowing until a metallic green sheen is formed
5. Allow to stand twice as long as step 2 (2-6 min.)
6. Rinse with tap water (air dry)

Diff-Quik Stain
1. Air dry slide
2. Dip in fixative 5 times (1 sec. each)
3. Dip in solution 1-5 times (1 sec. each)
4. Dip in solution 2-5 times (1 sec. each)
5. Rinse in distilled water (air dry)

Giemsa Stain
1. Air dry slide
2. Fix in methyl or ethyl alcohol (2-7 min.)
3. Air dry
4. Immerse in Giemsa stain (15-40 min.)
5. Rinse in tap water (air dry)

11

BIOCHEMISTRIES

Manfred Hochleithner

Properly evaluating a biochemical profile requires knowledge of the diagnostic sensitivities and specificities of tests, correct intervals for a specific test in a given species and a list of diseases that can induce the observed changes.

Nearly all routine hematologic and biochemical investigations can be performed with blood placed in lithium heparin, the anticoagulant of choice when dealing with most avian blood samples. The ability to use one single sample for numerous different tests limits unnecessary blood wastage, which can be an important consideration when dealing with small birds. The amount of blood needed to perform a specific diagnostic test depends on the equipment and technical capacity of the laboratory. When dealing with small birds, the use of micromethods is a necessity.

A blood smear should be made immediately after the blood is collected. A hematocrit-capillary tube is filled and the amount of blood needed for a total white cell count is collected in a diluting pipette. Immediately thereafter, the sample is centrifuged to separate the plasma. Any delay in separation may cause artificial changes of several plasma chemical variables.

The questions that laboratory results can answer generally fall into one of five categories:

1. Is an unapparent disease present? (screening)
2. Is a particular disease process occurring? (pathophysiology)
3. Is a tentative diagnosis correct? (confirmation)
4. What is the severity of a disease process? (prognosis)
5. Has therapy favorably altered the disease process? (monitoring)

Reference ranges established for a population of animals are statistically reduced to reference intervals to allow discrimination between health and disease.

Until reference intervals are established for birds free from subclinical infections (particularly viral diseases) and maintained on adequate diets for long periods, it will be impossible to define precise reference intervals on a population basis.

In interpreting clinicopathologic data, it should be noted that:

1. There are subtle changes that exist between health and disease. The concept of normality rarely exists.
2. Not all values from healthy individuals will fall within a normal reference interval (usually encompasses 95% of healthy individuals).
3. Some values from abnormal individuals will fall within the reference interval.

If data is normally distributed, 5% of the healthy population with values that are higher or lower than the defined 95% intervals are considered abnormal. With this test evaluation system, it is accepted that there are 2.5% (one out of 40) of the normal population that fall above or below the normal range even though they are clinically healthy.

Further, reference values established for a species may not be normal for an individual. The individual may regularly have a test value that is in the lower part of the normal range. If such a bird developed pathology, the test parameter could stay within the normal range for the species, even though it is elevated for the individual. Consequently, reference values established for an individual bird are more sensitive in detecting subtle abnormalities than comparing test results to reference intervals for a population.

Enzymology

When the integrity of a cell is disrupted, enzymes escape into the surrounding fluid compartment, where their activities can be measured as an index of cellular integrity.

It is important to realize that cells must be damaged before they release enzymes into the serum/plasma. Therefore, enzymatic-based tests are a measure of cell damage, and not necessarily a measure of organ function. Anoxia causes the cell membrane to lose its integrity so that soluble enzymes from the cytosol can leak into the serum/plasma.

Metabolites

Metabolites can be measured to provide information about the functional capacity of the organs that are involved in a particular metabolic pathway.

Electrolytes

Balances of electrolytes are essential for all living matter, and commonly measured electrolytes include potassium, chloride and sodium. Trace elements including magnesium may also be determined. The major electrolytes occur primarily as free ions. The trace elements exist primarily in combination with proteins.

Hormones

It has been suggested that hormone concentrations may be good indicators of disease in humans or mammals, but their analytic accuracy and precision are difficult to evaluate in birds. Nonspecific cross-reactions that occur when tests designed for mammalian hormones are used for bird plasma can lead to questionable results.

Table 11.1   Recommended Samples for Biochemical Tests

Tissue Enzymes	Sample
ALT	Hemolysis-free plasma or serum
AP	Heparinized plasma or serum
AST	Heparinized plasma or serum
CPK	Serum is preferred. Citrate and fluoride inhibit CK activity.
GGT	EDTA plasma or serum (see text)
GLDH	Heparinized plasma or serum
LDH	Hemolysis-free plasma or serum
Metabolites	**Sample**
Plasma Ammonia	EDTA (see text)
Amylase	Heparinized plasma or serum
Bile Acids	Heparinized plasma or serum
Bilirubin	Heparinized plasma or serum
Calcium	Heparinized plasma or serum
Cholesterol	Heparinized plasma or serum
Creatinine	Heparinized plasma or serum
Glucose	Heparinized plasma or serum
Iron	Heparinized plasma or serum
TIBC	Heparinized plasma or serum
Lipase	Heparinized plasma or serum
TP	Heparinized plasma or serum
Triglycerides	Heparinized plasma or EDTA plasma
Urea	Heparinized plasma or serum
Uric Acid	Heparinized plasma or serum
Electrolytes	**Sample**
Chloride	Heparinized plasma or serum
Potassium	Heparinized plasma or serum
Sodium	Heparinized plasma or serum

Enzymes

Alanine Aminotransferase ALT (GPT)

Diagnostic Value: Alanine aminotransferase activity occurs in many different tissues. Specific diagnostic value of these enzymes in birds is poor. In many cases, patients with severe liver damage have had normal ALT activities, reflecting a low level of enzyme activity in liver cells from certain species. Alanine aminotransferase activities often increase due to damage in many different tissues. In some avian species, normal ALT activities are below the sensitivity of many analyzers.

Pathologic Changes: Elevated activities are difficult to interpret, and this enzyme has limited usefulness in birds because it can be increased by pathologic changes in almost all tissues. Activity in erythrocytes is 1.6 times higher than in plasma, and hemolysis will cause elevated activities.

Alkaline Phosphatase - AP

Diagnostic Value: Alkaline phosphatase activities may be elevated due to irritation of the cells in different tissues. Increased activities have no specific importance.

Pathologic Changes: Elevations are most common with liver disease even though the level of activity in this organ is low. Enteritis has been described as a cause of higher AP activities but activity of this isoenzyme is labile and difficult to measure. Low AP activities have been linked to dietary zinc deficiencies.

Aspartate Aminotransferase - AST (GOT)

Diagnostic Value: High AST activity has been described in liver, skeletal muscle, heart, brain and kidney cells. The distribution of AST in avian tissues varies among the species. Elevated activities are usually indicative of liver or muscle damage. Aspartate aminotransferase activity provides the best information when combined with other more specific tests. Creatinine kinase activity can be used to exclude muscle damage as a cause of increased AST activity.

Pathologic Changes: In general, AST activities in birds greater than 230 U/L are considered abnormal. Abnormal activities have been linked to vitamin E, selenium or methionine deficiencies, liver damage (particularly psittacosis or Pacheco's disease virus), pesticide and carbon tetrachloride intoxication and muscle damage. Intramuscular injections of irritating substances may cause elevation of CK with no increases in AST activity. In other patients, both the CK and AST activities will increase post-injection.

Creatinine Kinase - CK (CPK)

Diagnostic Value: Elevations in activities are mostly seen because of muscle cell damage. This enzyme has value in distinguishing muscle from liver cell damage. However, the clinician should consider that muscle and liver cell damage can occur simultaneously from the same or different pathologic processes.

Pathologic Changes: Increase in CK activity has been linked to muscle cell necrosis, convulsions, intramuscular injections (depending on the volume and degree of irritation), vitamin E and selenium deficiencies, neuropathies, lead toxicity and occasionally chlamydiosis.

Gamma Glutamyl Transferase - GGT

Sample: EDTA plasma or serum can be used to determine GGT activity.

Diagnostic Value: Little is known about the significance of plasma GGT activity for the diagnosis of hepatobiliary disease in birds. In racing pigeons GGT has been found to be a specific indicator for liver disease. One investigator reported measurable activities in the kidney and brain of pigeons, and the kidney and duodenum of budgerigars. Another investigator concluded that GGT is not a sensitive test for the detection of liver disease in different avian species. Enzyme activity in normal birds typically falls below the sensitivity range of most analyzers.

Pathologic Changes: Elevations in GGT activity have been described in association with liver disease, but not on a regular basis. The highest levels of activity have been reported in the kidneys. However, elevations do not always occur with renal disease, probably because the enzyme is excreted in the urine.

Glutamate Dehydrogenase - GLDH

Physiology: Glutamate dehydrogenase is a mitochondrial enzyme found in numerous tissues.

Diagnostic Value: Significant amounts of this enzyme have been found in the liver, kidney and brain of chickens, ducks, turkeys and racing pigeons. In budgerigars, the highest enzyme activity has been reported in the kidney. Significant elevations have been observed in birds with liver disease, but few reference intervals are available for avian species.

Pathologic Changes: Activity in plasma or serum is increased in all conditions in which hepatocellular damage is present. As an exclusive mitochondrial isoenzyme, GLDH is released from cells that are necrotic or markedly injured. Therefore, activities are lower in inflammatory processes that do not result in cellular necrosis.

Lactate Dehydrogenase - LDH

Physiology: There are five LDH isoenzymes, each of which occurs in a wide variety of tissues, in particular skeletal muscle, cardiac muscle, liver, kidney, bone and red blood cells

Diagnostic Value: Although this enzyme is not specific for any organ, elevations are most common with hepatic disease in psittacines. Lactate dehydrogenase activities are thought to rise and fall more quickly than AST activities in birds with liver disease. These differences may provide information on the chronicity of liver disease.

Pathologic Changes: Elevated enzyme activity can be observed due to liver and muscle damage.

Nutrients and Metabolites

Plasma Ammonia

Sample: EDTA is the anticoagulant of choice. Lithium heparin can be contaminated with ammonium heparin, which will lead to falsely elevated values. Samples must be analyzed immediately because ammonia is released through the catabolism of various substances (eg, urea).

Diagnostic Value: Little data is available on the use of ammonia concentrations as a diagnostic test in birds.

Pathologic Changes: High blood ammonia concentrations may indicate reduced liver function or ammonia poisoning. Ammonia toxicity usually occurs from buildup of ammonia gases in poultry houses and has rarely been reported in companion birds. Atmospheric ammonia can contaminate a blood sample that is left open in room air.

Reference Value: Budgerigars - 36-74 μmol/L (Kodak Ektachem, 25°C).

Amylase

Physiology: Amylase occurs in plasma as a number of isoenzymes that are principally derived from the pancreas, liver and small intestine.

Diagnostic Value: Little information is available on amylase activity in birds.

Pathologic Changes: Increased enzymatic activity can be seen with acute pancreatitis. In these cases enzyme activity may exceed three times the upper limit of the reference interval. Activities less than twice the upper limit of the reference interval are sometimes seen in macaws with severe enteritis in the absence of pancreatic lesions.

Reference Values: Budgerigars (187-582 U/L); African Grey Parrots (211-519 U/L); Amazon parrots (106-524 U/L); macaws (276-594 U/L) (Kodak Ektachem, Amylopectin, 25°C).

Bile Acids

Physiology: The liver synthesizes the primary bile acids (cholic acid and chenodeoxycholic acid). It then excretes these acids as sodium salts into the bile. With the ingestion of food, bile is carried via the bile duct into the small intestine where the bile acids act principally as emulsifying agents in fat digestion and absorption. Most bile acids that enter the gastrointestinal tract are reabsorbed in the distal small and large intestines where they return, via the portal circulation, to the liver. They are then extracted from the blood and recycled. Only a small percentage of the total pool of bile acids is lost in the feces each day. A small quantity of the total bile acids reabsorbed from the gastrointestinal tract is not removed from the blood by the liver and reaches the general circulation. It is this fraction of unextracted bile acids that is measured. The quantity of bile acids in the plasma normally increases following the ingestion of food.

Diagnostic Value: If liver function is impaired, bile acids are not properly reabsorbed from the blood, and consequently the proportion of excreted bile acids reaching the peripheral circulation increases. Circulating bile acids can therefore be used as a sensitive indicator of liver function, and of the integrity of the circulation through the liver, biliary tract and intestines. It has been suggested that chronic liver disease that results in cirrhosis may decrease the production of bile acids with a subsequent decrease in the plasma. This may be particularly true in a post-prandial sample. Low bile acid concentrations are common in birds with microhepatia (as detected radiographically), poor feather formation and an overgrown, malformed beak.

Pathologic Changes: Elevations in bile acids have been shown to correlate with liver disease in pigeons, chickens and African Grey Parrots.

Reference Intervals: African Grey Parrots (18-71 μmol/L); Amazon parrots (19-144 μmol/L); cockatoos (23-70 μmol/L); macaws (25-71 μmol/L); pigeon (29-56 μmol/L).

Bilirubin

Physiology: In birds, the major bile pigment is biliverdin. The enzyme biliverdin reductase is absent, and biliverdin is not converted into bilirubin.

Diagnostic Value: The diagnostic value of bilirubin appears to vary among species. It has no value in chickens that cannot form bilirubin, but may be of value in other species.

Pathologic Changes: Bilirubin cannot normally be detected in plasma of normal psittacines. With severe hepatic disease (eg, chlamydiosis or Pacheco's disease virus) bilirubin concentrations up to 44.5 μmol/L have been reported.

Calcium

Diagnostic Value: Total calcium should always be interpreted along with albumin concentrations. Hypoalbuminemia will reduce the quantity of bound calcium and result in a decreased total calcium concentration without reducing biologically active calcium (ionized fraction).

Pathologic Changes: Decreased calcium concentrations are common in seizuring African Grey Parrots. This hypocalcemia syndrome has been described as a unique form of hypoparathyroidism in which calcium is not properly released from bone. Glucocorticoid therapy will decrease total calcium concentrations. Increased calcium concentrations have been reported with dietary excesses of vitamin D, osteolytic bone tumors and dehydration.

Cholesterol

Physiology: Cholesterol is a major lipid that is a precursor of all the steroid hormones and bile acids as well as a component of the plasma membrane of cells.

Diagnostic Value: Elevated and decreased cholesterol concentrations may occur from a number of physiologic influences and different diseases; however, the diagnostic value of this test in birds appears to be poor. Very high cholesterol concentrations usually accompany lipemia, especially in Amazon parrots, macaws and Rose-breasted Cockatoos with fatty liver degeneration.

Pathologic Changes: Elevations can occur because of hypothyroidism, liver disease, bile duct obstruction, starvation or high fat diets. High cholesterol concentrations have been reported in budgerigars with xanthomatosis. Decreased cholesterol levels have been associated with some cases of liver disease, aflatoxicosis, reduced fat in the diet, *Escherichia coli* endotoxemia and spirochetosis.

Creatinine

Diagnostic Value: There is a slim margin between the physiologic and pathologic levels of creatinine. For many analyzers, physiologic values are below the detectable range. This test parameter is very insensitive and is a relatively poor diagnostic test in birds.

Pathologic Changes: Severe kidney damage can lead to increased creatinine levels, especially if the filtration rate is decreased. Elevations have also been described in connection with egg-related peritonitis, septicemia (eg, chlamydiosis), renal trauma and nephrotoxic drugs.

Glucose

Diagnostic Value: Glucose is often a part of a laboratory panel even though pathologic changes in birds are seldom detected. Glucose should be evaluated in convulsing birds or those with glucosuria.

Pathologic Changes: Increases in plasma glucose levels are due to increased glucose production or release. Diabetes mellitus has been confirmed in budgerigars, cockatiels, Amazon parrots, Scarlet Macaws, Umbrella Cockatoos and a Toco Toucan. Transient elevations in glucose have been reported in cockatiels with egg-related peritonitis. Decreases in plasma glucose levels can be due to hepatic dysfunction (eg, Pacheco's disease virus), impaired glucose production or its excessive utilization (eg, septicemia, neoplasia, aspergillosis). Glucose concentrations can be artificially decreased during storage if the blood sample is contaminated with bacteria.

Phosphorus

Diagnostic Value: Changes in inorganic phosphorus concentration can occur with several diseases, but not on a consistent basis. The diagnostic value is poor.

Pathologic Changes: Increased plasma inorganic phosphate levels can be seen in some cases of severe kidney damage due to hypervitaminosis D, nutritional secondary hyperparathyroidism and hypoparathyroidism. False elevations will occur if samples are hemolyzed.

Iron

Diagnostic Value: The value of determining iron in different avian species has not been thoroughly investigated. A recent report shows a failure to correlate serum iron levels with liver biopsy and subsequent toxicologic analysis for iron.

Pathologic Changes: Severe and chronic loss of blood will increase iron values. Iron deficiency anemia has been described in raptors. Changes in plasma iron levels in mynah birds and toucans with iron storage disease are described in Chapter 47.

Total Iron-Binding Capacity (TIBC)

Diagnostic Value: Abnormalities in TIBC occur with some disorders of iron metabolism. Very little data from birds is available. This parameter appears to have little importance in diagnosing hemochromatosis, but insufficient research has been performed.

Lipase

Diagnostic Value: Lipase and amylase activities were high in a caique with clinical signs of pancreatic exocrine insufficiency when compared to the activities of these enzymes in the mate. Hemolysis inhibits enzyme activity.

Pathologic Changes: Although no reference values are currently available, birds do exhibit high lipase activity in severe cases of acute pancreatitis. For diagnostic purposes, a blood sample from a representative of the same species should be included for comparison.

Total Protein (TP)

Method: Total protein levels may be determined using a chemical method or a refractometer. The chemical method of choice is the biuret method. At protein concentrations < 3.5g/dL, refractometric results are likely to be inaccurate. Refractometry should be considered a rapid method for determining an estimate of the body fluid protein. Ideally, total protein concentrations have the most value when considered with the results of plasma protein electrophoresis.

Diagnostic Value: Total protein is often used as an indicator for the health status of a patient. Determination of plasma protein concentrations may be of value in diagnosing gastrointestinal, hepatic or renal diseases. Furthermore, plasma proteins will be abnormal in infectious diseases that cause a stimulation of the immune system.

Pathologic Changes (Dysproteinemia): Hypoproteinemia can reflect reduced synthesis caused by chronic hepatopathies, malabsorption caused by chronic enteropathies (enteritis, tumors, parasitism), increased loss caused by proteinuria due to renal disease, blood loss and malignant tumors (rarely seen in birds) or starvation and malnutrition. Hyperproteinemia may be induced by chronic infectious diseases that stimulate synthesis of gamma globulin. It also has been seen with chronic lymphoproliferative disease that resembles leukosis in chickens and myelosis in budgerigars. Dehydration should always be ruled out as a cause of hyperproteinemia.

Electrophoresis

Physiology: Most frequently used electrophoresis methods identify five main protein fractions in birds: albumin, α1-, α2-, β- and γ-globulins. A pre-albumin fraction has been described in pigeons and some parrot species. The α-globulins are acute phase proteins that typically increase with acute inflammation; β-globulins are composed of complement, hemopexin, ferritin, fibrinogen and lipoproteins. Some immunoglobulins, including IgM and IgA, also migrate in the β-globulin range. The β-globulins are also acute phase proteins. The γ-globulin fraction is mainly composed of immunoglobulins (IgA, IgM and IgG).

Diagnostic Value: In healthy birds the albumin fraction is the largest protein fraction. An inflammatory process will cause a rise in TP because of increased concentrations of α, β or γ globulin fractions. Often albumin concentrations are decreased in these situations. The combined effect of these changes is a decrease in the albumin/globulin (A/G) ratio. Often the TP concentration is within the reference range, while the A/G ratio is decreased. Therefore, the A/G ratio is of greater clinical importance than the TP concentration.

Serum or plasma protein electrophoresis can be used to monitor response to treatment. When the bird responds favorably, an increase in the albumin concentration and a decrease in the globulin concentration can be observed, which leads to normalization of the A/G ratio.

Pathologic Changes: Decreases in albumin concentration can occur from decreased synthesis due to chronic liver disease or chronic inflammation, increased albumin loss due to renal disease, parasitism or overhydration. A decrease in albumin causes edema because of a decrease in oncotic pressure. Increases are seen because of dehydration.

Increases in α- and β-globulins may be caused by acute nephritis, severe active hepatitis, systemic mycotic diseases (γ-) and the nephrotic syndrome. Increases in γ-globulins occur with acute or chronic inflammation, infection, chronic hepatitis and immune mediated disorders.

Triglycerides

Diagnostic Value: Triglyceride values have been insufficiently evaluated in birds.

Pathologic Changes: Egg-related peritonitis has been associated with high concentrations of triglycerides. High concentrations (2000-5000 mg/dL) were reported in Amazon parrots showing signs of hyperadrenocorticism. Because triglyceride values are determined based on enzymatically released glycerol, these values may be falsely elevated after exercise or following any event that causes increased levels of blood glycerol (eg, catching birds in an aviary).

Urea

Diagnostic Value: Urea is present in very small amounts in avian plasma, and determining urea levels has generally been considered of little value. However, recent investigations have shown good correlation between increased plasma urea concentrations and renal disease in pigeons. In other avian species, urea may have little value in detecting renal disease but can be used as a sensitive indicator of dehydration.

Pathologic Changes: High urea plasma levels can occur in all conditions that cause low urine flow, such as dehydration or bilateral ureteral obstruction.

Uric Acid

Physiology: In birds, uric acid is the major product of the catabolism of nitrogen. Synthesis occurs mainly in the liver and in the renal tubules. Approximately 90% of blood uric acid is eliminated by secretion into the lumen of the tubules. Only 50% of the healthy avian kidney is actually used for excreting protein waste, providing a large functional reserve.

Diagnostic Value: The evaluation of uric acid concentrations in plasma or serum is widely used in birds for the detection of renal disease. Species' differences in the ability of the avian kidney to compensate for damage before uric acid levels are elevated reduce the diagnostic value for this test. However, if reference intervals are available, hyperuricemia is a good indicator of renal disease. Normal uric acid concentrations do not guarantee that the kidneys are healthy.

Pathologic Changes: Hyperuricemia can be expected if the glomerular filtration is decreased more than 70-80%. Decreased filtration may occur from hypovitaminosis A-induced damage to renal epithelial cells, dehydration, intoxications or from some bacterial and viral (eg, Newcastle disease) infections. Uric acid levels may also be increased from the release of nucleic acids caused by severe tissue damage or starvation. If a toenail clip is used for blood collection and urates from the droppings contaminate the sample, the uric acid levels may be falsely elevated.

If the blood uric acid concentration exceeds its solubility it will be deposited in different locations in the body. High plasma or serum concentrations of uric acid are a prognostic indicator that gout may occur. Hypervitaminosis D_3-induced renal damage is frequently associated with gout and extremely high uric acid levels. This problem is particularly common in macaws. This has been described for aminoglycosides (gentamicin), and allopurinol in Red-tailed Hawks. Interestingly, in most species, allopurinol is effective in treating, not inducing, gout.

Electrolytes

Chloride

Diagnostic Value: Elevations in chloride concentrations rarely are detected.

Pathologic Changes: Hyperchloridemia can occur with dehydration. The role of chloride in maintaining acid-base balance has not been sufficiently evaluated in birds.

Potassium

Sample: Either heparinized plasma or serum is appropriate for detecting potassium. If ion-selective electrode methods are used, whole blood is also an effective sample. Potassium levels are usually higher in serum due to the release of potassium from thrombocytes damaged in the coagulation process. Hemolysis will elevate the plasma concentration of potassium (500-700%). Potassium concentrations were found to rapidly decline in pigeon and chicken plasma allowed to sit for two hours. For accurate results, plasma should be separated within minutes of collection. Hyperproteinemia and hyperlipemia will result in falsely low potassium levels caused by a decreased aqueous fraction of the total plasma volume.

Diagnostic Value: Alterations in potassium homeostasis have serious consequences. Decreased extracellular potassium is characterized by muscle weakness, paralysis and cardiac effects.

Pathologic Changes: Hyperkalemia can be caused by severe tissue damage, reduced potassium excretion by diseased kidneys, adrenal disease or because of redistribution of potassium from the intracellular to the extracellular fluid (acidosis). Dehydration and hemolytic anemia can also cause hyperkalemia.

Hypokalemia may be caused by decreased potassium intake, increased potassium loss due to chronic diarrhea or diuretic therapy (seldom used in birds) and the shift of potassium from the extracellular to the intracellular fluid (alkalosis).

Sodium

Diagnostic Value: Abnormal sodium levels that are not caused by technical failures are rarely seen in birds. If they do occur, they are good indicators of a pathologic situation. Salt poisoning, mainly from high salt foods, may occur more frequently in companion birds than is documented.

Pathologic Changes: Hypernatremia can occur from increased sodium intake (peanuts, crackers), excessive water loss or decreased water intake.

Hyponatremia may be due to increased sodium loss as in kidney disease or severe diarrhea. It may also be caused by overhydration as in psychogenic polydipsia or after intravenous fluid therapy with sodium-free or low sodium solutions. The relative overhydration, which follows a reduction in renal perfusion possibly because of decreased colloid osmotic pressure, may also cause hyponatremia.

Total Carbon Dioxide Content (Bicarbonate)

Physiology: Alterations of bicarbonate and CO_2 dissolved in plasma are characteristic of acid-base balance. For clinical purposes, the total CO_2 content is the same as the bicarbonate content.

Diagnostic Value: Bicarbonate levels are useful for establishing whether or not acidosis or alkalosis is present and, if so, the degree of severity.

Pathologic Changes: Increases are mainly due to metabolic alkalosis and decreases are due to metabolic acidosis. Reference intervals for most avian species are not available.

Reference Values for Adult Budgerigars: 21-26 mmol/L.

Blood Gases - pCO$_2$, pO$_2$ and pH

Sample: Venous heparinized blood is the most likely specimen that will be collected for blood gas analysis. Determination should be performed as quickly as possible (in house). When measuring blood gases and acid-base status in birds, it is necessary to collect blood samples in pre-cooled syringes and store the samples on ice to stop the metabolism of the erythrocytes. The nucleated avian erythrocytes possess virtually all the enzymes typical of metabolically active cells and consume oxygen seven to ten times faster than mammalian erythrocytes.

Diagnostic Value: Clinical significance in companion birds has not been thoroughly investigated.

Pathologic Changes: Acidemia (decrease in blood or plasma pH) has been reported in some birds with renal disease.

Reference Values for Budgerigars: pH (7.334-7.489); pCO$_2$ (30.6-43.2 mm Hg) (see Chapter 39).

Other Tests

Delta-Aminolevulinic Acid Dehydratase

Diagnostic Value: Delta-aminolevulinic acid dehydratase can be used to detect lead intoxication, and decreased plasma activity is pathologic.

Pathologic Changes: The activity can decrease depending on the dosage of lead and the species up to 50% of the normal value. Central nervous system changes have been reported if plasma activity is below 86 U/L (see Chapter 37).

Copper

Diagnostic Value: Elevation occurs with copper intoxication. In postmortem specimens, copper concentration in the liver provides the best diagnostic sample.

Urinalysis

Urinalysis is indicated if renal disease is suspected. Polyuria is a common clinical presentation in companion birds.

Volume, Color and Consistency

Urine evaluation should include a measurement of volume, a record of appearance (color, consistency) and determination of specific gravity. Normal companion birds produce a small quantity of urine, and if it can easily be collected it is generally abnormal (stress or disease). The urine is usually clear in most companion bird species, but in other birds, such as ratites and Anseriformes, it is normally opaque, cloudy or slightly flocculent.

Pathologic Changes: Lead intoxication in some species may result in chocolate milk-colored urine and urates. This hemoglobinuria is common and normal for some nervous birds. Severe liver disease, like that induced by chlamydia or Pacheco's disease virus, can increase the secretion of biliverdin, which results in yellow-green or mustard-colored urine and urates.

Specific Gravity

Normal: The specific gravity varies with the state of hydration and with the individual bird. In the polyuric bird, values from 1.005-1.020 are considered normal. A refractometer can be used for this determination. Water deprivation should be used to evaluate the kidney's ability to concentrate low levels, often due to psychogenic polydipsia.

Pathologic Changes: Increased loss of water without an increased loss of solute will create a low specific gravity. This situation can be caused by intravenous fluid therapy, hyperthyroidism, liver disease, pituitary neoplasia, progesterone or glucocorticoid therapy.

Specific Evaluation

Substances filtered by the normal kidney generally have a molecular weight of less than 68,000 (eg, water, uric acid, urea, glucose, electrolytes). Two substances that are on the border of this molecular weight cutoff are hemoglobin and albumin. Most other physiologic proteins have higher molecular weights. Most substances that are filtered by the kidneys are critical to normal bodily functions and are completely reabsorbed (eg, amino acids, glucose, vitamins).

Urinary pH and the concentration of some chemical constituents in the urine can be measured using commercial test strips designed for use with human urine. It should be noted that the sensitivity of these tests has been adjusted to detect what would be regarded as abnormal levels of certain substances in human urine. These sensitivities are not necessarily applicable to birds and the fact that a "higher" reading is obtained on an area of the test strip does not necessarily imply an abnormality. For example, alkaline urine can produce falsely elevated protein levels.

Normal pH: Most pet birds have a pH between 6.0-8.0, which is largely related to the diet. Birds fed large amounts of protein (carnivores) have an acidic urine, while grain-eating birds have more alkaline urine.

Pathologic Changes: Companion birds with urine pH lower than 5.0 are considered acidotic. Increased protein catabolism will cause a lower pH. Bacterial metabolism tends to cause an alkaline pH. Companion birds with papillomatosis and other disorders that typically cause tenesmus may have acidic urine.

Urinary Protein

Normal: Trace amounts of protein can be detected in the urine of 90% of birds tested.

Pathologic Changes: Many renal disorders will result in a mild to moderate proteinuria. Non-renal sources of proteinuria include hematuria, hemoglobinuria and hyperproteinemia, which are usually caused by an increase in the production of immunoglobulins. Inaccurate protein levels will be detected if the urine is alkaline or if the strip is *soaked* in urine (instead of briefly dipped), which leaches out the citrate buffer.

Glucose

Normal: Avian urine normally contains no glucose. Trace glucose readings may be detected in normal avian urine by using dip sticks.

Pathologic Changes: The threshold for glucosuria to occur varies with the species. Glucosuria will occur in most birds when the blood glucose level exceeds 600 mg/dL. In diabetes mellitus, birds may have blood glucose concentrations above 800 mg/dL.

Ketones

Ketones should be absent from the urine of birds.

Bilirubin

Bilirubin is not normally present in birds.

Urinary Urobilinogen

Normal readings are 0.0-0.1 in healthy birds. Pathologic changes would be expected in cases of intravascular hemolysis and severe liver disease, but are seldom reported.

Blood

Normal readings are negative or trace. Blood in the urine may originate from the cloaca or from the urinary, reproductive or gastrointestinal tracts. Hemoglobinuria can be due to intravascular lysis of RBCs (rare) or lysis of RBCs present in the urine.

Urinary Nitrite

This test is included on many commercial test strips and is used to screen for bacteriuria. It is an unreliable test for avian urine.

White and Red Blood Cells

The number of RBCs and WBCs in the sediment is reported as the number per high power field (HPF). Normal urine contains 0 -3 RBCs/HPF and 0-3 WBCs/HPF. More than 6 white or red blood cells per HPF is a cause for concern. All cells noted within the urine sediment may have origins within the cloaca or the urinary, reproductive or gastrointestinal tracts.

Epithelial Cells

Normal urine contains no epithelial cells.

Casts

Normally no casts are seen in avian urine. Casts are frequently noted in cases of renal disease. Granular casts are most common.

Bacteria

Gram-positive cocci and rods may be noted in the avian urinary sediment if the sample has been contaminated with fecal material.

Pathologic Changes: Reports of bacteria that are "too numerous to count" or numerous cocci and rods in reasonably clean urine samples should be viewed with suspicion.

IMAGING TECHNIQUES

Marjorie C. McMillan

With advancing technology, diagnostic imaging techniques available for avian patients now include ultrasound, fluoroscopy, computed tomography (CT) and nuclear scintigraphy; however, routine radiography remains the most frequently performed imaging modality in birds and frequently is diagnostic without the need for more sophisticated procedures.

Both risk and benefit to the patient should be considered when radiography is used as a screening procedure in an apparently normal companion bird. In general, radiography should be performed only when indicated by historical information, physical examination findings and laboratory data. Indiscriminate radiographic studies create an unnecessary risk to the patient and technical staff.

In general, image quality is controlled by:
- the production of the image—influenced by radiographic equipment, technical settings (kVp, mA, time), focal-film distance, part-film distance, focal spot size and collimation;
- the recording of the image—influenced by the type of film, cassette and screen combination;
- and the development of the image—influenced by the darkroom environment and type of processing equipment.

Radiographic detail depends on sharpness of the image and radiographic contrast. Sharpness, the ability to define an edge, is compromised by motion, uneven film-screen contact and a large focal spot. Radiographic contrast is controlled by subject contrast, scatter, and film contrast and fog. Detail is improved by using a small focal spot, the shortest possible exposure time (usually 0.015 seconds), adequate focus-film distance (40 inches), a collimated beam, single emulsion film and a rare earth, high-detail screen. The contact between the radiographic cassette and the patient should be even, and the area of interest should be as close as possible to the film.

Radiographic Technique

As a general rule, the clinician should choose the lowest kV, a high mA and a short exposure time. Usually, non-bucky techniques applicable for radiography of cats provide reasonable radiographic settings for medium to large psittacine birds.

In circumstances where single emulsion, rare earth, high-detail systems are used, kVp ranging from 60-75 at five mAs (300mA, 1/60th of a second) usually provides an appropriate scale of contrast and eliminates motion. In small Passeriformes, such as canaries and finches, reducing the focal-film distance by one-fourth (to 30 inches) and decreasing the mAs by one-half may improve the radiographic image.

Although the single-emulsion film and single screen, rare earth systems result in greater detail, they do require increased exposure when compared to double emulsion film-cassette combinations. Low-absorption cassette fronts may provide comparable detailed studies with less radiation exposure.

Restraint and Positioning

Poor positioning is the most frequently encountered factor that compromises a radiographic study and hampers interpretation of subtle lesions. Some birds can be adequately restrained for routine views with mechanical plexiglass devices and positioning aids such as sandbags, foam blocks, lead gloves, velcro, pipe cleaners and plastic and paper tape. Other patients will require isoflurane anesthesia to obtain the most diagnostic radiographs; however, it should be noted that anesthesia or chemical restraint for radiographic examination will decrease normal gastrointestinal motility and as such is generally contraindicated in studies to evaluate the function of this organ system. Anesthesia should be considered mandatory when radiographing strong, powerful birds or patients that are fractious, highly stressed, experiencing significant respiratory distress or those that have an injury that may be exacerbated by struggling.

If heavy metal intoxication is suspected in a critically ill bird, a quick radiographic screening for metal densities can be obtained by placing the bird in a bag and taking a DV radiograph.

The most frequently performed radiographic studies in companion birds are ventrodorsal (VD) and left-to-right lateral (LeRtL) whole body projections. For the VD view, the head is restrained and the wings are extended 90 degrees from the body and secured with sandbags, velcro straps or tape. The wings should be restrained close to the body to prevent iatrogenic fractures. The legs are pulled caudally and parallel to the body and secured at the tarsometatarsus with tape or velcro straps.

For the LeRtL view, the dependent wing is extended 90 degrees to the body and secured. A foam block or other soft material is placed between the wings, and the left wing is extended and restrained slightly caudally to the right. Placing a block of foam between the wings helps to prevent overextension and potential injury. Both legs are extended caudally with slight tension and secured individually at the tarsometatarsus. The dependent leg is positioned slightly cranially. Securing the legs individually helps to reduce rotation of the body, which is common if the legs are fastened together.

In a symmetrically positioned VD view, the spine and sternum will be superimposed, and the scapulae, acetabula and femurs will be parallel. In LeRtL projection, the ribs, coracoid, acetabula and kidneys will be superimposed, if the positioning is accurate.

The orthogonal view of the wing in the caudocranial projection requires horizontal beam radiography. In the lateral position, views of the pelvis, spine and legs can be achieved.

Radiography of the skull requires general anesthesia to ensure accurate positioning and to minimize motion. Complete evaluation of the skull requires LeRtL, RtLeL, VD, dorsoventral (DV) and rostrocaudal (RCd, frontal sinus) views. In evaluating skull trauma, left and right 75° ventrodorsal oblique views are recommended.

Radiographic Interpretation

Neonatal Radiography

Stress should be minimized when radiographing neonatal birds. The surface of the cassette should be warmed with a towel to avoid placing a young bird on a cold surface. Paper tape should be used for restraint to avoid damage to the numerous blood feathers. In some circumstances, proper positioning may be sacrificed in the best interest of the patient. Pressure must not be placed on a full crop to prevent regurgitation and subsequent aspiration.

The abdomen of neonates appears pendulous because the gastrointestinal tract is dilated, fluid-filled and blends with the other soft tissue organs, resulting in a homogenous appearance to the coelomic cavity and air sacs. The skeleton is incompletely mineralized and will have a reduced density, and fractures may be difficult to detect.

Radiographic Evidence of Skeletal Disorders

The important considerations in the radiographic evaluation of fractures include location, articular involvement, bone density, periosteal reaction, soft tissue involvement and whether the fracture is simple or comminuted and open or closed (see Chapter 42).

Accurate radiographs of the cervical spine require extension of the head and neck without rotation of the skull or body.

Diaphyseal fractures of the extremities are the most common traumatic injury. Acute fractures are characterized by sharp, well-defined margins, absence of periosteal response and concurrent soft tissue swelling. Chronic fractures are characterized by rounding, flaring and indistinct fracture ends, periosteal change and minimal soft tissue involvement or atrophy.

Osteolysis is the predominant radiographic change with infectious or neoplastic processes, and differentiation between these etiologies will require biopsy. Acute infection may show bone destruction with minimal periosteal reaction. Periosteal change is usually present with chronic infections.

Fungal osteomyelitis may cause pronounced periosteal reaction or increased medullary opacity due to granuloma formation. *Mycobacterium* spp. may also cause medullary granulomas as well as septic arthritis and bone lysis in the extremities.

With acute septic arthritis, joint effusion due to synovitis may be the only radiographic change, and arthrocentesis is necessary for diagnosis. Bacteria, mycoplasma, mycobacteria and parasites may be causative agents.

Primary bone neoplasia such as osteosarcoma is uncommon but has been reported in the proximal humerus, maxilla and wing tips. Bone neoplasia is frequently characterized by osteolysis with minimal periosteal change; however, osteoblastic tumors with marked periosteal reaction do occur. Most tumors involving bone occur secondary to soft tissue neoplasia. These tumors are frequently associated with soft tissue swelling, bone destruction and pathologic fractures, and biopsies are necessary to differentiate between tumors and osteomyelitis. Metastatic bone lesions are rare.

Normal pre-ovulatory hens will have an increased medullary bone density (polyostotic hyperostosis). Prolonged, abnormally elevated estrogen levels cause a diffuse, increased medullary bone density. The bones have a "marble" or mottled appearance, depending on whether bone deposition is uniform or patchy. Polyostotic hyperostosis has also been reported in hens with oviductal tumors and in cocks with sertoli cell tumors.

Hypertrophic osteopathy is rare, but has been reported in association with pericardial effusion. Radiographic lesions were characterized by extensive, fine, brush-like periosteal reaction involving most of the long bones.

Radiographic Evidence of Cardiac Disease

Congenital and viral diseases should be considered in juvenile birds with cardiac murmurs, exercise intolerance and cardiomegaly. Pericardial effusion is recognized radiographically as a symmetrical, globoid enlargement of the cardiac silhouette and may occur in birds with chlamydiosis, polyomavirus, tuberculosis and neoplasia.

With cardiomegaly, heart enlargement is usually asymmetrical. Cardiomegaly may be caused by cardiomyopathy secondary to poxvirus (reported in macaws), myxomatous valvular degeneration, endocarditis (particularly secondary to pododermatitis), hemochromatosis, chronic anemia and compression from extrinsic masses (see Chapter 27).

Microcardia is associated with hypovolemia due to acute volume loss or endotoxic shock. Whatever the etiology, microcardia suggests a critical state, and appropriate volume replacement should be instituted immediately.

Atherosclerosis with mineralization will result in prominence of the great vessels and may cause an increased density of the caudal lung field.

Radiographic Evidence of Respiratory Disorders

With pulmonary disease, the normal honeycombed pulmonary parenchyma may be enhanced by parabronchial infiltration causing prominent ring shadows obliterated by filling of the parabronchial lumen with fluid or caseous exudate or replaced by neoplastic or granulomatous infiltrates. Pneumonia often causes a prominent parabronchial pattern in the hilum and mid-portion of the lungs. As pneumonia progresses, the air-filled parabronchial lumen is replaced with caseous exudate, causing a blotchy mottled appearance to the lungs. This change is common at the caudal aspects of the lungs and is best detected on VD radiographs.

Pulmonary edema and hemorrhage have a more diffuse appearance. Discrete, well defined masses are usually abscesses, granulomas or tumors.

Radiographic changes indicative of inflamed air sacs include diffuse thickening, nodular infiltration or consolidation. Fine lines across the air sacs with mild increased opacity indicate thickening and are best detected on the lateral radiograph. Hyperinflation of the air sacs in combination with a radiolucent appearance suggest air trapping due to obstructed flow or abnormal compliance.

Subcutaneous emphysema may result from traumatic rupture of an air sac or as a complication of endoscopy. Fractures of the coracoid or ribs may penetrate the air sacs, causing emphysema.

Coelomic Cavity and Gastrointestinal System

Radiographic Anatomy

The proventriculus lies dorsal to the liver on the lateral view. The left lateral border of the proventriculus may be difficult to distinguish from the left lateral edge of the liver on the VD view. If the liver is of normal size, the proventriculus shadow will lie slightly lateral to the liver on the VD view.

Spleen

If detectable on the VD radiograph, the spleen will be noted as a slightly oblong, rounded structure to the right of midline between the proventriculus and ventriculus. On the lateral view, the spleen, if visible, overlaps the caudal end of the proventriculus and may be slightly dorsal to it. Suggested normal spleen sizes include: budgerigar = 1 mm, African Grey Parrot or Amazon parrot = 6 mm, Umbrella Cockatoo = 8 mm. The spleen of a pigeon is elongated or bean-shaped. In many other species it is spherical. Splenomegaly may be caused by infectious, neoplastic or metabolic diseases.

Liver

The liver does not normally extend beyond the sternum on the lateral radiograph. In psittacine birds, the liver should not extend laterally past a line drawn from the coracoid to the acetabulum. The size of the hepatic silhouette can best be determined by making measurements of a VD radiograph taken on inspiration. The distance is measured in millimeters from the mid-sternum to the lateral-most aspect of the ribs at the apex of the heart. This measurement is referred to as the sternal/rib distance (SR). This distance is divided by one-half and should be equal to the width of the right liver as measured at the apex of the heart. The size of the right liver is determined by measuring from the mid-sternum to the edge of the liver at the apex of the heart. If the actual measurement of the liver is greater than its anticipated size as determined by the SR value, then the liver is considered enlarged. If the actual measurement of the right liver is less than its anticipated size as determined by the SR value, then the liver is considered to be reduced in size.

The liver in macaws and cockatoos frequently appears to be reduced in size. The importance of this finding remains undetermined; however, many birds with microhepatia are being fed seed diets that may or may not be supplemented with fruits and vegetables.

The liver is frequently involved in systemic disease, and hepatomegaly is a common radiographic finding. Symmetrical enlargement of the liver lobes is most common and is usually associated with infectious and metabolic processes. Neoplasms and granulomatous diseases can cause asymmetrical enlargement of the liver.

Radiographic changes associated with liver enlargement are loss of hourglass waist in the VD view, rounding of liver lobe margins, compression of abdominal air sacs, extension of the liver lobes beyond the scapula/coracoid line, cranial displacement of the heart, dorsal elevation of the proventriculus and caudodorsal displacement of the ventriculus. A dilated, fluid-filled proventriculus may appear radiographically similar to hepatomegaly, and a careful assessment of the VD view can be used to differentiate between these lesions.

Pancreas

Radiographic changes involving the pancreas are rare, although diminished contrast in the right cranial abdomen due to sanguineous exudate from acute necrotizing pancreatitis has been reported.

Gastrointestinal Tract

Birds do not normally have gas in the intestinal tract, and any gas should be considered abnormal. Aerophagia can occur secondary to severe respiratory disease or is frequently seen as an artifact of gas anesthesia. Distended, fluid-filled bowel loops should be considered abnormal except in mynah birds and toucans.

Inflammation, infection, foreign bodies, parasites, intussusception, stricture, granuloma and neoplasia may cause intraluminal obstruction and segmental increases in the diameter of the gastrointestinal tract lumen secondary to excess gas and fluid accumulation. Extraluminal masses such as neoplasm, abscesses, eggs and cysts may compress the gastrointestinal tract and cause changes similar to intraluminal obstruction.

Uniform distention of the gastrointestinal tract is most commonly associated with functional ileus due to viral or bacterial infections, toxicity (eg, heavy metals), septicemia, hypoxemia, peritonitis or anesthesia. Distention of the ingluvies, proventriculus or ventriculus may be due to a localized process or obstruction within the intestines. A barium contrast study is indicated for complete evaluation of the intestinal tract.

The cloaca may be distended from a retained soft-shelled egg, papilloma, cloacalith, neoplasm or idiopathic atonic dilatation. Atonic distension of the cloaca may occur with spinal trauma and infiltrative neoplasms involving the sacral nerves.

Abdominal masses usually cause a change in the location of the gastrointestinal tract. Hepatomegaly usually causes dorsal displacement of the proventriculus and caudodorsal displacement of the ventriculus. Splenic, testicular, ovarian and renal masses compress the gastrointestinal tract ventrally and either cranially or caudally. Adhesions due to inflammatory or septic peritonitis from ruptured eggs or perforation can also result in displacement of the gastrointestinal tract.

Abdominal effusion is associated with liver disease, neoplasia, metabolic disorders, sepsis, inflammation and cardiac failure. Fluid results in a homogeneous appearance to the intestinal peritoneal cavity (IPC) and obscures visualization of specific organs. Consolidating air sacculitis can appear radiographically similar to fluid in the IPC in the lateral view, but differentiation is possible in the VD radiograph. If a pathologic process is occurring within the air sacs, specific organs within the intestinal peritoneal cavity will be definable in the VD view. If the fluid is within the IPC, there will still be a homogeneous appearance to the region of the viscera, and the air sacs will be compressed. Fluid accumulation in the IPC may compress the liver ventrally and displace the proventriculus and ventriculus cranially.

Urogenital System

The kidneys are attached to the synsacrum, are flattened dorsoventrally and have smoothly rounded cranial and caudal divisions.

The kidneys are best visualized in the lateral view. Because the renal silhouettes are superimposed, lateral oblique views may be necessary to distinguish each kidney. The cranial division of the kidney protrudes from the pelvic brim, and the caudal division may also be visualized on the lateral view. The kidneys are generally not visible on the VD view. The length of a normal African Grey Parrot kidney is about 3 cm on the lateral view. In the Umbrella Cockatoo, the suggested normal kidney size is 3 cm x 0.7 cm. The kidneys are normally surrounded by air, and loss of the air shadow indicates renal enlargement, dorsal displacement of abdominal organs or the presence of abdominal fat or fluid.

Bilateral symmetrical nephromegaly results in a diminished abdominal air sac space surrounding the kidneys and occurs with infection, metabolic disease, dehydration, post-renal obstruction and lymphoreticular neoplasia. Dehydration may also be associated with increased renal density. A localized enlargement with irregular borders is most commonly associated with a neoplasm, although abscesses may appear radiographically similar.

Biopsy is the only definitive way to differentiate cysts, neoplasms and abscesses. Intravenous excretory urography is necessary to confirm renal disease when severe nephromegaly obliterates the air space and creates a positive silhouette sign with other viscera.

Masses involving the spleen, oviduct, testicles, ovary and intestines may occupy space in the caudodorsal abdomen and mimic renal lesions. The testes of a reproductively active male are easily distinguishable and should not be misinterpreted as renal enlargement.

Hyperestrogen syndrome is common in budgerigars and is characterized by an enlarged, distended oviduct, medullary hyperostosis, diminished abdominal detail, visceral displacement, abnormal attempts at egg formation and abdominal hernia.

Egg-related peritonitis can be difficult to discern from other causes of abdominal effusion. Cessation of egg laying, weight loss and abdominal distention in a hen with a history of chronic egg laying are suggestive of egg-related peritonitis. Abdominocentesis and ultrasound can be used to differentiate between causes of abdominal fluid.

Gastrointestinal Positive and Double Contrast Procedures

Indications for barium follow-through examination are acute or chronic vomiting or diarrhea that is nonresponsive to treatment, abnormal survey radiographic findings suggestive of an obstructive pattern, unexplained organ displacement, loss of abdominal detail suggesting perforation, hemorrhagic diarrhea, history of ingestion of foreign material and chronic unexplained weight loss. Dehydrated birds should be rehydrated before administration of contrast media to prevent the material from forming concretions within the gastrointestinal tract.

Usually, a four-hour fast is adequate for emptying of the gastrointestinal tract without placing undue stress on smaller avian species. The gastrointestinal tract may be empty at the time of presentation in birds that are regurgitating.

Commercial barium sulfate suspensions provide the best studies. If perforation of the gastrointestinal tract is suspected, an organic iodine is recommended; however, these preparations are hypertonic and can cause dehydration, especially in small patients. Additionally, organic iodines are hydroscopic and are rapidly absorbed from the gastrointestinal tract. Dilution of the contrast medium with intraluminal fluid may compromise the study and interfere with defining the region of perforation. These agents do not coat the mucosa like barium does and are not recommended for routine gastrointestinal examinations.

The dose of barium sulfate varies depending on the species and presence or absence of a crop, and ranges from 0.025-0.05 ml/g body weight, with the lower dose range used in larger species.

The contrast media should be administered slowly until the crop is comfortably distended. Placing a finger over the distal portion of the cervical esophagus may help prevent reflux of barium sulfate while it is being administered. If any regurgitation occurs, the administration of contrast media should cease in order to reduce the risk of pulmonary aspiration. Barium has been used for bronchography in non-avian species because it is less irritating than other contrast agents. It is the volume of barium inhaled into the respiratory tract and not the agent itself that may cause problems.

In general, radiographs should be taken immediately after administration of contrast media and at 0.5-, 1-, 2-, 4-, 8- and 24-hour intervals. The temporal sequence may vary if a lesion is identified during the study.

Contrast Study Findings

Functional ileus occurs most frequently with neuropathic gastric dilatation and most often involves the proventriculus and ventriculus, although portions of the intestines may also be involved. Neurotoxins such as lead, inflammatory processes involving the coelomic cavity, severe enteritis and anesthetics may cause functional ileus.

Displacement of the gastrointestinal tract may occur with organomegaly, accumulations of fluid in the intestinal peritoneal cavity, adhesions or hernia. Hepatomegaly causes dorsal elevation of the proventriculus and caudal movement of the ventriculus. Splenic, gonadal and renal lesions may displace the intestines ventrally. Masses originating from the cranial division of the left kidney may push the ventriculus cranially. Adhesions associated with egg-related peritonitis may result in abnormal positioning of portions of the gastrointestinal tract, with a fixed appearance and changes in luminal diameter. Hernias, usually in hens, cause caudoventral displacement of the gastrointestinal tract.

Leakage of contrast media occurs most often with foreign body perforation, although metal feeding tubes or inflexible catheters can result in iatrogenic perforation of the gastrointestinal tract if improperly used. Mural erosion in association with neoplasm, abscess or granuloma are less frequent causes of perforation. If a perforation is suspected, an organic iodine contrast agent is recommended to prevent contamination of the coelomic cavity with barium.

Repeatability of a lesion on multiple views is important when attempting to identify intraluminal masses. Gas bubbles and ingesta can create artifacts that mimic mucosal defects and can lead to an incorrect diagnosis.

Table 12.3   Barium Sulfate Transit Times*

	Stomach	Small Intestines	Large Intestines	Cloaca
African Grey Parrot	10-30	30-60	60-120	120-130
Budgerigar	5-30	30-60	60-120	120-240
Racing pigeon	5-10	10-30	30-120	120-240
Indian Hill Mynah	5	10-15	15-30	30-90
Hawk	5-15	15-30	30-90	90-360
Amazon parrot	10-60	60-120	120-150	150-240
Canary	5	10-15	15-30	30-90
Pheasant	10-45	45-120	120-150	150-240

* Time in minutes for barium sulfate administered by crop gavage to reach and fill various portions of the GI tract.

Intravenous Excretory Urography

The primary indication for intravenous excretory urography is in defining mass lesions associated with the urinary tract or delineating the size and shape of the kidneys if they cannot be adequately visualized on routine radiographs. Excretory urography may also have some application for diagnosing functional disorders. Excretory urography should not be attempted in patients with dehydration or debilitation or if renal function is severely compromised.

Sodium diatrizoate (680 mg of iodine/kg), iothalamate sodium (800 mg of iodine/kg) or meglumine diatrizoate (800 mg of iodine/kg) have been used for urography in birds with no observable adverse effects. These organic iodines should be warmed prior to administration through the ulnar, jugular or medial metatarsal veins. Radiographs are taken immediately after contrast administration and at one-, two-, five-, ten- and twenty-minute intervals using the same technique developed for the survey radiograph.

Most diagnostic information is obtained within the first five minutes of the study. The aorta, heart and pulmonary artery will be visualized within ten seconds; kidneys and ureters in 30-60 seconds; and cloaca in three to five minutes after administering the contrast media. In the nephrographic phases of the study, there is an immediate, uniform opacification of the kidneys highlighting their size, shape and contour. In the normal kidney, the three divisions are readily discernible. There is no pyelographic phase.

Radiographic changes in the excretory urogram are most striking when the renal disease is unilateral because the unaffected kidney is usually hypertrophied. In contrast, obstruction of a ureter may increase the radiodensity of the ipsilateral kidney by delaying the washout from the kidney.

If one kidney appears to be non-functioning, it is important to consider the urinary protein concentration, cytologic features of sediment and the size of the contralateral kidney. In acute renal failure, the excretory function is rapidly and severely, but often reversibly, compromised. If the contralateral kidney is hypertrophied, the absence of function on the opposite side is probably chronic in nature (urolithiasis) and may even indicate agenesis of that kidney.

Positive Contrast Rhinosinography

A 15-20% organic iodine agent can be injected into the sinus, and the same views recommended under skull radiography are taken for evaluation. Reactions to the contrast agent include edema and periorbital swelling. At the end of the procedure, the media can be flushed out of the sinuses with sterile saline to decrease the amount of local irritation. Space-occupying masses such as neoplasms, abscesses or granulomas may cause an obstruction to the flow of contrast media. In normal psittacine birds, there should be communication between the infraorbital sinus, nasal cavity, opposite sinus, periorbital region and tympanic region. In some Passeriformes, the sinuses do not communicate.

Positive Contrast Tracheography and Bronchography

Contrast studies of the lower respiratory tract should be considered high risk because patients requiring these procedures are usually experiencing serious respiratory compromise. Tracheoscopy is preferable in patients of sufficient size (300 g). Focal lesions in the terminal trachea or at the tracheobronchial bifurcation that are difficult to visualize on survey radiographs may be defined by contrast tracheography.

Patients should be stabilized with oxygen therapy and a tube placed in an abdominal air sac to provide oxygen and anesthesia. Birds should be anesthetized for these studies. Contrast media is administered via a tube placed in the trachea. Small aliquots (approximately 0.1 ml) of a non-ionic agent or propyliodone should be given at a time, and radiographs taken to determine tracheal filling. A minimal amount of contrast media will be needed if fluoroscopy can be used to identify a foreign body.

Non-selective Angiography

Cardiac disease requiring definition by contrast studies is rare. Diseases such as cardiomyopathy, some congenital shunts and valvular disease may be defined by angiography in some larger birds; however, ultrasonography is being utilized with greater frequency in other species. Non-selective angiography has been used for defining the normal cardiac silhouette and major vessels. The same agents used for urography can be injected as a single, rapid, intravenous bolus in the jugular or ulnar veins to enhance visualization of the heart and great vessels. A rapid film changer, cine-fluoroscopy or videotaping is necessary to record the image.

Fluoroscopy

A fluoroscope can be connected via an image intensifier to a video camera that can be used to make real-time recordings of organ movement. In birds, fluoroscopy is the best way to monitor the motility of the gastrointestinal tract.

Ultrasound

Ultrasound studies in birds are somewhat limited by patient size and conformation and the presence of air sacs; however, in larger avian patients with abdominal effusion or organomegaly, ultrasound may be used to characterize lesions. Most studies can be performed without anesthesia. Patients may be held or secured with a plexiglass restraining device. Many birds that are minimally restrained in an upright position are extremely tolerant of the procedure. Feathers may be parted or removed, and a water-soluble, acoustic coupling gel is used to improve the transducer contact with the skin.

A 7.5 MHz end-fire mechanical sector scanner or phased array scanner is best in most birds, but 5.0 MHz and 10 MHz transducers may also be used. Higher frequency scanners provide less tissue penetration but finer resolution and are most useful in smaller species. Linear array transducers can also be used, but because of their shape, they do not conform well to the patient's body.

If the patient is in dorsal recumbency, the transducer is placed just caudal to the sternum and the beam is angled cranially. The liver has a uniform, slightly granular, echogenic pattern and is easily recognized. The right and left hepatic veins can be identified as anechoic channels on the dorsomedial aspect of the liver. A uniform, hyperechoic, hepatic parenchyma has been described in birds with fatty liver degeneration and hepatic lymphoma. Discrete hyperechoic masses throughout the liver may represent granulomas, abscesses or neoplasms.

Hepatomegaly should be suspected if the liver can be detected caudal to the sternum. Ultrasound is of little value in detecting acute or chronic hepatitis, and it is difficult to differentiate between cirrhosis and necrosis. Granulomas and neoplasms typically appear as focal hyperechoic walls with an echoic center. Hematomas and subcapsular bleeding will appear hypoechoic.

The liver may be used as a window to visualize the cardiac silhouette. Pericardial effusion and enlargement of cardiac chambers and valvular abnormalities can be detected in larger species. Pulmonary masses such as large granulomas have been defined using ultrasonography. A lateral approach can be used for visualization of the spleen, which is normally hyperechoic in comparison to the liver and is difficult to define unless enlarged.

Ultrasonographic visualization of the kidneys and gonads is not possible due to the presence of the air sacs, although large ovarian follicles can occasionally be defined. Ultrasound can be used to differentiate between soft-shelled eggs and egg-related peritonitis. Poorly mineralized eggs are often oval with a hyperechoic rim surrounding a hypoechoic content. With egg-related peritonitis, there is a heterogeneous hyperechoic appearance to the coelomic cavity. Effusion due to other processes is often anechoic or hypoechoic.

The presence of ingesta or gas will obscure portions of the gastrointestinal tract. Differentiation of the proventriculus, ventriculus and cloaca can be enhanced by administering water.

Ultrasound-guided biopsy can be used to collect diagnostic samples from the liver. The patient must be sedated or anesthetized. A variety of needles may be used for the biopsy. In larger species a 22 ga Westcott needle is used to obtain specimens for cytology, histology and culture.

Nuclear Scintigraphy

The potential value of nuclear medicine studies in avian patients remains unexplored. Unexplained abnormalities of the extremities, especially following trauma, would be most suitable for bone scintigraphy. Evaluation of the extent of osteomyelitis, joint disease, vascular compromise, impaired fracture healing and less commonly, bone neoplasia, is enhanced by nuclear medicine studies.

Computed Tomography

Computed tomography (CT) is superior to other modalities except magnetic resonance imaging for evaluation of head trauma and abnormalities involving the brain and spinal cord; however, the lack of availability and high cost often prevent the use of computed tomography in birds. Patients must be anesthetized to prevent any motion during the scan. Technical factors are inadequately studied in birds; however, slice section thickness ranging from 2-5 mm non-overlapping with varying window settings have been described for body scans. The value of CT in avian diagnostic radiology remains relatively uninvestigated, but characterization of lesions with CT should prove as valuable as in other species.

ENDOSCOPIC EXAMINATION AND BIOPSY TECHNIQUES

Michael Taylor

Equipment

Rigid Endoscope

Diameter Size: For diagnostic purposes, a 1.9 mm is the smallest diameter endoscope available with high quality optics. This endoscope is excellent for patients weighing less than 100 grams or in small anatomic sites (eg, sinus, trachea, oviduct). The major disadvantages of these very small endoscopes are their fragility, relatively small field of view and transmission of less light, which limit usefulness in larger body cavities. Because the 2.7 mm endoscope provides good light transmission capabilities with an adequate image size at a diameter that may be used in a wide range of birds, it is a good choice as the sole or principal endoscope in an avian practice. Endoscopes (4.0 or 5.0 mm) can be employed in larger patients or when documentation demands.

Length: For general avian endoscopy, a length of the endoscope in the range of 170-190 mm is recommended.

Angle of View: The final consideration when selecting an endoscope for avian diagnostics is the angle of view of the distal lens element. A 0° lens offset affords straight ahead viewing with a natural orientation. A 30° offset angles the field of view obliquely in the direction of the offset. This allows for improved viewing in confined areas, especially when the telescope is rotated. The beveled distal lens element necessary to achieve this viewing angle enables easier and less traumatic passage through air sac and peritoneal walls. For these reasons endoscopes with a 30° offset are recommended for general diagnostic purposes.

Flexible Endoscopes

Flexible endoscopes do provide a controllable distal tip, which allows manipulation that is not possible with a rigid rod-lens endoscope. They are most useful in examining tubular organs that are sinuous or folded.

Instrument Care

Torsional stresses upon the long axis of the endoscope must be avoided. It is particularly important that the operator be sensitive to the amount of force being applied to the telescope during a procedure. It is wise to clean the instrument immediately after a procedure is finished. In many cases, simply washing the telescope in distilled water is all that is needed. A lens paper is used to clean the lens surfaces. An alcohol flush chemically dries the endoscope before it is placed in a padded storage container that meets the manufacturer's recommendations. A simple but effective plastic endoscope sleeve is available to cover the shaft of the telescope for protection during transport and disinfection procedures.

Flexible endoscopes should also be handled with care. They should not be coiled tightly or have objects of any weight placed on the shaft, or the glass fiber bundles will be damaged. Instrument channels should be flushed thoroughly with warm soapy water to remove debris after use.

Sterilization

Two options provide safe yet consistently reliable sterilization for sensitive telescopes and light cables. Ethylene oxide gas is an extremely effective sterilant, but exposed materials must be aerated for a minimum of eight to twelve hours before use. Ethylene oxide is a human health hazard and must be used under carefully controlled conditions.

The most practical and safe alternative for the avian practitioner for office or field sterilization of sensitive endoscopic equipment is soaking in a two percent solution of glutaraldehyde. The solution must be used according to the supplier's directions for soaking telescopes, hand instruments and light cables. Minimum recommended soaking times in properly prepared glutaraldehyde solutions typically range from 15-20 minutes.

After the soaking cycle has been completed, the equipment must be thoroughly rinsed in sterile water to prevent tissue-damaging glutaraldehyde from contacting the patient. Glutaraldehyde is extremely irritating to most tissues and may cause local irritation, tissue death, delayed healing and peritoneal reaction. Rinsing the equipment in a sterile container of sterile water for three to five minutes is most effective. The instruments are drained, immersed in a second container of sterile water for three to five minutes and wiped dry. A final alcohol wash may be used to chemically dry the equipment.

Other types of disinfectant solutions such as quaternary ammonium compounds, chlorhexidine and povidone iodine are not acceptable alternatives for soaking endoscopic equipment.

Pre-endoscopy Considerations

Indications

Endoscopic examination is indicated whenever the visual inspection of an organ or site may yield additional diagnostic information. Diagnostic endoscopy is usually preceded by less-invasive examinations such as a complete blood count, biochemistries or radiology.

Diagnostic Uses: The endoscope and its light cable may be used to aid the physical examination. The light cable may be used singly to offer additional illumination, to transilluminate a structure such as the trachea, sinus or crop, to augment examination of the oral cavity or for back lighting of overexposed radiographs. Fine-diameter endoscopes can be used in a variety of external sites where the properties of magnification, illumination and small optic diameter enhance diagnostic visualization.

Table 13.2   Common Indications for Endoscopic Examination

- Loss or change in character of voice
- Acute or chronic dyspnea
- Acute or chronic sneezing
- Ingluvitis, crop burns or trauma
- Abnormal radiographic findings (plain or contrast); eg, lung, gastrointestinal tract, air sacs, organomegaly, granuloma
- Abnormal biochemical studies; eg, kidney (uricemia) or liver (elevated bile acids or liver enzyme activities)
- Persistent leukocytosis (nonresponsive to treatment)
- Acute or chronic systemic disease
- Reproductive system (suspected infertility)
- Polyuria, polydipsia
- Follow-up examination to check on lesion resolution ("second look")

A diagnostic endoscopy system for birds has been developed that greatly simplifies sample collection. The system incorporates a 2.7 mm, 30° view endoscope with a single instrument port in a special sheath. Various flexible instruments may be introduced into the sheath, passed alongside the endoscope and guided to a specific site with ease.

Contraindications

The general contraindications for endoscopy are those that would apply to general avian surgery and anesthesia. Moderate-to-marked obesity leading to the intra-abdominal deposition of fat is the most frequent cause of difficulty in endoscopic visualization.

The presence of ascites may cause difficulties if the peritoneum of the ventral hepatic peritoneal cavity (VHPC) or intestinal peritoneal cavity (IPC) is breached while entering the air sac. Fluid could drain from the peritoneal cavity into the air sac and from there into the lung, leading to aspiration and death. This is most likely to happen in a lateral approach to the caudal thoracic air sac. If ascites is suspected and an endoscopic examination of the liver is necessary, the ventral approach to the VHPC should be used. Fluid from the VHPC will drain from the incision site and can be safely suctioned without the concern for air sac involvement.

Left coelomic examinations should not be performed in the hen near the time of ovulation, as the ova greatly enlarges in size, virtually obliterating the abdominal air sac. The oviduct also increases in size and tortuosity, filling the left portion of the IPC. Use of the post-pubic approach to the abdominal air sac risks damage to the oviduct or an egg nearing oviposition. A left lateral coelomic approach is rendered less useful by the presence of large, developing ova that makes visualization difficult.

Complications

As part of the informed consent process, the client must be made aware of potential complications of the endoscopic process. Anesthesia-related incidents are described in Chapter 39. Organ trauma is one of the most serious intraoperative endoscopic complications. The proventriculus may be punctured using a trocar and cannula or similar entry device from a lateral approach. Failure to identify and repair this injury can result in a fatal peritonitis. Laceration of a blood vessel or organ such as the liver or spleen is possible and may lead to serious or fatal hemorrhage. Liver or kidney contusions can be caused by the endoscope tip during excessively vigorous manipulation. These are infrequently the cause of serious clinical problems. Subcutaneous emphysema is a potential (if rare) postoperative complication.

Air sac and peritoneal granulomas can occur by using instrumentation that has been improperly sterilized or in situations where poor technique or inadequate skin preparation has allowed contamination of the endoscope tip. The inability to perform proper sterilization of a single endoscope makes surgical sexing clinics obsolete. Transmission of viral infections (particularly Pacheco's disease virus and polyomavirus), resulting in the loss of numerous birds has been linked to "sexing clinics." The mixing of birds from multiple sources (particularly when an invasive procedure is performed) should be discouraged. It is possible, however, to safely perform endoscopy on several birds from a single client by utilizing two endoscopes, with one being sterilized while the other is in use.

Patient Preparation

Patients should be fasted a minimum of three hours. In some cases the length of the fast is extended, especially if the endoscopic examination will involve the gastrointestinal tract. Species that consume large boluses of whole foods (eg, raptors) may require fasting for 24-36 hours.

Surgical sites are prepared as for any avian surgery. Particular attention should be paid to the skin surface.

Anesthesia: Appropriate anesthesia is an essential part of good endoscopic practice. Consistency in positioning of the patient is mandatory for anatomic orientation. Maintaining position is neither possible nor humane using physical restraint only.

For endoscopic purposes, it is preferable to consider the cranial and caudal thoracic and the abdominal air sac pairs together. In the parrot, the cranial thoracic air sacs are the smallest of the group and are located ventral and cranial to the caudal thoracic air sacs. They are best accessed from the ventrolateral thoracic wall using the approach first described by Bush, who suggested an entry site caudal to the last sternal rib in the area of the lateral notch (a "V"-shaped depression palpable between the sternum and the last rib).

The patient is placed in lateral recumbency with the wings extended dorsally. The wings may be taped to a restraint surface or they may be affixed with a short loop of nonadhesive, self-adhering tape passed between the primary feathers and around the carpus. The landmarks are located and a small skin incision is made. The musculature of the body wall is bluntly separated and the endoscope is inserted in a craniodorsal direction. From this approach the pericardial sac and heart can be seen as well as the lobe of the liver and the caudal, ventromedial surface of the lung.

The traditional left lateral surgical approach takes advantage of the air sac anatomy to approach the gonads by either directly entering the abdominal air sac or by entering the caudal thoracic air sac first and then passing into the abdominal air sac through a small incision.

The patient is placed in true lateral recumbency with the wings extended dorsally. The upper leg is extended and held caudally. The point of insertion is located by palpating the triangle cranial to the muscle mass of the femur, ventral to the synsacrum and caudal to the last rib. The body wall may be penetrated by a trocar and cannula or by blunt separation. In Psittaciformes, this entry site has been demonstrated to occur between the seventh and eighth ribs (not the behind the last rib). With this approach, the tip of the endoscope enters the mid to caudal portion of the caudal thoracic air sac in most birds.

As an alternative approach to the caudal thoracic air sac, the bird is restrained in lateral recumbency except that the leg is extended cranially. The site of entry is the same as previously described in the upper part of the triangle formed by the proximal femur, the last rib and the cranial edge of the pubis.

The abdominal air sacs of most birds are the largest air sacs. They extend from the caudal surface of the lung to the craniolateral borders of the cloaca. Entry into the abdominal air sacs may be gained through one of the previously described caudal thoracic air sac approaches or by direct access through the caudal body wall. Lumeij was the first to describe a post-pubic approach to the caudal portion of the abdominal air sac. The entry point is situated dorsal to the pubic bone and caudal to the ischium. The endoscope generally first enters the most caudal portion of the intestinal peritoneal cavity and must penetrate through this thin membrane to enter the abdominal air sac. The endoscope can then be moved cranially up the length of the abdominal air sac. From the left approach a large number of structures may be examined including the kidney, adrenal, gonad and associated structures, spleen, proventriculus, ventriculus and intestine. The abdominal air sac may also be approached from a flank position. The entry site is located directly ventral to the acetabulum and just dorsal to the ventral border of the flexor cruris medialis muscle.

Reproductive Organs

The testicle of the adult male bird is ellipsoidal to bean-shaped. In most species it is creamy white although it may be more or less pigmented (gray to black) in others (eg, cockatoos, mynahs, toucans). Under the seasonal influence of hormones, the mass of the testicle may increase from 10 up to 500 times. The pattern of surface vessels increases and becomes more prominent. The epididymis enlarges, and the ductus deferens becomes very tortuous in preparation for storage and transportation of the spermatozoa.

In contrast, the ovary of the mature female has the appearance of tapioca pudding with many small follicles visible during the nonbreeding season. Under appropriate hormonal stimulation, a hierarchy of follicles develops and matures giving the ovary the appearance of a cluster of grapes. A follicle enlarges as it matures; simultaneously, the oviduct increases in size and becomes tortuous and folded in preparation to accept the ovum. A large ovum can be mistaken for a testicle, especially in an obese bird where other structures are difficult to see or where the surgeon fails to check related anatomic reference points.

The differences in the morphology of adult gonads are relatively distinct. In juvenile birds, gonadal tissue is less obvious and differentiation is more difficult.

In one study of juvenile macaws, differentiation of the sexes was uniformly possible as young as six weeks of age when gonadal and oviductal or ductus deferens morphology were considered together. Testicles were tubular to ellipsoidal with distinct, rounded cranial and caudal poles. A paired right testicle could usually be seen through the dorsal mesentery. The ductus deferens was a thin, white tubular structure, usually only one-third the diameter of the ureter.

The juvenile ovary was comma-shaped, dorsoventrally flattened and closely applied to the adrenal and cranial of the kidney. The surface texture of the ovary was dependent on the age of the bird. Very young ovaries had a faintly granular surface with fine sulci. As the birds aged, the sulci deepened, giving the ovary a furrowed, brain-like appearance. With the maturation of the primary oocytes, the ovary began to take on a distinctly granular texture with a more three-dimensional shape, and the sulci disappeared. The oviduct was pale white with a thicker, more substantial appearance than the vas deferens. The oviduct was generally two to four times the thickness of the ureter and on close inspection, fine, longitudinal, spiral bands were visible. The most interesting finding of this study was the presence of the supporting ligament of the infundibulum, which was clearly visible crossing the cranial division of the kidney. This structure is part of the dorsal ligament of the oviduct and is absent in juvenile males.

Caution should be exercised in estimating age, reproductive history or reproductive potential based upon a single endoscopic examination. During the nonbreeding times of the year, the adult gonads return to a quiescent state similar to those of the late adolescent bird.

During the endoscopic examination for gender determination, the endoscopist is able to evaluate the air sacs, liver, lung, spleen, kidney, adrenal gland, proventriculus, ventriculus and the visible portions of the intestines. A systematic examination that may suggest a subclinical health problem can provide data of value to the aviculturist. This information is not available using cytogenetic or molecular biological techniques of gender determination.

Ear Canal

The external auditory meatus is hidden by specialized covert feathers that lack barbules. There is no pinna. The opening is usually rounded but can vary in diameter from small (2.0-15.0 mm in passerine and psittacine birds) to very large (up to 6.0 cm in owls). The ear canal is straight and short. The tympanum can usually be visualized clearly. A 1.9 mm or smaller telescope is often needed to explore the deeper aspects of the canal. Unlike the dog and cat, birds infrequently suffer from otitis externa.

Oropharynx

The beak may be held open manually or with a speculum. In species with strong mandibular musculature (such as Psittaciformes) it is recommended that the patient be anesthetized for most oral examinations.

In the parrot, salivary glands are found along the roof and the floor of the mouth and on the tongue. The mucosa should be examined for adherent exudate, debris or ulcers, as may be seen in certain protozoal (eg, *Trichomonas* sp.), fungal (eg, *Candida albicans*) or viral (eg, poxvirus) diseases.

The choanal slit is visible as a median "V"-shaped cleft in the palate. The borders of the choanal slit are lined with sensory papillae. By entering the choanal slit with the scope and moving craniodorsally, the nasal septum and conchae can be examined. Just caudal to and on the midline of the choana is the small slit-like infundibular cleft. This is the common opening of the right and left pharyngotympanic tubes also referred to as the eustachian tubes.

The laryngeal mound is visualized at the base of the tongue on the midline of the caudal floor of the oropharynx. The paired, fleshy laryngeal prominences open and close to form the conspicuous glottis. There is no epiglottis.

Trachea

The tracheal mucosa consists of smooth, stratified squamous epithelium. The syrinx is the site of sound production and is located where the trachea bifurcates into the primary bronchi. The syringeal membrane may be the site of opportunistic bacterial and fungal infection (aspergillosis). Tracheoscopy to the level of the syrinx is possible in medium-to-large birds using a 180 mm long, 2.7 mm endoscope. Smaller patients may be examined with a 1.9 mm endoscope.

Tracheitis may be caused by bacterial or viral agents. Culture of the endoscope tip immediately after removal from the patient may be helpful in determining an etiologic agent.

Esophagus and Ingluvies

The esophagus is easily entered by passing the endoscope caudally into the pharynx and over the laryngeal mound. The surface of the esophagus is comprised of longitudinal folds that vary depending upon the dietary habits of the species.

It is a common misconception that all birds have an ingluvies. Galliformes, Psittaciformes, Columbiformes and some Passeriformes have a true crop. The ingluvies can be examined with either a flexible or rigid endoscope after passing the instrument through the cervical portion of the esophagus. Insufflating the crop with air will help with visualization. To do this, a small-diameter, flexible feeding tube, which has been attached to a 35 or 60 cc syringe, can be passed into the crop. Some pressure will need to be maintained around the proximal cervical esophagus to retain the infused air within the crop. With this technique the crop mucosa can be thoroughly examined and small foreign objects can be removed with grasping forceps. The grasping forceps can be endoscopically guided using either a flexible endoscope with an instrument channel or the rigid sheath with channel.

Proventriculus, Ventriculus

The proventriculus and the ventriculus may be examined using either flexible or rigid equipment. In a 250-600 g parrot it can be a difficult chore to guide a small-diameter, flexible endoscope down the cervical esophagus, across the crop and into the thoracic esophagus, although this equipment can be used successfully in larger parrots and in moderately large avian species that lack a crop (eg, owls and Anseriformes). A pediatric bronchoscope is required in smaller patients.

Preliminary studies using a midline ingluviotomy to enter the thoracic esophagus using the Storz 2.7 mm rigid endoscope and instrumented sheath have been performed. Birds were anesthetized, intubated and placed in dorsal recumbency.

Care was taken to avoid the passage of proventricular contents into the trachea or choana by inserting an absorptive gauze tampon into the cranial cervical esophagus and ensuring that the endotracheal tube was secure. Whenever possible, patients were fasted for five to six hours in order to empty the proventriculus.

Ventral Hepatic Peritoneal Cavities

The liver of the bird is encapsulated within two paired peritoneal cavities: the ventral and dorsal hepatic peritoneal cavities. The paired ventral hepatic peritoneal cavities (VHPC) are the largest and of greatest clinical significance. The right and left VHPC are separated by the ventral mesentery. The right lobe of the liver is larger in most birds.

The liver can be visualized from the cranial and caudal thoracic air sacs and indeed seems tantalizingly close in most birds. In reality, the liver is covered by a layer of peritoneum that is contiguous with the overlying air sac. To access the liver, the ventral hepatic peritoneal cavity (VHPC) must be entered either laterally from the caudal thoracic air sac or by a direct, ventral midline approach. The ventral approach is best for examining and sampling both lobes of the liver. A skin incision is made on the midline just caudal to the border of the sternum. The linea alba is incised and the caudal border of the VHPC is bluntly penetrated. A substantial fat pad may be present overlying the outer surface of the caudal border of the VHPC. Under conditions of health, the liver should not protrude past the caudal border of the sternum.

Intercostal Approach to Lungs

An intercostal approach to the lung for biopsy has been recently described in the pigeon. Entry was recommended through the dorsolateral portion of the third or fourth intercostal space where pulmonary tissue is the thickest in cross section. The third intercostal space is located by counting cranially from the last rib. The space is palpated just ventral to the scapula and a small skin incision is made. The intercostal muscles are bluntly separated to the level of the pleura.

An instrumented sheath and rigid endoscope are inserted into the incision and maneuvered carefully between the ribs so that the surface of the lung can be visualized. The rounded edges of the sheath aid in atraumatically positioning the instrument. A 5 Fr flexible forceps is advanced into the lung parenchyma, the jaws closed rapidly and removed. Post-biopsy hemorrhage may vary from mild to moderate but is usually controlled by pressure. Intercostal muscle and skin are closed routinely with simple interrupted sutures.

While it is not essential to utilize an endoscope to biopsy the lung from this site, it was found that the sheath and endoscope combination greatly aided the collection of quality pulmonary biopsies with less risk of trauma to the patient. Rigid cup biopsy forceps can be manipulated unaided through a similar intercostal incision, but trauma to the surface of the lung may be greater due to the short working distance and lack of magnification.

Intestinal Peritoneal Cavity

It is a single, midline potential space that extends from the level of the kidneys caudal to the vent. The gonads are actually suspended within the IPC and are not located within the abdominal air sac. The confusion in this positioning is understandable because the gonads are clearly visible from the abdominal air sac even though they are covered by the air sac wall and the confluent peritoneum.

Cloaca

Endoscopic examination of the three parts of the cloaca is complicated by the presence of feces and urates. Flushing the proctodeum with saline and then insufflating the structure while closing the vent lips around the telescope will enhance viewing.

Distal Oviduct (Uterus)

Endoscopic examination of the distal oviduct (uterus) is possible in reproductively active birds and may be a useful procedure for the sampling and diagnosis of oviductal disease.

Biopsy Techniques

Patient Considerations

Indications

Open (surgical) and percutaneous techniques for biopsy of the liver have been described in avian medicine. Other internal organs have occasionally been biopsied using open techniques. The ability to obtain precise target biopsies of specific organs is a natural extension of endoscopic examination and offers a far less traumatic method for obtaining diagnostic specimens.

Indications for biopsy may include abnormal radiographic findings or biochemical parameters, chronic respiratory disease, polyuria and polydipsia. The endoscopist should be prepared to collect biopsies during routine examinations. It is not uncommon to find unexpected lesions in patients presented for gender determination. Specimens from obvious lesions are easily collected from the border zone where abnormal meets normal tissue. If the patient's history, physical examination or biochemical findings suggest renal or hepatic abnormalities, biopsy of the kidney or liver is indicated.

The decision to biopsy the liver or kidney is frequently made too late in the disease process to be truly helpful to the patient and client. Sampling the end stage liver is seldom illuminating beyond confirming a poor prognosis that should be otherwise clinically evident. Many birds with early cases of hepatic disease demonstrate few clinical signs. Recent advances in avian clinical biochemistry procedures, particularly the measurement of bile acids, promise to improve the clinician's ability to detect liver disease at an early stage. Histologic changes are seen in the livers of patients with persistent increases in the bile acids of two times or greater the normal reference intervals. A liver biopsy is recommended in cases where the bile acids measurement remains elevated following the completion of therapy for a systemic disease (eg, chlamydiosis) or where continued elevation of two weeks or more is confirmed.

Renal disease can also be challenging to recognize and diagnose in its early stages. Polyuria is frequently noted. Kidney biopsy is recommended when uric acid levels are consistently above reference values or show evidence of an increasing trend or where polydipsia and polyuria persist without clinical explanation.

Air sac and pulmonary biopsies are indicated when clinical examination, radiographic studies or auscultation reveal persistent, nonresponsive respiratory disease.

Biopsies of the spleen are indicated in persistent systemic diseases where an etiologic diagnosis is lacking, in cases of unexplained splenomegaly and in granulomatous inflammation of the spleen. Samples of the ventricular serosa and muscularis that include nerve tissue can be valuable in the definitive antemortem diagnosis of neuropathic gastric dilatation (NGD). A minimum of two specimens is obtained from the caudoventral surface of the ventriculus. A site near a branching blood vessel is chosen in an attempt to harvest nervous tissue. Ventricular biopsies are preferred for the diagnosis of NGD over proventricular biopsies because the serosa of the ventriculus can be harvested much more safely with less risk of perforation due to the thicker muscularis.

Small, precise biopsies of the testicle may be useful in the documentation of reproductive failure due to dysfunction of the testes.

Contraindications

The specific contraindications for biopsy relate to blood clotting. Biopsy collection should be delayed in any avian patient that shows evidence of abnormalities of the hemostatic system. This usually becomes evident at the time of blood collection. Most birds should show clot formation in one to two minutes. Deficiency of vitamin K is the most common coagulation disorder, for which vitamin K_1 is administered presurgically. The blood film should be examined for the presence of adequate thrombocyte numbers.

Instrumentation

A rigid cup biopsy forceps originally designed for otolaryngology can be guided along the shaft of the endoscope to the visual field. Biopsies of the liver, kidney, spleen, air sacs, lung and testes can be obtained under direct observation. This instrument should not be used in birds under 200 g. This forceps in combination with a 2.2 or 2.7 mm telescope has been the most widely utilized and accepted method for collecting optically guided biopsies in the avian patient. The forceps is "walked" into position along the shaft of the endoscope until it can be visualized.

In an effort to improve the usefulness of endoscopically guided biopsies, an endoscope and sheath set has been developed in cooperation with Karl Storz Endoscopy. An instrument channel permits the use of implements up to 5 Fr (1.7 mm) diameter. Flexible forceps for biopsy and grasping as well as aspiration and infusion cannulas can be placed into the port of the channel and guided easily to the tip of the sheath and into the viewing field of the endoscope.

Preparation of Small Biopsies

The biopsies obtained with the types of forceps previously mentioned are small and must be handled with care so that they are not lost or damaged. The specimens can be placed into a small stoppered blood collection container without anticoagulant.

This system is simple and effective, allowing the technician to clearly visualize the sample(s). No more than two to three specimens should be placed in each clearly labelled container. If biopsies cannot be processed immediately, the specimens can be stored in a solution of 97% methyl alcohol after fixation in order to ensure sample quality.

NECROPSY EXAMINATION

Kenneth S. Latimer
Pauline M. Rakich

Maximum necropsy information can be obtained only by following a systematic approach and using ancillary support services as needed to establish a definitive diagnosis. Ancillary support services include histopathology, clinical pathology, microbiology, parasitology and toxicology.

Medical Precautions

Zoonotic diseases of special concern include chlamydiosis, mycobacteriosis, salmonellosis and campylobacteriosis. Therefore, appropriate protective measures such as surgical masks, eye protection, gloves and disinfectants are recommended. Wetting the carcass with soapy water or disinfectant solutions decreases the possibility of aerosol exposure to potential pathogens and irritating feathers or dander. Ventilation hoods or downdraft necropsy tables provide an ideal environment for pathogen containment during avian necropsies; however, such equipment is seldom available in a private practice setting.

Equipment and Supplies

An assortment of instruments including scissors, poultry shears, scalpels, rongeurs, thumb forceps and hemostats will aid in tissue incision, dissection and specimen procurement. Instruments that are sterilized in chemical disinfectants should be rinsed thoroughly before use to avoid killing pathogens in tissues intended for culture.

Ancillary equipment may include sterile swabs and sealable plastic bags to obtain microbiologic and parasitologic specimens; sterile collection tubes for blood, serum or body cavity fluids; and glass slides, stains and a microscope to examine cytologic and blood smear specimens.

A printed necropsy form should be available to record important observations. Indelible marking pens should be used to legibly identify all specimen containers concerning patient identification and origin of the specimen(s).

Euthanasia

Acceptable methods of euthanasia include carbon dioxide or anesthetic gas administration, intravenous barbiturate administration (jugular vein or cerebral sinus) or anesthetic gas administration followed by exsanguination.

Handling the Carcass Prior to Necropsy

Rapid autolysis of avian carcasses is the result of a normally high body temperature, body conservation of heat by insulating feathers, and use of incubators, heating pads or heating lamps to increase environmental temperatures of neonates and ill patients. Autolysis may be retarded by soaking the carcass thoroughly in cool soapy water, placing it in a thin plastic bag and storing the body under refrigeration before performing a necropsy or shipping the body to the diagnostic laboratory on ice.

A carcass intended for necropsy *should not be frozen.* Placing a carcass directly on ice or dry ice during shipping also may result in freezing of the entire carcass or that portion in contact with the ice.

External Examination of the Carcass

Carcass identification should be verified by visual inspection based upon signalment (age, species and color) as well as leg band, tattoo or microchip implant data. Leg band numbers and other identifying marks should be recorded on the necropsy form. Palpation of the carcass may reveal fractures; swellings involving subcutaneous air sacs; masses of the skin, subcutis or underlying tissues; or physical deformities. An evaluation of general body condition also should be made, and body weight recorded. The integument including skin, mucocutaneous junctions, plumage, beak and nails should be examined carefully.

All body orifices (eyes, external auditory meatus, nares, oral cavity and vent) should be examined for discharges, masses, foreign bodies, ulcers and plaques. At this time, swabs of the choanal slit and vent may be taken for microbiological culture if desired. After cursory external inspection, the feathers may be wetted with soapy water to reduce feather dust and debris. The feathers subsequently may be removed to reveal subtle cutaneous pathology such as wounds or hemorrhages. Plucking feathers from the ventral cervical, thoracic and abdominal areas also facilitates further dissection and will avoid obscuring internal lesions.

When external examination of the carcass is complete, survey radiographs may be taken if heavy metal toxicosis is suspected. These radiographs may assist the clinician in localizing metal densities that may be collected for analysis during the necropsy.

Initial Dissection

The bird is placed in dorsal recumbency for initial dissection. With very small birds, the wings and legs may be pinned to a dissecting tray or board to immobilize the carcass. With larger birds such as ducks or geese, the coxofemoral joints may be disarticulated by incising the skin, adductor muscles of the medial thigh and coxofemoral joint capsule. The knees are then forced craniolateral. Using a scalpel and scissors, a ventral midline incision is made from the intermandibular area to the pelvic area, encircling the vent. The skin is reflected by blunt dissection to reveal the underlying cervical musculature, trachea, crop, keel and pectoral and abdominal musculature. The musculature should be examined for hemorrhage, penetrating wounds, pallor, pale streaking or loss of total mass.

Exposure of the Thoracoabdominal Cavity

An incision is made through the abdominal musculature at the distal tip of the sternum. The incision is continued left and right through the pectoral musculature lateral to the sternum, which can be lifted craniodorsal to expose the thoracic and abdominal air sacs. If air sacs appear opaque or contain accumulations of fluid or exudate, appropriate specimens should be obtained for microbiological culture or cytology before the field is contaminated. Air sac tissues collected for histopathology should be placed on a small piece of paper before fixation.

The sternal plate is removed by continuing to incise the thoracic musculature and transecting the ribs, coracoid bones and clavicles using scissors, rongeurs or poultry shears (large pruning shears may be necessary for ratites). The midline incision is extended caudally through the abdominal musculature proximal to the vent; care should be taken to prevent incising the cloaca. The pectoral musculature of the sternal plate may be incised and examined; any abnormal tissue is collected for cytologic imprints and histopathologic evaluation. Abdominal wall musculature is then removed as necessary to expose the viscera within the body cavity.

Examination of Thoracoabdominal Viscera *In Situ*

Several gross observations should be made before the viscera are disturbed. The presence of fluid, exudates or fibrin tags within the thoracoabdominal cavity should be noted (minimal fluid is present in health). A small amount of fat may be observed normally in the abdomen, around the cloaca and within the coronary groove. Excessive fat may be present in obese companion birds, while serous (gelatinous) atrophy of fat may occur with inanition. The pericardial sac should be relatively transparent and contain little measurable fluid. White streaks occasionally are present on the pericardial sac and epicardium following euthanasia by intracardiac injection. Petechial epicardial hemorrhages may represent septicemia or be observed as an agonal event.

The liver is mahogany brown and bilobed, extending around the left and right margins of the heart. In psittacine birds, the right lobe is larger, occasionally giving it an asymmetric appearance. The gallbladder should be examined if present (some birds lack a gallbladder), and the patency of the common bile duct should be determined if possible.

The heart and great vessels are examined next. The epicardium should be examined for petechiation. The heart is roughly triangular with length slightly exceeding width. Any alteration in the size or shape (eg, globose shape) of the heart should be noted.

As the great vessels are examined, any changes in the size of the thyroid and parathyroid glands also should be recorded. These glandular structures are located at the thoracic inlet lateral to the syrinx and adjacent to the jugular veins and carotid arteries. Normal thyroid glands are small, oval and reddish-brown. The parathyroid glands are very small and best distinguished microscopically.

A small portion of the ventriculus may be observed ventral to the liver. Much of the caudal portion of this organ is obscured by the duodenal loop and pancreas. The proventriculus is located beneath the left liver lobe and may not always be visible unless severely dilated.

Gas-filled intestinal loops and discoloration due to altered intestinal contents or hemorrhage should be noted. On rare occasions, gastrointestinal lesions may be quite striking. Examples include gastrointestinal tract obstruction and impaction in pheasants with proliferative typhlitis secondary to *Heterakis isolonche* infestation, severe nematode or trematode infestations, surgically-induced visceral adhesions, marked proventricular distention in birds with neuropathic gastric dilatation and severe egg-related peritonitis.

In hens, the viscera are reflected on the left side of the dorsal thoracoabdominal cavity to examine the communication of the colon and oviduct with the cloaca. The cloacal bursa may be partially visualized, especially in juvenile birds.

Removal and Examination of the Viscera

The heart is removed by transecting the great vessels. At this time the thyroid and parathyroid glands also may be collected while they are easily identified. The epicardial surface should be examined for changes in size, shape and color. The heart of small birds may be transected near the apex and placed whole in formalin solution. In larger birds, the heart may be opened to inspect the valves and chambers; sections of tissue may be taken for formalin fixation.

The tongue and oral mucosa should be inspected for erosions, ulcers, plaques or masses. The tongue is freed by transecting the hyoid apparatus and pharyngeal tissues in the intermandibular region. Gentle traction is applied to remove the tongue, esophagus, crop, trachea and thymus with attached large vessels. The thymus may appear as pale tan to gray lobules of tissue extending along the cervical fascial planes adjacent to the trachea. This organ undergoes involution as sexual maturity is reached. The distal trachea is transected below the syrinx, leaving the lungs for later dissection. The esophagus is transected just below the syrinx and lifted upward. The ligamentous attachments, air sacs, blood vessels and ureters (including the oviduct if present) are transected and the vent area is excised with an intact margin of skin. The entire gastrointestinal tract, along with the liver and spleen, is removed from the carcass. The adrenal glands, gonads and kidneys remain in the carcass.

The spleen may be found dorsally in the angle between the ventriculus and proventriculus. It appears as a variably-sized, round to elongate, red-brown structure. It should be removed and examined. Swelling and tan discoloration suggest inflammation or infection. Cytologic imprints may be made and a small portion removed for microbiological culture; the remainder is fixed in formalin solution.

The liver, gallbladder (if present) and patency of the bile duct connections to the duodenum should be examined. Excess accumulation of bile may cause gross distention of the bile ducts. The liver is removed, and its color, size and texture are examined in more detail. The parenchyma is examined by making several transverse slices through the organ with a sharp knife or scalpel. Lesions are imprinted and appropriate specimens are fixed for histopathologic examination, and fresh tissue is retained for other ancillary tests (microbiologic culture or toxicologic analysis) as necessary.

Lobules of thymic tissue, if present, are preserved for histopathologic examination. The esophagus, crop and trachea should be opened and the luminal surfaces and contents examined. Any abnormalities such as hemorrhage, erosion or ulceration and plaques or masses should be noted and appropriate portions of tissue imprinted, preserved in formalin solution and retained for other analyses. The crop contents should be examined carefully, especially in cases of unexplained death where poisonous plants may have been ingested. Crop contents may be collected for analysis if toxicosis is suspected.

The proventriculus and ventriculus are opened and examined for surface erosions or ulcers and foreign bodies. The ventriculus of seed-eating and omnivorous birds has a thick muscular wall, and the mucosa has a koilin lining (thick horny material) that is often bile-stained. In carnivorous and piscivorous birds, the ventriculus may be fusiform, thinner-walled and blend with the proventriculus.

The intestine may be opened in large birds and inspected for luminal hemorrhage, erosions, ulcerations or parasites. Direct visualization of parasites is noted and intact organisms may be preserved in appropriate fixatives for later identification (see Table 14.4). Wet mounts of intestinal contents and mucosal scrapings should be examined microscopically to identify protozoa (giardia, cryptosporidia), parasite ova or merozoites (coccidia). In large birds, various portions of the intestinal tract may be excised and preserved for histopathologic examination. In tiny birds, the intestine may be fixed *in toto* without gross examination, but it should be cut into multiple sections to allow adequate penetration of the formalin fixative. Portions of intestine also may be retained in a sealable plastic bag for microbiologic culture.

The terminal colon and cloaca should be examined externally and internally. Patency of the colon, ureters and oviduct, if present, should be determined. In some species of birds, such as pheasants and peafowl, the ceca should be examined for the presence of inspissated exudates, masses, parasites or other lesions.

The bursa of Fabricius generally may be found associated with the dorsal wall of the cloaca. Grossly, this organ may resemble a large lymph node in young birds. In older individuals, the bursa may have involuted and will be difficult to identify. Histopathologic examination of formalin-fixed cloacal tissue may allow identification of bursal remnants following involution.

In juvenile hens, the reproductive tract will be minimally developed. The ovary will be small and have a slightly granular appearance. Adult hens that are sexually quiescent or severely stressed may experience atrophy of the reproductive tract, resembling a juvenile hen. In sexually active hens, the oviduct is a prominent, large, off-white, flaccid, vascular, hollow tubular organ with a rugose luminal surface. Egg binding may induce inflammation wherein the distal wall of the oviduct will appear thickened. The oviduct also may be the origin of adenocarcinoma, especially in budgerigars. Hens that have undergone stress may have the uterus and ovaries reduced in size to that of juveniles due to alterations in hormonal secretions.

Removal of the majority of the viscera permits inspection of the lungs *in situ*. Normal lungs are deep pink. The lungs should be examined for areas of discoloration or other abnormalities. A dark red, wet appearance of the lungs suggests pulmonary edema and hemorrhage, which may accompany acute pulmonary sarcocystosis, polytetrafluoroethylene (eg, Teflon®) toxicosis, inhalation of noxious gases, carbon monoxide asphyxiation or necrotizing bacterial pneumonia. Fungal pneumonia may present as cavitating nodules, the walls of which have a velvety green lining.

Because avian lungs are attached to the dorsal rib-cage, removal requires gentle traction along with blunt and sharp dissection (see Chapter 22). The lung parenchyma should be transected at 0.5 cm intervals (as with the liver) to look for occult lesions such as bronchial exudates, particulate debris and areas of consolidation or cavitation. In small birds, use of a magnifying loupe may facilitate identification of particulate debris in aspiration pneumonia.

Next, the kidneys, gonads and adrenal glands are inspected *in situ*. These organs are removed as a single unit by careful dissection, especially in regard to removing the kidneys from the renal fossae of the synsacrum. The sacral plexus is embedded within the kidney, which makes removal of the kidneys difficult. Normal kidney tissue is dark red-brown. The renal parenchyma is examined for discoloration, pallor, swelling or masses or linear white foci that may indicate renal gout. Removal of the kidneys may be impossible in some small birds; however, this portion of the synsacrum may be removed from the carcass and fixed *in toto*. The tissue subsequently may be decalcified, processed, embedded in paraffin and sectioned *en bloc*.

The testes are elongate to cylindrical organs near the anterior portion of the kidneys. In adults the testes appear large and are commonly white with a vascular surface. Some species have melanistic testicles.

Only the left ovary normally persists in psittacine hens. In some species (eg, some raptors), the ovaries are frequently bilateral.

The adrenal glands are identified as small, round, yellow structures to the left and right of the midline at the cranial pole of the kidneys.

Examination of Special Organs and Tissues

Examination of the nervous system and associated tissues is governed by the presence or absence of neurologic or ocular disease. Although the brain and ischiatic (sciatic) nerves are routinely obtained for histologic evaluation, the spinal cord, brachial and sacral nerve plexuses and eyes are obtained only if pathology is present.

Brain

The brain may be removed by plucking the feathers from the head, incising the scalp and reflecting it. A sagittal incision is made through the calvarium using a pair of blunt-sharp scissors. Using a forceps or rongeurs, the bony calvarium is removed as necessary to expose the brain.

Before removing the brain from the calvarium, it should be inspected for congestion or hemorrhage. Depending upon the rapidity of death or method of euthanasia, agonal hemorrhage may be observed in birds following severe terminal motor activity. Agonal hemorrhage must be distinguished from antemortem head trauma if possible. Greenish bruising is more typical of old hemorrhage. The brain may be removed from the calvarium by severing the cranial nerves from rostral to caudal. The optic tectum (a bony plate that covers the large optic lobes) may present a problem in removing the brain from psittacine birds. In hatchlings, the calvarium is soft and may be transected through the midline with a scalpel. The halves of the calvarium may be fixed *in toto* or one-half of the calvarium may be retained for culture.

Vertebral Column

If neurologic disease involves spinal cord or nerve roots, appropriate sections of the vertebral column or synsacrum may be identified, removed *en bloc* and fixed in formalin solution. The pathologist subsequently can decalcify these tissues and section them with a knife or scalpel to discern subtle gross lesions. These tissue sections can be processed and examined microscopically to evaluate nervous tissue, bone and attached soft tissues.

Brachial Plexus

The brachial plexus lies lateral to the thyroid gland in the vicinity of the subclavian artery. Although the plexus commonly is inspected at necropsy, dissection and collection of tissues is limited except in cases of suspected neurologic damage from penetrating wounds, inflammation, neoplasia or trauma resulting in avulsion of the plexus.

Sacral Plexus

The sacral nerve plexus should be examined carefully in instances where pelvic limb paresis or paralysis has been noted. This plexus is best inspected when removing the adrenal glands, gonads and kidneys because it is embedded in the midportion of the kidney just anterior to the ischiatic artery. The ischiatic nerve, which innervates the pelvic limb, may be damaged in severe nephritis or renal neoplasia where compression or infiltration of the nerve occurs.

Ischiatic (Sciatic) Nerve

In instances of pelvic limb paresis or paralysis, the ischiatic nerve should be examined grossly and histologically. The ischiatic nerve can be found beneath the medial thigh muscles caudal to the femur.

Removal of the Eyes

If intraocular disease is present, the eye(s) should be removed from the orbit(s) for histologic evaluation. This process is slightly more difficult in birds because of the relatively large size of the eye. The eyeball is removed by sharp and blunt dissection of orbital soft tissues and transection of the optic nerve.

Other Cranial and Skeletal Tissues

The nares, cere, beak, choanal slit, infraorbital sinus and ears should be examined. Abnormal tissues can be collected for formalin fixation or ancillary testing. Joints of the wings, legs and feet should be opened and examined. Articular surfaces should be off-white, smooth and glistening. If exudates are present, appropriate specimens should be taken for cytologic and microbiologic examination. White, chalky deposits may represent urate deposition. The presence of urate crystals can be confirmed by microscopic examination of cytologic preparations. Urate crystals will appear as refractile needles.

Collection of Bone and Bone Marrow

In the case of fractures, osteomyelitis and arthritis or synovitis, the tissues of interest may be localized with the assistance of survey radiographs. Blunt and sharp dissection will allow gross observations of these tissues. Callus formation, if present, should be noted, and specimens for culture or cytology can be taken after the site is exposed by dissection. Cytology preparations will be useful to characterize inflammatory infiltrates, identify pathogens or identify urate crystals.

Joints can be disarticulated with a scalpel, knife or scissors. The joint capsule, ligaments and tendons can be inspected grossly. Articular surfaces should be examined for erosions of cartilage, eburnation of sub-chondral bone, tags of fibrin or the presence of exudates or hemorrhage. Rongeurs or a small dove-tail saw can be used to excise portions of bone *en bloc* for histopathologic examination.

If the bird is anemic based upon laboratory studies or gross necropsy examination (pale liver and kidneys suggest anemia) or has a blood cell dyscrasia, bone marrow also should be examined. The tibiotarsus or vertebral rib(s) should be used for collection.

Whole Carcass Submission

In instances where the entire carcass is extremely small, such as embryos, nestlings or very small adult birds, the entire carcass may be submitted for histologic examination. This is best accomplished by opening the thoracoabdominal cavity, gently separating the viscera and fixing the entire carcass in formalin solution.

Ancillary testing often is essential to confirm or establish a definitive diagnosis. Tissue specimens should be collected routinely for histopathologic evaluation; however, additional specimens (eg, swabs for bacterial culture, fresh tissues for bacterial culture and virus isolation, crop contents for toxicologic analysis) are obtained as necessary based upon historical, clinical and necropsy findings. These latter specimens can be submitted along with the formalin-fixed tissues if the need for additional laboratory testing is obvious or they may be held under appropriate conditions for later submission if required.

Hematologic and Cytologic Specimens

Smears of blood or exudates may be prepared in a routine manner by the wedge technique. Tissue scrapings may be smeared onto a clean glass slide, or squash preparations may be made if particles of tissue are present. Tissue imprints are prepared by blotting the tissue specimen on an absorbent surface to remove excess blood and tissue fluid. The tissue specimen is then gently touched to a clean glass slide several times or vice versa. Imprints of liver and spleen can be prepared on a single slide and submitted for special stains (eg, Macchiavello's or Gimenez staining for chlamydiosis, acid-fast staining for mycobacteriosis or fluorescent antibody staining for chlamydiosis or herpesvirus infection). Intestinal mycobacteriosis also may be diagnosed using cytologic imprints. Swab specimens are properly prepared by gently rolling the swab the length of the glass slide. All specimens are air-dried before staining or heat fixing.

Table 14.1	Tissues Routinely Collected for Histopathology	
Skin (including feathers, follicles)	Crop	Pancreas
Trachea	Proventriculus	Ovary and Oviduct (female)
Lung	Ventriculus	Testis (male)
Air sac	Small intestine	Pectoral muscle
Heart	Large intestine	Bone marrow
Kidneys	Ceca (if present)	Cloacal bursa
Thyroid glands	Cloaca	Thymus
Parathyroid glands	Spleen	Brain
Adrenal glands	Liver	Ischiatic nerve
Esophagus	Gall bladder (if present)	

Selection of additional tissues will depend upon gross lesions observed at necropsy.

Microbiology

Microbiology includes culture and identification of bacteria, viruses and fungi as well as certain serologic assays to detect the presence of or exposure to these pathogens. Specimens may include culture swabs, fresh tissues, body fluids or exudates, cytology smears and imprints and serum. These specimens are perishable and should be shipped to the laboratory without delay. Fresh tissues submitted for bacterial culture should be at least two cubic centimeters to yield accurate results.

Fresh tissues (especially liver, spleen, kidney, lung and brain) are collected for viral isolation. The selection of tissues for viral isolation depends in part upon the organ system affected. Tissue specimens may be placed in sealable plastic bags and frozen prior to shipment to the laboratory. If tissues are not sent to the laboratory immediately, they may be stored in the freezer until needed for diagnostic testing.

Tissue specimens for fungal culture and identification may be collected, placed in sealable plastic bags and refrigerated or frozen until analyzed.

Parasitology

Fecal specimens may be taken for analysis at necropsy, especially in those patients with diarrhea, where protozoal infection is a consideration. Also, intact parasites such as cestodes, trematodes, nematodes or arthropods may be taken for specific identification when encountered in exotic birds or observed in unusual locations. Preferred fixatives for preservation of fecal material and parasites are detailed in Tables 14.3.

Wet mounts of feces or a feces-saline slurry should be examined within minutes of death to detect organisms such as *Giardia* sp., which are identified by their characteristic rolling movement. Following initial examination, a small drop of Lugol's iodine can be added to kill and stain protozoa and their cysts for more detailed examination.

Toxicology

A veterinary toxicologist or diagnostic laboratory should be contacted to ensure that the proper samples are collected and submitted for analysis.

Heavy Metals

Heavy metal toxicosis is most frequently associated with ingestion of zinc by companion or aviary birds and lead by foraging waterfowl. Suspicion of heavy metal toxicosis may be based upon observing metallic foreign bodies in the crop and gizzard on routine survey radiographs or at necropsy.

Quantitation of lead requires submission of 250 μl of blood in heparin or one-half gram each of liver and kidney. Quantitation of zinc requires 250 μl of serum (avoid hemolysis) or one-half gram each of liver and kidney. The above specimens may be submitted refrigerated or frozen. Blood and serum should be submitted in screw-cap plastic containers or stoppered test tubes.

Aflatoxins

Aflatoxins B_1, B_2, G_1 and G_2 are metabolites of *Aspergillus flavus*. They may be identified in feed or tissue specimens using thin-layer chromatography or high performance liquid chromatography. An ELISA test is available for identification of aflatoxin B1. Identification of aflatoxin in foodstuffs requires submission of 50-100 g of feed. Detection of aflatoxin residues in tissues requires 100 g of fresh or frozen liver. Samples for analysis should be placed in sealable plastic bags.

Poisonous Plants and Chemicals

Suggestion of plant-induced toxicosis may be based upon the medical history and observation of crop contents. Diagnosis of plant alkaloids or chemical-induced toxicosis should be pursued on an individual basis. A veterinary toxicologist should be consulted concerning appropriate specimens and handling prior to analysis.

Table 14.2   Fixative Solutions for Tissue Specimens

- **Neutral-buffered 10% formalin solution:** This solution is used as a common fixative to preserve tissue specimens for histologic examination. Proper fixation requires a ratio of one part tissue to 10-20 parts fixative solution.
  Concentrated formaldehyde (37%) . . . . .100 ml
  Distilled water . . . . .900 ml
  Sodium phosphate monobasic, monohydrate . . . . .4.0 g
  Sodium phosphate, dibasic, anhydrous . . . . 6.5 g

- **Carson's modified Millong's phosphate-buffered formalin:** This solution may be used for routine preservation of tissue specimens for both histopathology and electron microscopy. Proper fixation requires a ratio of one part tissue to 10-20 parts fixative solution.
  Concentrated formaldehyde (37%) . . . . .100 ml
  Deionized water . . . . .900 ml
  Sodium phosphate monobasic . . . . .18.6 g
  Sodium hydroxide . . . . 4.2 g

Table 14.3   Fixative Solutions for Fecal Material

The following fixatives are intended for preservation of fecal material for storage or mailing to the diagnostic laboratory. Comments on the usefulness of each fixative solution follow.

- **PVA fixative:** This fixative is recommended because stained preparations of fecal material subsequently can be made for identification of protozoa.
  PVA, Elvanol 71-24 . . . . .10.0 g
  95% ethanol . . . . .62.5 ml
  Mercuric chloride, saturated aqueous . . . . .125.0 ml
  Glacial acetic acid, concentrated . . . . .10.0 ml
  Glycerin . . . . .3.0 ml

  Mix all liquid ingredients thoroughly. Add the PVA powder without stirring and allow to soak overnight in a sealed beaker. Heat solution slowly to 75°C, remove from heat and swirl for 30 seconds until a homogeneous, slightly milky solution is observed. Using applicator sticks, mix approximately 1g feces with 7-9 ml fixative and store in a labeled brown bottle.

- **10% formalin solution:** This fixative is used primarily to preserve ova for identification. Stained smears cannot be made for identification of protozoa.
  Concentrated formaldehyde (37%) . . . . .100 ml.
  Deionized water or 0.85% saline . . . . .900 ml

  Best preservation is achieved by mixing 1 part feces with 10-20 parts of hot (60°C) fixative.

- **MIF preservative:** Fecal specimens may be stored indefinitely in MIF solution and ova may be harvested by common concentration techniques. This fixative is useful for large surveys where fecal materials are collected from many animals over a long period of time.

  Solution A (store in a brown bottle):
  Distilled water . . . . .50 ml
  Concentrated formaldehyde (37%) . . . . .5 ml
  Thimerosal (tincture of merthiolate, 1:1,000) . . . . .40 ml
  Glycerin . . . . .1 ml

  Solution B (Lugol's solution; good for several weeks in a tightly capped bottle):
  Distilled water . . . . .100 ml
  Potassium iodide crystals . . . . .10 g
  Iodine crystals (after above crystals dissolve) . . . . .5 g

  Combine 9.4 ml of solution A with 0.6 ml of solution B just before use in a small vial. Add feces (up to 1 g) and mix thoroughly. If the suspension is allowed to sit undisturbed for 24 hours, 3 well-defined layers will be apparent. The microscopic specimen is collected from the interface and bottom layers using a disposable Pasteur pipette.

Table 14.4 Fixative Solutions for Specific Parasites

• **Trematodes and Cestodes:** Platyhelminths may be fixed in 10% neutral-buffered formalin solution or alcohol-formalin-acetic acid mixtures. The parasites should be flattened under a slide and coverslip during fixation. Fixatives are best used hot (60°C) for more rapid penetration.

Alcohol-formalin-acetic acid fixative (Galigher's fixative):
    Concentrated formaldehyde (37%) . . . . .10 ml
    95% ethanol . . . . .70 ml
    Distilled water . . . . .15 ml
    Glacial acetic acid, concentrated . . . . .5 ml

• **Nematodes:** Living nematodes should be placed in boiling (60-63°C) alcohol glycerin fixative to rapidly kill the parasites and prevent contraction of the specimen. Nematodes can remain in this fixative indefinitely.

Alcohol-glycerin fixative:
    95% ethanol . . . . 70 ml
    Distilled water . . . . .25 ml
    Glycerin . . . . .5 ml

• **Arthropods:** Arthropods can be preserved in 70% ethanol or 70% isopropyl alcohol solutions (formalin is unsatisfactory for arthropod fixation).

SUPPORTIVE CARE AND EMERGENCY THERAPY

Katherine E. Quesenberry
Elizabeth V. Hillyer

Knowledge of the principles and techniques of supportive care and emergency medicine is necessary for the successful medical management of avian patients.

Because certain syndromes are more common in certain species and at certain ages, the signalment of the bird is helpful in establishing a rule-out list. Recently obtained birds frequently present with acute infectious problems, including chlamydiosis and viral diseases. Neonates that are being hand-fed commonly suffer from management-related problems (eg, crop burns, nutritional deficiencies) and certain fungal, bacterial and viral diseases such as candidiasis, gram-negative ingluvitis and avian polyomavirus. Birds that are long-term companion animals are more likely to have chronic infectious diseases such as aspergillosis, chronic nutritional diseases or toxicities.

The bird should be observed carefully in its enclosure before handling, to assess the depth and rate of breathing. If respiration is rapid or difficult, the bird should be placed immediately in an oxygen cage. While the bird is allowed to stabilize, a complete history can be obtained from the owner, and a diagnostic and therapeutic plan based on the history, clinical signs and initial physical findings can be formulated.

If the bird can be weighed without undue stress, an accurate pretreatment weight should be obtained. Otherwise, drug dosages are calculated based on an estimate of the body weight for the species.

Some veterinarians prefer to use isoflurane anesthesia when treating very weak, dyspneic or fractious birds. For gradual induction in critically ill patients, low isoflurane concentrations (0.25%) are slowly increased to 1.5% or 2.5% over two to five minutes. Once the bird is anesthetized, lower maintenance concentrations (0.75-2%) can be used. Birds can be maintained with a face mask or intubated.

The use of anesthesia allows several procedures to be performed within a few minutes, including collection of a blood sample, placement of a catheter or air sac tube and radiographs. For each bird, the risk of anesthesia must be considered and weighed against the risks of stress associated with manual restraint.

Pretreatment blood samples are valuable if appropriate to obtain. If intravenous fluids are given, a sample can be obtained through a butterfly catheter in the jugular vein immediately before fluid administration. If the conjunctiva and mucous membranes appear pale, the packed cell volume (PCV) should be determined by taking a small blood sample from a toenail clip. If the PCV is 15% or less, collecting blood for a full biochemistry analysis or complete blood count can be life-threatening. Collecting a pretreatment blood sample is usually too stressful in extremely dyspneic birds unless anesthesia is used for restraint.

Radiographs are usually postponed until the bird is stable. If radiographs are essential for establishing a correct diagnosis and initiating treatment, isoflurane anesthesia can be used.

Fluid Replacement Therapy

Fluid Requirements

The daily maintenance fluid requirement for raptors and psittacine birds is estimated at 50 ml/kg/day (5% of body weight).

An estimate of hydration status is based on the clinical signs and history. The turgescence, filling time and luminal volume of the ulnar vein and artery are good indicators of hydration status. A filling time of greater than one to two seconds in the ulnar vein indicates dehydration greater than seven percent. Severely dehydrated birds (ten percent) may have sunken eyes and tacky mucous membranes. The skin of the eyelids may tent when pinched.

Most birds presented as emergencies have a history of inadequate water intake and can be assumed to be at least five percent dehydrated. An estimation of the fluid deficit can be calculated based on body weight:

Estimated dehydration (%) x body weight (grams) = fluid deficit (ml)

Half of the total fluid deficit is given over the first 12-24 hours along with the daily maintenance fluid requirement. The remaining 50% is divided over the following 48 hours with the daily maintenance fluids. Lactated Ringer's solution (LRS) or a similar balanced isotonic solution warmed to 100.4-102.2°F (38-39°C) is recommended for fluid replacement and shock therapy.

Hemodilution is the primary limitation to crystalloid fluid therapy, making administration of colloids or blood necessary for effective shock therapy. Synthetic colloid solutions (dextran, hetastarch) have not been used to any extent in birds. These solutions contain large molecules that do not cross the endothelium and remain in the intravascular fluid compartment. Colloid solutions draw fluid from the interstitial fluid compartment into the intravascular space and are more effective blood volume expanders than crystalloids. They are particularly useful in restoring circulating blood volume without aggravating hypoproteinemia or causing pulmonary edema in animals with low oncotic pressure and hypoproteinemia.

There is evidence that hemorrhagic shock does not occur in birds. Severe blood loss is tolerated much better in birds than in mammals, especially in flighted birds.

Route of Fluid Therapy

Fluids can be given orally for rehydration and maintenance in birds that are mildly dehydrated. In pigeons, administration of an oral five percent dextrose solution has been shown to be more effective for rehydration than oral administration of lactated Ringer's solution. For effective rehydration, oral fluids need to be readministered within 60-90 minutes of the first treatment. Mixing oral fluids with psyllium may increase fluid and calcium absorption from the intestinal villi. Oral fluids should not be given to birds that are seizuring, laterally recumbent, regurgitating, in shock or have gastrointestinal stasis.

Subcutaneous administration is used primarily for maintenance fluid therapy. The axilla and lateral flank areas are commonly used for injection. The intrascapular area is preferred by some clinicians in young birds that may be difficult to restrain for flank injection. The area around the neck base should be avoided because of the extensive communications of the cervicocephalic air sac system. A small (25-27 ga) needle is used to prevent fluids from leaking from the injection site. The total volume of fluids should be given in several sites (5-10 ml/kg/site) to prevent disruption of blood flow and subsequent poor absorption. If ventral abdominal edema is noted, subcutaneous fluid administration should be decreased or discontinued.

Intravenous fluids are necessary in cases of shock to facilitate rapid rehydration. Intraosseous cannula or use of the right jugular vein is the best access point to the peripheral circulation. Dyspneic birds and those with distended, fluid-filled crops should be carefully handled to prevent regurgitation and aspiration. Injection of a large fluid volume into the ulnar or metatarsal veins is difficult and frequently results in hematoma formation.

A butterfly catheter (25 ga) with 3.5-inch tubing is ideal for fluid administration in medium-sized to large birds. A 27 ga needle can be used in small birds. Drug dosages and fluids should be prepared before the bird is restrained.

The amount of fluid that can be administered at one time depends on the size of the bird. Injections of ten ml/kg given slowly over five to seven minutes are usually well tolerated. The bolus injections can be repeated every three to four hours for the first twelve hours, every eight hours for the next 48 hours, and then q12h.

Intravenous catheters (24 ga in medium to large birds) can be placed in the jugular, ulnar or medial metatarsal vein of most birds for continuous fluid administration.

An intraosseous cannula (see Figure 15.4) can be used for administration of fluids, blood, antimicrobials, parenteral nutritional supplements, colloids, glucose and drugs used for cardiovascular resuscitation in birds. Continuous fluid administration by intraosseous cannula is less stressful than repeated venipunctures.

A cannula may be placed in the distal ulna in medium-sized to large birds that will require several days of therapy. The proximal tibia is ideal in birds that will require shorter terms of therapy. Pneumatic bones such as the humerus and femur cannot be used. In medium-sized or larger birds, an 18-22 ga, 1.5-2.5 inch spinal needle can be used as the cannula. In smaller birds, a 25-30 ga hypodermic needle is used.

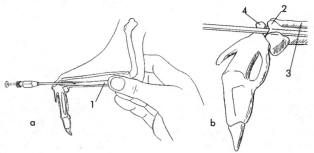

FIG 15.4 Technique for placing an intraosseous cannula in the distal ulna. If fluid or drug administration will be restricted to a single dose or a short period (eg, surgery), it is easier to place a catheter in the tibia. An intraosseous catheter placed in the ulna is easier to maintain if several days of continuous IV therapy are necessary. **a)** The thumb is placed in the center of the 1) ulna as a guide. **b)** The cannula is inserted slightly ventral to the 2) dorsal condyle of the distal ulna. The 3) radius and 4) radial carpal bone can be used for orientation.

For placement in the ulna, the feathers from the distal carpus are removed and the area is aseptically prepared. Using sterile technique, the needle is introduced into the center of the distal end of the ulna parallel to the median plane of the bone. The entry site is ventral to the dorsal condyle of the distal ulna. The needle is advanced into the medullary cavity by applying pressure with a slight rotating motion. If resistance is encountered, the needle may have entered the lateral cortex. The cannula should be flushed with a small amount of heparinized saline, which should flow without resistance. Initial fluids should be administered slowly to check for subcutaneous swelling, which would indicate improper placement of the cannula. The cannula is secured in place by wrapping a piece of tape around the end and suturing the tape to the skin or by applying a sterile tissue adhesive. A figure-of-eight bandage is used to secure the wing.

Tibial cannulas are seated in the tibial crest and passed distally, similar to the technique used for obtaining a bone marrow aspirate. A light padded bandage or lateral splint is used to secure the cannula in place.

Fluids are administered through the cannula using an infusion pump, buretrol or Control-a-Flow regulator. A flow rate of ten ml/kg/hr is suggested for maintenance.

Intraosseous cannulas are most successful in birds if used during the first 24-48 hours for initial rehydration and shock therapy. Cannulas can remain in place for up to 72 hours without complications if placed aseptically and maintained with heparinized flushings every six hours.

Antibiotics

Septicemia and bacteremia should be considered in any bird that is severely depressed. Antibiotics are not necessary in all emergencies. Birds with simple closed fractures, uncomplicated heavy metal toxicity, hypocalcemia and other noninfectious problems may not require or benefit from the use of antibiotics. However, in many emergency patients the history and clinical signs are vague and inconclusive, and antibiotics may be indicated on a precautionary basis. Parenteral antibiotics are recommended for the initial treatment of birds that are weak, sick, debilitated or in shock.

Intravenous administration is recommended if septicemia is a primary concern. Intravenous drugs can be given during the initial fluid bolus or through an indwelling or intraosseous cannula. Intravenous drugs should be given slowly to avoid circulatory shock.

Intramuscular administration of antibiotics is used routinely for maintenance therapy. A small gauge needle (26-30 ga) is used to minimize muscle trauma. The pectoral muscles should be used for most injections.

Subcutaneous administration of drugs is less traumatic to the muscle and is often used for maintenance therapy. Subcutaneous injections may be preferred in very small or cachectic birds with limited muscle mass and in birds with suspected coagulopathies. Disadvantages of subcutaneous injections include the possibility of leakage from the injection site and poor absorption.

Birds with suspected gram-negative septicemia should be treated with a bactericidal antibiotic effective against the most common avian pathogens, including *Escherichia coli, Enterobacter* spp., *Klebsiella* spp. and *Pseudomonas* spp. Antibiotics commonly used for initial treatment of septicemia include piperacillin, cefotaxime, enrofloxacin, trimethoprim-sulfa, doxycycline and amikacin.

If chlamydiosis is suspected, the bird should be treated with a parenteral doxycycline to rapidly establish therapeutic blood concentrations and stop the shedding of the organism. After initial parenteral therapy (IV doxycycline in the United States, IM doxycycline in the rest of the world), the patient can be switched to oral medication for continued therapy.

Other Drug Therapy

Bicarbonate replacement therapy has been recommended in birds if severe metabolic acidosis is suspected, but because it is not usually feasible to measure blood gases in birds, bicarbonate deficit must be estimated. A dose of 1 mEq/kg given IV at 15- to 30-minute intervals to a maximum of 4 mEq has been recommended. If administered too rapidly or given in excessive amounts, alkalemia, hypercapnia, hypocalcemia, hypernatremia, hyperosmolality, hypokalemia and paradoxical CNS acidosis may occur.

Stress causes release of catecholamines, which have hyperglycemic effects. Consequently, birds with traumatic wounds or chronic, nonseptic diseases may have normal to increased blood glucose concentrations and do not need initial supplemental glucose. Hypoglycemia is most common in sick hand-fed babies, septicemic birds, raptors or extremely cachectic birds in which body stores of glycogen have been depleted. In birds that have been determined to be hypoglycemic, an IV bolus of 50% dextrose at 2 ml/kg body weight can be given with fluids to restore blood glucose concentrations. Glucose can then be added to maintenance fluids in a 2.5-10% solution given intravenously or intraosseously.

Birds that are on poor diets or are chronically ill should receive a parenteral multivitamin on initial hospitalization. Vitamin A and D_3 should be administered with care in patients on formulated diets to prevent toxicities from oversupplementation. Vitamin B complex is suggested both initially and on a daily basis in anorectic or anemic birds. Iron dextran therapy is also recommended in anemic birds. Vitamin K_1 will improve clotting time and is important in birds with suspected hepatopathies or birds that may require surgery. Vitamin E and selenium should be considered in patients that have neuromuscular disease. Supplementation of calcium and iodine may be indicated in some cases.

An injectable amino acid supplement (PEP-E) has been marketed for use in birds. The product has been recommended for use as an immune stimulant and a nutritional supplement in anorectic and compromised birds. Although no scientific studies have been conducted, some veterinarians report improvement in birds after using this product at recommended doses, and no detrimental side effects have been reported.

Corticosteroids

The use of corticosteroids in the treatment of shock is controversial. Experimentally, pharmacologic doses of steroids have anti-shock effects in laboratory animals. These include improved microcirculation, organelle and cell membrane stabilization, improved cellular metabolism and gluconeogenesis and decreased production of endogenous toxins. Hydrocortisone, prednisolone, methylprednisolone and dexamethasone are recommended in the treatment of hypovolemic and septic shock. There is no definitive evidence of one drug being superior to another.

Complications of steroid use include immunosuppression, adrenal suppression, delayed wound healing and gastrointestinal ulceration and bleeding. Except for immunosuppression, which may occur with one dose of dexamethasone, other negative side effects are primarily associated with chronic therapy using high dosages.

Corticosteroids are used in birds in the treatment of shock, acute trauma and toxicities. Clinically, birds receiving corticosteroids for head trauma and shock therapy seem to improve; however, clinical improvement may result from supportive care and fluid therapy rather than corticosteroid use.

Secondary fungal and bacterial infections are common in birds receiving steroids for longer than one week. These findings suggest that birds are very susceptible to the immunosuppressive effects of corticosteroids; therefore, corticorsteroids should be used in birds on an infrequent, short-term basis.

Nebulization

Nebulization therapy may be beneficial in birds with bacterial or fungal respiratory infections, particularly those limited to the upper respiratory system. In effect, nebulization provides topical, localized treatment of the internal air sacs and is not dependent on absorption. Because of the anatomy of the avian respiratory tract and the lack of physical activity in the sick bird, nebulized drugs probably reach only 20% of the lung tissue and the caudal thoracic and abdominal air sacs.

Ultrasonic nebulizers are most effective in producing small particle size and are recommended for use in birds.

In general, most parenteral antibiotics formulated for intravenous use can be used for nebulization. Bactericidal antibiotics appear most successful in nebulization therapy. With air sacculitis caused by an unidentified bacteria, the authors prefer to use cefotaxime (100 mg in saline) or piperacillin (100 mg in saline) for nebulization. The suggested protocol is to nebulize for ten to thirty minutes, two to four times daily for five to seven days. Saline is preferred as the nebulizing fluid. Mucolytic agents should be avoided due to their irritant properties. If amikacin is used, the patient should be carefully monitored for signs of polyuria. The effectiveness of treating mycotic air sacculitis with nebulization is not known. In some cases, medications can be injected directly into the trachea or a diseased air sac.

Nutritional Support

There are two main routes for providing nutritional support. Enteral feeding uses the digestive tract and is the simplest, while parenteral feeding bypasses the digestive tract by supplying amino acids, fats and carbohydrates directly into the vascular system.

Enteral nutritional support is generally provided in companion and aviary birds using a tube passed into the crop. Necessary equipment includes 10-18 ga stainless steel feeding needles with rounded tips, rubber feeding catheters of various diameters, plastic catheter adapters, oral beak specula and regular and catheter-tipped syringes. Raptors are usually hand-fed pieces of prey.

Parenteral medications and fluids should be administered before gavage feeding. If given afterwards, there is a risk of regurgitation during restraint for the subsequent treatments. Oral medications can often be administered with the enteral feeding formula.

The crop should be palpated before each feeding to determine if residual feeding formula remains. Birds with ingluvitis or gastrointestinal stasis frequently have slow crop emptying times. If residual food remains, the crop should be flushed thoroughly with a warm, dilute chlorhexidine solution. The crop may need flushing for several days before motility returns to normal. "Crop bras" are sometimes used to support slow-moving, pendulous crops and will often improve crop emptying (see Chapter 30).

The total volume that can be given depends on the size of the bird (Table 15.3).

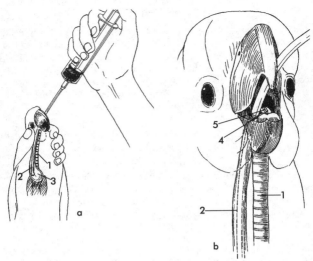

FIG 15.6 a) For tube-feeding or crop aspiration, the bird is held in an up-right position with the neck in extension. **b)** The tube is passed through the left side of the oral cavity and down the esophagus in the right side of the pharyngeal cavity. The tip of the tube should be palpated to ensure that it is in the crop before delivering fluids or feeding formula. 1) trachea 2) esophagus 3) crop 4) laryngeal mound 5) rima glottis and 6) tongue.

Table 15.3 Suggested Volumes and Frequency for Tube Feeding Anorectic Birds

	Volume	Frequency
Finch	0.1-0.3 ml	Six times/day
Parakeet	0.5-1.0 ml	q6h
Cockatiel	1.0-2.5 ml	q6h
Conure	2.5-5.0 ml	q6h
Amazon	5.0-8.0 ml	q8h
Cockatoo	8.0-12.0 ml	q12h
Macaw	10.0-20.0 ml	q12h

If reflux of formula occurs at any time during the tube-feeding process, the bird should be released immediately to allow it to clear the oral cavity on its own. Attempting to swab the oral cavity or turning the bird upside down will cause undue stress and may increase the possibility of aspiration.

Most hospitalized birds are tube-fed two to four times daily according to their clinical condition and caloric needs. Neonates and small birds may need to be fed more frequently.

If the crop or upper gastrointestinal system is dysfunctional (eg, crop stasis, crop burns, proventricular dilatation or ventricular impaction), a bird can be provided enteral nutrition by injecting food directly into the proventriculus or lower gastrointestinal tract through an esophageal gastric tube (pharyngostomy tube) or duodenal catheter. The first method involves placing a soft feeding tube into the esophagus at the base of the mandible, through the esophageal opening at the crop base and into the proventriculus.

A second method for supporting enteral alimentation while bypassing the crop is the placement of a duodenal feeding catheter. A small Foley catheter is surgically placed in the proximal duodenum and exited through the lower abdominal wall. The end of the tube is secured to the dorsum or intrascapular area with tape or sutures. An easily absorbed liquid diet is infused into the proximal small intestine. The volume of liquid formula that can be infused at one time is small, and frequent feedings (as often as every one to two hours) are necessary to meet caloric requirements. Alternatively, food can be infused at a constant rate using an infusion pump.

Total Parenteral Nutrition

Potential indications for the use of total parenteral nutrition (TPN) in birds include gastrointestinal stasis, regurgitation, some gastrointestinal surgeries, severe head trauma that precludes oral alimentation, malabsorption or maldigestion.

Difficulties associated with parenteral nutrition in birds include placing and maintaining a catheter, the necessity of multiple intermittent feedings to supply caloric requirements and potential metabolic complications associated with parenteral nutrition (hypophosphatemia, hypo- or hyperkalemia, hyperglycemia and liver function abnormalities). Sepsis or bacteremia can occur from bacterial contamination of the catheter. Continuous infusion is the preferred method for administration of TPN, allowing for rapid dilution of the hypertonic solution, which minimizes irritation to the vascular endothelium.

The intraosseous cannula or a vascular access device can be used for parenteral alimentation.

Typically a 10% amino acid solution, a 20% lipid solution and a 50% dextrose solution are used. The amino acid solution provides 100 mg protein/ml, the lipid solution provides 2 kcal/ml, and the dextrose solution, 1.7 kcal/ml. These three solutions can be mixed under clean conditions as a three-in-one TPN solution. A 1000 ml bag of five percent dextrose solution is connected to an IV drip set and aseptically emptied. One day's supply of amino acid solution is injected through the port into the bag. The 50% dextrose solution is then added and mixed by inverting the bag. The lipid solution is added last. It should be added and mixed slowly over a two-minute period. This mixture should be used within 24 hours and should be stored in the refrigerator.

Nutritional Requirements

Release of catecholamines, glucagon and glucocorticoids increases the rate of gluconeogenesis and glycogenolysis. Blood glucose concentrations are increased. Intravenous infusion of isotonic glucose has little sparing effect on body proteins, and may actually be detrimental by increasing the release of insulin. The antilipolytic action of insulin may decrease the use of fat stores and increase body protein break-down.

Protein demand is high during periods of hypermetabolism. Proteins are necessary for tissue repair, white and red blood cell production, maintenance of blood proteins (albumin, fibrinogen, antibodies) and enzyme production.

The basal metabolic rate (BMR) is the minimum amount of energy necessary for daily maintenance. An estimate of the BMR for birds can be made based on metabolic scaling:

$$BMR = K(W_{KG}^{0.75})$$
$$\text{Passerine birds K} = 129$$
$$\text{Non-passerine birds K} = 78$$

The K factor is a theoretical constant for kcal used during 24 hours for various species of birds, mammals and reptiles. The maintenance energy requirement (MER) is the BMR plus the additional energy needed for normal physical activity, digestion and absorption. The MER for adult hospitalized animals is approximately 25 percent above the BMR. In passerine birds, MER varies from 1.3-7.2 times the BMR, depending on the energy needed for activity and thermoregulation during different times of the year. With growth, stress or disease, animals are in a hypermetabolic state with daily energy needs that surpass maintenance. The amount of increased demand depends on the type of injury or stress and varies from one to three times the daily maintenance requirement (Table 15.4).

Table 15.4	Adjustments to Maintenance for Stress (as multiples of MER)
Starvation	0.5-0.7
Elective Surgery	1.0-1.2
Mild Trauma	1.0-1.2
Severe Trauma	1.1-2.0
Growth	1.5-3.0
Sepsis	1.2-1.5
Burns	1.2-2.0
Head Injuries	1.0-2.0

Enteral Nutritional Formulas

Commercial enteral nutritional formulas marketed for humans are widely available. These diets are usually liquid formulations sold in 250 ml containers. The diets vary in caloric density, protein, fat and carbohydrate content and osmolality (Table 15.5). Formulas vary from meal replacement formulas, which require some digestion, to monomeric diets, which require little or no digestion. Almost all diets are lactose-free and are approximately 95 percent digestible. Formulas range from less than 1.0-2.0 kcal/ml. With a calorie-dense formula (2.0 kcal/ml), the total volume of liquid can be given in two to four feedings per day. Maintaining adequate hydration is important in birds when using calorie-dense formulas. Once opened, enteral formulas can be refrigerated for two to three days. For feedings, the formulas can be heated gently, such as in a syringe under hot running water.

Table 15.5	Commercial Enteral Products: Nutrients per 100 kcal Energy (kcal = calories)			
Product	Protein (g)	Fat (g)	Carbos (g)	kcal/ml
Isocal	3.4	4.4	13.3	1.0
Isocal HCN	3.8	5.1	10.0	2.0
Traumacal	5.5	4.5	9.5	1.5
Pulmocare	4.2	6.1	7.0	1.5
Ensure Plus	3.6	3.5	13.0	1.5

Formula may curdle in the crop of birds with ingluvitis and gastrointestinal stasis, probably because of changes in the pH of the crop. Flushing the crop with warm water while gently massaging the crop will cause the curdled formula to break apart, allowing aspiration and removal. Multiple feedings of small amounts of an isotonic or diluted formula should be given until the crop motility is normal.

Commercial enteral formulas marketed for use in birds are available. These diets are either dry powders or liquids. They are consistent in nutritional content, easy to prepare and use and relatively low in cost. In general, these diets are relatively high in carbohydrate content when compared to human products.

Following the bird's weight on a daily basis (in grams) is the best evaluation of enteral feeding.

Oxygen Therapy

An oxygen enclosure is highly recommended as standard equipment in an avian practice. Most are designed as incubators with controls for heat and monitors for humidity. Administration of oxygen by face mask is effective for short-term treatment if an oxygen enclosure is not available, or during restraint while treatments or diagnostic tests are performed. If there is upper air-way obstruction, oxygen can be infused through an air sac tube.

Clinically, dyspneic birds appear to stabilize when placed in an oxygen enclosure and maintained at 40-50% oxygen concentration. Oxygen can be supplemented in small animals at levels up to 100% for less than 12 hours without complications. Canaries and budgerigars given continuous supplemental oxygen at concentrations of 82-100% and 68-93%, respectively, showed signs of lethargy, anorexia, respiratory distress and death after three to eight days.

Birds that are severely anemic or in circulatory shock need adequate volume expansion and red blood cell replacement for improved tissue oxygenation to occur.

Air Sac Tube Placement

Placement of an air sac tube is beneficial in birds with tracheal obstructions, or when surgery of the head is necessary. In companion birds the tube is normally placed in the caudal thoracic or abdominal air sac, allowing direct air exchange through the tube into the air sac. An alternative site for air sac cannulation used in raptors is the interclavicular air sac.

A shortened endotracheal tube, trimmed rubber feeding tube or plastic tubing from an IV extension set can be used for an air sac tube. The tube can be placed in the lateral flank area in the same anatomic location as for lateral laparoscopy, or caudal to the last rib with the femur pulled forward (Figure 15.10).

If placed correctly, the bird will immediately begin breathing through the tube. If anesthetized, the bird will become light unless the end of the tube is occluded or attached to the anesthesia machine. The air sac tube can be left in place for three to five days. The effect of direct exchange of room air into the air sac and the

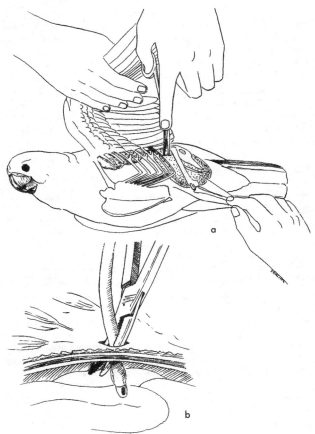

FIG 15.10 Placement of a tube in the abdominal air sac can be used to provide oxygen or isflurane anesthesia. **a)** The tube is placed by making a small skin incision caudal to the last rib. **b)** A pair of hemostats is passed through the body musculature and the air sac tube is inserted between the jaws of the hemostats.

potential for introduction of contaminants and infectious organisms into the cannulated air sac are unknown.

An air sac tube allows many treatment techniques to be performed that would otherwise be impossible in a dyspneic bird. Liquid medications can be instilled directly into the trachea for the treatment of bacterial or fungal tracheitis. The bird can be anesthetized through the tube for surgery or endoscopy of the trachea or head, and the tube can be used for positive pressure ventilation or resuscitation. Birds can be nebulized with the air sac tube in place, possibly increasing the concentration of antimicrobials in the air sacs. If apnea occurs, a needle can be used in place of a tube for providing a rapid source of oxygen.

Heat

Floor heating elements may occasionally cause hyperthermia when debilitated birds are forced to stand or lie on the enclosure floor or in direct contact with the heating surface. Alternatively, heat can be provided by a hot water bottle or well insulated heating pad (preferably water). Small, heated rooms that hold two to three enclosures allow birds to be treated in a temperature-stable environment, reducing the stress associated with being removed from a warm incubator to a cooler treatment area.

Ambient temperature for adult birds should be 85°F and humidity should be approximately 70%. Unfeathered baby birds less than ten days old need an ambient temperature of 94°F. Older chicks can be maintained at 90°F. Birds in heated enclosures should be monitored for hyperthermia, which is clinically suggested by panting and holding the wings away from the body.

Housing

Many sick birds are too weak to perch. These birds should be placed in a smooth-sided enclosure or incubator without perches. Many sick birds will not eat unless food and water are easily accessible. Seeds, fruits and vegetables can be spread around the bird to encourage eating. If the bird is still perching, food and water containers should be placed next to the perches to encourage food consumption. Millet spray is an attractive food item for many smaller species.

Although abrupt diet changes should not be attempted while the bird is sick, offering the bird a balanced diet in addition to any food it is accustomed to eating is appropriate, and may offer therapeutic benefits because of improved nutrient value.

Birds with leg fractures or paralysis are best maintained in a wire enclosure on thick cage paper or toweling. These birds will grasp the wire siding with their beak to steady themselves. If perches are provided, they should be close to the enclosure floor to prevent injuries.

Cardiovascular System

Bleeding and Anemia

Anemia in birds may be caused by blood loss, decreased red blood cell production and increased red blood cell destruction.

The most common cause of blood loss in birds is trauma. Other causes include gastrointestinal (GI) bleeding, genitourinary bleeding, hemolysis and idiopathic hemorrhage. intestinal ulcers, coagulopathies, liver disease and GI foreign bodies. Cloacal bleeding may be caused by cloacal papillomas, cloacitis, egg laying, or cloacal or uterine prolapse. Heavy metal toxicity can cause hemolysis, which may result in dramatic hemoglobinuria in some birds, especially Amazon parrots. Conures may present for a sudden onset of weakness, ataxia, epistaxis, bloody regurgitation, bleeding from the oral cavity, hematochezia, hemorrhagic conjunctivitis or muscle petechiation.

Anemias resulting from decreased red blood cell production are common in birds, possibly because of the relatively short life-span

(28-45 days) of the avian erythrocyte. "Depression anemias" are usually caused by chronic infectious, toxic or nutritional disease. A rapidly fatal nonregenerative anemia seen in two- to four-month-old African Grey Parrots is suspected to be of viral etiology. Some birds with this problem have been shown to have polyomavirus or PBFD virus antigens in the bone marrow.

Diagnosis of anemia is based on clinical signs and documentation of a decreased PCV. Weakness is the most common clinical sign. Severely anemic birds may have a dull, almost dazed demeanor. Tachypnea and tachycardia may also be present. On physical examination, pallor of mucous membranes is evident in the oral cavity, palpebral conjunctiva and cloaca.

CBC and reticulocyte count, serum or plasma biochemistry analysis, blood heavy metal concentration and whole body radiographs should be considered in cases of anemia of unknown origin. Further testing might include chlamydia screening and a bone marrow aspirate. If an intraosseous cannula will be necessary for stabilizing the patient, a bone marrow sample can be obtained through the cannula at the time of placement. If the mucous membranes are pale, the PCV should be determined before drawing more blood. If the PCV is below 15%, further blood collection is inadvisable. It should be noted that the volume of serum or plasma relative to the volume of whole blood will be increased due to the anemia; the minimum amount of blood necessary to perform the desired diagnostic tests should be drawn.

If the bird is actively bleeding on presentation, localization of hemorrhage and hemostasis are the first priorities. Developing feathers are called "blood feathers" because of the rich vascular supply within the shaft. When one of these feathers is broken, it may continue to bleed until it is removed from its follicle. For removal, the base of the damaged feather is identified by parting the surrounding feathers. The base is grasped firmly with hemostats, and the feather is removed from its follicle by gently placing opposing pressure on the structure around the feather base. If any bleeding occurs from the dermis, it can be controlled by applying pressure to the area or packing the follicle with surgical gel. Chemical or radiosurgical cautery should not be used inside the feather follicle because the subsequent inflammation and tissue damage can cause abnormal feather regrowth, resulting in the formation of feather cysts.

Persistent bleeding from soft tissue wounds is less common. If such bleeding occurs, it can be controlled by applying pressure to the area or through the use of bipolar radiosurgery. Surgical tissue adhesive is often useful. Hemorrhage from oral and tongue lacerations may be difficult to control. Complete evaluation and suturing of these lacerations usually require general anesthesia.

Nonspecific treatment for blood loss includes volume replacement by subcutaneous or intravenous fluids, and the administration of iron dextran and B vitamins (see Chapter 18). Birds on an all-seed diet can be assumed to be nutritionally deficient and will benefit from an injection of vitamin K_1.

In birds with idiopathic hemorrhage, such as in conure bleeding syndrome, injectable vitamin K_1, vitamin D_3, calcium and antibiotics are indicated. If hemoglobinuria is present, treatment should be initiated with calcium disodium edetate (CaEDTA) for possible heavy metal toxicity (see Chapter 37). If clinical signs are being caused by heavy metal toxicity, there will usually be clinical improvement within six hours of initiating CaEDTA therapy.

The benefits of blood transfusions in birds are controversial. In pigeons that lost 70% of blood volume, it was determined that fluid replacement with LRS was more effective in resolving anemia than iron dextran, homologous blood transfusions or heterologous blood transfusions. All study birds had a normal PCV within six days following acute blood loss. Until a controlled study is performed, it is probably valid to assume that homologous blood transfusions are preferable to heterologous, and that in most instances, a blood transfusion will not greatly increase the survival rate in acute blood loss. However, in the authors' experience, even heterologous blood transfusions appear to be clinically beneficial to birds suffering from chronic anemia. The goal of the transfusion is to stabilize the patient while diagnostic tests can be used to determine the etiologic agent of the anemia. A transfusion volume of roughly 10-20% of calculated blood volume is ideal. A rough crossmatch can be performed by mixing red blood cells from the donor with serum from the recipient; the absence of gross agglutination or hemolysis suggests compatibility.

Shock

Clinical signs include weakness, pallor and poor perfusion of peripheral vessels. Vascular perfusion can be estimated by occluding the ulnar vein proximally on the medial surface of the wing and evaluating turgescence and filling time. Decreased turgor and a filling time greater than 0.5 seconds are indications of reduced circulatory volume. Septic shock is a possibility in debilitated birds, and is clinically recognized as severe depression, particularly in birds with known exposure to infectious diseases.

Therapy for shock includes intravenous administration of fluids to expand the circulating blood volume and rapidly acting corticosteroids. Intramuscular corticosteroids and subcutaneous fluids are beneficial but take more time to enter the circulation. Metabolic acidosis may be present, and bicarbonate replacement therapy should be considered. Parenteral bacteriocidal antibiotics are given if bacterial infections are suspected.

Cardiac Failure

Suspicious clinical signs of cardiac failure include weakness, anorexia, tachypnea, dyspnea, coughing and abdominal distension due to hepatomegaly and ascites. The diagnosis is suggested by an arrhythmia or murmur on auscultation, and by radiographic changes including cardiomegaly, hepatomegaly and ascites. A single IM dose of furosemide, low-dose subcutaneous fluids and an oxygen-rich environment are indicated. Electrocardiography and ultrasonography may confirm cardiac disease and guide the selection of other cardiac medications (see Chapter 27).

Cardiopulmonary Resuscitation (CPR)

Avian CPR follows the same "ABC's" as mammalian CPR: Airway, Breathing and Circulation. In a bird that has stopped breathing, an airway must be established by placing an endotracheal or air sac tube. To avoid the danger of zoonotic disease, it is preferable to ventilate the bird in this fashion; alternatively, mouth-to-mouth respirations can be given by cupping the mouth over the bird's nares and beak opening. Positive pressure ventilation should occur once every four to five seconds. Once ventilation has been started, the heart beat or peripheral pulse should be determined. If neither is present, the heart should be massaged by firm and rapid compression of the sternum. Epinephrine and doxapram are given as necessary. The intratracheal, intracardiac or intraosseous routes (even spray into the thoracic cavity if open) for emergency drug administration should be considered when peripheral vascular access is not possible.

Cardiopulmonary resuscitation should always be attempted in previously healthy birds that have collapsed; however, CPR is rarely successful in birds that are debilitated from long-standing, chronic disease.

Gastrointestinal System

Crop Burns and Injuries

Thermal burns of the crop are seen in hand-fed neonates, particularly psittacine birds. The presence of a fistula is alarming to most owners; however, it is a true emergency only if the fistula is so large that all formula drains out of the crop, leaving the bird in danger of dehydration and starvation. The frequency of feedings may have to be increased in the interim in order to replace the formula lost through the fistula. If the burn is discovered soon after it occurs, the crop area should be monitored daily. The use of anti-inflammatories (eg, corticosteroids) represents more of a risk than a benefit in young birds (see Chapter 41). Some periesophageal burns, lacerations and other injuries may not result in fistula formation and are recognized clinically as crop stasis. In some cases, the feeding instrument may have punctured the crop, and the food is deposited between the skin and the crop wall. This is a true emergency because the bird can suddenly become toxic, exhibit massive edema and die.

Gastrointestinal Stasis

Multiple factors that may affect GI motility in young birds include infectious disease, poor sanitation, low environmental temperature, low formula temperature and low humidity. Causes of GI stasis in adult birds include gastroenteritis (leading to ileus), neuropathic gastric dilatation, heavy metal toxicity and obstruction (see Chapter 19).

Delayed crop emptying is the most common presenting sign of GI stasis. Regurgitation or vomiting may occur also. Fecal output is reduced. Chronic cases in debilitated birds can be difficult to manage and treat effectively, and the client should be advised that therapy may be lengthy and that the prognosis is poor.

Physical examination begins with an assessment of hydration status and thorough palpation of the crop for the presence of foreign bodies or inspissated food material. Some crop foreign bodies, particularly linear ones, can be removed by carefully manipulating them back up the cranial esophagus and into the oropharynx, where they are visualized and grasped with forceps. Removal of other foreign objects and inspissated food material is most easily accomplished via ingluviotomy. The bird is anesthetized with isoflurane and intubated to reduce the danger of aspiration. A small incision is made over the left lateral pendulous crop to ensure that the incision is not damaged should the bird require tube-feeding. The incision is closed in two layers using a 6-0 absorbable suture. Postoperative feedings should be small and frequent, beginning with clear liquids and gradually increasing the strength and amount of formula over the next 24-48 hours until a normal feeding schedule has been resumed.

If a crop foreign body cannot be palpated, food and water should be withheld until the crop is empty or the crop can be drained by the clinician. Usually it is difficult to empty the crop via gavage tube because crop contents tend to become thickened when the crop is static. Flushing the crop with 0.05% chlorhexidine solution is often beneficial. After flushing, a small amount of LRS, followed in three hours with dilute formula or Isocal, should be administered by gavage tube.

Radiographs and a barium series are indicated if impaction or extraluminal obstruction is suspected, particularly in adult birds. Before the series is begun, the crop contents should be removed and the anesthetized bird should be held upright until the esophagus can be packed with moist gauze. A finger placed over the cranial esophagus will help prevent reflux from entering the pharyngeal area.

A minimum database should include cytology of the crop contents and fecal wet mounts. Samples can be collected by crop lavage or by passing a flexible swab directly into the crop. Culture and sensitivity of the crop contents and feces are indicated if bacterial infection is suspected. An in-house blood glucose determination is important if the bird is weak.

Restoring and maintaining hydration with subcutaneous, intravenous or intraosseous fluids is important, and should be considered prior to performing surgery or other stressful procedures. Parenteral antibiotics and metoclopramide are often indicated (see Chapter 18). Oral medications are mostly ineffective because of slow passage into the intestinal tract. Oral aminoglycosides, however, may be beneficial in cases of bacterial overgrowth because they act locally with minimal absorption or side-effects. Parenteral feeding or placement of a duodenal feeding tube should be considered in critically ill birds (see Chapter 41).

Budgerigars with goiter often present with crop stasis and a history of regurgitation due to pressure of the enlarged thyroid glands on the caudal esophagus. These birds may also have a squeaky voice or an audible click with each respiration; tachypnea and tail-bob may be present. Diagnosis of goiter is based on clinical signs and history of an iodine-deficient diet. These birds should be hospitalized for parenteral fluids, steroids, antibiotics and iodine therapy.

Regurgitation and Vomiting

Regurgitation to a "mate" (often the owner) or mirror is a normal part of breeding behavior; this is seen most commonly in budgerigars and cockatiels but can occur in any psittacine bird. A clinical history that includes intermittent regurgitation when the bird is being handled or talked to will help differentiate this normal behavior from a pathologic problem. Pathologic regurgitation in birds is caused by primary GI problems, metabolic problems and toxicities that induce nausea. Primary GI problems include infection (bacterial, viral, fungal and parasitic) and both intraluminal and extraluminal obstruction. Metabolic problems include hepatic and renal disease (see Chapter 19). Toxins that may cause vomiting include ingestion of some plants, pesticides and heavy metals such as lead or zinc. Some birds will regurgitate from stress or from motion sickness (such as during a car trip).

Birds that are regurgitating will make a head-bobbing and neck-stretching type of motion. A bird will often shake its head when regurgitating, depositing the regurgitus about the face and head. Goiter is the most common pathologic cause of regurgitation in budgerigars over two years of age. Bloody regurgitation may be seen in conure bleeding syndrome.

Initial diagnostic testing should include swabbing or flushing the crop for a wet mount, cytology, Gram's stain and culture. Fecal examination by wet mount and Gram's stain is often informative also. Other diagnostic tests to consider include a CBC, biochemistry profile and blood heavy metal concentration. Whole body radiographs, a routine barium series, or a double contrast study of the upper GI tract may be useful (see Chapter 12).

Initial stabilization of the regurgitating patient involves parenteral fluid therapy, removal of foreign bodies or toxins, specific toxin antidotes and appropriate antimicrobials if bacterial or fungal infections are suspected. Flushing the crop with 0.05% chlorhexidine reduces local bacterial levels in cases of ingluvitis.

Severe Diarrhea, Hematochezia and Melena

Stools may "normally" be loose from stress, excitement, over-consumption of dairy products and ingestion of foods with a high water content (vegetables and fruits). Pathologic diarrhea usually results from bacterial, viral, fungal, chlamydial or parasitic gastroenteritis. The presence of a foreign body in the GI tract can also cause diarrhea. Pancreatic or liver disease and ingestion of some toxins may cause diarrhea. The differential diagnosis list for the emergency patient with diarrhea includes gram-negative enteritis, hepatopathy, chlamydial infection and heavy metal toxicity.

Physical examination of the bird with diarrhea should begin with careful evaluation of the hydration status and gross evaluation of droppings for evidence of blood, mucus, undigested food, plant material or gravel. Melena may be noted with problems of the upper GI tract (enteritis, foreign bodies, parasites, ulcers).

Hematochezia may be present with disease of the colon or cloaca. Cytology or a dip stick for fecal occult blood should always be used to document GI bleeding before aggressive and unnecessary therapy is instigated. The cloacal mucosa can be examined by prolapsing it gently with a well lubricated cotton swab. The presence of yellow or green urates suggests involvement of the liver. Brown, pink, red or rust-colored urates are seen most commonly with acute heavy metal toxicity, particularly in Amazon parrots. Birds consuming heavily pigmented fruits (eg, blueberries, blackberries) may have dark feces that mimics melena or hematochezia.

The database for diarrhea includes fecal examination by wet mount, Gram's stain and culture. Cytology for *Giardia* sp., *Trichomonas* sp. or other protozoa should be considered. Other valuable diagnostic tests include a CBC, biochemistry profile, radiographs, blood heavy metal concentration and screening for chlamydia.

Parenteral fluids should be administered to meet maintenance levels and replace estimated fluid volume lost to diarrhea. Debilitated birds may benefit from intravenous or intraosseous fluids and one dose of rapidly acting corticosteroids. Parenteral administration of a bacteriocidal antibiotic with a broad gram-negative spectrum is indicated because bacterial enteritis is common with diarrhea either as a primary cause or as a secondary problem.

Cloacal Prolapse

Prolapse of the cloacal mucosa is associated with masses within the cloaca, neurogenic problems or conditions causing tenesmus (eg, enteritis, cloacitis or egg-binding). Idiopathic prolapses are seen also.

The history should include questions about diarrhea, straining or previous egg laying. Abdominal palpation for a mass and checking for prolapse of the ureters or uterus should be a priority during the physical examination. Cloacal tumors, such as adenocarcinomas, tend to be single and discrete. An irregular, "raspberry-like" appearance of the mucosa suggests cloacal papillomatosis.

Diagnostics and treatment are best performed with the bird relaxed under isoflurane anesthesia. Fecal retention is a problem with long-standing prolapses and with neurogenic etiologies. Manual massage of the caudal abdominal and cloacal regions promotes fecal evacuation. Parenteral fluid therapy and treatment for septic shock should be used in these cases.

A complete examination of the cloacal area must be performed. In larger birds, a vaginal speculum and strong light source permit examination deep into the cloacal region. Diagnostic tests to consider include fecal wet mount, Gram's stain, culture and radiographs. If cloacal papillomatosis is suspected, tissue excision with biopsy is necessary to confirm the diagnosis. A prolapsed cloaca caused by papillomas does not require a purse-string suture preoperatively. In fact, purse-string sutures in birds with cloacal papillomas may result in blockage of the cloacal opening and are thus contraindicated. Solitary tumors should be biopsied by excision if possible.

Prolapsed mucosa should be protected from damage and desiccation. The tissues should be flushed with saline and covered with a sterile lubricating jelly or ointment. The need for a retention suture will vary depending on the individual bird and the clinician's preferences. Retention sutures may complicate the prolapse by exacerbating straining and should be avoided if at all possible. If a retention suture is placed, it must not interfere with evacuation of the cloaca. A cloacapexy may be necessary in some birds that chronically prolapse (see Chapter 41). It is important to treat any possible underlying cause of prolapse such as hypocalcemia or other nutritional or metabolic problems.

Liver Disease

Clinical signs of hepatitis are often nonspecific, including lethargy, inappetence, polyuria, polydipsia, diarrhea and ascites. Birds with ascites are often tachypneic or dyspneic. The presence of yellow or green urates is an indicator of probable liver disease. On physical examination, an enlarged liver may be palpable or, particularly in passerine birds, may be visible through the skin.

The basic database includes a complete blood count, serum biochemistry profile, bile acids, fecal Gram's stain, fecal culture, cytology of the abdominal fluid, whole body radiographs and chlamydial testing.

While laboratory tests are pending, treatment for suspected liver disease includes basic supportive care, broad-spectrum antibiotics, oral lactulose and at least one dose of parenteral vitamin K_1. Doxycycline is the drug of choice for chlamydiosis. Metronidazole, cephalosporins and the penicillins are the antibacterials of choice for small mammal hepatic infections.

Pancreatic Disease

Primary pancreatitis is seldom diagnosed in birds, but is occasionally found at necropsy. Bacterial, viral and chlamydial infections of other organs may spread to the pancreas causing secondary problems.

Clinical signs of pancreatitis may include inappetence, lethargy, weight loss, polyuria, polydipsia, abdominal distension and abdominal pain. Pancreatic exocrine insufficiency results in polyphagia, weight loss and bulky, pale droppings.

A CBC and a biochemical profile that includes amylase and lipase levels are indicated. In cases of acute pancreatitis, a radiograph may demonstrate a hazy or fluid-filled abdomen. Initial treatment should include aggressive parenteral fluid therapy and broad-spectrum antibiotics. One dose of rapidly acting corticosteroid may be beneficial in some birds. Plant enzymes (rather than canine pancreatic enzymes) can be added to the tube-feeding formula to help with digestion (see Chapter 18). Vitamin E and selenium should also be given, and the bird tested for zinc toxicosis.

Urogenital System

Egg Binding

Egg binding is most common in hens that are on a poor diet, are first-time egg layers or are prolific layers. Problems are most common and most severe in smaller species such as cockatiels, budgerigars and finches. Lack of sufficient dietary calcium, protein and trace minerals such as vitamin E and selenium will predispose to egg binding by resulting in soft-shelled eggs and uterine atony. Hypovitaminosis A is often a contributing factor due to alteration of mucosal integrity.

On physical examination, the hen may appear weak and quiet. Tachypnea is common. Unilateral or, less commonly, bilateral leg lameness or paresis occurs if the egg is pressing on the ischiatic nerve as it runs through the pelvic region. In most cases an egg is palpable in the abdomen. If the egg is poorly calcified, it may not be palpable but the abdominal region will be moderately swollen and soft. The cloacal region is often swollen also. Whole body radiographs can be used to confirm the diagnosis. Medullary bone formation, also termed hyperostosis or osteomyelosclerosis, occurs under the influence of female reproductive hormones and is seen especially in the femur, tibiotarsus, radius and ulna.

Occasionally, the presence of an egg with a non-calcified shell may be difficult to distinguish radiographically from egg-related peritonitis or an abdominal mass. In this case, a repeat radiograph approximately one hour after the administration of barium may aid in localizing internal structures. An alternative is to administer supportive care, calcium, vitamins and antibiotics, and then to repeat the radiograph one to two days later, assuming that an egg would have calcified or passed in that time period. Uterine rupture is possible, and will negate this last assumption (see Chapter 41).

Conservative medical treatment for egg binding is often successful and should always be given a chance to work before more aggressive therapy is instigated. Decisions regarding therapy should be based on the bird's clinical condition, but in most cases, it is best to allow up to 24 hours of medical therapy before initiating more aggressive steps. Even with paresis of a leg, it is best to attempt medical therapy first because the paresis usually resolves once the egg is passed. Small birds such as finches may require earlier intervention. The real emergency associated with a retained egg is that it may place excessive pressure on internal pelvic structures, such as the caudal poles of the kidneys, where ischemic renal necrosis may occur. In contrast, some birds are not clinically ill from egg binding. An example is an egg-bound budgerigar that the authors treated medically for six months because the owners refused surgery.

Medical therapy for egg binding includes fluids, lubricating the cloaca, supplemental heat and parenteral calcium, vitamin A and vitamin D$_3$. If the bird is anorectic, oral dextrose or a small gavage feeding may be given, and the bird should be placed in a warm, moist environment such as an incubator containing wet towels. (An old-fashioned, sometimes successful, therapy for egg binding is to submerge the caudal portion of the bird in a bowl of warm water for five to ten minutes!) After one or two doses of calcium, an injection of oxytocin may promote egg passage. Prostaglandin may be more effective in facilitating the passage of an egg than oxytocin (see Chapter 29).

If the egg has not passed in 24 hours, or if the bird appears to be weakening, two nonsurgical techniques can be considered. The first works best if the egg is low in the abdomen. With the bird under isoflurane anesthesia to achieve full relaxation, the egg may be manually pushed caudally so its tip is visible through the uterine opening into the cloaca (see Chapter 29).

An 18-22 ga needle is inserted into the egg, the egg contents are withdrawn, the egg is carefully imploded and the egg shell fragments are withdrawn using a small hemostat.

The second technique is transabdominal aspiration of egg contents using a large gauge needle (see Chapter 29). The egg is manipulated to the ventral body wall and the egg contents are removed with a syringe. The egg is then gently imploded, relieving pressure on pelvic structures. Supportive care and calcium are continued until the bird delivers the egg shell on its own. Some clinicians flush the uterus for several days to prevent feces from contaminating the traumatized uterus. The disadvantage of this technique is that occasionally a hen does not pass the egg shell fragments, necessitating a hysterectomy.

Surgical removal of the egg via laparotomy is necessary if the uterus is ruptured, if an egg cannot pass due to adhesions or other causes, or if there are multiple eggs (see Chapter 41).

Uterine Prolapse

Uterine prolapse containing an egg is common, particularly in budgerigars. Occasionally the uterus will prolapse without the egg. Both conditions probably result from constant straining coupled with muscle weakness due to nutritional deficiencies or physical exhaustion.

The bird is anesthetized with isoflurane to allow careful examination of the prolapsed tissue. While the bird is anesthetized, SC or IV fluids, parenteral calcium, vitamins A and D_3 and a broad-spectrum bacteriocidal antibiotic are administered. One dose of a rapidly acting corticosteroid is appropriate if the bird appears to be in shock. The ureters, rectum and cloaca will sometimes prolapse with the uterus. The prolapsed tissue should be flushed with sterile saline and replaced with a lubricated blunt probang, sterile swab or other sterile, blunt instrument.

Oxytocin or prostaglandin (see Chapter 29) applied directly to the uterus will help reduce swelling and control bleeding. If an egg is in the prolapsed tissue, the open end of the prolapse should be identified and the egg contents aspirated with a needle to gently collapse the egg. The egg is usually tightly adhered to the fine, transparent uterine tissue, which should be liberally moistened with warm sterile saline. A moist, sterile swab will help gently peel the uterine tissue from the egg without tearing. The prolapsed tissue should be flushed again and replaced as described. The need for a retention suture in the cloaca is based on clinical judgment.

The prognosis for recovery depends on the extent of tissue trauma. In the authors' experience, many hens respond well to therapy even if the replaced uterine tissue appears severely desiccated or inflamed. Antibiotic therapy for five to seven days is recommended. Any remaining necrotic areas should be exteriorized and amputated. The necrotic areas are sutured with 4-0 or 5-0 absorbable suture material, being careful to avoid the ureters. Most birds will temporarily cease egg laying after the trauma and illness associated with uterine prolapse. After the bird is stable, a hysterectomy may be necessary to prevent future egg-related problems.

Egg-related Peritonitis

Egg-related peritonitis is thought to occur because of a failure of the ovum to enter the infundibulum. The peritonitis that occurs is usually sterile, but may be complicated by secondary bacterial infection. The condition is seen most commonly in cockatiels, lovebirds and budgerigars, but can occur in any hen.

The history usually includes a gradual onset of lethargy, weakness, inappetence, tachypnea and dyspnea. Nesting or egg-laying behavior often precedes the onset of illness. Occasionally, a bird will show no clinical signs other than tachypnea or dyspnea related to fluid accumulation in the abdomen. The clinical presentation of egg-related peritonitis varies with the species. Ascites is most common in cockatiels.

On physical examination, the bird is found to have a fluid-filled, distended abdomen. If the bird is dyspneic, it should be placed in an oxygen-rich environment prior to diagnostics and treatment. Abdominocentesis is performed with a 23 or 25 ga butterfly catheter or an appropriately sized needle and syringe (see Chapter 10). Only a sufficient volume of fluid to relieve the dyspnea should be removed. The needle is passed into the abdomen just below the end of the keel. Care should be exercised to prevent laceration of the liver if hepatomegaly is suspected. More than one abdominocentesis may be necessary. Some veterinarians prefer to place a Penrose drain to allow a continuous port for fluid removal.

Fluid analysis and cytology, a CBC and whole body radiographs should be performed. Radiographic changes are characterized by a fluid-filled abdomen with loss of detail. Increased ossification in the long bones suggests that calcium is being stored for impending ovulation. Parenteral fluids, a broad-spectrum antibiotic and an anti-inflammatory dose of corticosteroid should be administered. Although corticosteroids should be used with caution in birds, low-dose corticosteroid therapy for two to five days in conjunction with antibiotics appears to be beneficial in birds with egg-related peritonitis. A course of medroxyprogesterone acetate is a common companion therapy to steroids (see Chapter 29). A laparotomy and abdominal lavage may be necessary in birds with severe or nonresponsive egg-related peritonitis (see Chapter 41).

Renal Failure

Possible causes of renal failure include some toxicities, ureteral obstruction and trauma (such as occurs with egg binding) and bacterial, viral, fungal or parasitic infections.

Clinical signs include polyuria, polydipsia, inappetence, depression and dehydration. Uric acid deposits may be visible on joint surfaces. The basic database consists of a CBC, biochemistry analysis, urinalysis, fecal Gram's stain and fecal culture. Radiographs are useful to evaluate the size and density of the renal shadows. Uric acid deposits are radiolucent but renal mineralization will be visible on radiographs.

Emergency treatment consists of subcutaneous or intravenous fluids, antibiotics and a multivitamin injection. The latter would be contraindicated if hypervitaminosis is suspected (eg, vitamin D toxicosis in macaws).

Respiratory System

Dyspnea

Dyspnea in birds is characterized by open-mouthed breathing, prominent abdominal excursions and tail-bobbing with respiration. Causes of dyspnea can be divided into two categories: primary respiratory and extra-respiratory disease. Primary respiratory disease occurs in the trachea, lungs or air sacs and may be caused by viral, bacterial, fungal, parasitic, chlamydial and mycoplasmal infections, inhaled toxins or foreign body aspiration. Extra-respiratory diseases can cause dyspnea by interfering with normal air flow patterns through the respiratory tree or by limiting expansion of the lungs and air sacs. This category includes thyroid enlargement, abdominal masses, abdominal fluid and oral masses such as papillomas. Birds with severe rhinitis, impacted nares, choanal atresia or sinusitis may also show open-mouthed breathing and a tail-bob because they cannot breathe through the nares. Anemia may also induce dyspnea (see Chapter 22).

A thorough history should include questions regarding the possibility of exposure to other birds or to airborne toxins, the possibility of foreign body aspiration and recent evidence of crop stasis or ileus, which may lead to aspiration. Before a dyspneic bird is handled, it should be carefully observed for conjunctivitis, swollen sinuses, nasal discharge and respiratory sounds. Budgerigars with goiter may have a high-pitched voice or a squeak with each respiration. These birds are also prone to crop-emptying problems and may have a dilated crop. Mynah birds and toucans may develop cardiomyopathy or iron-storage hepatopathy, resulting in ascites and dyspnea. Egg binding or egg-related peritonitis should be considered as a cause of dyspnea if the bird has a history of egg laying. The bird should be placed in an oxygen-rich environment while diagnostic and treatment plans are being formulated.

Some birds may benefit from immediate placement of an air sac tube while diagnostic tests are performed. If a bacterial pneumonia or air sacculitis is likely, antibiotics may be administered by nebulization in order to minimize handling. Alternatively, the bird may be anesthetized with isoflurane to collect diagnostic samples and initiate therapy. Initial diagnostic tests should include radiographs, CBC, biochemistry profile, abdominal fluid analysis (if present) and tracheal wash. Birds with ascites or egg-related peritonitis will often improve once the abdominal fluid is removed. Early in the course of therapy, enough fluid should be withdrawn to relieve dyspnea and provide a diagnostic sample. In theory, sudden withdrawal of too much fluid can cause hypovolemia and shock; however, in practice, the authors have not experienced this problem.

A tracheal wash should be performed just before the bird recovers from anesthesia. A sterile catheter or tube is passed into the tracheal opening. With the bird held parallel to the floor, sterile saline (up to 10 ml/kg) is infused into the trachea and immediately aspirated. Cytology and bacterial and fungal culture can be used to evaluate the aspirated material.

Acute Dyspnea

Acute onset of dyspnea in a previously healthy bird is usually due to one of three causes: 1) inhalation of a toxin, 2) plugging of the trachea by dislocation of an infectious plaque from the choana or tracheal bifurcation or 3) inhalation of a foreign body such as seed or bedding material. Inhalation of small seeds by cockatiels is common.

When a blockage of the upper respiratory tract is suspected, an air sac tube will provide immediate relief of dyspnea. The bird can be anesthetized by administering isoflurane through the air sac tube, making it possible to examine the trachea endoscopically. In smaller birds, transillumination of the trachea may be used to identify tracheal foreign bodies. Radiographs often demonstrate the site of obstruction and will allow for evaluation of the lungs and air sacs. Removal of a tracheal foreign body is accomplished using suction or a biopsy forceps. In some cases it may be necessary to perform a tracheotomy by incising between tracheal rings just distal to the foreign material. The foreign body is retrieved with biopsy forceps or pushed up and out of the trachea using a blunt probang.

Air Sac Rupture

Rupture of an air sac often results in a balloon-like deformity of the skin. While the clinical appearance is quite alarming to owners, the problem is rarely a true emergency. Rupture of a cervicocephalic air sac in small birds is most common. The rupture is usually acute, but gradual onset is seen also. Most birds are reported to be otherwise normal and the cause of the rupture is not identified.

A medical workup should be considered if the bird is showing clinical signs of illness, particularly those associated with respiratory disease.

Initial treatment for air sac rupture involves making a percutaneous fistula to allow for continued drainage of air. This relieves pressure on the site of rupture to allow for healing. A rapid, simple technique is to use a hand-held ophthalmic cautery to make a one to two centimeter opening in an avascular area of skin over the swelling, causing rapid deflation. Occasionally the swelling may recur when the fistula closes and the technique must be repeated, making a larger fistula. Surgical repair may be necessary in some birds if initial treatment fails (see Chapter 41).

Neurologic System

Head Trauma

Birds frequently recover from seemingly severe head trauma. Examination should include visual assessment for alertness and neurologic signs, an evaluation for shock, and examination of the cranium, eyes, nares and ears for evidence of fractures, hemorrhage or bruising. If the trauma is recent, treatment consists of IV or IM rapidly acting corticosteroid and placement of the bird in a dark environment maintained at a comfortable (cool) temperature. A warm environment may potentiate intracranial vasodilation. If the bird is in shock, IV fluids are given at one-half to two-thirds of the normal volume to avoid overhydration and cerebral edema. Mannitol or furosemide may be beneficial if the bird does not respond to initial therapy. Short-term monitoring consists of neurologic evaluation and measurement of blood glucose.

If the trauma occurred over 24 hours previously, an empirical course of antibiotics and short-term corticosteroids can be attempted, but this is usually ineffective. Neurologic impairment may be permanent if the injury is several days old and no improvement is noted following 48 hours of therapy. Long-term corticosteroid therapy should be avoided in such birds.

Seizures

Several different types of seizure activity are seen clinically. Mild seizures are characterized by a short period of disorientation with ataxia and inability to perch. Generalized seizures are characterized by a loss of consciousness, vocalizing, wing flapping and paddling. Partial seizures are characterized by persistent twitching or motor activity of the head or one of the extremities. They can be continuous and chronic.

Causes of seizures in birds include primary central nervous system (CNS) disease resulting from trauma, hyperthermia, vascular accidents, infection or neoplasia, and metabolic problems such as hypocalcemia, hypoglycemia, hepatoencephalopathy, toxin exposure and fat emboli. Idiopathic epilepsy, a diagnosis of exclusion, has been reported in Peach-faced Lovebirds, Red-lored Amazon Parrots, Double Yellow-headed Amazon Parrots and mynah birds. A syndrome of hypocalcemia causing weakness and seizures occurs in African Grey Parrots. Cockatiels and lovebirds may show neurologic signs with an undiagnosed, fear-induced mild flapping of the wings, or occasionally with chlamydiosis. Egg-laying birds often have severe lipemia and may develop fat emboli with resultant neurologic abnormalities including seizures and paralysis. Hypoglycemic seizures occur most commonly in raptors and neonates of other species.

The history should include questions regarding diet, egg laying and possible toxin exposure. Owners rarely can verify heavy metal exposure although it is common in psittacine birds due to their propensity for chewing on toys and household objects. If the bird is not actively seizuring, a full physical and neurologic examination including a CBC, biochemical analysis and blood metal concentration should constitute the minimum database in most cases (see Chapter 37). Radiographs are useful to evaluate bone quality and screen for metallic particles in the gastrointestinal tract. If the bird is weak or actively seizuring, an in-house blood glucose test should be performed. Abnormal values are less than 50% of the published normal reference interval for the species (see Appendix).

If the bird is seizuring on presentation, the first goal of therapy is to stop the seizure activity with IM or IV diazepam. Intravenous phenobarbital should be underdosed and used with caution in birds. If lead or zinc poisoning is a possibility, treatment with CaEDTA should begin immediately. Hyperthermia should be evaluated and treated, and hypoglycemia should be corrected with IV dextrose. Suspected chlamydiosis or other infectious diseases should be treated accordingly.

Seizure activity associated with hypocalcemia is most common in African Grey Parrots and young birds on a poor diet. The African Grey hypocalcemic syndrome is thought to occur because of a lack of compensatory mechanisms to maintain serum calcium levels. The syndrome may actually represent a deficiency of vitamin D_3; however marginal dietary calcium levels seem to play a role. These birds can have a serum calcium concentration as low as 2.5 mg/ml. Radiographically, the skeletal mineralization appears normal, indicating an inability to mobilize skeletal calcium. Other species that develop hypocalcemia will show decreased bone density, folding fractures and pathologic fractures. Treatment for hypocalcemia consists of parenteral calcium, vitamin D_3 and supportive care.

Coma

Coma can result from head trauma, toxin ingestion, hyperthermia, CNS infection or neoplasia, cerebral ischemia due to a vascular accident, or severe metabolic disease such as hepatic encephalopathy or uric acidemia. The history should include questions related to the onset of clinical signs and possible trauma, toxin ingestion or inhalation (carbon monoxide) and exposure to viruses or parasites (eg, *Sarcocystis* spp. , *Baylisascaris* sp.).

Ensuring a patient's airway and adequate ventilation are of primary importance. Establishing an airway with a tracheal or air sac tube and placing the bird in an oxygen-rich environment or applying positive pressure ventilation may be necessary. The bird should be given dextrose IV if an in-house test indicates hypoglycemia. Emergency treatment consists of IV fluids (low dose if cerebral edema is a possibility), parenteral corticosteroids and treatment for hyperthermia as necessary. The use of IV diuretics such as mannitol or furosemide should be considered in birds with head trauma and hyperthermia. Bacteriocidal antibiotics or doxycycline for chlamydiosis may be indicated in some patients. The bird should be placed in a dark, cool environment after treatment to discourage cerebral vasodilation and edema.

Supportive care should include lubrication of the eyes and frequent turning of the recumbent bird as necessary.

Paralysis of Acute Onset

Possible causes of leg paresis include soft tissue trauma, fractures, osteoporosis, neural infections or vertebral trauma or neoplasia. Fractured leg bones are usually associated with reversible paresis of the foot and toes. Another cause of unilateral or, less commonly, bilateral leg paresis is pressure on the pelvic portion of the ischiatic nerve caused by egg binding or renal or gonadal tumors. Paresis of a wing is indicated by a wing droop. This is most commonly caused by soft tissue or bony trauma. Occasionally lead or other heavy metal toxicity will cause peripheral neuropathy resulting in wing or leg paresis.

Muscles may undergo atrophy in the affected limb. The feathers should be parted with alcohol in order to examine the skin for evidence of bruising or wounds. This technique is useful for detection of fractures. The skin overlying the skull and spine should also be examined.

Radiographs may be useful to detect or assess intra-abdominal masses, metallic densities in the GI tract, coxofemoral luxations, or fractures of the spine, long bones or shoulder girdle. If heavy metal poisoning is a possibility, blood levels of lead or zinc can be determined.

Treatment is tailored to the specific condition. Egg binding and fractures are managed routinely. Paretic toes must be taped in the proper perching position to avoid knuckling and resultant damage to the top of the foot. One to three days of corticosteroid therapy may be indicated in cases of head or vertebral trauma. In general, birds have a good capacity for return to function after the cause of the paresis or paralysis is resolved. It is impossible to predict the possibility of recovery with most avian neurologic injuries.

Chronic Disease With Acute Presentation

The most common avian emergency presented to avian clinicians is a chronically ill bird that has decompensated to the point where the owner finally becomes aware of the illness. These birds are usually debilitated, dehydrated and cachectic. It is important with these patients to minimize stress (eg, loud noises, bright lights and excess handling). These birds generally require therapy for severe dehydration and cachexia. Emaciated birds are frequently anemic. Some birds begin to eat on their own within a short time after the initiation of therapy. Birds that refuse to eat should receive an easily digestible enteral preparation such as Isocal-HCN.

Occasionally a cachectic bird will be presented that is alert and relatively active with a good appetite. The owner may not be aware of the weight loss and may have brought the bird in for another problem. This is a common presentation in birds with tuberculosis and some neoplasias. Although the bird may appear strong, its body fat and glycogen stores are depleted and it may decompensate as easily as birds that appear weaker. Prognosis for cachectic birds is grave.

Physical Injury

Animal Bites

Bite-induced injuries are typically of the crushing and tearing type, often necessitating surgical repair or debridement of damaged tissue (see Chapter 16). These are true emergencies and require immediate attention due to the pathogenic oral bacteria that are introduced deep into bite wounds. Cat attacks, in particular, are especially dangerous because many cats carry *Pasteurella multocida* on the gingival tissue and teeth.

Shock therapy is instituted if necessary. For a carnivore bite, treatment with a bacteriocidal antibiotic should begin immediately. Penicillins are the antibiotics of choice for cat bites because of their efficacy against *P. multocida*. All wounds must be flushed with copious volumes of warm sterile saline or 0.05% chlorhexidine.

Burns

The most common burns in birds occur on the legs and feet. These result when free-flighted birds land in hot cooking oil, hot water or on a hot surface. Burns to the oral mucosa and tongue may occur when birds bite on electric cords.

The treatment for burns involves basic supportive care, topical therapy and prevention of secondary infection while the wounds are healing. Secondary invaders are typically *Staphylococcus intermedius,* streptococci, coliforms and *Pseudomonas* spp. Systemic antibiotics and corticosteroids should be avoided during initial therapy because their use may predispose the patient to immunosuppression and nosocomial infection.

Diligent topical therapy is the key to burn management. The burned areas should be flushed with copious amounts of cool water or saline. Feathers surrounding the wounds should be removed to allow for aeration. Water-soluble, topical antibacterial creams such as silver sulfadiazine should be used instead of greasy or oily medications. If the wound is not infected (Gram's stain of cleansed wound negative for organisms), a hydroactive dressing is beneficial to prevent water loss and promote granulation tissue (see Chapter 16). Wounds should be flushed twice daily and debrided once a day.

Gram's staining and culture and sensitivity of burned tissue may be indicated to monitor for infection. Systemic antibiotic therapy is initiated based on positive culture results.

Glue Traps

Removing a bird from a glue trap entails gentle restraint of the body while freeing one extremity at a time. Feathers may be cut or gently removed. Shock therapy and supportive care should be given as needed. A commercial automobile protectant is nontoxic and can be rubbed gently on affected feathers to remove the glue. This material can be rinsed away with warm water. These agents should be used with caution because some products contain lead (see Chapter 37).

Exposure

Oil

The goals of treating oil-soaked birds are to reverse shock, prevent or treat hypothermia, provide basic supportive care and remove the oil from the feathers, nares and oral cavity. The bird is wrapped in a towel or thermal blanket to conserve body heat, and shock therapy is initiated if needed. The eyes are lubricated and oil is removed from the nares and oral cavity with a swab. Depending on the bird's tolerance for restraint, it may be necessary to alternate rest periods in a dark, heated environment (95°F) with warm baths (100-105°F) to remove the oil. A commercial dish-washing detergent is a safe and effective solvent and is used in decreasing concentrations in sequential baths with thorough warm water rinses in between. When the feathers are clean, the bird is dried with a blow-dryer and placed in a warm environment.

Hyperthermia

Panting and holding the wings away from the body indicate hyperthermia in birds. Birds do not have sweat glands and do not dissipate heat efficiently. If allowed to progress, hyperthermia results in ataxia, seizures and coma.

The first goal of emergency therapy is to reduce body temperature by placing the feet and legs in cool water and wetting the feathers down to the skin with water or alcohol. If the bird is severely overheated, cool water can be infused into the cloaca, taking care not to induce hypothermia by overzealous cooling. Flunixin meglumine may be used to reduce hyperthermia rapidly and safely. A bird in shock should be given low doses of IV or SC fluids, and one dose of rapidly acting corticosteroid. Mannitol or furosemide may help control cerebral edema.

Frostbite

If the injury is recent, the frozen tissues appear pale, dry and avascular, sometimes with a swollen area proximally. If left untreated, the frozen tissue will become necrotic with an erythematous line of demarcation separating it from viable tissue.

Treatment of a recent frostbite injury involves gradual warming of the extremity by placing the affected tissue in circulating water baths and increasing the water temperature over a 20- to 30-minute period. If the tissue becomes necrotic, it can be surgically amputated at a later date (see Chapter 41).

General Emergency Principles of Toxin Exposure

Toxins that may enter by the alimentary route include lead, zinc and other heavy metals, various plants, rodenticides and some foods like chocolate (see Chapter 37). Birds are also very sensitive to aerosolized toxins, which include overheated polytetrafluoroethylene (Teflon® or other nonstick coatings), tobacco smoke, hair spray, pesticides, paint fumes, naphthalene, ammonia and carbon monoxide.

Ingestion of prey animals or contaminated water may expose free-ranging birds to potential toxins, the most common being organophosphates, botulism toxin and lead.

Occasionally a bird will be exposed deliberately or allowed unrestricted access to substances such as chocolate, alcohol or marijuana. Careful and specific questioning is usually necessary to delineate potential toxin exposure.

The first step in treatment of any toxin exposure is to stabilize the patient as necessary with shock and anticonvulsant therapy. If a known toxin was recently ingested, a crop lavage is the quickest method of removal. An ingluviotomy may be necessary to remove solid toxins (see Chapter 41). If more than one-half hour has passed since ingestion, a poison control center should be contacted (see Chapter 37).

Most often, an exposure to a specific toxin cannot be identified. A CBC and biochemistry analysis, blood lead and zinc concentrations and radiographs are indicated. Nonspecific treatment for suspected toxicosis includes decreasing further absorption of the toxin from the GI tract, hastening elimination of the toxin and providing supportive care. If heavy metal toxicity is a possibility, treatment with CaEDTA should be initiated.

If the ingested toxin is still in the GI tract, lavage is performed with saline or activated charcoal. Crop, proventricular and ventricular lavage are best performed with the bird intubated and under isoflurane anesthesia. A tube is passed into the proventriculus per os or a small crop incision is made and a red rubber tube is passed distally. The bird can be held with the head tilted down, and foreign objects and toxins can be retrieved by flushing. The administration of activated charcoal helps to bind toxins and decrease GI absorption.

Saline and osmotic cathartics are used to speed elimination of toxins. Saline cathartics (eg, sodium sulfate [Glauber's salt]) will precipitate heavy metal in the GI tract, decreasing absorption. Psyllium is an osmotic cathartic. For specific toxin therapies see Chapter 37.

Quick Reference for Emergency Therapy

ANIMAL BITES
  Parenteral penicillin ASAP
  Clean wounds
BLOOD LOSS/ANEMIA
  Stop bleeding
  Volume replacement (IV or IO
    fluids)
  Iron dextran
  B vitamins
  Vitamin K_1
  Blood transfusion (PCV <20%)
BURNS
  Gently remove feathers
  Clean wounds
  Antimicrobial creams
  Hydroactive dressing if not
    infected
CACHEXIA
  Fluids - IV or IO
  5% dextrose IV or IO
  Oral or parenteral
    alimentation
COMA
  Ensure patent airway
  Oxygen-rich environment
  Low dose fluids if dehydrated
  Single-dose corticosteroids
  Mannitol or furosemide
CPR
  Establish airway - air sac tube
  Ventilate every 4-5 secs
  Rapidly press on cranial
    sternum
  Epinephrine and doxapram IC,
    IO, IT
DIARRHEA
  Fluids (IV, IO)
  Bactericidal antibiotics
  Shock therapy if necessary
DYSPNEA
  URD - air sac tube
  Oxygen-rich enclosure
  Removal of some ascitic fluid
  Remove tracheal foreign bodies
    (suction or surgery)
EGG BINDING
  Medical therapy initially:
    Subcutaneous fluids
    Lubricate cloaca
    Prostaglandin
    Parenteral calcium, oxytocin
    Dextrose oral (50%) SC (5%)
    Vitamins A and D_3

  Supplemental heat
  If medical therapy fails:
    Assisted cloacal delivery
    Percutaneous ovocentesis
    Ventral laparotomy
FROSTBITE
  Gradual warming in water
    bath
  Increase temperature
HEAD TRAUMA
  Corticosteroids - IV, IO
  Dark, cool environment
  Minimal fluids - correct shock
    only
HYPERTHERMIA
  Wet with cool water
  Flunixin meglumine
  Mannitol
  Single dose corticosteroids
  Dry and keep at 85°F
LIVER DISEASE
  Fluids (IV, IO)
  Lactulose
  Vitamin K_1
  Doxycycline - if susp. chlamydia
  Parenteral penicillin - if susp.
    bacteria
OIL
  Shock therapy
  Prevent hypothermia
  Bathing in warm detergent
PANCREATITIS
  Fluids (IO)
  Bactericidal antibiotics
  Single-dose corticosteroids
  NPO if possible
PROLAPSED CLOACA
  Keep tissues moist and clean
  Replace cleansed tissue
  Correct underlying urogenital
    or GI problem
  Retention suture if necessary
PROLAPSED UTERUS
  Clean with sterile saline
  Topical oxytocin or prosta-
    glandin to reduce swelling
  Lubricate with water-soluble gel
  Replace with blunt probang
  Retention suture if necessary
REGURGITATION
  Fluids (IV, IO)
  Remove foreign bodies or toxins
  Gastric lavage

Specific toxin antidotes
Appropriate antimicrobials
SEIZURES
Diazepam - IV or IM
Supportive care
African Grey Parrots - calcium
and vitamin D_3
Raptors and neonates - glucose
if needed
SHOCK
Fluids (IV or IO)
Corticosteroids (IV or IO)
Bicarbonate if acidotic
Bactericidal antibiotics if septic

SUPPORTIVE CARE
Fluids
Heat
Vitamin/mineral supplements
Nutritional support
TOXINS
Treat for shock
Remove ingested foreign bodies
Oxygen for inhaled toxins
Specific antidotes (see Chap. 37)

TRAUMA MEDICINE

Laurel A. Degernes

16

Proper management of traumatic injuries in birds significantly decreases complications and wound-healing time. An understanding of wound healing is important in order to devise a treatment plan for optimal results.

Inflammatory Phase: Immediate vasoconstriction to control hemorrhage is followed by vasodilation within 30 minutes. Polymorphonuclear leukocytes and monocytes infiltrate the margins of the injured and necrotic tissue within the first 2-6 hours, causing active phagocytosis of necrotic cellular debris and bacteria.

By 12 hours post-injury, the ratio of polymorphonuclear to mononuclear cells shifts toward a predominance of mononuclear cells. During the next 36 hours, necrotic leukocytes that were active in phagocytosis accumulate at the periphery of the necrotic tissue and are phagocytized by macrophages and multinucleated giant cells. Fibroblasts appear in the wound during this period and continue to proliferate during the next few days, signaling the end of the first phase of the healing process.

Collagen Phase: Beginning the third or fourth day, fibroblasts synthesize collagen in the form of microfibrils, which aggregate into larger fibers over time. During this phase, which lasts approximately two weeks, capillaries develop from bud-like structures from nearby vessels and penetrate the wound. Wound contraction occurs, and epithelial cells proliferate and migrate across the wound surface.

Maturation Phase: The final phase of wound healing may take weeks to months, and is marked by remodeling of the collagen bed and a decrease in the number of fibroblasts. The weak, poorly developed collagen is replaced by thicker, stronger collagen fibers, which become oriented relative to the normal tension on the wound margins (see Chapter 40).

Principles of Wound Management

Impediments to Wound Healing

Dehydration, starvation, severe protein deficiency and chronic anemia may have adverse effects on wound healing. Necrotic tissue or blood clots may harbor bacteria and physically impede epithelial cell migration. Infection by pathogenic bacteria may significantly delay wound healing. Dirt, debris, dead bone and even suture material may cause host reaction leading to the development of fistulous tracts.

Tissue destruction resulting from desiccation, severe trauma (eg, crushing or projectile injuries) or poor surgical technique will delay healing. Wounds of the distal extremities (reduced vascular supply) and non-immobilized injuries over joints, the axilla and the patagia tend to heal more slowly.

Initial Assessment

Traumatized birds often have multiple injuries and may be further compromised by dehydration, malnutrition and other problems, especially if there has been a delay (hours to days) between injury and presentation. Shock, fluid and nutritional therapy are critical in the early management of traumatized birds. Over-zealous wound and fracture treatment before stabilization of the patient may result in the patient's death. Anesthesia may be necessary with fractious birds or in birds with extensive soft tissue or orthopedic injuries. However, if the bird is not stable, partial wound management and bandaging may have to suffice until more thorough treatment can be safely completed.

Surface Preparation and Wound Treatment

The initial goal in treating contaminants or infected wounds is the removal of devitalized tissue, foreign material and bacteria. The feathers surrounding the wound should be gently plucked or trimmed to allow more thorough cleansing and to prevent feather matting during the healing phases.

Wound lavage using a curved tip irrigating syringe will remove foreign material, reduce bacterial numbers and rehydrate soft tissues. Sterile isotonic saline with or without 0.05% chlorhexidine or 0.5-1.0% povidone iodine solution is recommended for wound lavage. Cultures should be obtained after surface contaminants have been removed and before any antiseptics have been applied. Hydrogen peroxide has been shown to be ineffective for bacterial infections, but may be effective as a sporicide in cases of suspected clostridial infections, or for initial cleansing of dirty wounds.

Wound debridement following lavage involves removal of as much of the devitalized and necrotic tissue as possible until viable, vascularized tissue is recognized. In complicated or older wounds, the debridement process may have to be repeated over a period of a few days.

Topical medications in certain wounds may be beneficial; however, use of non-water-soluble medications should be avoided due to loss of insulation with soiled feathers. Bacitracin, neomycin and polymyxin are effective against a wide spectrum of bacteria. One percent silver sulfadiazine is effective for thermal burns and other wounds. Topical use of hemorrhoid creams containing live yeast cell derivatives (LYCD) has been shown to stimulate epithelialization and collagen synthesis in human and canine wounds. LYCD has been successfully used in raptors with granulating wounds and pododermatitis (bumblefoot) lesions.

Products that have been shown to retard wound healing in mammals include nitrofurazone, which slows epithelialization, and gentamicin sulfate, which impairs wound contraction.

After lavage and debridement, the wound should either be sutured, managed by second intention healing or managed as an open wound with delayed closure. Wounds less than eight hours old and not heavily contaminated, or wounds that were surgically created under sterile conditions should be sutured. Older, infected or more complicated wounds should be managed as open wounds and allowed to heal by second intention.

Bandaging Principles

The functions of bandages are to:
- Apply pressure to reduce dead space, swelling, edema and hemorrhage
- Protect the wound from pathologic microorganisms
- Immobilize the wound and underlying fractures, if present
- Protect the wound from desiccation and additional trauma from abrasions or self-mutilation
- Absorb exudate and help debride the wound surface
- Provide comfort for the patient.

The three layers of a bandage are the primary layer (or dressing that is in contact with the wound), the secondary layer for absorption and the tertiary layer, which serves to hold the other layers in place.

Primary Layer

This layer should be sterile, remain in place even with patient movement, provide a moist wound environment and assist with the debridement process

The two basic groups of dressings include adherent and nonadherent dressings. Adherent dressings such as fine mesh or open weave gauze pads are indicated during the initial phase of wound treatment when there is a large amount of necrotic debris that cannot be surgically debrided, or with excessive exudate production. Wet-to-dry bandage techniques involve the application of sterile saline-soaked, warm gauze pads over the wound surface. The exudate and necrotic debris will be mechanically removed with daily dressing changes during the first few days of treatment, at which time the type of dressing used can be changed to a nonadherent one.

Traditional nonadherent products commonly used in veterinary wound management include cotton film dressings and petrolatum-impregnated fine mesh gauze pads.

Increased understanding of wound healing processes has resulted in the development of many new synthetic adhesive, nonadherent dressings for use in humans. These new dressings keep the wound surface moist and prevent scab formation, which significantly increases the rate of re-epithelialization, compared to air-exposed and wet-to-dry gauze dressings.

Hydrocolloid dressings or hydroactive dressings (HAD) are semiflexible, opaque membranes that are impermeable to moisture vapor and oxygen, and absorb fluid and exudate to develop a moist, gelatinous cover over the wound. These dressings adhere to normal skin and not wounds, but generally require additional bandaging material to be held in place.

Moisture vapor permeable (MVP) dressings are thin, flexible, transparent polyurethane membranes that are oxygen permeable, impermeable to water and bacteria, allow accumulation of fluid and exudate under the dressing and are adhesive to normal skin but not wounds. The maintenance of a moist, aerobic environment under the dressing promotes leukocyte debridement of the wound surface, prevents desiccation and scab formation and reduces pain associated with desiccation of raw nerve endings. Epithelialization is more rapid when scabs are not present to impede cell migration from the wound margins.

Both MVP and hydrocolloid dressings are indicated for a variety of avian wounds, but MVP dressings are more suited to areas that are impossible to bandage (eg, head wounds) because of the superior adhesive quality and flexibility of the material. The dressings are changed every two to three days initially, or more often if excessive exudate production results in fluid leakage from underneath the dressing. Once a healthy granulation bed is established, dressings can be changed weekly. Wounds treated with these dressings appear to heal more rapidly and with fewer complications compared to conventional nonadherent dressings.

Secondary Layer

The functions of the secondary bandage layer are to absorb fluids and wound exudate, pad the wound from trauma, and immobilize the wound and underlying fracture during the healing phases. Conforming gauze material or cast padding is most commonly used.

Tertiary Layer

The tertiary or outer layer serves to hold the other layers of the bandages in place. Self-adherent bandages are excellent for birds because they are lightweight and breathable, are well tolerated by most birds, and the material adheres to itself cohesively without problems associated with tape residues on feathers.

Band Injuries

Band injuries should be prevented by anticipating potential problems, especially with open bands that have large gaps and with inappropriately sized bands (too small or too large). Prophylactic band removal or crimping to reduce the gap is preferable to treating a band injury (see Chapter 1). Once an injury or associated problem with a band is recognized, extreme caution should be exercised with band removal to avoid additional injury to the bird. The owner should always be warned of potential risks to the bird whenever a band is removed, even when the procedure is elective and not associated with trauma. Complications may include fractures, dislocations and lacerations. If a wound is already present, avascular necrosis may complicate the band removal procedure. Specific treatment options following band removal involve wound debridement and cleansing, surgical closure if indicated and coverage with appropriate dressing and bandaging material as needed.

Feather, Toenail and Beak Injuries

For broken blood feathers, a first-aid home procedure involves putting flour over the bleeding feather stub. This conservative treatment may be adequate in some cases, but most broken blood feathers require timely removal. The feather should be grasped at the base with a hemostat (needle-nosed pliers can be used on large birds) or fingers and pulled from the follicle while applying counter pressure to the area surrounding the follicle, to prevent tearing the skin.

It is critical to remove the entire feather shaft from the follicle and continue to apply pressure over the follicle until the hemorrhage stops. Products intended for hemorrhage control during nail and beak trims, such as silver nitrate and ferric subsulfate powder should never be used in a feather follicle to stop bleeding, due to the irritation caused by these products and the possible foreign body reaction that may occur (granuloma or feather cyst formation). Radiocautery should also not be used to blindly cauterize the interior of a follicle. Broken or torn toenails can be managed by trimming the exposed portion with a nail trimmer to make a smooth surface, and packing ferrous subsulfate or silver nitrate into the exposed nail bed pulp cavity. If the keratin sheath of the toe nail has been pulled off to expose the underlying bone, direct pressure should be applied to control hemorrhage. The exposed bone can be protected with liquid bandage products, or light bandaging.

Beak injuries occur most often from bites from other psittacines, or from collisions during flight. Head trauma is common with mate aggression and may be associated with beak fractures, punctures or avulsion of the maxillary or mandibular beak, in addition to soft tissue trauma. Hemorrhage may be controlled with direct digital pressure or by applying clotting products such as silver nitrate or ferric subsulfate. For specific beak repair see Chapter 42.

Self-mutilation

A thorough diagnostic workup to rule out predisposing factors should be considered. Appropriate antibiotic, antifungal or anthelmentic treatment is combined with soft tissue wound management and protection of the wounds from further trauma.

Application of moisture vapor permeable dressings is very effective in promoting rapid wound healing, and is well tolerated by most avian species including psittacines. In severe cases of self-mutilation, an Elizabethan collar or neck brace collar may be indicated to protect the wounds from further trauma.

Burns

The most common thermal burns occur in the crop of neonates fed improperly heated hand-feeding formula (microwaved without proper stirring). Further discussion of medical and surgical management of crop burns is covered in Chapter 30. Accidental burns may occur when pet birds come in contact with hot liquids, hot surfaces or electrical wires. Treatment action to be taken includes immediate cooling and rinsing of the affected areas, followed by supportive care, topical wound management and systemic antibiotic therapy. Topical medications may include DMSO for acute inflammation and silver sulfadiazinec cream for antibacterial protection.

Chemical burns secondary to contact with caustic solutions, acids or other irritants may be seen occasionally. The affected areas should be thoroughly washed and the compound neutralized by either sodium bicarbonate solution for acidic compounds, or dilute vinegar for alkaline compounds.

Bumblefoot

Bumblefoot or pododermatitis is a general term for any inflammatory or degenerative condition of the avian foot and may range from very mild redness or swelling to chronic, deep-seated abscesses and bony changes. Considerations for prevention of bumblefoot include proper perches (size, shape and texture), flight pen or cage construction (wall components, substrate, perch arrangements), nutrition, general health of the bird and sanitation of facilities.

Classification and Causes of Bumblefoot

A classification scheme grading from minor early clinical signs progressing to severe lesions is proposed (Table 16.1).

Grade I to III lesions may not be recognized in raptors that are commonly presented with Grade IV or V lesions. Older budgerigars and cockatiels (five to ten years old) may have a Grade V to VI lesion if precipitating factors are not corrected early. Bony changes and osteomyelitis may be present. Prognosis for full recovery of Grades I to IV is usually more favorable than Grade V to VI lesions.

Grade I to III lesions are common in Psittaciformes and Passeriformes that are on all-seed or over-supplemented fruit and vegetable diets, overweight, have no exposure to sunlight or are kept on improper perches (covered with sandpaper, too small or too large, no variance in size). With proper husbandry and nutrition, most cases recover. Substrate, perch size, shape and covering material may all influence the bird's weight distribution on the toes and metatarsal pad and the amount of skin wear on the plantar surface. For example, a perch that is too wide and flat may cause excessive weight-bearing on the toe pads, while one that is too small may cause excessive weight-bearing on the metatarsal pads.

Table 16.1	**Clinical Grades of Bumblefoot**
Grade I	Desquamation of small areas of the plantar foot surfaces represented clinically by the appearance of small, shiny pink areas peeling or flaking of the skin on the legs and feet.
Grade II	Smooth, thinly surfaced, circumscribed areas on the plantar metatarsal pads of one or both feet with the subcutaneous tissue almost visible through the translucent skin. No distinct ulcers are recognized.
Grade III	Ulceration of the plantar metatarsal pads. In some birds a peripheral callus may form.
Grade IV	Necrotic plug of tissue present in ulcer. Most species with ulcers and accumulation of necrotic debris exhibit pain or mild lameness.
Grade V	Swelling and edema (cellulitis) of the tissues surrounding the necrotic debris. The digits or foot may also be edematous. Necrotic debris may start to accumulate in the metatarsal area, suggesting infection of the tendon sheaths. Severe lameness is common. The entire metatarsal pad may be affected. This is generally a chronic lesion.
Grade VI	Necrotic tendons recognized clinically as swelling in the digits and ruptured flexor tendons. Ankelosis and nonfunctioning digits usually present in recovery.
Grade VII	Osteomyelitis.

Prevention and Treatment

Prevention of bumblefoot involves constant vigilance for early signs of hyperkeratosis, baldness, flaking of the skin of feet and legs, redness or swelling and correction of the underlying causes. The walls of an enclosure should be designed with vertical bars or solid barriers to minimize the tendency for hanging from the wire. Selection of proper perch size, shape and cover for a particular species of bird is very important. Perches wrapped with hemp rope or covered with Astroturf work well for most raptors. Falcons do best on flat shelf or block perches covered with short Astroturf or cocoa mats. Strict sanitation of the facilities and feet is important to minimize bacterial infections. Feeding some formulated diets and providing fresh water for bathing prevents or reverses early bumblefoot in Psittaciformes.

The goals of advanced bumblefoot treatment are to reduce inflammation and swelling, ensure an adequate diet, establish drainage if needed, begin an antibacterial therapy to eliminate underlying pathogens, manage the wound to promote rapid healing and address dietary deficiencies. Surgical excision of the abscess or amputation of a severely traumatized digit may be indicated. Treatment for Grade V to VI lesions must be vigorous, and the prognosis is guarded. Treatment for Grade IV should include drainage, irrigation and closing the wound when the infection has been resolved. The prognosis is fair. Grade I to III lesions generally respond to keeping the foot clean and correcting underlying management or nutritional deficiencies. With Anseriformes, this frequently involves changing the dimension, shape and surface of the enclosure, including the addition of adequate swimming areas.

Conservative treatment options may include changing the diet and padding the perches, applying topical medications and, if needed, bandaging. Many topical products have been used, such as softening agents (udder balm or lanolin-based lotions) for dry, scaly feet; topical dimethylsulfoxide (DMSO) for acute inflammation and swelling; hemorrhoidal ointment with live yeast cell derivative for granulating wounds; and liquid bandage products for minor skin cracks or torn talon sheaths.

Moisture vapor permeable dressings or hydrocolloid dressings should be applied topically to enhance wound healing for open, granulating wounds or postoperative incisions. Bandaging of affected Psittaciformes may go on for several months until the bird responds to the new diet. Bandaging options include simple toe bandages, interdigitating bandages and ball bandages.

In raptors, therapy for Grade IV to V lesions include a DMSO preparation that is made by combining piperacillin (1 g) with dexamethasone (4 mg) and DMSO to make a 10 ml mixture. This is refrigerated and discarded after one week. Resolution of Grade IV to VI lesions is slow, and complete healing may take several months. Initial treatment also includes systemic antibiotics for seven to ten days. The entire foot should be cleaned with surgical scrub and any scabs should be soaked free without applying pressure to the wound. A swab taken from deep within the abscesses should be cultured for bacteria and fungus. *E. coli*, *Staphylococcus* and *Candida* are commonly isolated pathogens. The wound should be flushed with copious quantities of one percent povidone iodine solution and allowed to soak for five minutes. The wound should then be flushed with large quantities of sterile saline, the defect packed with a sterile gauze 2 x 2 soaked in povidone iodine solution and a large soft bandage applied. On the second day, the flushing of the wound, gauze pack and bandaging are repeated. Most can be done without anesthesia.

On the third day, swelling may be reduced and much of the exudate gone. Any fibrotic material is removed and the foot is prepared for sterile surgery. A wide exposure of the affected area is made and the abscess wall is dissected out. Any devitalized ligaments or tendons must be removed in their entirety. A tourniquet may be required to control hemorrhage. The wound should be vigorously irrigated with povidone iodine followed by sterile saline. If hemorrhage returns after removing the tourniquet, pressure, epinephrine or selective radiocautery may be used for control, and the wound should be flushed to remove all free blood. The wound is partially sutured shut to allow for drainage, packed with a seton soaked in saline and rebandaged with a large soft wrap. If hemorrhage was poorly controlled, the bandage should be changed in four to six hours.

The bandage should be removed daily and the foot scrubbed and flushed with iodine solution and sterile saline until a "dry socket" is obtained. This may take a week or more. Then the bandage can be changed at two- to three-day intervals. Each time the bandage is changed, the wound should be flushed and kept open as long as there is serum seepage. Mechanical debridement of the wound with a sterile swab will prevent premature closure. The wound may be sutured closed when there is no apparent infection or drainage. Appearance of granulating tissue around the edges of the wound indicates healing is occurring, which may take up to two to five weeks. A week after closure, bandaging can be reduced to only a light wrap. After healing is complete, the foot may still be tender for several weeks. Prevention of trauma and maintaining the patient on soft footing are important to prevent recurrence. Waterfowl should be returned to water as soon as possible to prevent other problems.

Nonsurgical Immobilization of Fractures

The following bandages and splints have been developed and modified to meet specialized anatomic requirements for avian limb immobilization. Specific indications, contraindications and application techniques will be discussed for each type of bandage or splint.

Fracture Stabilization

To be effective, an external coaptation device must immobilize the joint above and below a fracture. Once in place, bandages should be carefully monitored for tissue abrasions, slipping, seepage or swelling in the distal part of a limb, all of which would indicate that the bandage needs to be replaced.

Figure-of-Eight Wing Bandage

The indications for figure-of-eight wing bandages include wing fractures distal to the elbow, luxations of the elbow or carpal joint and soft tissue wounds in these areas that require bandaging and immobilization. In general, external coaptation in the form of a figure-of-eight wing bandage can be considered for the following fractures: most closed fractures of the ulna and radius, when the fragments are relatively well-aligned; most fractures of the major and minor metacarpals; fractures that are too close to a joint or too comminuted to surgically repair; fractures in birds that may not require full return to flight capability; fractures in small or very young birds; and following most orthopedic surgeries of the wing. It is contraindicated to apply a figure-of-eight wing bandage for a humerus fracture without also immobilizing the shoulder with a wing-body wrap.

Application of a figure-of-eight wing bandage is shown in Figure 16.13. It is important to incorporate the scapular or tertiary covert feathers in the bandage and apply the bandage as high in the axillary region as possible to prevent the bandage from slipping below the elbow. The bandage should not extend more than approximately one-half bandage width beyond the elbow joint and should not be applied too tightly. If the primary and secondary flight feathers have a criss-crossed appearance following bandaging (instead of lying parallel), the bandage is too tight. It may be advantageous to tape the tips of the primaries to the tail feathers in birds with long primary feathers.

The length of time a wing bandage is left on is determined by the underlying problem. Most fractures require three to five weeks of bandaging, and soft tissue wounds may require a few days to two weeks of immobilization. Complications of prolonged bandaging are joint stiffness, bony changes, disuse muscle atrophy and occasionally sloughed flight feathers. Weekly bandage changes with physical therapy on the wing, proper bandage application and removal of the bandage as soon as possible after healing will minimize these problems.

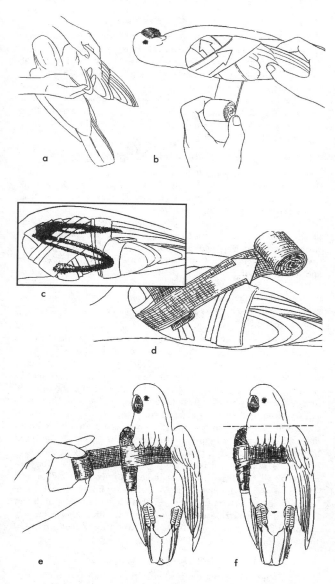

FIG 16.13 a,b,c) Rolled cotton padding is used for the initial layer of a figure-of-eight bandage **d,e)** followed by the application of a self-adherent bandage material. **f)** If the bandage is properly applied, the carpus of the injured wing will be positioned neither higher nor lower than the unbandaged carpus. In addition, the primary and secondary feathers will be in a normal anatomic association. If the primary tips are medial to the secondary feathers, the carpus is being excessively flexed and the bandage is too tight.

Wing-Body Wrap

Fractures or luxations involving the humerus, coracoid, furcula or scapula should be immobilized with a wing-body wrap. Humerus fractures are often immobilized with both figure-of-eight and wing-body wrap bandages, and most of these fractures require orthopedic repair. The legs should be extended to pull the stifle joints away from the keel, and the wing should be folded in a normal flexed position and held to the body using a self-adherent bandage or adhesive tape that does not harm feathers (masking tape or Durapore tape).

Schroeder-Thomas Splint

The use of a Schroeder-Thomas splint is limited to fractures of the tarsometatarsus and the distal one-third of the tibiotarsus. Indications for these splints include fractures of the tarsometatarsus in psittacine birds in which the bone is too small to apply any form of orthopedic repair, fractures too close to the tibiotarsal-tarsometatarsal (hock) joint or foot, uncomplicated fractures in small birds, and following internal surgical fixation of distal tibiotarsal fractures. Contraindications for Schroeder-Thomas splints include all fractures of the femur and proximal two-thirds of the tibiotarsus, because the extreme flexion at the ileal-femoral joint and the wide inguinal skin web in birds results in the proximal portion of the splint acting as a fulcrum and interfering with immobilization.

The wire or rod material of the splint should be made with two right-angle bends next to the ring at the top so that the splint is parallel to the long axis of the leg. The leg should be positioned with some flexion at the hock joint, with the splint angles bent to conform to the angles of the leg. The splint should be slightly longer than the partially flexed leg and extended toes. The leg is lightly bandaged with gauze and tape and is suspended within the splint by alternating strips of tape placed cranially and caudally with the toes extended to the end of the splint. The splinted leg is then covered with bandaging material. Weekly or bimonthly bandage changes with passive physical therapy should be conducted until the fracture heals in four to six weeks. The bird should be provided a low perch so that the splinted leg can hang below or be propped on the perch. With all leg injuries, bumblefoot lesions in the contralateral, weight-bearing foot should be prevented through the use of soft flooring materials, adequate nutrition and, in some cases, ball bandages.

Robert Jones Bandage

The Robert Jones bandage should be limited to simple fractures of the distal one-third of the tibiotarsus and tarsometatarsus, injuries involving the hock joint, soft tissue wounds of the tibiotarsus or tarsometatarsus, or following orthopedic repair of the distal two-thirds of the leg. These heavily padded leg bandages can be used with or without additional splinting material, such as tongue depressors, aluminum splints or orthopedic casting material. Fractures involving the tarsometatarsus should be combined with a ball bandage to immobilize the foot. The Robert

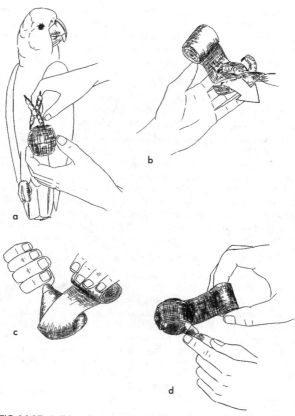

FIG 16.17 Ball bandages can be used to protect foot injuries while they heal. A stack of gauze pads or a piece of cardboard cut to fit the bottom of the foot is covered with cotton padding and placed on the plantar surface of the foot. The foot is then wrapped with a layer of rolled cotton padding and covered with a self-adherent bandage material.

Jones bandage is contraindicated for leg fractures of the femur, proximal two-thirds of the tibiotarsus and in larger birds (eg, over 500 g) because of inadequate immobilization.

A thick layer of casting material is wrapped from the top of the foot to the most proximal point of the leg. The leg is slightly flexed, conforming gauze material is tightly wrapped around the cast padding, additional splinting material is incorporated into the bandage and tape or self-adherent bandaging material is used to cover the bandage. The toes should be monitored for swelling and discoloration if they are not incorporated within the bandage.

Spica Splint

Spica splints may be used for simple, aligned fractures of the femur in smaller birds, but generally need to be combined with orthopedic fracture repair in larger birds (eg, over 300 g). Splint material can be molded from orthopedic casting material or padded aluminum finger splints. This splint is a modification of the Robert Jones bandage, except that the padded, molded splint extends from the tibiotarsus proximally and over the bird's pelvis in an inverted U-shape to immobilize the femur against the body of the bird.

Ball Bandage

Indications for ball bandages include moderate to severe forms of pododermatitis (bumblefoot), toe fractures and other soft tissue injuries involving the toes or feet in perching birds.

The toes should be conformed around a stack of gauze sponges, and wrapped snugly with conforming gauze material to form a teardrop-shaped bandage. There should be adequate padding and support around the distal tarsometatarsus to allow the bird to be able to stand upright on the bandaged foot. It is also important to make sure that the bandage is not applied too tightly around the tarsometatarsus at the top of the bandage, which can cause vascular compromise of the foot. Birds with one or both feet in ball bandages should be placed in an enclosure with a padded surface.

Other Leg and Foot Bandages and Splints

Toe fractures can be immobilized by taping two toes together, by splinting with a padded tongue depressor or cardboard in a modified "snowshoe" splint using two or more toes, or by using thermoplastic coated casting materials to mold a "shoe splint" to fit the entire foot. For small birds, hydrocolloid dressings can be used as splint material for tibiotarsal and tarsometatarsal fractures. The hydrocolloid dressing should be covered by another bandage material to prevent chewing, and should be changed on a daily basis if it becomes moist. When the wound is dry, the dressing can be left in place for up to ten days.

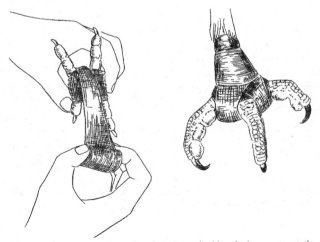

FIG 16.19 An interdigitating bandage is applied by placing gauze on the metatarsal pad and wrapping it in place with cotton padding, which is then covered with a self-adherent bandage.

Soft tissue wounds involving the plantar surface of the foot can be effectively bandaged with an interdigitating bandage that leaves the toes exposed for perching. It is important to avoid applying the bandage too tightly, or using too much bandaging material between cranial digits. The lightest possible bandage would be used in finches and other small birds to prevent loss of balance.

ANTIMICROBIAL THERAPY

Keven Flammer

Published avian drug doses are often based on clinical experience or data extrapolated from other species. Suggested doses may or may not be optimal, and avian veterinarians should be attentive to the possible toxic effects or lack of efficacy when treating birds with empirically derived doses. Subtherapeutic dosing can result in treatment failure and encourage the development of microbial resistance. Excessive drug treatment may be toxic and damage the kidneys or liver. In particular, care should be extended when treating rare birds in which the effects of a specific drug have not been investigated.

Table 17.1 General Approach to Treatment of Bacterial Diseases

1. **Identify** the pathogen and location of infection.

2. **Determine** the antimicrobial susceptibility of the isolate if the susceptibility cannot be predicted.

3. **Select** an antimicrobial drug based on susceptibility, ability to reach the site of infection, available routes of administration, required frequency of administration and minimal toxicity to the host.

4. **Determine** if it is feasible for the bird owner to complete the treatment regimen.

5. **Treat** with appropriate antibiotics.

6. **Maintain** host defenses by reducing stress and maximizing supportive care.

7. **Find** and **eliminate** the source of bacteria.

8. **Decontaminate** the bird's environment.

Antimicrobial Spectrum

Some microbial organisms have predictable susceptibility. For example, all strains of chlamydia are presumed to be susceptible to tetracyclines. Unfortunately, the most common infectious agents in psittacine birds (gram-negative bacteria, streptococcus and staphylococcus) have unpredictable antimicrobial susceptibilities, and an *in vitro* susceptibility test is required to aid drug selection.

Antimicrobial susceptibility tests using dilution methods determine the minimal inhibitory concentration (MIC) of the antibiotic. Since the MIC is quantitative, it allows the clinician to select the drug to which the organism is most susceptible and provides a better prediction of treatment success.

In a severely ill patient, or in one that has an infection in an area that is difficult to culture, it may be necessary to start treatment without the benefit of a culture and susceptibility test. In these cases it is helpful to know the common causes of infection and the antimicrobial drugs most likely to be effective.

The most common causes of primary and secondary microbial infections in psittacine birds are gram-negative bacteria, chlamydia and yeast. Gram-negative bacteria are frequently resistant to routine antibiotics (eg, ampicillin, tetracycline, chloramphenicol and erythromycin); however, most isolates are susceptible to trimethoprim/sulfa combinations, enrofloxacin, amikacin, and the advanced generation cephalosporins (eg, cefotaxime) and penicillins (eg, piperacillin). Yeast are usually confined to the alimentary tract. Most are susceptible to treatment with nystatin, ketoconazole or fluconazole. Chlamydia are susceptible to treatment with tetracyclines.

Less common infectious agents of psittacine birds are gram-positive bacteria (*Staphylococcus aureus* and some *Streptococcus* spp.), mycoplasma, systemic fungi and mycobacteria. Many of the *S. aureus* and streptococcus isolates tested by the author are susceptible to cephalexin or cephalothin. Mycoplasma are presumed to be susceptible to enrofloxacin, tetracyclines and tylosin. Systemic fungal infections are difficult to treat under any circumstances and require multiple drug therapy with amphotericin B and itraconazole, fluconazole or flucytosine. Mycobacteria are extremely difficult to eliminate. *Mycobacterium avium* can cause fatal infections in immunosuppressed humans, and therapeutic management must be considered with caution (see Chapter 33).

Clinical Applications

- Prolonged tetracycline therapy may be catabolic, cause immunosuppression, reduce normal gut flora or render a bird more susceptible to secondary pathogens.

- Nystatin must come in direct contact with yeast to be effective. If nystatin is delivered by gavage tube, infections in the mouth will not be treated.

- Medicated food and water are traditionally favored routes for poultry but seldom achieve therapeutic drug concentrations in companion and aviary birds.

- Birds receiving antibiotics should be monitored for secondary infections with cloacal cultures and fecal Gram's stains.

- Trimethoprim/sulfadiazine is often effective for treating gram-negative infections in nestling birds.

- Critically ill birds should be treated via parenteral routes to establish effective drug concentration quickly.

- Given orally, the IM formulation of enrofloxacin produces therapeutic plasma concentrations.

Pharmacodynamics of the Drug

Most bacteria remain extracellular while causing infection; however, there are a few notable exceptions (eg, salmonella, mycobacteria, some staphylococci). Treatment of intracellular infections may require drugs that are highly lipophilic and can penetrate cells (eg, chloramphenicol). Polar drugs (eg, the beta lactams, aminoglycosides) are often excluded from pharmacologically privileged spaces such as cerebrospinal fluid (CSF) and ocular fluids.

The pharmacokinetics of the drug are also important. With bacteriostatic drugs, it is desirable to maintain the concentration of drug above the bacterial MIC for at least half of the dosage interval, and preferably throughout the interval, if this is attainable and not toxic. With most bacteriocidal drugs, it is not necessary to maintain the drug above the MIC for the entire dosage interval; however, if concentrations drop below the MIC for too long, the bacteria will multiply, and a "break-through bacteremia" may occur. Although allometric scaling has validity for some compounds, veterinarians should be aware of its limitations. Evaluation of drug excretion and potential metabolic pathways are important, as numerous exceptions to scaling exist — some with potentially toxic results.

Route of Administration

Factors to consider when selecting a route include: 1) The severity of the infection. Critically ill birds should be treated with parenteral medications to establish effective drug concentrations quickly. 2) The number of birds to be treated. Medicated food or water may be the only practical way to treat multiple-bird flocks. 3) The availability of appropriate drug formulations. 4) The frequency of administration, resultant stress to the bird and the labor involved in completing the treatment regimen. 5) The ability of the owner to complete the treatment regimen.

Water-based Drug Administration

There are some specific drugs and therapeutic situations where water-based administration may be successful. Enrofloxacin may successfully treat highly susceptible gram-negative bacteria (MIC <0.05 mg/ml). Sulfachlorpyridizine may be effective against alimentary tract infections caused by highly susceptible strains of *Escherichia coli*. Spectinomycin may be effective against alimentary tract infections caused by highly susceptible strains of *E. coli*. Nitrofurazone may slow the spread of salmonella within a flock. Aminoglycosides (eg, gentamicin, neomycin and amikacin) are not absorbed but may have a local effect against pathogens in the gut. Tetracyclines may slow the spread and alleviate clinical signs in birds with chlamydiosis but will not consistently clear birds of infection. Tetracyclines degrade rapidly in water. Chlorhexidine may inhibit the spread and severity of candida infections of the alimentary tract.

Food-based Drug Administration

Powders, ground tablets and oral suspensions can be added to a palatable food vehicle such as cooked mashes, rolled corn, canned and frozen vegetables or fruit mixtures. A cooked mash containing 13% dry oatmeal and 29% each cooked kidney beans, rice, and corn is nutritious and well accepted by many psittacine birds. If a favorite treat food is well accepted and quickly consumed, it may be possible to lace it with the divided daily drug dose and offer it several times daily.

Formulated diets containing chlortetracycline are commercially available and can be used to treat chlamydiosis. Chlortetracycline-impregnated millet seed is also available and is readily accepted by budgerigars and finches. These products sustain chlortetracycline blood concentrations of 0.5-1.5 mg/ml when fed with diets containing < 0.7% calcium. It is also possible to prepare a medicated mash using powdered chlortetracycline.

Oral Medication

It is surprisingly difficult to force psittacine birds to accept oral medications. Bird owners may initially be able to administer the drug, but as treatment progresses the bird may become more difficult to medicate. Sometimes the stress of handling exceeds the benefits of the drug itself. Acceptance can be improved if the drug is mixed with a palatable vehicle such as lactulose syrup or fruit juice. Oral suspensions and solutions are appropriate for use in all birds; tablets and pills are probably not appropriate for use in birds with a crop. Capsules that rapidly dissolve can be used in those birds that are "pillable" (eg, pigeons, waterfowl and gallinaceous birds).

Intramuscular Injection

Intramuscular injection is often the quickest and least stressful method of directly administering drugs to companion birds. Most bird owners can be taught to perform this procedure. The proximal two-thirds of the pectoral muscles provide the optimal injection site. Drugs injected into the muscles of the legs may pass through the renal portal system first, clearing the drug before it can reach the systemic circulation.

Intramuscular injection may not be feasible in all birds. Nestling birds of all species have relatively little pectoral muscle mass, and it is easy to pierce the sternum, which is non-ossified at this age. Ratites, even as adults, lack large pectoral muscles. Owners of racing pigeons, raptors and some game birds may refuse to give medications IM in the breast because they fear muscle damage will interfere with flight or normal activity.

The injection volume in relation to body size must also be considered. For example, on a body weight basis, a 0.05 ml injection in a canary is equivalent to a 40 ml injection in a 25 kg dog. Injection volumes in psittacine birds should be small but permit accurate measurement of the medication.

Subcutaneous Injection

The subcutaneous route is not ideal but can be used for irritating drugs when muscle necrosis or injection trauma is to be avoided. This site is often used by pigeon and game bird breeders.

Intravenous Injection

The right jugular, superficial ulnar, basilic vein on the ventral humerus and superficial plantar veins are most accessible. Intravenous catheters are available but are potentially dangerous to leave in unattended birds. Intravenous fluids can be delivered as a slow bolus at a dose of 10 ml/kg without pulmonary compromise.

Intraosseous Injection

A cannula can be inserted and used for repeated fluid or drug administration. If properly bandaged, psittacine birds will usually tolerate cannulas for short periods of time. Intraosseous cannulas are well tolerated in raptors, pigeons, waterfowl and other less temperamental species. The distal ulna and proximal tibia are the best locations for cannulation.

Only fluids or nonirritating drugs should be delivered via intraosseous cannulas. Sterility is critical, as infection may result in osteomyelitis.

Nebulization

Nebulized antibiotics are useful for pulmonary, sinus and trachea infections, and are often combined with mucolytic and penetrating agents (eg, DMSO) to break down caseous material and increase antibiotic uptake. Simple humidification of the lungs is also helpful.

Topical Medications

Skin: Oily and toxic compounds should be avoided, as they will mat the feathers and be ingested when the bird preens. If it is necessary to use greasy compounds, the site should be bandaged or the bird collared to prevent preening and ingestion.

Eye: Liquid eye drops retard corneal healing less than ointments but must be given more frequently. Ointments should be applied very sparingly, as excess ointment will cause matting and loss of feathers surrounding the eye. Misting the eye with a water-soluble, topical spray may also be effective. Subconjunctival injections may be considered for delivering repository drugs.

Nasal Flushes: Antibiotics can be added to flushing solutions, but in many cases unmedicated saline works as well.

Infraorbital Sinus Injection: Sinus injection is useful for flushing and delivering medication into the infraorbital sinus in birds with sinusitis. The injection is made at the level of the commissure of the beak, just ventral to the zygomatic arch, the same site as for cytologic sampling (see Chapter 10). If sinusitis has resulted in blockage of the outflow tracts, low volumes of fluid must be slowly injected to prevent exophthalmus. Only nonirritating drugs should be used.

Intratracheal (through the glottis): This is an effective route for delivering amphotericin B to birds suffering from tracheal and pulmonary aspergillosis.

Toxicity and Adverse Effects of Antimicrobial Therapy

All antimicrobial drugs have the potential to harm the host. Direct toxic effects and the reduction of normal alimentary tract flora can occur even when antibiotics are used properly, requiring that birds should be monitored during treatment. Treatment failure and the development of resistant strains of bacteria occur most often when drugs are used improperly. Routine prophylactic treatment of birds without a clear indication of infection is not suggested in any circumstance.

Direct Toxic Effects

Beta lactam antibiotics have relatively few direct toxic effects. The aminoglycosides are nephrotoxic at therapeutic doses and should be used with extreme caution in juvenile and dehydrated birds. Sulfa drugs should also be used cautiously in birds that are uricemic, because they are potentially nephrotoxic in dehydrated animals and are metabolized via the same metabolic pathway in the liver as uric acid. The fluroquinolones cause defects in the articular cartilage of some species of growing animals (eg, dogs, pigeons and horses) but not others (eg, cats). To date, toxic effects have not been proven in psittacine birds treated with recommended doses of fluroquinolones.

Adverse Effects on Normal Alimentary Tract Flora

Most of the antibiotics used in avian practice are broad spectrum and their use will reduce or eliminate normal alimentary tract flora. Eliminating normal flora may render the bird more susceptible to colonization by potential pathogens such as yeast, viruses and gram-negative bacteria. Birds receiving antibiotics should be monitored for secondary infections with cloacal cultures and fecal Gram's stains.

It may be advisable to culture the cloaca prior to antimicrobial treatment of all birds, even if the alimentary tract is not the primary site of infection. If potential pathogens are isolated, the treatment regimen should include a drug that will be effective for these organisms as well as the primary pathogens; otherwise minor alimentary tract pathogens may proliferate and cause illness if the competition from normal flora is eliminated. Young and immunocompromised birds should be monitored every day during antimicrobial therapy to prevent potential yeast infections.

Treatment Failure

It is important to establish a correct diagnosis and implement an effective treatment plan early in the disease process because there is seldom time to simply try a drug and see what happens. If the wrong drug or route of administration is selected, or if the problem is not due to a microbial infection, the bird may die while waiting to determine if prophylactic therapy is successful.

Some pet stores may sell over-the-counter (OTC) antibiotics with label claims that they are beneficial for treating a variety of avian respiratory and gastrointestinal complaints. Most of these products contain tetracycline, erythromycin or a sulfa drug, and are compounded for water administration. These products are seldom effective at the doses and routes recommended, and many bird owners waste valuable time attempting treatment with these products before consulting an avian veterinarian. By the time the bird receives appropriate care, it is usually too late. Bird owners should be educated to avoid these useless medications and to use more effective diagnostic and therapeutic methods with their pets.

Development of Resistant Strains of Bacteria

Bacteria develop resistance to drugs by two primary methods: transfer of plasmids and chromosomal mutation. These methods may: 1) induce production of an enzyme that degrades the antibiotic; 2) alter membrane permeability and therefore prevent the antibiotic from penetrating the bacteria; or 3) create an alternate metabolic pathway that bypasses the action of the antibiotics. Resistance is most common among gram-positive and gram-negative bacteria and less common in anaerobes, chlamydia and yeast.

Sub-therapeutic treatment can encourage the development of resistant bacteria.

Antibacterial Therapy

Fluoroquinolones

Pharmacology

The fluoroquinolones are a relatively new class of antimicrobial drugs that inhibit bacterial gyrase, the enzyme responsible for coiling DNA within the bacterial nucleus. They are bactericidal, widely distributed to tissues and the extracellular space, and are excreted primarily through renal tubular secretion and glomerular filtration. Fluoroquinolones are generally well tolerated, although gastrointestinal upset and anorexia have been occasionally reported, and they may induce seizures in seizure-prone animals.

Use in Companion Avian Medicine

Enrofloxacin: Enrofloxacin has excellent activity against mycoplasma, some gram-positive bacteria and most gram-negative bacteria. Resistance of *Pseudomonas* spp. is occasionally seen. Enrofloxacin is highly active against most Enterobacteriaceae recovered from psittacine birds. It reduces clinical signs in birds infected with *Chlamydia psittaci*, but anecdotal comments indicate that enrofloxacin treatment does not routinely clear the carrier state.

Combination therapy in Senegal Parrots treated with enrofloxacin-medicated drinking water (100 ppm) and ketoconazole (30 mg/kg PO q24h) for 10 days produced evidence of renal toxicity. Recommended doses are 5 mg/kg, q12h IM, PO or SC, or 100-200 ppm (0.1-0.2 mg/ml) in the drinking water for highly susceptible bacteria. Enrofloxacin and ciprofloxacin have been widely used in psittacine nurseries without reports of side effects. However, the drug should be used with caution in growing birds since toxic effects are species-specific and dose-related, and the drug has not been studied in all species. There have been scattered, anecdotal reports of aggressive, irritable behavior in adult Amazon parrots treated with quinolones.

Penicillins

The penicillins are beta lactam antibiotics. They inhibit the formation of the bacterial cell wall and are bactericidal for growing and dividing organisms.

Penicillins are widely distributed to the extracellular space but poorly penetrate the CSF. Excretion is rapid (half-lives are usually less than 60 minutes) and is accomplished primarily through renal tubular secretion and glomerular filtration. Procaine penicillin may cause adverse reactions in small patients due to the procaine component. Penicillins have reduced efficacy in the presence of overwhelming numbers of organisms ("inoculum effect"). Penicillins are synergistic when combined with aminoglycosides, and this combination can be used to treat severe infections, especially those caused by *Pseudomonas* spp.

Use in Companion Avian Medicine

Natural Penicillins: They are rarely used in avian medicine due to the availability of more effective drugs.

Ampicillin/Amoxicillin: Many gram-positive bacteria are susceptible to ampicillin and amoxicillin, but most gram-negative isolates are resistant at concentrations achievable in birds.

Ticarcillin: The pharmacology of ticarcillin is similar to that of carbenicillin; however, it is often two to four times more active against *Pseudomonas* spp. It is available for parenteral administration only.

Piperacillin: It is widely used by avian veterinarians to treat systemic gram-negative bacterial infections. Doses up to 1000 mg/kg did not induce clinically apparent toxic effects. Doses of 75-100 mg/kg IM administered three to six times daily have been recommended. Higher and more frequent doses should be used in more severe infections.

Clavulinic Acid: When combined with a penicillin, it inhibits beta-lactamase, a bacterial enzyme that inactivates many penicillins. Reports of use in birds are rare, but this drug may offer safe, effective activity against gram-negative and gram-positive pathogens.

Cephalosporins

Pharmacology

Cephalosporins are beta lactam antibiotics. They are widely distributed in the extracellular space, but most products poorly penetrate the cerebrospinal fluid and other pharmacologically privileged spaces. Excretion is primarily through renal tubular secretion and glomerular filtration. They are classified into first, second and third generation products. In general, first generation products are effective against many gram-positive and some gram-negative bacteria, while increasing generations demonstrate enhanced gram-negative activity but reduced activity against gram-positives. Like the penicillins, cephalosporins also suffer from the "inoculum effect".

First Generation Agents (eg, cephalexin and cephalothin): The antimicrobial spectrum of first generation agents includes most gram-positive cocci, some gram-negative bacteria and some anaerobes.

Second generation agents (eg, cefoxitin and cetaxitin) have increased gram-negative activity and are available primarily in parenteral formulations. There are few reports of their use in birds.

Third generation agents (eg, cefotaxime and ceftriaxone) have an expanded gram-negative spectrum (including increased activity against *Pseudomonas* spp.) and variable activity against gram-positive bacteria. Cefotaxime is unusual among cephalosporins because it penetrates the CSF in effective concentrations. Doses of 75-100 mg/kg IM given three to six times daily should maintain effective plasma concentrations.

Aminoglycosides

Pharmacology

Aminoglycoside antibiotics interfere with bacterial protein synthesis and are bactericidal. They are not absorbed from the GI tract and must be administered parenterally. Aminoglycosides are confined to the extracellular space and poorly penetrate the eye and cerebrospinal fluid. Excretion is almost exclusively by glomerular filtration. Aminoglycosides must penetrate the bacterial cell wall to interfere with protein synthesis. This process requires oxygen, so aminoglycosides are not active against anaerobes or at sites with low oxygen tension (eg, large abscesses).

Nephrotoxicity and ototoxicity are relatively common. The nephrotoxicity associated with recommended dosage regimens and short-term treatment is usually reversible once treatment stops. Chronic renal dysfunction occurs when high-dose or prolonged therapy is attempted. Aminoglycosides should be used with caution in dehydrated patients. Neuromuscular synaptic dysfunction and paralysis can occur if the drug is given intravenously at a rapid rate.

Use in Companion Avian Medicine

Gentamicin: Gentamicin is effective against many gram-negative and gram-positive bacteria. It is more toxic than amikacin, and signs of nephrotoxicity (eg, polyuria and polydipsia) are often encountered even when birds are treated with low doses. A dosage of 2.5 mg/kg IM q8h is recommended for psittacines and raptors. Previously recommended doses (10 mg/kg IM q8h) are excessive and may cause severe toxicity and death.

Tobramycin: The pharmacology of tobramycin in mammals is similar to that of gentamicin, but it has greater activity against *Pseudomonas* spp. and some other gram-negative bacteria. In dogs and humans, tobramycin is considered slightly less toxic than gentamicin but more so than amikacin. The estimated dose for tobramycin is 2.5-5 mg/kg IM q12h.

Amikacin: Amikacin has excellent activity against many gram-negative bacteria, including some strains that are resistant to gentamicin and tobramycin. Amikacin causes fewer toxic side effects and is the aminoglycoside of choice for use in birds.

Amikacin doses of 10-15 mg/kg IM administered q8-12h should provide effective plasma concentrations for most susceptible gram-negative bacteria. In dehydrated birds and those with compromised renal function, the dose should be reduced or a less toxic drug selected.

The aminoglycosides are excellent drugs for treating resistant gram-negative bacterial infections in birds. They are active against *Pseudomonas* spp., especially when combined with a third generation cephalosporin (eg, cefotaxime) or late generation penicillin (eg, piperacillin). However, these two agents must not be combined in the same syringe.

Tetracyclines

Pharmacology

Tetracyclines interfere with bacterial protein synthesis and are bacteriostatic. Tetracyclines are primarily used to treat chlamydiosis and mycoplasmosis. Tetracyclines are lipid soluble and are widely distributed to tissue. Oral absorption is generally good except in the presence of cations such as calcium or magnesium. Tetracyclines will chelate calcium in the teeth and bone. GI upset and photosensitization have been reported. Prolonged treatment may have catabolic and immunosuppressive effects, reduce normal gut flora and render the animal more susceptible to opportunistic infections.

Chlortetracycline: Diets containing 1% chlortetracycline are recommended for treating psittacine chlamydiosis in the United States. Diets containing 0.5% chlortetracycline have been shown to be effective in Europe. Powdered chlortetracycline can be added to a cooked mash, or medicated pellets are commercially available. Although medicated diets may be successful in reducing the clinical signs of chlamydiosis, common sequelae to treatment include diet refusal, starvation, treatment failures and secondary microbial infections.

Minocycline: This drug has an extended half-life in mammals. It has been used experimentally to coat millet seeds and treat chlamydiosis in small psittacine birds.

Doxycycline: Doxycycline has a prolonged half-life and differs from conventional tetracyclines because it is more lipophilic. The half-life varies with the species. At oral doses of 50 mg/kg, the half-life averages ten hours in cockatiels and Amazon parrots and greater than 20 hours in cockatoos and macaws.

This is the drug of choice for treating chlamydiosis, and oral dosage recommendations are: 40-50 mg/kg PO q12h in cockatiels and Blue-fronted and Orange-winged Amazons; 25 mg/kg PO q12h in African Grey Parrots, Goffin's Cockatoos and Blue and Gold and Green-winged Macaws. In untested species it is impossible to precisely extrapolate dosages; however, 25-30 mg/kg is the recommended starting dose in cockatoos and macaws, and 25-50 mg/kg is recommended other species.

If regurgitation occurs, the dose should be reduced by 25% or divided and administered q12h. Hepatotoxicity, as detected by elevated AST and LDH tests, may occur in macaws. Dosage recommendations for treating chlamydiosis in psittacine birds with injectable doxycycline (Vibravenös formulation only!) is 75-100 mg/kg IM every five to seven days. In macaws, the lower dose and more frequent administration should be administered in the last three weeks of treatment. There have been anecdotal reports of use of pharmacist-compounded injectable doxycycline products; however, kinetic studies are lacking and it is impossible to extrapolate dosage schedules from one formulation to another.

Trimethoprim/Sulfonamide Combinations

Pharmacology

A combination of trimethoprim and a sulfonamide is synergistic, as both drugs interfere with microbial folic acid synthesis. This combination has good efficacy against many gram-positive and gram-negative bacterial pathogens, with the exclusion of *Pseudomonas* spp. Use of these drugs in combination has largely replaced use of either component alone for treatment of systemic bacterial infections. The sulfa drugs are primarily distributed to the extracellular space, while trimethoprim is more lipophilic and has good tissue penetration. Excretion is primarily renal.

Empirical doses of 16-24 mg/kg trimethoprim/sulfonamide (oral solution) administered q12h, and 8 mg/kg IM (40 mg/ml trimethoprim + 200 mg/ml sulfadiazine) q12h have been widely used clinically with good success.

Trimethoprim and sulfonamide combinations have few toxic effects, but many birds (especially macaws) suffer GI upset and will regurgitate one to three hours after an oral dose. The incidence of GI upset can be reduced if the drug is added to a small amount of food or if the dose is reduced. Sulfonamides form crystals and damage renal glomeruli in dehydrated birds and those with compromised renal function. The injectable product may cause irritation and necrosis at the site of injection.

Trimethoprim/sulfadiazine is an excellent broad-spectrum bacteriostatic drug. It is often the drug of choice when using the oral route to deliver antibiotics (eg, treating gram-negative infections in nestling birds).

Macrolides and Lincosamides

Pharmacology

The macrolides and lincosamides interfere with bacterial protein synthesis, are bacteriostatic and share similar pharmacology. Their spectrum of action includes gram-positive bacteria, pasteurella, bordetella, some mycoplasma and obligate anaerobic bacteria. All are well distributed to tissues and eliminated primarily by hepatic metabolism.

The primary uses for the macrolides are to treat gram-positive infections in finches, suspected or confirmed mycoplasma in psittacine birds and gram-positive or anaerobic osteomyelitis. These drugs are also active against *Campylobacter* spp. and *Clostridia* spp. Clindamycin is the most active of the listed drugs.

Tylosin: Effective pulmonary concentrations were achieved with nebulization of 1 gram tylosin in 50 ml dimethyl sulfoxide (DMSO) for one hour. Treatment of conjunctivitis in cockatiels with a tylosin and water spray has been suggested.

Erythromycin: Erythromycin is rarely used in companion and aviary birds.

Clindamycin: Clindamycin is the most active of the macrolides mentioned. It is used to treat anaerobic infections and osteomyelitis caused by susceptible gram-positive pathogens.

New Macrolides (eg, azithromycin, clarithromycin): The disposition and safety of these drugs in birds remain to be investigated.

Lincomycin: Lincomycin is usually combined with spectinomycin and has been used in finches to treat respiratory and alimentary tract infections caused by gram-positive bacteria and mycoplasma in other species.

Chloramphenicol

Pharmacology

Chloramphenicol interferes with bacterial protein synthesis and is bacteriostatic. Its antimicrobial spectrum includes many gram-positive and some gram-negative bacteria. It will inhibit chlamydial growth and alleviate clinical signs in infected birds, but will not routinely clear a bird of infection. Oral absorption is highly erratic. Chloramphenicol is highly lipid-soluble and is widely distributed to most tissues, including the central nervous system.

Potential toxic effects include reversible dose-related bone marrow depression, inhibition of hepatic microsomal enzyme synthesis, inhibition of host protein synthesis resulting in decreased wound healing and decreased immunoglobulin synthesis. In a small percentage of the human population, non-dose-related, irreversible, aplastic anemia may occur, even with mild cutaneous contact. For this reason, clients are instructed to handle this drug carefully and wear gloves when treating birds. Doses of 50 mg/kg IM q8h of the injectable formulation are recommended for most psittacine birds.

Use of chloramphenicol has been largely replaced by other antibiotics. Chloramphenicol is still useful for treating infections caused by susceptible intracellular bacteria (eg, salmonella) and where penetration into the central nervous system is desired. Chloramphenicol is bacteriostatic and is probably not the drug of choice for initial treatment of severe, life-threatening infections.

Antifungal Therapy

Nystatin

Pharmacology

Nystatin is a polyene antimicrobial that disrupts the fungal cell membrane by substituting for ergosterol. It is effective against most strains of candida and some other yeasts, although clinical evidence suggests resistant yeast strains may occur in some psittacine nurseries. It is not absorbed from the GI tract and is available for oral or topical use only. It must come in direct contact with the yeast to be effective. Treatment failures may occur if the nystatin is delivered via a tube or syringe to the back of the oral pharynx, bypassing more rostral sites of infection in the mouth.

If resistance or a non-alimentary tract infection is encountered, a systemically active antifungal should be used.

Individual birds can be treated with 300,000 IU/kg orally q8-12h for five to ten days. Nystatin can also be added to hand-feeding formulas for prophylactic treatment in nurseries experiencing chronic yeast problems.

Amphotericin B

Pharmacology

Amphotericin B is a polyene antimicrobial drug that disrupts the fungal cell membrane by substituting for ergosterol. It is active against most of the yeast and fungi of medical importance. Resistance by some strains of *Aspergillus* spp. has been reported in man and other animals. Clinical data demonstrating improved efficacy when amphotericin B is combined with flucytosine or an azole antifungal are conflicting, but combination therapy is a common practice for treating serious fungal infections in humans. Amphotericin B is not well absorbed after oral administration and is too irritating for intramuscular or subcutaneous injection; thus, it must be delivered intravenously or used topically. It is widely distributed to tissue and extracellular spaces where it is metabolized and slowly excreted in the urine.

It has been used in combination with flucytosine in raptors and swans with fair results. A new, orally active azole, itraconazole, may offer similar activity or may potentiate the effects of amphotericin B.

Amphotericin B can be nebulized or injected into an affected air sac for respiratory infections. It can also be injected through the glottis or administered transtracheally to treat tracheal and syringeal aspergillosis. A topical cream in a plasticized base is available for treatment of topical lesions and oral candidiasis.

Doses of 1.5 mg/kg IV q12h are recommended. The drug may be safer in avian than mammalian species. However, until more information on avian use is available, patients receiving this drug should be monitored for signs of nephrotoxicity (polyuria and uricemia).

Flucytosine

Pharmacology

This drug is excreted almost entirely unmetabolized in the urine, and dosage modifications are necessary in patients with reduced renal function. Dose-related, reversible bone marrow depression is the major toxic change seen in humans, presumably due to the conversion of flucytosine into 5-fluorouracil by GI tract bacteria. Hepatotoxicity and GI toxicity are occasionally reported in mammals.

Flucytosine has been used singly as a prophylactic treatment to prevent aspergillosis in highly susceptible avian species undergoing stress (eg, hospitalization of swans) and in combination with other drugs to treat respiratory aspergillosis. *In vitro* susceptibility of eleven strains of *Aspergillus fumigatus* indicated that flucytosine doses of 20-30 mg/kg q6h would maintain inhibitory plasma concentrations. Because reported *in vitro* susceptibility data varies greatly, a combination of flucytosine, amphotericin B and rifampin has been suggested for treating respiratory *Aspergillosis* in raptors. Clinically, doses of 50 mg/kg orally q12h for two to four weeks appears to prevent aspergillosis when prophylactically administered to swans. Flucytosine has been safe for long-term use (two to four weeks) in raptors and waterfowl. Successful treatment of esophageal and subcutaneous aspergillosis in a cockatoo has been reported using a combination of flucytosine (65 mg/kg orally q12h) and ketoconazole (20 mg/kg orally q12h) for approximately one month.

Ketoconazole

The use of the azole antifungals in veterinary medicine has been reviewed. They inhibit synthesis of the primary fungal sterol, ergosterol, which is important in fungal cell membrane integrity. Potential toxic effects of interfering with vertebrate P_{450} enzymes include decreased synthesis of cholesterol, cortisol and reproductive steroid hormones. All three azoles are fungistatic and several days of therapy are needed to achieve steady-state concentrations.

Pharmacology

Ketoconazole is effective against many of the yeast and fungi of medical importance, but *Aspergillus* spp. are often resistant. It is widely distributed to tissues but is highly protein-bound and does not significantly penetrate into the cerebrospinal or ocular fluids. Reports of toxicity are rare in birds.

Ketoconazole is available in 200 mg tablets. Crushed tablets can be compounded with 0.15% methylcellulose into an oral suspension that is stable for six months if refrigerated.

Ketoconazole is currently the most widely used, least expensive, orally available and systemically active antifungal. It is useful for treating resistant yeast infections and yeast infections where systemic drug delivery is required. It is not usually effective against aspergillosis alone, but may have a synergistic effect when combined with other antifungals. It appears to be safe and effective when administered 20-30 mg/kg q12h, PO, up to 30 days.

Itraconazole

Pharmacology

Itraconazole is similar to ketoconazole but has 5-100 times greater potency, better *in vitro* and *in vivo* activity against *Aspergillus* infections and meningeal cryptococcoses, and fewer side effects. It is insoluble in water, highly lipophilic and is well absorbed if taken with a meal. It is poorly distributed to CSF, ocular fluids and plasma. It is degraded by hepatic metabolism, and the primary route of elimination is via the bile.

Fluconazole

Pharmacology

In vitro potencies of fluconazole up to 100 times greater than ketoconazole. Most yeast and fungi of medical importance are susceptible to fluconazole *in vitro*. *In vivo*, it has excellent activity against yeast and variable activity against *Aspergillus*. In contrast to ketoconazole and itraconazole, fluconazole is highly water soluble and is readily absorbed from the GI tract regardless of acidity or food intake. It is not highly protein-bound and penetrates the CSF, brain tissue, ocular fluids and sputum. It is eliminated primarily by the kidney. The dose should be modified if renal function is impaired. The manufacturer recommends giving a double loading dose during the first 24 hours, because five to seven days are needed to achieve steady-state concentrations in man.

It is probably the drug of choice in situations where penetration into the CSF is desirable.

Juvenile psittacine birds treated with fluconazole were found to be fecal negative for yeast as determined by Gram's stain; clearance of yeast required 48 hours. Based on this limited study, dosage recommendations of 2-5 mg/kg/day were suggested. Transient regurgitation, increased AST and LDH levels were observed in some birds. Further studies are needed to establish the safety and efficacy of fluconazole in birds.

Summary of Anitfungal Treatment

Nystatin is the drug of choice for uncomplicated yeast infections of the alimentary tract. It is inexpensive and virtually nontoxic. Resistant or severe yeast infections can be treated with ketoconazole or fluconazole. Systemic yeast infections can be treated with either ketoconazole, fluconazole or itraconazole, depending on the site of infection.

Cutaneous aspergillosis is probably best treated with fluconazole or itraconazole. Topical administration of enilconazole or miconazole may also be effective. Severe pulmonary or disseminated aspergillosis carries a poor prognosis for recovery regardless of the treatment program. Amphotericin B is the primary drug of choice for chronic infections and infections in immunocompromised patients because it rapidly develops fungicidal concentrations. Based on human clinical studies, it is probably most effective to use amphotericin B in combination with itraconazole for initial treatment, and then continue long-term treatment for months with itraconazole alone. Flucytosine also has substantial anti-aspergillus activity and may be preferable if there is CNS involvement. Intratracheal administration of amphotericin B is very useful when treating syringeal or tracheal infections. Systemic infections caused by other fungi (eg, mucormycosis and cryptococcosis) can be treated in the same manner as systemic aspergillosis.

Table 17.2   Susceptibility of Common Avian Infectious Agents to Antimicrobial Therapy, in Decreasing Order

Gram-negative bacteria	Amikacin, 3rd generation Cephalosporins, Trimethoprim/Sulfa, Enrofloxacin, Gentamicin
Pseudomonas	Amikacin, 3rd generation Cephalosporins, Gentamicin
Gram-positive bacteria	1st generation Cephalosporins, Macrolides (Tylosin, Clindamycin), New Macrolides, Trimethoprim/Sulfa, Amikacin, Ampicillin/Amoxicillin, Chloramphenicol, Enrofloxacin, Gentamicin
Mycoplasma	Enrofloxacin, Tetracycline
Chlamydia	Tetracycline
Anaerobes	Macrolides (Tylosin, Clindamycin), New Macrolides
Yeast	Amphotericin, Flucocytosine, Fluconazole, Itraconazole, Nystatin
Aspergillus	Itraconazole, Amphotericin, Fluconazole
Other Fungi	Amphotericin, Flucytosine, Itraconazole

FORMULARY

Branson W. Ritchie
Greg J. Harrison

This chapter provides an overview of the unique characteristics of various drugs used in avian species. All suggested drug uses are for companion (non-food) birds only. Complete reviews of all the drugs discussed in this book are available through a variety of desk references and product information forms provided by the manufacturers. The clinician is referred to these references for a review of the general pharmacology and specific contraindications of any drug discussed. The suggestions of the manufacturer should always be followed. A drug should never be used for which the clinician is not fully aware of the indications, contraindications and potential side effects. Some drugs administered concurrently will potentiate toxicity, and the clinician should review any potential drug interactions before placing a bird on more than one drug at a time.

In this chapter, commonly used drugs and their associated doses are provided in table form for easy reference. The information concerning the use of the drugs listed in the table should be reviewed before administering any therapeutic agent. If a drug is not discussed, either insufficient data is available to warrant its use in birds, or it has been used but has little applicability.

The doses and material presented for each drug have been compiled from numerous reference sources, including the various chapters in this book and have been updated as of 10-96. Some of the recommended doses are based on pharmacokinetic information, and some are based totally on observation. Although every effort has been made to ensure accuracy (particularly drug doses), it is the responsibility of the clinician to critically evaluate the material. Notes on any adverse drug reactions should be forwarded to Wingers Publishing (P.O. Box 6863, Lake Worth, FL 33466) to keep colleagues informed of any problems that occur with commonly used therapeutic agents. Representative manufacturers listed in the formulary are for reference purposes only. Other manufacturers may produce similar products of equal efficacy.

Table 18.2 Therapeutic Agents

Drug	Route	Dosage	Comments
Acetic acid (apple cider vinegar)	PO	15 ml/qt drinking water	For asymptomatic birds with gram negative rods and/or yeast detected in cytology sample from the mouth or cloaca
Acetylsalicylic acid (5 gr tab)	PO	1 tab/250 ml water (change 2 x day); 5 mg/kg q8h	Analgesic, antipyretic, anti-inflammatory, anticoagulant, uricosuric; efficacious for egg yolk-related embolisms and peritonitis; don't combine with tetracycline, insulin or allopurinol
ACTH (stimulation test)	IM	Baseline at 0 hr: give 16-26 IU; sample at 1-2 hr	May not be valid in birds because of the stress of handling and venipuncture
Activated charcoal	Oral	200-800 mg/kg as needed	Antitoxin; may cause constipation; chronic use depletes vitamins, esp. B
Acyclovir (200 mg capsule/tab; 50 mg/ml suspension)	PO, IV, IM	80 mg/kg q8h; up to 240 mg/kg food (400 mg/qt food); 20 mg/kg PO q12h x 7d; 50 mg/4 oz H_2O x 21d	Has antiviral activity against some avian herpesviruses; potentially nephrotoxic
Allopurinol (100 mg tab)	Oral (water)	Budgerigar: Crush 1 tab in 10 ml water; give 1 ml/30 ml water, fresh several times daily	Gout; possible hepatotoxicity; monitor uric acid levels weekly; reduce use if bird appears nervous
Aloe vera (solution)	Topical	0.5 ounce/pint of water, use as spray; formula: 0.5 oz aloe vera oral liquid with 1 tsp ammonia solution, 2 drops mild detergent, 1 pt water	Solution for treating pruritic skin lesions; caution when using any solution containing soap; avoid in birds that show post-use depression
Amikacin (50 mg/ml and 250 mg/ml)	IV, IM, SC	10-15 mg/kg q8-12h; cockatiels: 15-20 mg/kg q8-12h	Can be nephrotoxic; make sure hydration is maintained
Aminopentamide hydrogen sulfate (Centrine® 0.5 mg/ml)	IM, SC	0.05 mg/kg q8-12h x 3d with tapering dose; 5 dose maximum	Antiemetic; cholinergic blocker; do not use with GI obstruction. See notes on atropine
Aminophylline (25 mg/ml)	IV, PO	10 mg/kg IV q3h; after initial response can be given orally	Diruetic; vasodilator; cardiac stimulant; For lung edema

Table 18.2 Therapeutic Agents

Drug	Route	Dosage	Comments
Amitryptiline HCl	PO	1-2 mg/kg q24h	Tricyclic antidepressant; do not use if on thyroid replacement, or with impaired liver function; see notes on doxepin
Ammonium solution (Penetran®ointment)	Topical	As needed	Analgesic, antipruritic, anti-inflammatory; reduces swelling and relaxes muscles; can be used on fresh wounds; avoid overuse
Amoxicillin (250 mg/ml injectable)	IM	150 mg/kg q6-8h	Use to prevent pasteurellosis from animal bites - may require other antibiotics if bite is severe (eg, IV cefazolin)
Amoxicillin w/ clavulanic acid	PO	125 mg/kg q12h	Don't use with allopurinol; may have variable absorption
Amoxicillin	PO	200-400 mg/L in drinking water; 300-500 mg/kg in soft food	Canaries
Amphotericin B (5 mg/ml)	IV	1.5 mg/kg q8-12h for 3-7d	Fungal infections; nephrotoxic; maintain diuresis; caution: extravascular reactions can be severe; will precipitate out in saline; once diluted with sterile water, freeze in 10 ml aliquots at -20°C. Dilute 1:50 with 5% dextrose prior to IV or nebulization use (final concentration 0.1 mg/ml)
	In trachea, air sac	1 mg/kg q8-12h	
	Nebulize	1 mg/ml sterile water (15 min q12h)	
Amphotericin B (3% cream)	Topical	q12h	
Ampicillin	PO, IM	100-200 mg/kg q8h-q6h; chicken: 150 mg/kg PO q6h; Blue-naped Amazon: 50-100 mg/kg IM q48h; Emu, cranes: 15-20 mg/kg IM q8h; Gallinules: 25 mg/kg IM q8h	Erratic absorption orally; this form is of little value for avian diseases
	PO	1000-2000 mg/L in drinking water; 2000-3000 mg/kg in soft food	Canaries
Ampicillin (100 mg/ml)	IM	Psittacines: 100-150 mg/kg q4h	To prevent pasteurellosis from animal bite; may require other antibiotics if wounds are severe (eg, IV cefazolin)

Table 18.2　Therapeutic Agents

Drug	Route	Dosage	Comments
Amprolium (Corid® 9.6% solution)	Water	2-4 ml/gallon for 5 days	Coccidiostat; birds may not drink medicated water
Arginine vasotocin	IV	Physiological chicken dose: 40 ng/kg; Desert quail: 10 ng/kg; reduces GFR about 50%	Antidiuretic, causes shell gland contraction, possibly causing premature ovulation and oviposition; may cause hypertension from fluid overload; freeze small volumes in sterile vials for long term storage
Ascorbic acid (vitamin C) (250 mg/ml)	IM	20-40 mg/kg, daily to weekly	Support for patients with infectious or debilitating metabolic diseases; augments conversion of folic acid to its active form; increases iron absorption (caution in those prone to hemochromatosis); may cause diarrhea; do not use if oxalate crystals in urine
Atropine (0.5 mg/ml or 15 mg/ml)	IM, SC	For organophosphate toxicity: 0.1-0.5 mg/kg until cessation of clinical signs; repeat as needed; To increase heart rate: 0.01-0.04 mg/kg	Anticholinergic for organophosphate or carbamate toxicosis; may cause increased viscosity to respiratory secretions; decrease in gut motility; make sure well oxygenated; normally not used as avian preanesthetic
Azithromycin (250 mg capsules)	Oral	(Solution: 250 mg capsule per 0.25 oz lactulose) Sig: 1 drop solution/100 g BW q12h x 14 days; 50-80 mg/kg q24h; Stable refrigerated for 3-4 weeks	For mycoplasma: on 3d off 4d for 21 days; chlamydia: on 3d off 4d for 6 wk; may promote overgrowth of clostridium in GI tract; don't use with hepatic or renal impairment; may cause GI upset; expensive drug
Benzathine penicillin G	IM	100 mg/kg q24-48h (turkeys)	May cause death if administered IV
Butorphanol tartrate - Torbugesic® (1,5,10 mg); Torbutrol® (10 mg/ml & 2 mg/ml)	PO, IV	1-4 mg/kg PRN not to exceed q4h	Synthetic opiate used for abdominal and post-surgical pain

Table 18.2 Therapeutic Agents

Drug	Route	Dosage	Comments
Calcitonin	IM	4 IU/kg q12h x 2 wk	Treatment of hypercalcemia secondary to neoplasia or cholecalciferol analogs (rodent poison) toxicity. Monitor calcium levels; diurese; may also require steroids, and activated charcoal for toxicity
Calcium disodium versenate (CaEDTA 200 mg/ml)	IM	35 mg/kg q12h for 5 days; off 3-4 days, then repeat if needed	For chelation of heavy metal toxicosis: beryllium, copper, cerium, iron, zinc, lead; may add 2% Metamucil® in peanut butter to help remove metal particles; keep hydrated; caution in patients with renal or hepatic impairment
Calcium gluconate	Water	5 ml/30 ml of water	Used as calcium supplement
Calcium gluconate (50 mg/ml), Calcium lactate (50 mg/10 ml)	IM	5-10 mg/kg q12h as needed	When giving calcium, hydration must be maintained to avoid renal failure and/or soft tissue calcification; be careful when administering lactate - a properly functioning liver is necessary to break lactate down to bicarbonate
Calcium gluconate	IV - diluted	50-500 mg/kg slowly to effect	For hypocalcemic tetany; maintain hydration
Capricillic acid (325 mg)	Oral	1/4 capsule/300 g BW	Empirical use in birds; positive clinical results seen when administered with antifungals for aspergillosis in parrots; contains calcium, magnesium and zinc caprylates
Carbaryl (5% powder)	Topical	Dust lightly or add to nest box litter	Used to control mites and ants, only when necessary; remove after 24h
Carbenicillin	IM, IV, PO	100-200 mg/kg IM, IV q6-12h; 200 mg/kg PO q12h	Good frozen for 30 d; active against some *Pseudomonas* sp. and *Proteus* sp; renally excreted; may cause GI upset
Carnidazole (10 mg tablet)	PO	30-50 mg/kg once	Trichomoniasis, hexamitiasis, histomoniasis, cockatiels with giardia; may need to be repeated in 10-14 days

Table 18.2 Therapeutic Agents

Drug	Route	Dosage	Comments
Cefazolin (Ancef®)	IM, IV	25-50 mg/kg q12h	(All cephalosporins below: excreted by kidneys; reduce dose with renal impairment; good for *Staph* sp., *Strep* sp. and some gram neg bacteria; may cause diarrhea, secondary candidiasis, increase in hepatic and renal blood values); Stable for 10d in refrigerator, 48h room temp, can be frozen
Cefotaxime sodium (Claforan® - 10-300 mg/ml)	IM, IV	75-100 mg/kg q4-8h; Blue-front: 100 mg/kg IM q6-8h; 50-100 mg/kg q8h	Broad-spectrum; penetrates CSF; may be frozen for 13 wk (thaw at room temperature), refrigerate for 5d
Cefoxitin sodium (Mefoxin® - 10-400 mg/ml)	IM, IV	50-100 mg/kg q8-12h	
Ceftriaxone (10-250 mg/ml)	IM, IV	75-100 mg/kg q4-8h	May prolong bleeding times
Cephalexin oral suspension (Keflex® - 25-100 mg/ml)	PO	Psittacines: 50-100 mg/kg q8h; emus, cranes: 35-50 mg/kg q6h; 50-100 mg/kg q8h; quail, ducks: 50-50 mg/kg q2-3h	Varied efficacy for many gram-negative bacteria
Cephalothin (100 mg/ml)	IM, IV, PO	100 mg/kg q6h; quail, ducks: 100 mg/kg q2-3h	
Cephradine (25 or 50 mg/ml)	PO	35-50 mg/kg q4h	
Chloramphenicol (succinate 100 mg/ml, suspension, palmitate 30 mg/ml)	IM, PO, SC	80 mg/kg q12h or q8h parenteral; 30-50 mg/kg PO q6-8h; cranes: 100 mg/kg SC q8h	Good tissue penetration; broad spectrum bacteriostatic antibiotic; cause blood dyscrasias in humans, not reported in birds; wear gloves when handling
	IM, IV	102 mg/kg q6h	Chinese spot-billed ducks
	IM	50 mg/kg q6h	Macaws, Nanday Conures, Sun Conures
	IM	50 mg/kg q12h	Budgerigars, turkeys, chickens, Egyptian Geese
	IM	50 mg/kg q24h	Peafowl, eagles, hawks, owls
	PO	100-200 mg/L drinking water; 200-300 mg/kg soft food	Canaries

Table 18.2 Therapeutic Agents

Drug	Route	Dosage	Comments
Chlorhexidine solution, 2%	Oral, topical	10-25 ml/gallon; for wound flush: 1 ml to 39 ml sterile water	Do not use with finches (topical can be fatal in nun and parrot finches)
	Water	10 ml/gal for 7-14 days, 5-10 mg/kg; dissolve 1/4 tab (200 mg) in 0.2 ml 1 N HCL and 0.8 ml water	Psittacines - to help control amplification of susceptible viruses
Chloroquine (Aralan®)	PO	Dissolve 500 mg tab in 5 ml H_2O: Human dose: 10 mg/kg PO once, then 5 mg/kg PO at 6, 24, 48h	For acute plasmodium infections (erythrocytic forms) and extra-intestinal amoebiasis. Will suppress extra erythrocytic forms; may cause visual impairment (irreversible) or seizure, vomiting; many strains are resistant; accumulates in the liver - caution in liver impairment. Control mosquitos
Chloroquine + primaquine	PO	Combine 500 mg chloroquine + 25 mg primaquine in 333 ml H_2O. Give 10 ml/kg PO x 7d for prevention. For treatment: give at 0, 6, 24 & 48 hours; (0.75 mg/kg primaquine + 15 mg/kg chloroquine)	For plasmodium infection; Stable in refrigerator for 2 wk
Chlortetracycline (25 mg tab)	PO	95 mg/kg q6h, 190 mg/kg q8h	
Chlortetracycline	Feed	1% in pelleted feed; only food source for 45d	Psittacines; initiate concurrent treatment for yeast infections
	Feed	0.5% in millet; only food source for 45 days	Small psittacines, finches; initiate concurrent treatment for yeast infections
	PO	1000-1500 mg/L drinking water; 1500 mg/kg soft food	Canaries; treat for 30 days for chlamydiosis
Chlorsulon 8.5% (Curatrem®)	PO	20 mg/kg, 3 times, two weeks apart	For flukes
Cimetidine (200, 300, 400 800 mg tabs; 60 mg/ml suspension; 60 mg/ml, 150 mg/ml inj solution)	PO, IM, IV	(Mammal dose): 2.5-5 mg/kg q6-12h IV (very slow infusion over 30-40 min)	Use for gastric ulcerations; decreases cloacal acidity; aids in tenesmus, cloacal papillomatosis; may potentiate anti-seizure drugs and tricyclic antidepressants; may cause drowsiness

Table 18.2 Therapeutic Agents

Drug	Route	Dosage	Comments
Ciprofloxacin (250, 500, 700 mg tab; 200, 400 mg/ml injectable)	Oral, IV	20-40 mg/kg q12h	Most anaerobes, *Pseudomonas* sp. and *Streptococcus* sp. are resistant - these may overgrow; chlamydia and mycoplasma only moderately susceptible
Cisapride (Propulsid® 20 mg/tab)	PO	0.5-1.5 mg/kg q8h	Gastrointestinal stimulant; high therapeutic index
Clazuril (Appertex®)	In feed	Sand Hill Cranes: 1.1 ppm in feed for 5 days	
Clortrimazol (Lotrimin® 1% solution)	Nebulizing	30-45 min q24h x 3 d, off 2 days; may need for 1-4 mo	Fungicidal; for patients with aspergillosis that are stable and out of respiratory distress
Colchicine (0.5 mg tab; 0.5 mg/ml injectable)	Oral, IV	0.04 mg/kg q24h, gradually go to q12h	Uricosuric; may prevent hepatic fibrosis; will inhibit tubular excretion of penicillins; may cause hypertension, hypothermia; potentiates CNS depressants
Copper sulfate (51% powder)	Topical	q24h	Not for deep wounds; very caustic; destroys granulation bed; if ingested, causes gastric irritation and possible copper toxicity
Cyanocobalamin (vitamin B$_{12}$ 1,	IM	250-500 μ g/kg once/week	
Danofloxacin	Water	50 ppm for 3d (day old chicks)	Superior to tylosin for treating *M. gallisepticum*
Deferoxamine mesylate (Desferal® 500 mg/vial; reconstitute to 250 mg/ml)	SC, PO	100 mg/kg q24h (may take 3 mo)	Iron chelation in hemochromatosis; suggest monthly biopsies to quantitate liver iron; may give reddish color to urine; don't use if renal impairment; offer only low-iron foods
Desoxycorticosterone acetate	-	4 mg/kg q24h	For confirmed Addisonian (ACTH test)
Derm caps liquid	PO	0.1 ml/kg q24h	May aid in feather picking; anecdotal efficacy
Dexamethasone	IM, IV	0.5-2 mg/kg q24h	Use with caution; egg-related peritonitis

Table 18.2 Therapeutic Agents

Drug	Route	Dosage	Comments
Dextrose (5% = 50 mg/ml; 50% = 500 mg/ml)	IV	50-100 mg/kg, slowly	Should measure blood glucose level prior to use; for seizuring birds caused by hypoglycemia
Diazepam (5 mg/ml injectable; do not dilute)	IM, IV	0.5-1 mg/kg q12h, q8h	For seizures; cimetidine delays clearance; may cause hypotension; rapid IV can exacerbate seizures; increase intracranial and intraocular pressure; caution in renal and liver impairment
	Oral	2.5-4 mg/kg as needed	For calming effect
Diatrozoate sodium 37% iodine (Renografin-76®)	IM	122 mg/kg	For goiter in budgies
Digoxin solution (0.05-15 mg/ml)	Oral	0.02-0.05 mg/kg q24h	For congestive heart failure; conures, parakeets; positive inotrope, negative chronotrope; caution in patients with impaired renal function (give lower dose); monitor closely
Dimercaprol (BAL)	IM	2.5-5.0 mg/kg q4h x 2d, then q12h x 10d or until recovery	For arsenic and gold; mercury if ingestion <2hr; with CaEDTA helps in lead excretion
Dimethyl sulfoxide 90% (DMSO)	Topical	1 ml/kg q4-5d or weekly	For edema, pain, swelling; paint a thin film over the area; wear glove when applying; absorbed cutaneously and distributed systemically; causes vasodilation and histamine release
Dimetridazole (Emtryl®)	Oral (gavage)	Budgerigar stock solution = 1 tsp/pint water; dose: 0.5 ml/30 g repeat at 12 and 24 h	Giardia, anaerobes; not available in the US; extremely hepatotoxic; can cause death
Diphenhydramine HCl (Benadryl® 25, 50 mg cap; 2.5 mg/ml oral; 10 or 50 mg/ml injectable)	Oral, IM, IV	0.5 tsp/8 oz water or 2-4 mg/kg q12h	Has calming effect in some anxious birds; do not give with monoamine oxidase inhibitors (see atropine precautions); may cause hypotension

Table 18.2 Therapeutic Agents

Drug	Route	Dosage	Comments
Doxepin (Sinequan®, Adapin®)	PO	0.5-1.0 mg/kg q12h	Tricyclic antidepressant; rotating trials in feather picking birds; may temporarily increase liver enzymes; may increase intraocular pressure, cause urinary retention and seizures; do not use with MOA inhibitors, cimetidine, anticholinergics; discontinue in a tapering dose
Doxycycline	PO	0.1% in diet	Amazons, cockatoos, African grey parrot
	PO	25-50 mg/kg q24-48h	Green-winged Macaws, Amazons, Cockatiels
	PO	25 mg/kg q24h	African Greys, Goffin Cockatoos, Blue and Gold Macaws, Pigeons
	PO	25 mg/kg q12h	Senegal parrots
	PO	250 mg/L water; 1000 mg/kg soft food	Canaries: treat for 30 days for chlamydiosis
	PO	8 mg/kg q12-24h	Nectar eaters
Doxycycline (Vibravenös®)	IM	75-100 mg/kg SC or IM q7d x 4 then q6d x 2	May cause injection site hemorrhage and necrosis in all IM or SC dosing; only available in Europe and Canada
Doxycycline (Vibramycin® calcium syrup 10 mg/ml)	PO	50 mg/kg q24h	Cockatiels, Orange-winged Amazons, Blue-fronted Amazons
Doxycycline (Vibramycin® hyclate 10 mg/ml)	IV	25-50 mg/kg	Use once to get peak dose in critical cases (psittacines)
Doxycycline (75 mg/ml - Mortar & Pestle)	IM	75 mg/kg q7d x 3 (cockatoos); 100 mg/kg q7d x 3 (others)	Individually compounded and sold to veterinarians only per valid perscription
d-penicillamine (125, 250 mg caps; 250 mg tabs)	PO	17-55 mg/kg q12h on 1-2 wk, off 1 wk, repeat as needed	For heavy metal toxicity, esp. copper, lead, zinc, mercury; often used with EDTA until asymptomatic; give with empty crop & proventriculus

Table 18.2 Therapeutic Agents

Drug	Route	Dosage	Comments
Echinacea	PO	Mix 15-28 drops with ½ oz. lactulose. Sig: 1 drop/100g q12h (<200g BW), 1 drop/300g q12h (>200g BW)	Immunostimulant, anecdotal efficacy; use alcohol-free
Enrofloxacin (Baytril® 22.7 mg/ml injectable)	IM, PO	7.5-15 mg/kg q12h; finches: 100-200 mg/L drinking water x 5-10d; Senegals: 15 mg/kg IM q8-12h (not effective if MIC is >30); budgies, African Greys, cockatoos: 15 mg/kg q12h	African Greys, Amazons, cockatoos; can use injectable orally; should not be used with liver or renal impairment; do not use in growing animals; may be ineffective against some *Pseudomonas* sp. and cause *Strep.* sp. and *Clostridium* sp. overgrowth
Enrofloxacin	Feed	500 mg/kg mixed with cooked corn x 14d; 200 ppm for 14 d	Chlamydiosis therapy in psittacines
Enrofloxacin	PO	200 mg/L drinking water; 200 mg/kg soft food	Canaries; in case of chlamydiosis, treat for 21 days
Erythromycin (powder)	Water	500 mg/gallon drinking water; finches for mycoplasma: 300 mg/L H_2O x 10d	Will form L-bodies esp. when treating salmonellosis; don't use with hepatic impairment; hepatotoxic, concentrates in the liver; may not have good absorption in birds; don't use with lincomycin or clindamycin, theophylline
Erythromycin (100-200 mg/ml injectable)	Nebulize	200 ml/10 ml saline, 15 min q8h	Nebulize with caution as vehicle is polyethylene glycol; can cause severe necrosis IM; cannot be given IV
Erythromycin (40 mg/ml)	Oral	45-90 mg/kg q12h x 5-10d	May cause GI upset
Erythromycin	PO	125 mg/L drinking water; 200 mg/kg soft food	Canaries
Ethambutol (100-400 mg tab)	Oral	15 mg/kg q12h	Controversial therapy for TB; caution with renal or hepatic impairment; may cause visual impairment, carditis, GI upset
Fenbendazole (100 mg/ml suspension)	Oral	For ascarids: 20-50 mg/kg, repeat 10 days; For flukes and microfilaria: 20-50 mg/kg q24h for 3 days; For capillaria: 20-50 mg/kg q24h for 5 days; Ratites: 15 mg/kg PO, 80-100 mg/kg of nectar; Finches: 50 mg/L drinking water x 3d	Dangerous in canaries, possibly ibis, California quail and pigeons; do not use during a molt or in pin feather stage; do not use in cockatiels; low margin of safety

Table 18.2 Therapeutic Agents

Drug	Route	Dosage	Comments
Ferric subsulfate	Topical	As needed	Restrict use to hemorrhage of beak and nails as it will cause tissue necrosis
5-Fluorocytosine	Gavage	250 mg/kg q12h or 120 mg/kg q8h	Antifungal; Psittacines: caution with renal or liver impairment; excreted by kidneys; may cause anemia & GI upset
Flucytosine	Oral (feed)	50-250 mg/kg feed	Psittacines and mynahs
	PO	African Grey: 50 mg/kg q8h or 60-100 mg/kg q12h; Psittacines: 150-250 mg/kg q12h or 75-120 mg/kg q12h x 2-4 wks	
Fluconazole (50, 100, 200 mg tab; 2 mg/ml injectable)	Oral, IV	May dissolve 200 mg in 1 ml HCl then add 99 ml sterile H_2O; Cockatoo, African Grey, Amazon: 20 mg/kg PO q48h; For cryptococcus in psittacines: 8 mg/kg PO q24h x 30d; For *Candida* in psittacines: 10 mg/kg PO q24h x 10-30d	May cause regurgitation
Flunixin-meglumine (50 mg/ml injectable)	IV, IM	1-10 mg/kg	Analgesic, anti-inflammatory, antipyretic (hyperthermia); can cause GI ulceration; do not combine with other NSAIDs or steroids
Furazolidone	Oral	100-200 mg/L water; 200 mg/kg soft food	Canaries
Furosemide (50 mg/ml inj.)	IV, IM	0.15-2 mg/kg, q12-24h	Diuretic, low therapeutic index; lories very sensitive; watch potassium levels; will increase nephrotoxicity of aminoglycosides and should not be used to treat anuria secondary to aminoglycoside toxicities; do not use with steroids (inc. K+ loss); caution with liver impairment
Gentamicin	IM	Cockatiels: 5-10 mg/kg q8-12h	Only for resistant infections; maintain hydration; nephrotoxic
Gentian violet (powder, 16 mg/ml solution)	Feed, topical	0.5-1.0 g/kg of feed; paint lesions with 0.25-0.5%	Resistant candida strains; caution when using in feed; may cause ulceration of mucous membranes and mucosa, laryngeal paralysis; other anti-fungal may be safer

Table 18.2 Therapeutic Agents

Drug	Route	Dosage	Comments
Glipizide	PO	1.25 mg/kg q24h	In mammals stimulates insulin secretion; metabolized in liver; do not use if ketoacidotic; efficacy not established in birds
Guanidine	PO	15-30 mg/kg	As adjunct therapy for treatment of botulism
Haloperidol (50, 100 mg/ml injectable)	IM	1-2 mg/kg every 2-3 weeks	Seldom used
Haloperidol (2 mg/ml solution)	Oral	0.2 mg/kg q12h for birds <1 kg; 0.15 mg/kg q12-24h for birds >1 kg	For compulsive/obsessive behavior; commonly fails; may work because increases prolactin levels; may cause hypotension, anorexia
Hemicellulose (psyllium, sterilized by autoclave)	Oral	<1% of diet or handfeeding formula	Improves calcium absorption, hypercholesterolemia, bulk laxative to remove GI metal; caution: gel may form in crop of some birds and act as foreign body in neonates (day 1-7); use with caution in cockatiels: may promote onset of renal disorders
Heparin (1000 IU/150 mg aloe vera)	Topical	PRN	Treatment for sores; shown to have anti-inflammatory properties
Hetastarch (6% in 0.9% NaCl)	IV	Use at fluids doses	Blood replacement; stop use when total solids acceptable
Human chorionic gonadotropin (HCG - 10,000 IU/10 ml vial)	IM	500-1000 IU/kg (generally effective)	At press time, this dose was used for sexual feather plucking in female birds; may need to be repeated every 3-6 weeks; used for egg-laying; more research needs to be done on exact mechanisms of action in reproductive hormone axis of birds. Use with caution and consult more current references
Human gamma globulin (Gammar)	IV	150 mg/kg q7d for 4 wk then q4wk for 5 mo	Efficacy in birds unknown, anecdotal, anaphylactic reactions may occur
Hyaluronidase (Wydase®) 1500 IU/10 ml vial	Oral	1 ml/L fluids	Mix freshly weekly; store in refrigerator; for rapid administration of fluids administered SC

Table 18.2 Therapeutic Agents

Drug	Route	Dosage	Comments
Hydrochloric acid (1 M/L solution)	Water	30 ml/gallon drinking water for 10 days	Enterobacteriaceae, megabacteria, candida in asymptomatic birds; use alone or in combination with lactulose, hemicellulose and pharmaceuticals in ill birds
Hydroxyzine HCl syrup	PO	2.2 mg/kg q8h or 4 mg/4 oz drinking water	Lowers the threshold for seizures, hypotensive, anti-anxiety, antipruritic and antihistamine action; do not use with CNS depressants
Insulin NPH U40	IM	Cockatiel: 1.4 units/kg q12-24h; Toco Toucan: 0.01 to 0.1 units/kg q12-24h; Budgie: 0.3 to 3.0 units/kg q12-24h	Must monitor with glucose curve; use appropriate insulin diluents; many birds have normal insulin and high glucagon levels; may not be effective
Interferon (Actimmune®)	SC	1-2 IU q24h on 7d off 7d	Caution with liver impairment; anecdotal efficacy
Iron dextran (100 mg/ml)	IM	10 mg/kg, repeat in 7-10 days if needed	Used in malnourished and iron deficient birds; contraindicated in mynahs, toucans and other potential hemachromatosis birds
Isoniazid (300 mg tab)	Oral	15 mg/kg q12h	Controversial for TB treatment; may cause fatal hepatitis, peripheral neuropathy and vomiting
Itraconazole (100 mg caps)	Oral	Stable in 0.1 N HCl for 7d; 5-10 mg/kg q12h; candida in cockatiels: 5 mg/kg q24h; Double Yellow-head: 5-20 mg/k q12h x 10d; dissolve in 2 ml 0.1 NHCl then dilute further for gavage	Aspergillosis, candida, cryptococcus in Psittaciformes, Anseriformes, penguins; reported side effects in parrots; caution in African Greys: may cause hepatitis, hypokalemia and bone toxicity
Ivermectin (10 mg/ml injectable)	IM, oral, topical	200 μ g/kg, repeat 10-14 days; except in budgies, use:	Nematodes, lice, mites; reported toxicity in finches & Orange-cheeked waxbills
Ivermectin (10 mg/ml injectable)	PO	0.8-1.0 mg/L H$_2$O (not water soluble)	Canaries
Ketoconazole (200 mg tab)	Oral	Gavage or by dropper; 20-30 mg/kg q12h for 21 days	Mix with lactulose; hepatotoxic in mammals

Table 18.2 Therapeutic Agents

Drug	Route	Dosage	Comments
Ketoconazole (200 mg tab)	Oral	Psittacines: 30 mg/kg q12h; for candidiasis in swans: 12.5 mg/kg q24h x 30d	Hepatotoxic
	PO	200 mg/kg soft food	Canaries
Lactobacillus (avian)	Oral	1 pinch/day/bird or 1 tsp/quart of hand-feeding formula	Avian *Lactobacillus* sp; probiotic for stimulation of autochthonous bacterial colonization
Lactulose (667 mg/ml suspension)	Oral	0.3-0.7 ml/kg q8-12h	To reduce toxins, restore GI flora in liver-damaged birds, carrier for oral meds; overdose causes diarrhea; can use for 7 days to months; decrease dose if diarrhea occurs; caution in birds with diabetes mellitus
Levamisole (136.5 mg/ml injectable, 20 mg tab)	Oral (gavage)	Australian parakeets: 15 mg/kg, repeat in 10 days; Anseriformes: 20-50 mg/kg; Ratites: 30 mg/kg PO q10d; immune modulator: 2 mg/kg IM q14d x 3 Tx	Low therapeutic index; seldom used; metabolized in the liver and renally excreted; lethal in White-faced Ibis
	Oral (water)	5-15 ml/gallon, 1-3 days; Finches: 80 mg/L drinking water x 3d	
	IM, SC	2 mg/kg IM q14d x 3 doses	Most dangerous route; restores depressed immune system
Levothyroxine (0.1, 0.2, 0.3, 0.5, 0.8 mg tabs; 0.4 mg/ml suspension)	Oral	20 μ g/kg q24h-q12h	For true hypothyroidism, chronic disorders (respiratory, dermal); use is controversial; can cause hypertrophic cardiomyopathy if levels are above euthyroid levels; hypothyroidism must be diagnosed with a TSH stimulation test
Lincomycin	Oral	100-200 mg/L water; 200 mg/kg soft food	Canaries
Lugol's iodine	Water	2 ml/20 ml water for stock sol; Give 1 drop/250 ml water	For goiter; excess may cause thyroid hyperplasia; unnecessary if on formulated diet

Table 18.2 Therapeutic Agents

Drug	Route	Dosage	Comments
Mannitol (20 or 180 mg/ml)	IV	0.5 mg/kg slowly q24h	Brain edema, osmotic diuretic; caution if intracranial hemorrhage
Mebendazole (40 mg/g soluble powder; 33.3 mg/ml suspension)	Oral	Psittacines: 25 mg/kg q12h for 5 days; Anseriformes: 5-15 mg/kg q24h for 2 days.	For nematodes; may need to repeat monthly; may not work for ventricular/proventricular parasites; reports of toxicity in finches, psittacines, pigeons (12 mg/kg); necrotic enteritis in penguins, cormorants, pelicans.
Medroxyprogesterone acetate (100 mg/ml injectable; 2.5, 5, 10 g tabs)	IM, SC	5-25 mg/kg, every 4-6 weeks	May increase or decrease LH depending on time in cycle given or increase or block ovulation; if given to a bird without an oviduct, ovulation into the coelomic cavity may occur; seldom used due to side effects, primarily obesity, diabetes mellitus, salpingitis, molt, PU/PD, lethargy, thromboemboli, liver impairment, prolonged bleeding times, hypothyroidism
Meperidine (Demerol®)	IM	1-4 mg/kg	Do not use with other CNS depressants; hypotensive; decreased respiratory effort, increases airway resistance. May aggravate cardiac arrhythmias and seizure activity; caution with renal impairment, hepatic impairment, hypothyroidism
Methocarbamol (Robaxin-V®)	IV, PO	Swans, Demoiselle cranes: 50 mg/kg slow IV, avoid extravasation; 32.5 mg/kg PO q12h	For capture myopathy; CNS depressant; do not use injectable with renal impairment (polyethylene glycol vehicle)
Methylprednisolone acetate (20, 40 mg/ml injectable)	IM, Oral	0.5-1 mg/kg	To control allergies (eg, Amazon foot necrosis); orally once a week, then taper off to once a month, then stop
Metoclopramide (Reglan® - 10 mg tabs; 1 mg/ml syrup; 5 mg/ml injectable)	IM, IV, Oral	0.5 mg/kg q8-12h	Limited success with GI stasis; do not use if GI obstruction/ hemorrhage or hypertension present; do not use in epileptics (lowers the threshold for seizures); caution in the renally impaired; antagonized by narcotics; do not use with monoamine oxidase inhibitors

Table 18.2 Therapeutic Agents

Drug	Route	Dosage	Comments
Metronidazole (250 or 500 mg tabs; suspension from Mortar & Pestle)	Oral	10-30 mg/kg q12h for 10 days	For limited success treatment of giardia, hexamita, anaerobic bacteria; caution in renal or hepatic impairment; may cause seizures, peripheral neuropathies, anorexia or GI upset; may enhance candidiasis; toxic in finches
Metronidazole (5 mg/ml inj)	IM	10 mg/kg q24h for 2 days	Toxic in finches
	PO	100 mg/L drinking water or /kg soft food	Canaries
Miconazole (10 mg/ml injectable; 1-2% ointment/cream)	IV, Topical	20 mg/kg q8h; can nebulize diluted 15-20 min q12h	Candida, cryptococcus, coccidiomycosis, pseudoallescheriosis and paracoccidioidomycosis; IV must be given diluted in 0.9% NaCl and very slowly or death may occur; do not use with rifampin, hypoglycemic agents, anticoagulants; caution with CNS-active drugs; adverse reactions include death, phlebitis, pruritus, nausea, fever, rash; metabolized in liver, excreted in urine
Midazolam	IM	Amazons: 2-3 mg/kg; waterfowl: 4-6 mg/kg; ratites: 0.3 mg/kg, most birds 1.5 mg/kg	See diazepam
Monensin	In feed	Sand Hill Cranes: 100-400 ppm in feed (low dose best)	For control of *Eimeria* sp; wear rubber gloves, protective clothing and mask when mixing; make sure feed is thoroughly mixed
Naloxone	IV	2 mg q14-21h if needed	Antagonist for opiates and to some degree agonist-antagonists (butorphanol); repeat if necessary; some narcotics have longer t1/2 than naloxone
Neomycin (50 mg/ml solution)	PO	80-100 mg/L drinking water; 100 mg/kg soft food	Canaries; not absorbed from GI tract
Neomycin ointment	Topical	q6-12h	Caution: ointments may grease feathers; best to use under a bandage; use on small superficial wounds only; may be absorbed systemically and cause ototoxicity and nephrotoxicity

Table 18.2 Therapeutic Agents

Drug	Route	Dosage	Comments
Norcuronium ophthalmic prep	Topical	2 drops q15min x 3 in eye for pupillary dilation	Takes about 60 min; should return to normal by 7 hr; watch for toxicity - muscle relaxation
Nortriptyline HCl syrup (2 mg/ml)	Oral	2 mg/4 oz water	Tricyclic antidepressent; do not use with cardiac disease; discontinue on a tapering dose (see notes for doxepin)
Nystatin (1000,000 IU/ml suspension)	Oral (gavage)	Psittacines: 3000,000 IU/kg q8-12h x 7-14d; passerines: 100,000 IU/L and 200,000 IU/kg soft food	Not absorbed from gut, only good when in contact with yeast; for oral candida, must apply to oral cavity; resistance common; rarely causes nausea or diarrhea; canaries: treat *Candida albicans* for 3-6 weeks
Oxytetracycline	IM	50 mg/kg q12h	Psittacines other than Amazons; caution: some injectables contain lidocaine; renal impairment may lead to excessive systemic accumulation and lead to hepatotoxicity; may cause photosensitization and myonecrosis; when give SC may lead to an area of skin necrosis which heals with or without treatment in about 3 wk
	IM, SC	Cockatoos: 50-100 mg/kg, every 2-3 days	
Oxytetracycline (Long-acting 200 mg/ml)	IM	Amazons: 58 mg/kg, q24h; pheasants: 43 mg/kg q24h	Initial chlamydia treatment; secondary yeast infection common
Oxytocin (20 U/ml injectable)	IV, IM, SC	5 U/kg once	For egg expulsion, to stop uterine bleeding; should not be used with a closed utero-vaginal sphincter; may cause cardiac arrhythmias
Pancreatic enzymes (Viokase®, Prozyme®, Pancrezyme® 2400 g tab)	Oral	2400-4800 g/kg of food	To dissolve plant-based foods and fibers; many are made from pork pancreas (eg, Viokase); if in mouth may cause digestion of tissues; don't inhale; high doses may raise uric acid levels; safest to mix with food and let stand 30 min

Table 18.2 Therapeutic Agents

Drug	Route	Dosage	Comments
PGF$_{2\alpha}$ (Lutalyse® 5 mg/ml)	IM (systemic effects)	.000004-.00004 ml/g (.00034 ml/g - cockatiel)	Although Lutalyse has successfully expelled eggs if used early in egg binding, it does not relax the vagina.
Phenobarbital (16.2 mg tab; 3 mg/ml elixir; 4 mg/ml solution)	Oral	1-5 mg/kg q12h; Red-lored Amazon: 5 mg/kg q12h or 8 mg/120 ml H_2O; lovebird (50-75 g BW): 0.08-1.8 ml/60 ml H_2O	For controlling seizures; will diminish oviduct contractions; may cause osteomalacia; regular hepatic function test should be performed; caution in the liver impaired; addictive; shortens half-life of doxycycline
Phenylbutazone (200 mg/ml injectable; 100 or 400 mg tab)	IV, Oral	3.5-7 mg/kg q8-12h	NSAID; GI ulcers, blood dyscrasia; do not use if liver, kidney or cardiac abnormalities exist
Pimaricin (Natamycin® 5% ophthalmic solution)	Ophth.	1 drop q6h; after 14-21 days, taper off	For ocular mycosis; do not use with steroids; expensive; surgery may be more beneficial
Piperacillin (200 mg/ml injectable)	IM, IV	100-200 mg/kg q6-8h; Budgerigars: 200 mg/kg q8h; Blue-fronted Amazons: 100 mg/kg q6h	Excellent clinical antibiotic alone or when combined with amikacin (never in the same syringe); effective against many gram-negative, gram-positive, anaerobes, *Pseudomonas* sp.; increase t1/2 in renal impairment; excreted in urine & bile; good for liver infections, dog bite wounds; may be contraindicated in neonates; reconstituted good for 24h at room temp, 7d in refrig, 30d at -10 to -20°C
Piperazine	PO	100-500 mg/kg q10-14d	Not effective in psittacines; good for poultry for *Toxocara leonina*; do not use with kidney impairment
Polymyxin	PO	50,000 IU/L drinking water or /kg soft food	Canaries
Polysulfated glycosamine glycan (Adequan®)	IM, PO	5 mg/kg	Cartilage precursor used for arthritis

Table 18.2 Therapeutic Agents

Drug	Route	Dosage	Comments
Potassium chloride	IV	0.1-0.3 mEq/kg	Potassium replacement in conjunction with ECG & electrolyte analysis
Pralidoxime chloride (Protopam®)	IM, IV slow	10-30 mg/kg q24h or until cessation of clinical signs; repeat as needed	For organophosphate toxicities; use with atropine (use lower dose in conjunction w/atropine) and oxygen therapy; reduce dose with renal impairment; cholinesterase reactivator; may increase carbamate toxicity; good for up to 36 hours after exposure
Praziquantel (Droncit® 23 or 34 mg tab; 56.8 mg/ml injectable)	Oral	10-20 mg/kg; repeat 10-14 days; toucans for flukes: 10 mg/kg q24h x 14d PO then 6 mg/kg q24h x 14d	For tapeworms, flukes
Praziquantel	IM	For flukes: 9 mg/kg q24h x 3d then PO x 11d; for tapeworms: 9 mg/kg once, then repeat in 10 days	Metabolized in liver; toxic to finches; caution in neonates and juveniles (esp. African Greys)
Prednisolone sodium succinate (10 or 50 mg/ml injectable solution)	IM, IV	Anti-inflammatory: 0.5-1 mg/kg once; Immunosuppressive: 2-4 mg/kg; appropriate for shock (dog shock dose: 5-20 mg/kg IV)	IM injections may cause myonecrosis at site of injection; may cause GI ulcers
Prepidil® gel (PGE$_2$) 0.5 mg/3.0 g (2.5 ml)	Topical	± 1 ml/kg applied to utero-vaginal sphincter; as little as 0.05 ml/kg may be sufficient (in chickens, 1 µ g PGE$_2$	Dilates sphincter; allows for expulsion of egg
Primaquine (15 mg tab = 26.3 mg primaquine phosphate)	PO	Most birds: 0.75 mg/kg; game birds: 0.03 mg/kg q24h x 3	For treatment of *Plasmodium* sp; metabolized in liver; usually used with chloroquine
Probucol (Lorelco® 250 mg, 500 mg tabs)	Oral	250 mg/0.25 oz lactulose: 1 drop q12h/300 g BW for 2-4 mo	To lower cholesterol, control lipemia & lipomas; contains iron - use with caution in those birds that are susceptible to hemachromatosis; may increase bile acids when assayed; should only be used in birds with primary LDL-cholesterolemia; all birds should be on a low fat, low cholesterol diet with adequate exercise

Table 18.2 Therapeutic Agents

Drug	Route	Dosage	Comments
Procaine penicillin G (aqueous formula best)	IM only	100 mg/kg q24-48h	Turkeys; drug of choice for *Clostridium tetani* infections; slowed excretion with renal impairment; many birds are sensitive to procaine; procaine should never be used in parrots or passerines!
Propranolol (1 mg/ml injectable)	IM	0.2 mg/kg	For tachycardia; do not use with ventricular tachycardia secondary to A-V block; causes broncho constriction, hypotension; use with supraventricular arrhythmias, atrial flutter or fibrillation; do not use in diabetics or when hypoglycemia is present; decreases myocardial oxygen consumption
Propranolol	IV	0.04 mg/kg slowly	Monitor with ECG during and for several hours after administration
Pyrantel pamoate (Nemex-2® 4.5 mg/ml suspension)	Oral	4.5 mg/kg, repeat 10-14 days	GI nematodes
Pyrethrins (0.150%)	Topical	PRN	Kitten flea spray for resistant lice; avoid contact with eyes; some sprays may cause pneumonitis when inhaled
Pyrimethamine (25 mg tab)	Oral	0.5 mg/kg q12h	Plasmodium, toxoplasmosis, sarcocystis; competes for folic acid; when combined with sulfonamides the treatment of toxoplasmosis is enhanced; may help for sarcocystis infections; should not be used for acute plasmodium infection; use chloroquine or quinine; caution with liver or kidney impairment; sulfas with pyrimethamine may cause bone marrow suppression; decrease dose if vomiting; discontinue if rash or hematologic disorders observed (see chloroquine)
Pyrimethamine + trimethoprim/sulfadiazine (TMS)	PO	Pyrimethamine: 0.5 mg/kg q12h (may drop to 0.25 mg/kg after 2-4); TMS (combined mg): 30 mg/kg IM q12h	For sarcocystis treatment for at least 30 days; re-biopsy q4-8wk

Table 18.2 Therapeutic Agents

Drug	Route	Dosage	Comments
Quinacrine (Atabrine® 100 mg tab)	Oral	5-10 mg/kg, q24h for 7 days	For giardia, tapeworms, plasmodium; don't use with primaquine; many *Plasmodium* sp. are resistant; concentrates in liver, caution with liver impairment; may cause yellow color to skin, seizures; give with food
Rifampin (150 or 300 mg capsule)	Oral	10-20 mg/kg q12h	*Mycobacterium* sp, *Haemophilus influenza*, *Staph. epidermis*, *Neisseria* sp.; rifampin has numerous drug interactions; never use halothane; side effects are numerous and associated with most body systems; hepatotoxic - do not use with liver impairment; usually use with other drugs to treat myobacterium; resistance occurs rapidly; absorption reduced with food
Selenium	IM	0.06 mg/kg q3-14d	Cockatiels
Silver sulfadiazine 1%	Topical	Apply q12-24h	For burns, ulcers, under bandage; good to help rehydrate wounds when applied under a transparent dressing; if used over large areas, make sure hydration is maintained
Sodium bicarbonate (1 mEq/ml)	IV	1-4 mEq/kg slowly over 15-30 minutes	Do not exceed 4 mEq/kg; do not use with hypochloremia (vomiting); don't use with calcium-containing fluids; best to use only when blood pH values are known
Spectinomycin	PO	200-400 mg/L H_2O; 400 mg/kg soft food	Canaries
Spiramycin	PO	200-400 mg/L H_2O; 400 mg/kg soft food	Canaries
Stanozolol (Winstrol® - 2 mg tablet, 50 mg/ml injectable)	Oral, IM	0.5-1.0 mg/kg IM q3-7d	Synthetic derivative of testosterone; schedule drug; do not use with renal impairment; repeat use with caution; consider adverse effects as with humans

Table 18.2   Therapeutic Agents

Drug	Route	Dosage	Comments
STA solution (salicylic acid, tannic acid in ethyl alcohol)	Topical	As needed	Moist & fungal dermatitis; may burn; tannic acid is caustic & drying
Streptomycin	IM	Large birds 10-30 mg/kg q8-12h	More nephrotoxic than most aminoglycosides; provide fluids when using; not for use in psittacines, passerines
Sucralfate (1 g tab)	Oral	25 mg/kg q8h (maximum)	For upper GI bleeding; should be given 1 hr before food or other drugs, 2 hr prior to H2 blockers; may cause constipation
Sulfachlorpyrizidine (5 g packet)	Water	1/4 tsp powder/L for 5-10d; canaries: 150-300 mg/L drinking water	Most species; don't use sulfa drugs in birds laying eggs
Sulfamethazine (12% solution)	Oral	Mix to 30 mg/oz drinking water; for coccidia in chickens: 128-187 mg/kg q24h x 2d than 1/2 dose for 4d	For *Coccidia, Haemoproteus, Pasteurella, Salmonella* in small psittacines; make sure hydration is maintained
Sulfadimethoxine (Albon®)	PO	50 mg/kg q24h for 5d; off 3d repeat for 5d	
Sulfadimidine	PO	150 mg/L drinking water	Canaries
d-tubocurarine in 0.025% benzalkonium Cl ophthalmic prep	Topical	Mix fresh, apply 3 drops to eye q15 min	For dilation of pupil; watch for toxicity - muscle relaxation
Testosterone (10 mg or 25 mg tab, 200 mg/ml inj)	Oral, IM	8 mg/kg, weekly as needed	Anabolic steroid; lymphocytotoxic
Tetracycline (soluble powder, 250 mg caps, suspension)	Water	0.25-1 tsp/gallon	Seldom used; birds may not drink sufficient water
Tetracycline	Oral	50 mg/kg q8h	Psittacines
Thiabendazole (4 mg/30 ml suspension)	Oral	Ascarids: 250-500 mg/kg, repeat 10-14 days; for *Syngamus:* 100 mg/kg q24h for 7-10 days	Possibly toxic in ostriches, ducks, cranes; may have CNS side-effects, nausea, hypotension, hyperglycemia, crystaluria, leukopenia

Table 18.2 Therapeutic Agents

Drug	Route	Dosage	Comments
Thyroxine (Synthroid® - best quality, less fluctuation in mg/tab)	PO	0.02 to 0.04 mg/kg q24h in confirmed hypothyroidism. Check blood levels: 4 hr post meds =- 3 mg/dl; 12 hr post med = 2 mg/dl	May cause recrudescence of thymus in adults; toxic levels cause hypertrophic cardiomyopathy and heart failure
Ticarcillin (30-40 mg/ml injectable)	IM, IV	150-200 mg/kg q6-8h	Effective against many gram-positive and gram-negative organisms including *Pseudomonas* sp. and some anaerobes; synergistic with aminoglycosides (do not mix together); resistance may develop rapidly
Tiletamine HCl / zolazepam HCl (Telazol®)	IV	Ratites: 2-8 mg/kg; induction 15 sec; duration = 20-40 min.; may add 0.5 mg/kg xylazine IV and carfentinil 0.015 mg/kg IV	Monitor heart rate (xylazine can cause A-V block) May pretreat with Azaparone IM or post-induction for smoother recovery at 1-2 mg/kg; Do not use Telazol with cardiac, pancreatic, renal, pulmonary disease. Eyes remain open so apply ointment to eyes. Very similar to ketamine. Good for 14 days in refrigerator once reconstituted. Do not use with psittacines, passerines.
Tobramycin (40 mg/ml injectable)	IM	2.5-5 mg/kg q12h	Oto and nephrotoxic; hydrate while using; do not use furosemide; caution with renal impairment; dose by lean body weight
Trimethoprim + sulfadiazine (Tribrissen®, Di-Trim® 24% suspension)	IM	0.22 ml/kg q12-24h	Don't use sulfas in birds laying eggs or those with hepatic or renal compromise; maintain hydration
Trimethoprim + sulfamethoxazole (Bactrim® = 8 mg trim + 40 mg sulfa/ml suspension, Septra®)	PO	25 mg/kg q12h; 50 mg/kg q24h	GI and respiratory infections in neonates (use lower dose in neonates because of incompetent kidneys); may cause vomiting esp. in Blue and Gold Macaws
Trimethoprim + sulfamethoxazole	Oral	25 mg/kg q24h	Toucans, mynahs for coccidia
	PO	50-100 mg/L drinking water (trimeth part)	Canaries

Table 18.2 Therapeutic Agents

Drug	Route	Dosage	Comments
Trimethoprim + sulfaquinoxaline 1:3 ratio	Oral	30 mg/kg/day (186 mg/L ad lib water or 332 mg/kg feed);	Chickens: >0.25% in feed or 0.012% sulfaquinoxaline for 72 hr may cause death
Trimethoprim + sulfachloropyridazine Na (1:5 ratio)	Oral	0.04% in feed	Geese
Trimethoprim + sulfachloropyridazine Na and sulfamethoxazole (1:5 trim to combined sulfas)	Oral	0.04% in feed	Geese
TSH (thyroid stimulating hormone)	IM	1 IU/bird	Difficult to get but can be obtained; take 0 time blood sample and 4-6h post TSH blood sample; normal = 2x baseline
Tylosin (50 or 200 mg/ml injectable)	IM	Poultry: 10-40 mg/kg q6-8h; quail, emus: 15-25 mg/kg q6-8h; cranes: 15 mg/kg q6-8h	Good for some *Mycoplasma* sp, *Pasteurella* sp, *Fusobacterium* sp. *Actinomyces pyogenes*; may cause diarrhea
Tylosin (soluble powder or inj)	Eye spray	Mix 1 ml injectable with 100 ml sterile water: apply q8-12h; or 1:10 powder to water	Discontinue immediately if pain or redness occurs after instillation
Tylosin (250 mg/8.81 oz soluble powder)	Water	2 tsp/gallon	Many sick birds do not drink sufficient water
Tylosin	PO	250-400 mg/L drinking water; 400 mg/kg soft food	Canaries
Tylosin	Nebulize	1 hr q12h; mix 200 mg with 50 ml DMSO	See DMSO notes.
Tyrode's solution	PO	8.00 g NaCl, 0.13 g CaCl₂, 0.20 g KCl, 0.10 g MgCl₂, 0.05 g Na₂HPO₄, 1.00 g NaHCO₃, 1.00 g glucose: add to 1 liter drinking water.	Useful in restoring renal medullary gradient in PU/PD cockatiels; should see improvement in 4 days if sole source of drinking water
Ultralente insulin	IM	2 IU/bird	See Insulin notes; longer acting insulin

Table 18.2 Therapeutic Agents

Drug	Route	Dosage	Comments
Vitamin A, D_3, E (compounded injectable)	IM	0.3-0.6 ml/kg q7d (large birds); 0.02 ml/kg (finches, canaries)	Not to be used in birds on formulated diets; vitamin A stored in the liver; carotene may be better in birds; never give IV; vitamin A toxicity in humans includes: lethargy, anorexia, vomiting, premature growth plate closure, increased intracranial pressure, dry cracking of skin and hepatosplenomegaly; vit D_3 may not be the active metabolite in birds; compounded by Mortar and Pestel and sold only to veterinarians per valid prescription
Vitamin B complex	IM	10-30 mg/kg thiamine q7d	Most birds
Vitamin B complex	PO	1-2 g/kg food; raptors, cranes, penguins: 1-2 mg/kg q24h	Daily
Vitamin B_{12}	IM	200-500 g/kg q7d	Do not combine in same syringe with anything other than saline or water diluent
Vitamin E/selenium (1 mg Se, 50 mg vit E per ml)	IM, SC	0.05-0.1 ml/kg q14d	IM best
Vitamin K_1	IM	0.2-2.5 mg/kg, as needed; warfarin poisoning: 0.2-2.5 mg/kg q12h x 7d; other vit K_1 inhibitors: x 21d	For anticoagulant rodenticide toxins; don't give IV; can give prior to liver biopsy
Yeast cell derivatives (Preparation H®, cream only)	Topical	q24h with bandage change	For healing wounds; avoid ingestion or contact with eyes

Table 18.1 Conversions and Formulas for Drug Dose Calculations

mg/g X wt divided by mg/ml = dose in ml

(wt in g/1000) X (mg/kg) divided by mg/ml = dose in ml

1 ppm (dry weight) = 1 mg/kg

1 ppm (liquid) = 100 mg/dl

1 oz (dry) = 28.35 g

1 oz (liquid) = 29.5 ml

1 lb = 454 g

1% = 10 mg/ml

16 oz = 480 ml = 1 pint

1 cup = 8 oz = 237 ml

1 TBS = 15 ml

1 tsp = 5 cc

1 oz = 30 ml

1 ml = 1 cc

GASTROENTEROLOGY

J. T. Lumeij

Diseases of the alimentary tract occur frequently in birds. Nonspecific clinical signs of gastrointestinal diseases may include anorexia, dysphagia, regurgitation, vomiting, constipation, diarrhea and tenesmus. With polyuria, the feces are normal and are surrounded by a large volume of clear fluid, while with diarrhea the feces are abnormal. The composition and quality of food and ingestion of bedding material, poisonous plants or chemicals may influence gastrointestinal signs. Weight loss and generalized weakness are characteristic of chronic diseases.

Fecal evaluation, hematology, blood chemistry, radiology and esophago-ingluvio (gastro) scopy or laparoscopy are considered indispensable diagnostic tools in avian gastroenterology. Diseases that may affect the gastrointestinal system are listed in Table 19.1.

Cytologic examination of a fresh ingluvial aspirate is best for detecting flagellates (*Trichomonas* spp.). Examination of freshly voided feces is essential to detect *Histomonas meleagridis, Hexamita* spp., *Giardia intestinalis, Cochlosoma* sp. and *Chilomastix gallinarum*. Direct microscopic examination of feces may reveal helminthic ova and protozoal oocysts. Flotation and sedimentation techniques are best for detecting the low number of eggs or oocysts that occur in an early parasitic infection (see Chapter 36). Parasites infecting the liver, kidney, uterus and pancreas can deposit ova or oocysts that can be detected in the feces. Parasite ova originating from the respiratory tract may be coughed up, swallowed and found in the excrement.

Bacteriologic cultures of the gastrointestinal tract must be interpreted with respect to the normal flora. Gram-positive microorganisms including lactobacilli, staphylococci, streptococci and *Bacillus* spp. are common in the oropharynx of healthy psittacine birds. *Mycoplasma* spp. and *Aspergillus* spp. are sometimes encountered. Enterobacteriaceae are normally not found in the feces of Psittaciformes and Passeriformes, where gram-positive organisms, especially *Corynebacterium* sp. and *Bacillus* sp., predominate. The isola-

**TABLE 19.1   Differential Diagnosis of Clinical Signs Associated
with the Gastrointestinal Tract**

Regurgitation or Vomiting in Adults
- Iatrogenic - apomorphine, levamisole, trimethoprim/sulfadiazine (macaws), ketoconazole, doxycycline suspension (particularly macaws and Amazons)
- Fear and excitement (vultures, pelicans, penguins)
- Courtship behavior (male psittacines)
- Crop milk feeding in pigeons
- Physiological cast formation - (raptors)
- Goiter (particularly budgerigars)
- Callus formation after coracoid fracture
- Neuropathic gastric dilatation (NGD)
- Food allergies
- Motion sickness
- Viral diseases - looping ill virus, Pacheco's disease virus, pigeon herpesvirus, avian polyomavirus, avian viral serositis (togavirus), poxvirus (diphtheritic form)
- Bacterial diseases - megabacterial infection, most Enterobacteriaceae, *Pasteurella*, *Serratia*
- Mycotic diseases - candidiasis, aspergillosis
- Helminths (oropharynx/ingluvies/esophagus) - capillariasis, serratospiciliasis
- Protozoal disease - trichomoniasis of upper digestive tract, *Plasmodium* (penguins, gyrfalcon)
- Poisoning - alcohol, arsenic, copper, lead, organochlorine (lindane), organophosphate, carbamate, organomercurial, rotenone, phosphorus, polytetrafluoroethylene (Teflon), sodium chloride, thallium, zinc
- Plants - Yew (*Taxus baccata*), *Philodendron* spp., *Rhododendron* spp. (azalea), Solanaceae (green berries and roots)
- Obstructed alimentary tract - stricture, foreign body, neoplasia, intussusception, volvulus, hernia, stenosis, impaction, paralytic ileus
- Organopathy - renal disease, hepatopathy, pancreatitis, peritonitis, egg binding, electrolyte disturbances

Regurgitation in Neonatal Psittacines (Sour Crop)
- Overgrowth of bacteria or yeast (improper food storage)
- Overheated formula
- Underheated formula
- Crop burns
- Foreign body ingestion (eg, substrates)
- Improper formula consistency
- Over-stretching the crop
- Aerophagia
- Fear and excitement
- Infectious agents: Avian polyomavirus, Avian viral serositis, *Candida* spp., Gas-producing bacteria

Diarrhea
- Use of antibiotics
- Dietary changes
- Bowel obstruction
- Toxins
- Obstruction
- Foreign bodies
- Organopathy - hepatopathy, renal disease, pancreatitis
- Viral diseases - Newcastle disease virus, paramyxovirus type 3, influenza, adenovirus, astrovirus, calicivirus, coronavirus, enterovirus, Pacheco's disease virus, pigeon herpesvirus, duck virus enteritis, herpesvirus (Ciconiidae), herpesvirus (gruiformes), Marek's disease virus, orthoreovirus, parvovirus, reovirus, rotavirus, togavirus-like agent, retrovirus (leukosis/sarcoma group)
- Bacterial diseases - borreliosis, spirochaetosis, most Enterobacteriaceae, *Campylobacter* spp., *Streptococcus* spp., *Erysipelothrix rhusiopathiae*, *Listeria monocytogenes*, megabacteria, *Clostridium* spp., *Mycobacterium avium*, *Yersinia pseudotuberculosis*, *Aeromonas hydrophila*, *Pasteurella multocida*, *Pasteurella anatipestifer* (new duck disease)
- Chlamydia
- Mycoplasma
- *Candida albicans*
- Protozoa - *Histomonas meleagridis*, *Hexamita* spp., *Giardia* spp, *Cochlosoma* sp., *Chilomastix gallinarum*, coccidiosis
- Helminths - nematodes, trematodes, cestodes

Hematochezia
- Cloacal papillomas
- Egg laying
- Ulcers
- Hepatitis
- Infectious enteritis - bacterial, viral, parasitic
- Aflatoxicosis
- Coagulopathies
- Heavy metal intoxication
- Foreign bodies
- Cloacal neoplasias

Passing Undigested Food
- Gastric foreign body
- Gastrointestinal dysfunction
- Neuropathic gastric dilatation
- Enteritis - bacterial, viral, parasitic
- Pancreatitis
- Use of antibiotics
- Food allergies
- Hepatitis

Tenesmus
- Egg-laying problems (binding)
- Abdominal mass
- Goose venereal disease
- Cloacal pathology
- Prolapse
- Papilloma
- Stricture
- Cloacolith
- Cloacitis
- Intestinal obstruction (eg, constipation)
- Uterine prolapse
- Rectal prolapse
- Enteritis - diarrhea
- Bacteria
- Parasites
- Fungi
- Viruses
- Toxins
- Decreased bacteria (eg, indiscriminate antibiotic use)

tion of a large number of Enterobacteriaceae in pure culture from Psittaciformes or Passeriformes is suggestive of a primary or secondary infection. *E. coli* and other Enterobacteriaceae are normal inhabitants of the gastrointestinal tract in Galliformes, Columbiformes, Falconiformes, Strigiformes and Corvidae.

Routine bacteriologic examination of the feces may fail to reveal some important microbes that can cause diarrhea, including mycobacteria, campylobacter and chlamydia. A technique for identifying mycobacteria is described in Table 19.2. Detection of campylobacter can be augmented by the use of Hemacolor; the bacteria appear S-shaped or in gull-wing form. Chlamydia is best detected using an antigen capture system.

Table 19.2   Detection of Acid-fast Bacteria in Feces

- Combine 4 grams of feces and 12 ml of 15% sputofluol (Merck)
- Gently mix for 30 minutes
- Centrifuge for 5 minutes 10,000 rpm
- Make smear of sediment
- Stain with Ziehl-Neelsen

The Beak and Oropharynx

Beak Diseases

A variety of congenital and acquired defects, including scissor beak and mandibular prognathism, can interfere with normal beak function. In gallinaceous birds, a deformed upper mandible has been associated with embryonic deficiencies of folic acid, biotin or pantothenic acid. Crusty, scab-like lesions in the corners of the mouth are considered a definite sign of biotin or pantothenic acid deficiency in these birds.

Any bacterial, mycotic, viral or parasitic pathogen that damages the germinative layers of the beak can cause developmental abnormalities. Examples include *Candida albicans*, psittacine beak and feather disease virus, *Knemidokoptes* spp. in Psittaciformes or *Oxyspirura* spp. in cranes. Rhinothecal overgrowth in psittacines, especially budgerigars, has been associated with liver disease. The rhinotheca may overgrow in hardbills maintained in an indoor environment and provided soft foods. "Rubber bill," caused by insufficient mineralization of the upper beak, has been described with vitamin D and calcium deficiencies. Necrotic lesions at the commissure of the beak have been described with trichotecene mycotoxicosis, avian poxvirus and trichomoniasis (cockatiels).

Chronic rhinitis may lead to permanent defects in the adjoining germinative layer of the rhinotheca. Dysphagia, which may be recognized clinically as an accumulation of food under the tongue, can be an indication of rhamphothecal dysfunction.

Oropharyngeal Diseases

Poxvirus

Poxvirus may cause proliferative caseous lesions (diphtheritic form) in the mouth and esophagus in a variety of avian species. Diagnosis can be achieved by identifying elementary bodies (Bollinger bodies) in impression smears prepared from lesions and stained with Wright's stain or by the Gimenez method. Trichomoniasis lesions may have a similar gross appearance.

Pigeon Herpesvirus Infection (Smadel's Disease)

Pigeon herpesvirus (PHV) infection has been associated with pharyngeal and esophageal diphtheritic membranes, which are attached to the underlying tissues. Lesions are most severe when secondarily infected with *Trichomonas* spp. Other clinical signs include dyspnea, mucopurulent rhinitis and conjunctivitis. Histologic identification of basophilic and eosinophilic intranuclear inclusion bodies is suggestive.

Granulomas

Granulomas caused by *Mycobacterium* spp. or other bacterial or fungal agents frequently occur in the oral cavity. A diagnosis can be made by staining suspected material with the Gram's or Ziehl-Neelsen methods (see Table 19.2). Surgical removal in conjunction with appropriate antimicrobial agents is usually effective in resolving nonmycobacterial-induced granulomas.

Nematodes

Various *Capillaria* spp. may infect the mucosa of the tongue, pharynx, esophagus and ingluvies of Falconiformes, Psittaciformes, Galliformes, Passeriformes and Anseriformes. Characteristic lesions include hemorrhagic inflammation in the commissure of the beak and diphtheritic membranes in the pharynx and tongue. Parasites can be found embedded in inflammatory material. Typical bipolar eggs may be found in esophageal smears or ingluvial washings. In Strigiformes, *Synhimanthus (Dyspharynx) falconis* has been reported in the oropharynx.

Spirurid infections have been reported in diurnal and nocturnal birds of prey. Lesions containing the adult nematodes can be found in the mouth, esophagus and crop. The embryonated eggs are thick-walled. Ascarides belonging to the genus *Contracaecum* have been found in fish-eating birds, and severe infections of the oral cavity have been documented in young Pelecanidae. In birds of prey, *Seratospiculum amaculatum* can cause lesions that resemble those of oral trichomoniasis. The adult worms are found in the air sacs. Eggs may be found in the oral mucus or feces.

Hypovitaminosis A

In psittacine birds, a typical clinical sign of hypovitaminosis A is metaplasia of the submandibular or lingual salivary glands and clubbing of the choanal papillae. Affected birds are usually fed all-seed diets with a large percentage of sunflower seeds. Treatment should include parenteral vitamin A and the use of a formulated diet. Keratogenic cysts in the lingual salivary glands should be differentiated from lingual abscesses by biopsy.

Lesions associated with hypovitaminosis A in gallinaceous birds first appear in the pharynx and are largely confined to the mucous glands and their ducts. Small, white, hyperkeratotic lesions (up to 2 mm in diameter) may be seen in the nasal passages, mouth, esophagus, pharynx and crop.

Sialoliths in Pigeons

Mucosal lesions that appear similar to those caused by hypovitaminosis A have been described on the palate of pigeons and are referred to as sialoliths. The etiology of sialoliths remains unknown. However, based on their histologic, histochemical, chemical and physical characteristics, they are not thought to be caused by hypovitaminosis A. An association with pigeon herpesvirus infection has been suggested and seems plausible.

Foreign Bodies

Clinical signs of foreign bodies in the upper GI tract can include respiratory distress, head shaking, scratching the head with the feet, dysphagia or anorexia.

A string looped around the base of the tongue and passing down the esophagus has been associated with dysphagia and respiratory distress in gallinaceous birds. Ring-shaped foreign bodies (eg, tracheal rings of prey eaten by raptors) can become lodged around the tongue, causing avascular necrosis. Fish bones may lodge in the pharynx or proximal part of the esophagus causing dysphagia. Plant hairs that lodge in the oral or esophageal mucosa can cause granulomas.

Stomatitis

Stomatitis in birds has been associated with the consumption of hot foods, ingestion of oil and ingestion of caustic substances. Birds that chew on silver nitrate sticks may have extensive chemical burns of the oropharynx and crop. Use of bipolar radiosurgery is superior to silver nitrate sticks for controlling hemorrhage of the beak and nails. Stomatitis may occur secondary to food accumulations caused by beak deformities (eg, PBFD). Beak necrosis has been described in pigeons and gallinaceous birds fed a finely ground, high-gluten food.

Many trichotecenes, notably T_2 toxin, can cause caustic injury to the alimentary mucosa. Yellow erosive and exudative plaques with underlying ulcers located near the salivary duct openings on the palate, tongue and buccal floor are characteristic lesions. Thick crusts of exudate may accumulate along the anterior margin of the beak. Anorexia is probably caused by the painful lesions in the beak.

Lacerations of the Tongue

Anesthesia, magnification and radiocautery are usually necessary to control bleeding and repair tongue lacerations.

Glossitis Gelatinosa Circumscripta

A gelatinous mass may be found on the dorsal aspect of the tongue in five- to twelve-week-old ducklings and goslings. The precise etiology is undetermined, but a multi-deficient diet has been suggested.

The Esophagus and Crop

In Galliformes and Falconiformes, the crop forms a ventral enlargement of the esophagus at the thoracic inlet. In Psittaciformes, the crop is stretched transversely across the neck. In canaries and ducks, the crop is absent, but there is a spindle-shaped swelling of the esophagus at the thoracic inlet. In pigeons, the ventral diverticulum of the esophagus that forms the crop is divided into two large lateral sacs. The esophagus is lined with partly keratinized stratified squamous epithelium. Mucous glands are located in the lamina propria, and are numerous in the thoracic esophagus.

Investigative Methods

Clinical signs of esophageal or ingluvial disorders may include dysphagia, anorexia, retching, regurgitation or vomiting. In budgerigars, vomiting may be accompanied by a rapid flick of the beak, which frequently deposits vomitus on top of the bird's head. A history of recent drug administration, assisted feeding, poor hygiene or access to toxic compounds may suggest an etiology for esophageal problems.

The skin and feathers overlying the crop should be examined for abnormalities. Wetting of the feathers will help in visualizing lacerations, discolorations or necrosis of the crop. Hypermotility or hypomotility may occur with crop disorders. In domestic fowl, peristaltic waves occur in the cervical esophagus at intervals of 15 seconds and in the thoracic esophagus, at intervals of about one minute. A psittacine crop that is partially filled with food should average one or two contractions per minute.

An enlarged crop with a dough-like consistency that fails to empty is suggestive of a crop impaction. Occasionally, large deposits of fat, and in some cases lipomas, can occur near the crop and should not be misdiagnosed as a full or impacted crop. The improper placement of feeding cannulas can result in esophageal lacerations, with food being deposited into the subcutaneous, periesophageal tissues. Discolored necrotic areas, swelling and edema are common clinical findings.

For diagnostic purposes, an esophageal or ingluvial aspirate can be obtained by inserting a catheter and washing the mucosa with sterile isotonic saline solution. Luer-lock syringes should always be used when tube-feeding or collecting samples from psittacine birds to prevent them from swallowing the tube. Immediate microscopic examination of a wet mount slide is best for diagnosing trichomoniasis. Material aspirated from the crop should be centrifuged, and microscopic examination of the sediment may reveal nematode eggs or *Candida* spp. Air-dried smears can be stained with Diff-Quik, Gram's stain, Wright's stain, Hemacolor or other stains for specific cytologic examination (see Chapter 10).

A fecal flotation and crop aspirate should be performed to detect parasite ova that might indicate an esophageal or ingluvial nematode or trematode infection. Flotation is more likely to detect low concentrations of eggs than a direct smear. Endoscopy is useful for examining the gastrointestinal mucosa and for removing some foreign bodies.

Diseases of the Esophagus and Crop

Trichomoniasis

Trichomonas gallinae infections commonly occur in pigeons and raptors, and may also occur in Passeriformes (particularly canaries and Zebra Finches) and Psittaciformes (particularly budgerigars and cockatiels). In pigeons, the proliferative necrotic lesions caused by trichomoniasis are called "canker," while in falcons the disease is called "frounce." Trichomoniasis lesions appear similar to those caused by poxvirus; however, in cockatiels, poxvirus infections are uncommon.

Samples for detecting *T. gallinae* can best be collected by introducing a slightly moistened cotton-tipped applicator into the esophagus, and moving it up and down several times against the mucosal lining. The cotton tip is then compressed between the thumb and index finger to produce one drop of fluid, which is placed on a slide for direct examination.

Trichomoniasis can cause inflammation of the upper intestinal tract and mouth resulting in dysphagia or vomiting, and may be an underdiagnosed cause of ingluvitis in budgerigars. The intracellular occurrence of trichomoniasis has not been reported in other avian genera, and this unique feature of infection in budgerigars may contribute to the underdiagnosis of trichomoniasis as a cause of morbidity and mortality in Psittaciformes.

Nitroimidazole drugs like metronidazole, ronidazole, dimetridazole and carnidazole are usually effective in treating trichomoniasis; however, nitroimidazole-resistant strains of trichomoniasis occur in The Netherlands because of the improper use of these drugs by pigeon fanciers.

Nematode and Trematode Infections

Many nematodes including *Capillaria* spp., *Echinura uncinata*, *Gongylonema ingluvicola* and *Dyspharynx nasuata* can invade the esophageal or crop mucosa. The thorny-headed worm (*Oncicola canis*) has been reported in turkeys.

Ingluvial/Esophageal Stasis and Dilatation

The suggestive causes of crop stasis include heavy metal toxicity, crop impaction, callus formation after a coracoid fracture, thyroid enlargement, atonic crop, sour crop, overstretching of the crop, esophagitis (candidiasis, trichomoniasis, capillariasis, serratospiciliasis), ingluvioliths and esophageal stenosis. If the fluid in the crop remains stagnant, it will decay and have a foul odor (often referred to as sour crop). Regurgitation of proventricular fluid may be a contributing factor. Feeding a liquid formula to granivorous birds can induce crop stasis, possibly as a result of a lack of mechanical stimulation.

Crop Impaction

Impacted material in the crop can be softened by the administration of warm water followed by massaging the crop. However, an ingluviotomy will generally be the method of choice for removing impacted material. Foreign bodies may be removed endoscopically. Expressing the ingluvial contents through the mouth by turning the bird upside down is a dangerous procedure that may lead to irritation of the nasal mucosa, sinusitis or aspiration pneumonia. Packing the choana with cotton and intubating with an endotracheal tube will help eliminate this problem.

Ingluvioliths

Urate (excreta) calculi with seed husk centers were described in the crops of several budgerigars. Other ingluvioliths have been found to contain potassium phosphate, oxalate and cystine, and were not considered to have occurred secondary to urate ingestion.

Foreign Bodies

Any ingested foreign body, including rubber or metal feeding tubes, should be removed immediately from the ingluvies before it has an opportunity to align with the thoracic esophagus and pass into the (pro)ventriculus.

Crop and Esophageal Lacerations and Fistula

Penetration of the pharynx or esophagus by feeding cannulas, or esophageal-ingluvial burns caused by ingestion of overheated feeding formulas or caustic materials can result in deposition of food subcutaneously and lead to extensive foreign body reactions. A feeding tube can be passed from the esophagus directly into the proventriculus to allow enteral feeding while the esophagus and crop heal (see Chapters 15, 16 and 41).

Esophageal strictures may also occur secondary to burns or foreign body ingestion. A cockatoo with severe self-mutilation syndrome damaged the periesophageal skin to such a degree that the esophagus was occluded and the bird died from asphyxiation.

The Proventriculus and Ventriculus

Proventricular and Ventricular Diseases

Megabacterial Proventriculitis

"Going light" syndrome in budgerigars, a disease characterized by emaciation, weakness, high morbidity and low mortality, has been described in canaries and budgerigars. Vomiting of slimy material is seen in advanced stages of the disease. Postmortem findings include proventriculitis and proventricular dilatation. Histologically, gram-positive, PAS-positive, acidophilic (with Giemsa), rod-shaped bacteria can be identified, especially in the area between the proventriculus and ventriculus.

A diagnosis can be made by cytologic demonstration of the organisms in a proventricular washing. The pH of the proventriculus is markedly elevated in affected birds. The pH of the proventriculus from normal canaries was found to range from 0.7-2.4 compared to severely infected canaries in which the pH was 7.0-7.3. In birds with moderate numbers of megabacteria, the pH of the proventriculus ranged from 1.0-2.0. The most important differential diagnosis is trichomoniasis.

Proventricular and Ventricular Nematodes

Many nematode species have been reported to occur in the proventriculus (*Echinura uncinata, Gongylonema ingluvicola, Cyrnea* spp., *Dyspharynx nasuata* and *Tetrameres* spp.). *Amidostomum* spp., *Cheilospirura spinosa* and *Epomidiostomum uncinatum* are found under the horny layer of the ventriculus. Lesions vary considerably depending on the host and the parasite, and may be quite extensive (see Chapter 36). Clinical signs may be absent or include emaciation, anemia and mortality. Diagnosis can often be made by detecting parasite eggs using a fecal flotation technique. Treatment can be attempted with levamisole (20 mg/kg orally, or 10 mg/kg parenterally) or ivermectin (200 μg/kg parenterally). It should be stressed that experience with ivermectin in many avian species is absent. Acute death has been reported after the use of ivermectin in some mammalian and reptilian species.

Neuropathic Gastric Dilatation and Encephalomyelitis of Psittacines

Many psittacine species can be affected, including macaws, cockatoos, conures, African Grey Parrots, Senegal Parrots, Amazon parrots, Eclectus Parrots, Thick-billed Parrots and cockatiels.

Clinical signs are related to (pro)ventricular and sometimes neurologic dysfunction, and may include anorexia, regurgitation, undigested seeds in the feces and weight loss. The occurrence of neurologic signs is variable. In advanced cases, proventricular dilatation can be visualized on abdominal radiographs, with or without contrast media. In the clinical patient, a tentative diagnosis of NGD can be made based on clinical signs and radiographic findings. It should be stressed that other diseases can mimic NGD and should be ruled out before a definitive diagnosis is considered. NGD can be confirmed by histologic identification of characteristic lesions in the splanchnic nerves from a ventricular biopsy. However, a negative result derived from a small biopsy of the ventricular wall does not rule out NGD.

Table 19.6 Differential Diagnosis of Neuropathic Gastric Dilatation
• Heavy metal poisoning
• Fungal infection of ventriculus or koilin mycosis
• Nematode infection of the (pro)ventriculus
• Megabacteria infection of the proventriculus
• Gastric impaction
• Pyloric obstruction by a foreign body
• Ventriculus perforation by a foreign body
• Myoventricular dysgenesis
• Proventricular foreign body
• Koilin dysgenesis
• Myoventricular calcinosis
• Intestinal papillomatosis
• Proventricular and ventricular neoplasia
• Vitamin E and selenium deficiencies

Although the etiology is presently unclear, a viral etiology has been suggested because of epidemiologic histories of affected aviaries and the demonstration of intranuclear and intracytoplasmic inclusion bodies in affected tissue of some birds.

Affected animals invariably die after a more or less protracted course of the disease. General therapy including supportive care, a liquid diet, vitamin supplementation and treatment of secondary diseases has been recommended. It has been suggested that birds can survive on a liquid diet, but no case reports could be found that document long-term survival of birds confirmed by ventricular biopsy to have NGD. Treatment of NGD should be considered with caution, given that the disease may be caused by an infectious agent.

It has been suggested that a virus may induce an autoimmune reaction that would be responsible for the lesions observed in NGD. The inciting virus would no longer be present when the disease became clinically obvious or was diagnosed at necropsy. If this scenario is true, then administration of an anti-inflammatory dose of corticosteroids might be indicated.

Ganglioneuritis and Encephalitis in Geese

Proventricular impaction with nonsuppurative encephalomyelitis and ganglioneuritis morphologically similar to NGD in psittacine birds has been reported in two Canada Geese.

Gastric Impaction and Gastric Foreign Bodies

Gastric impaction is common in psittacine babies that consume bedding material such as crushed walnut shell, ground corncob, shredded paper pulp, Styrofoam packing, kitty litter and excess grit. These bedding materials should not be used with neonates.

Ventricular impaction secondary to litter ingestion has been reported to cause high mortality during the first three weeks of life in turkey poults.

Although poorly documented in birds, emetics might be useful to remove foreign bodies that would not damage the gastrointestinal mucosa during the regurgitation process. Apomorphine induced emesis in 55% of treated birds and in another study, a 0.5% solution of tartar emetic was effective.

Metallic Foreign Bodies: Traumatic Gastritis, Heavy Metal Poisoning

Ingestion of metallic foreign bodies is relatively common in Galliformes, Anseriformes, Columbiformes, Gruiformes, Pelecaniformes, Psittaciformes and ratites. In captive Psittaciformes and free-ranging Anseriformes, ingestion of lead is extremely common. Paralysis of the intestinal tract from nerve damage may occur secondary to lead poisoning. In Anseriformes, this is clinically recognized as esophageal and proventricular dilatation. In the other orders, ingestion of ferrous metal objects, such as nails, wire, hairpins and needles, account for the majority of cases. This is particularly common in gallinaceous birds.

Ingestion of ferrous objects may cause perforation of the ventriculus (majority of cases) or proventriculus, leading to an acute, generalized, purulent peritonitis or to a local peritonitis with abscess formation on the serosal surface of the (pro)ventriculus or duodenum.

In the racing pigeon, passing undigested seed is considered pathognomonic for a traumatic gastritis. In chronic cases, anorexia, weight loss and a palpable abscess on the left side of the abdominal wall may be noted. Radiology is the method of choice to confirm a tentative diagnosis.

Noninvasive treatments for removal of gastric metal foreign bodies should be attempted before (pro)ventriculotomy. Ferrous metals may be removed from the (pro)ventriculus using a powerful magnet of neo-dymium-ferro-borium alloy (The Magnet Store 1-800-222-7846) attached to a small-diameter polyvinyl catheter with a removable steel guide wire. The size of the polyvinyl probe and magnetic disk can be varied according to the size of the animal. Fluoroscopy or endoscopy can be used to guide grasping forceps in the removal of gastric foreign bodies. Most cases of lead and zinc ingestion can be managed medically and do not require surgery.

Vitamin E and Selenium Deficiencies

Vitamin E and selenium deficiencies may cause degenerative lesions in the smooth muscle of the ventriculus of domestic and free-ranging Anseriformes.

Gastric Ulceration, Ventriculus Erosion, Gastritis, Koilin Dysgenesis

Idiopathic proventricular ulcers do occur in psittacine birds. Many affected animals are "high strung" or live in what could be called stressful environments.

High dietary levels of certain types of fish meal or finely ground, low-fiber diets can cause erosions and ulcers in the koilin layer of gallinaceous birds.

Infectious and parasitic agents may damage the ventricular wall causing dysfunction. Penetration of foreign bodies may cause localized lesions. Zoalene (DOT) toxicosis may cause gastric erosion. Ventriculus erosion with a heavy infiltration of heterophils has been reported with zinc poisoning.

Copper Poisoning

Excessive dietary copper leads to roughening and thickening of the koilin layer.

Neoplasias

Clinical signs of neoplasias may include weight loss, vomiting, passing of whole seeds in the feces, regenerative anemia, hypoproteinemia and melena. Although hypoproteinemia may occur, the albumin/globulin ratio is not affected, which together with the anemia and melena is strongly indicative of gastrointestinal blood loss. Death usually ensues when massive gastric bleeding occurs following erosion of a major vessel. Contrast radiography using both positive and negative contrast may be helpful in outlining the (pro)ventricular neoplasm. Endoscopic-guided biopsy may be used to confirm a tentative diagnosis.

Tumors are frequently located at the isthmus on the boundary between the proventriculus and ventriculus. Gross lesions in the (pro)ventriculus may be subtle, and histologic examination is needed to differentiate tumors from other causes of ulceration or hypertrophy.

Presently, no reports of successful treatment of (pro)ventricular tumors have been published, but it has been suggested that early diagnosis and surgical excision are feasible.

The Small and Large Intestines

Intestinal Diseases

Enteritis

Many infectious agents can cause enteritis. Table 19.1 lists some infectious causes of diarrhea. Infectious stunting syndrome (ISS) in chickens (probably of viral etiology) is associated with an enteritis and inflammation of the pancreatic ducts. Most affected birds recover completely after a period of diarrhea. However, some birds develop exocrine pancreatic deficiency secondary to blockage of the pancreatic ducts.

Ileus

Ileus can be defined as a condition wherein the passage of intestinal contents is arrested or severely impaired. The cause of intestinal obstruction may be physical or it may be due to impaired motor function (paralytic ileus). Occlusion of the intestinal lumen may be caused by foreign bodies, enteroliths or parasites. Intestinal wall lesions that have been reported to cause stenosis in birds include tumors, granulomas and strictures. Extraluminal compression may occur from intussusception, volvulus mesenterialis, volvulus nodosus, incarcerated hernia mesenterialis, pseudoligaments and adhesions due to tumors or peritonitis.

Vascular causes of ileus include embolism and thrombosis of a splanchnic artery or vein with infarction of a bowel segment.

Neurogenic causes (paralytic ileus) include lead poisoning, peritonitis, neuropathic gastric dilatation and enteritis.

Once the intestine is obstructed it dilates, and fluid is collected in the intestinal lumen and lost from the circulation. Clinical signs depend on the site and severity of the obstruction. The birds become rapidly dehydrated and are severely depressed. In many conditions ischemic necrosis of the intestinal wall occurs, leading to increased permeability and protein loss into the intestinal lumen. Resorption of intestinal contents, including endotoxins released from gram-negative bacteria, can cause shock. Usually complete intestinal obstruction in birds caused by intussusception or volvulus is fatal within 24-48 hours. A more protracted course is common with other causes of intestinal obstruction. Vomiting is usually present in complete mechanical obstruction, although this sign may be absent when the obstruction is in the caudal part of the intestinal tract. The passage of feces is diminished or absent. Diarrhea may be present with partial obstruction. Emaciation is seen when the obstruction occurs gradually from a progressive disease.

Plain radiographs may show the extent and location of the gas-filled intestinal loops. A barium enema or upper GI contrast study may be used to determine the exact location of the obstruction. The use of double contrast techniques facilitates visualization of lesions in the intestinal wall. Early diagnosis and rapid surgical correction may successfully resolve many intestinal obstructions. Birds should be stabilized with fluids and antibiotics before surgery.

The Cloaca

Clinical Examination

Clinical signs indicative of cloacal disorders may include flatulence, tenesmus, soiled pericloacal area, protruding tissue from the cloaca and foul-smelling feces. Examination of the cloaca should start with the feathers and skin around the vent. Normally these structures should be clean, and there should be no signs of inflammation. An abnormal acidic smell can be a sign of cloacitis, which is often associated with cloacal papillomatosis.

A prolapse involving the cloaca may contain intestines, oviduct and one or both ureters. The appearance of smooth, glistening, pink tissue is an indication that the cloaca has prolapsed, which may be caused by sphincter problems, chronic irritation of the rectum or tenesmus. A cloacal prolapse may cause severe constipation and toxemia.

Acute cloacal prolapse associated with egg laying generally responds to manual reduction, followed by application of two simple transverse stay sutures perpendicular to the vent. Postoperative straining can be prevented by applying xylocaine gel in the cloaca q12h. The cause of the straining or increased abdominal pressure should be corrected to prevent further prolapsing.

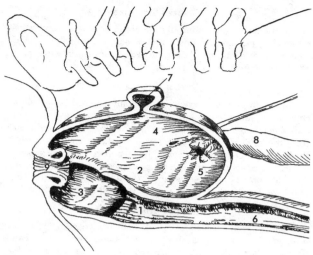

FIG 19.16 The cloaca is composed of the 1) coprodeum, 2) urodeum and 3) proctodeum. The 4) openings of the ureter and 5) vagina can be seen in the urodeum. Other structures associated with the cloaca include the 6) rectum, 7) cloacal bursa, 8) oviduct and 9) vent.

In cockatoos, chronic cloacal prolapse may be associated with sexual behavior in the presence of the owner, or can be caused by idiopathic straining. A combination of ventral cloacopexy and cloacal mucosal "reefing" has been used to correct chronic cloacal prolapse (see Chapter 41).

Cloacitis

A sporadically occurring, chronic inflammatory process of the cloaca with a very offensive odor, commonly known as "vent gleet," may occur in laying hens and occasionally in males. A yellow diphtheritic membrane may form on the mucosal surface, and urates and inflammatory exudate contaminate the skin and feathers around the vent. The cause is unknown. Treatment consists of cleaning the area and applying a local antibiotic ointment.

Neisseria, Mycoplasma spp. and *Candida albicans*

Bacteria (especially *Neisseria* and *Mycoplasma* spp.), and *Candida albicans* have been associated with a venereal disease affecting ganders. It seems likely that the cloacitis observed in drakes has a similar etiology, but an association has not been confirmed.

Phallus Prolapse and Venereal Disease in Anseriformes

The phallus may not retract into the cloaca in some sexually mature drakes. The problem is usually associated with an extensive infection in the erectile tissue at the base of the phallus. It has been suggested that the etiology of this condition is traumatic, because the incidence is higher under conditions where the drakes have to mate with the females out of the water. Drakes with females that have cloacitis may have a phallus infection, suggesting that an infectious agent can play a role in phallus prolapse.

Cloacal Stricture

Infections, surgical manipulation of the cloaca (particularly for removal of papillomas) and trauma may cause stricture of the vent, requiring surgical recreation of an opening and appropriate aftercare to prevent a recurrence.

Cloacal Impaction

Cloacal impaction may occur from foreign bodies (eg, potato chunks in Galliformes), fecaliths, concrements of urates and retained necrotic eggs. Uroliths can vary from six to eight millimeter-thick concrements on the cloacal wall to solid masses the size of a chicken egg. In any case of cloacal impaction, passing excrement is difficult or impossible and can cause congestion of the ureters and dilatation of the intestines as far proximal as the duodenum. Renal failure and visceral gout may occur if the ureters are blocked.

Cloacal Papillomatosis

Cloacal papillomatosis is a well known disease in psittacine birds and is recognized clinically as a glistening red or pink cauliflower- or strawberry-like mass rising from the cloacal orifice. Early lesions are characterized by a rough-appearing mucosa at the mucocutaneous junction of the cloaca. Other presenting signs may include tenesmus, melena, foul-smelling feces, flatulence, pasting of the vent and cloacoliths. The abnormal odor is likely to be caused by bacterial proliferation in the crypts caused by the papillomas. The incidence of disease is higher in New World parrots, but Old World parrots may also be affected. The condition is frequently misdiagnosed as a cloacal prolapse. Applying an acetic acid solution (apple cider vinegar) to cloacal epithelium will change the color of papillomatous tissue to white. A definitive diagnosis can be made after histopathologic examination of a biopsy. Cloacal papillomas are often associated with similar lesions in the oropharynx, choana, esophagus, crop, proventriculus, ventriculus and occasionally mucosa of the eye and nose. The etiology is presently unknown. There seems to be a high correlation between neoplasia of bile ducts and pancreatic ducts and papillomatosis in psittacine birds.

Various techniques have been used to treat cloacal papillomas, including cryosurgery, chemical cautery, radiosurgery and autogenous vaccination, but the reported spontaneous remissions and intermittent nature of the disease makes evaluation of the various treatments difficult. The introduction of birds with papillomas to a breeding facility should be prevented by performing a thorough physical examination at the beginning and end of the quarantine period. Of 41 papillomatous lesions, growth was benign in 40, but one single case was diagnosed as carcinoma *in situ*. Other tumors should be considered in the differential diagnosis. Papillomas are most easily removed from the cloaca with careful, staged cauterization with a silver nitrate stick. The silver nitrate must come in contact only with the tissue intended to be removed to prevent severe burns of normal cloacal mucosa.

The Pancreas

Diagnostic Considerations

The pancreas has both endocrine and exocrine functions. The former are discussed in Chapter 23. Many postmortem lesions have been reported in avian pancreata. There are two major clinical manifestations of pancreatic disease. If no pancreatic enzymes are available in the duodenum, maldigestion and passing of feces with excessive amylum and fat will occur. Affected animals may have voluminous, pale or tan, greasy feces. Fat in the feces can be demonstrated by Sudan staining. Interpretation of microscopic examination of feces for undigested food such as fat, starch grains and muscle fibers is complicated by variation in diets and by changes due to intestinal causes of malabsorption. Measurement of fecal proteolytic activity can be performed in several ways. The X-ray film gelatin digestion test is an unreliable assay of fecal proteolytic activity. A test for fecal proteolytic and amylase activity is probably more reliable for use in birds.

Pancreatic Diseases

Acute Pancreatic Necrosis/Acute Pancreatitis

The pathogenesis of acute pancreatitis involves the activation of pancreatic enzymes in and around the pancreas and in the bloodstream, resulting in coagulation necrosis of the pancreas, and necrosis and hemorrhage of peripancreatic and peritoneal adipose tissue. Affected birds may be in shock, and radiographs may show loss of abdominal detail due to peritonitis and fluid accumulation in the peritoneal cavity. Dilatation of the small intestine may be visible due to an accompanying ileus. Increased plasma amylase activity (secondary to destruction of exocrine pancreatic cells) has been reported in chronic active pancreatitis in birds. Elevated plasma amylase may also occur with occlusion of the main pancreatic duct, and might be a component of the infectious stunting syndrome in chickens. Lipemia may be present. A diagnosis of pancreatitis can be confirmed by endoscopy or exploratory laparotomy.

Obesity seems to be a predisposing factor of pancreatitis in birds. Treatment should include withholding food and oral medication for 72 hours, correction of fluid and electrolyte balance and prophylactic use of antibiotics. Dietary fat intake should be restricted to decrease the secretory load of the pancreas.

Chronic Pancreatic Fibrosis/Chronic Pancreatitis/ Pancreatic Exocrine Insufficiency

A decrease in pancreatic glandular tissue or fibrosis may occur as the result of a chronic inflammatory process and cause clinical changes suggestive of pancreatic exocrine insufficiency (PEI). Further studies on the relation between pancreatic disease and plasma amylase and plasma lipase activities in birds are needed to facilitate clinical diagnosis; however, birds with a malabsorption syndrome and high amylase and lipase levels may respond to therapy with pancreatic enzymes, suggesting PEI. Frequently, the cause of PEI is undetermined. Pancreatic fibrosis was reported in two psittacine birds with chronic chlamydiosis.

High dietary levels of zinc may cause dilation of acinar lumina and degenerative changes in acinar cells including depletion of zymogen bodies, cytoplasmic vacuolization, the presence of hyaline bodies and other electron-dense debris, necrosis of individual acinar cells and fibrosis. Excess levels of zinc also interfere with exocrine pancreatic function.

Pancreatic atrophy and fibrosis accompanied by impaired fat digestion have been reported in chickens on a selenium-deficient diet. It has been shown that addition of 0.1 ppm selenium to the diet could reverse the clinical signs and cause complete pancreatic acinar regeneration.

Paramyxovirus Infections in Psittaciformes and Passeriformes

Paramyxovirus type III is a common infection in *Neophema* spp. and *Platycerca* spp., and is also encountered in some passerine birds, especially Estrildidae. Torticollis, other neurologic signs, cachexia and death are common. Some infected birds develop a yellow-to-white chalky stool that contains large amounts of starch. In almost all cases, a pancreatitis can be detected. Histologically, the lesions can vary from a few lymphoid follicles to massive infiltration with lymphocytes and plasma cells. In some cases, this is clinically manifested as pancreatic exocrine insufficiency.

Campylobacter infections in Estrildidae cause similar discoloration of the feces. Histologically, atrophy of the microvilli of the small intestine, which may cause a malabsorption syndrome, can be found.

Pancreatic Tumors

A high correlation between neoplasia of bile ducts and pancreatic ducts and internal papillomatous diseases in psittacine birds has been suggested.

The Pleuro-peritoneum

Ascites

Ascites is defined as the accumulation of serous fluid within one or more of the peritoneal cavities and may be caused by peritoneal and extraperitoneal diseases. Accumulation of fluid in one or more peritoneal cavity can result in abdominal distention. Large amounts of ascitic fluid may compress the pulmonary air sac system, causing dyspnea. During physical examination, abdominal distention can be recognized by the increased distance from carina to pubic bones. A bird with ascites should be handled carefully to prevent rupture of the air sacs, which can lead to immediate asphyxiation. Clinical signs may or may not occur with abdominal fluid accumulations. In liver disease, yellow or green feces may be seen. In neoplastic or liver disease, palpable masses may be present in the abdomen.

In ascites associated with liver disease (including hepatic congestion due to cardiac disease), increased portal venous hydrostatic pressure and decreased portal venous colloid osmotic pressure are important factors. Increased subperitoneal capillary permeability, decreased peritoneal lymphatic drainage and leakage from disrupted abdominal viscera (bile, urine) may cause non-liver related ascites. Sometimes the definition of ascites is restricted to noninflammatory transudate, but the distinction between transudate and exudate is not always clear under clinical conditions. Conditions where an inflammatory exudate is present can be defined as peritonitis.

Although it has been suggested that chylous ascites (ascites due to the presence of lipoproteins and chylomicrons in the peritoneal cavity) can occur in birds, current information on avian physiology suggests that the absorption of fat from the intestine in birds is different from what occurs in mammals. The lymphatic system is not as well developed in birds as in mammals. The lymphatic vessels are small, the largest being hardly more than 1 mm in diameter, and the thoracic duct is only 1.5 mm across. Because there is no functional intestinal lymphatic system in birds, absorbed lipids enter the portal system as large, very low-density lipoproteins. These lipoproteins have been defined as "portomicrons" in contrast to "chylomicrons" (the fat-rich particles that are absorbed by mammals). Chylous peritonitis, which occurs in mammals secondary to rupture of the lymphatic vessels or lymphatic congestion, is therefore theoretically not possible in birds.

Blockage of lymph drainage can be an important factor in the development of ascites in birds. For example, implantation of oviduct carcinoma on the intestinal peritoneal cavity rapidly induces ascites from portal hypertension secondary to pulmonary hypertension. Right ventricular failure with valvular insufficiency results in increased pressure in the vena cava where the lymph ducts connect to the circulatory system.

Pseudochylous ascites is the condition whereby turbid or milky abdominal fluid is seen. This may be caused by cellular debris and is associated with abdominal malignancies and infections.

Edema may occur in organs and tissues in conjunction with ascites caused by hypoalbuminemia. It may be recognized clinically as edema of subcutaneous tissues of the abdomen or pitting edema on the feet (ducks with amyloidosis).

Diagnostic Methods

Radiographically, ascites is characterized by a diffuse, ground-glass haziness in the abdomen, and specific organs are often impossible to delineate. Administration of furosemide for several days or abdominocentesis will increase the diagnostic value of the radiographs. The cardiohepatic silhouette may appear widened, and the air sacs may appear narrowed laterally on the ventrodorsal view. Occasionally, ileus or enlargement of the heart, liver, spleen or other abdominal organs may be detected, providing information with respect to the primary disorder. Ultrasonography is a noninvasive technique that is valuable in the differential diagnosis of abdominal enlargement and ascites (see Chapter 12).

Abdominocentesis provides diagnostic information in birds with ascites (see Chapter 10).

Clinical Biochemistry and Hematology

Laboratory investigations in birds with ascites should include plasma chemistries for hepatic and renal disease (AST, CPK, LDH, bile acids, protein electrophoresis, uric acid, urea). Renal protein loss should be evaluated by a quantitative determination of protein in the urine. Additionally, a PCV and total WBC and differential are indicated. When peritonitis is present, a marked leucocytosis can be observed, with the predominant cell type being heterophilic leukocytes. Juvenile heterophils (band cells) are normally not present in the peripheral blood and indicate severe inflammation. Granulomatous diseases and avian tuberculosis are often associated with monocytosis.

In neoplastic disease, exfoliated neoplastic cells may be encountered. Hemorrhagic effusions may have the appearance of peripheral blood and have leukocyte and erythrocyte numbers comparable to peripheral blood. Chronic hemorrhagic effusions may show signs of erythrophagocytosis. Urine in the abdominal cavity can be recognized by the presence of spherical urate crystals.

Differential Diagnosis

Abdominal enlargement due to ascites should be differentiated from other causes of abdominal enlargement such as obesity, neoplasia, herniation, egg-related peritonitis, granuloma, gravid uterus, gastrointestinal dilatation, hepatomegaly, splenomegaly and renomegaly. A cystic right oviduct can also pose a diagnostic challenge to the clinician because these fluid-filled cysts may reach a size up to 10 cm in diameter and may compress the abdominal viscera, mimicking ascites.

Chronic liver disease can cause ascites through intrahepatic portal hypertension due to hepatic fibrosis (aflatoxicosis, coal tar poisoning, plant toxins from *Crotalaria* spp. or rapeseed, bacterial or viral cholangiohepatitis). The accompanying hypoalbuminemia contributes to ascites formation.

Ascites may occur as part of generalized edema secondary to hypoalbuminemia caused by chronic liver disease, nephrotic syndrome and protein-losing enteropathy.

Congestive heart failure (with right ventricular failure), from various causes, may cause ascites.

Exposure to chlorinated biphenyls, dioxin (toxic fat syndrome), creosol and coal tar products can damage the endothelial lining of blood vessels, causing hydropericardium and ascites.

Viral infections such as Marek's disease tumors may occur in the heart, and viruses of the leukosis-sarcoma group can cause various tumors associated with ascites (hemangioma and hemangiosarcoma of mesentery, erythroblastosis, mesotheliomas). Other viruses including avian polyomavirus and avian viral serositis can cause myocarditis and pericarditis leading to RVF and ascites.

Mycobacterium spp. infections can cause blockage of lymph drainage in some cases. Acid-fast (Ziehl-Neelsen) staining organisms may be noted in ascitic fluid.

Penetrating or nonpenetrating trauma to the abdomen can cause urate ascites, bile ascites, pancreatic ascites and hemoperitoneum (rupture of liver, spleen or kidney). Enlargement of an organ or other space-occupying masses can block lymph drainage, resulting in ascites.

Cystic right oviduct occurs if the right Muellerian duct does not regress normally. The oviduct remnant is attached to the cloaca by a narrow stalk. Ultrasonography can differentiate between free fluid and fluid encapsulated within a cyst.

Therapy for ascites should be aimed at the primary disorder. Therapeutic removal of ascitic fluid is indicated only if ascites is accompanied by a life-threatening dyspnea. If hypoproteinemia is present, abdominocentesis will remove protein from a bird that may have compromised liver or kidney function. Diuretic therapy (furosemide) can be administered to effect. Low-sodium diets may be helpful.

Accumulation of fat in the peritoneal cavity can cause dyspnea through compression of the thoracic and abdominal air sacs. Obesity is commonly seen in parrots, cockatoos and pigeons on high-energy diets with restricted exercise, but many other species can be affected.

Ventral abdominal hernias are common in budgerigars and racing pigeons (particularly hens). A causal relationship with hyperestrogenism, which causes weakening of the abdominal muscles, has been suggested. The hernia may contain fat, loops of bowel or other abdominal organs. Incarceration of the intestinal tract is a rare but possible complication. A diagnosis can be made by physical examination and radiology. Treatment involves surgical closure of the abdominal hernia. Removal of excess fat that is primarily located between the sheets of the posthepatic septum facilitates the procedure. A perineal hernia containing a persistent right oviduct was observed by the author in a budgerigar.

The most common causes of peritonitis in birds are foreign bodies (from alimentary tract or through abdominal wall) and egg-related peritonitis.

HEPATOLOGY

J. T. Lumeij

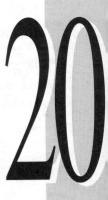

The avian liver is bilobed and relatively large in comparison to the size of the bird. The left hepatic duct connects to the duodenum. The right hepatic duct connects to the gall bladder in those species that have this organ (gallinaceous birds, ducks, geese). If the gall bladder is absent (pigeons, parrots, ostriches), the right hepatic duct drains directly into the duodenum. If this duct dilates, it may appear as though a gall bladder is present. Birds have no mesenteric lymph nodes, and patients with chronic enteritis may also have periportal hepatitis. The liver in a normal Psittaciforme rests ventrally against the sternum, wraps cranially around the base of the heart and wraps dorsally along the lateral margins of the proventriculus. Bile acids secreted by the liver function to emulsify fats and activate pancreatic lipase and amylase, all of which aid in digestion. The liver also metabolizes fats, proteins and carbohydrates and detoxifies metabolites and ingested toxins.

Diagnostic Considerations

Physical findings associated with liver disease are often nonspecific, and are generally not sufficiently diagnostic to establish a clinical diagnosis. A green coloration of the urine and urate fractions in the excreta is a strong indication of liver disease. Dyspnea is a common finding in birds with hepatomegaly or ascites. Occasionally, an enlarged liver can be palpated and in the smaller Passeriformes, an enlarged liver may be visible through the transparent abdominal wall. Abnormal coloration of the liver is also sometimes visible, particularly in small species and neonates. Polydipsia and vomiting are sometimes associated with liver disease. Pruritus occurs commonly in icteric humans and is thought to be caused by the deposition of irritant bile salts in the skin. Clinical signs suggestive of pruritus and feather picking have been reported in birds with liver disease. Other integumentary disorders that are loosely discussed in association with liver disease include feather pigment changes, abnormal molting and softening, flaking and overgrowth of beak and nails.

Because liver diseases may be associated with many physical findings and may even be asymptomatic, fecal examination, hematologic examination (PCV, WBC and differentiation, buffy coat for parasites), total protein, plasma protein electrophoresis (A:G ratio), AST, LDH, bile acids and a total body radiograph are considered the ideal database for evaluating a sick bird. The history should involve questions concerning contact with birds outside the premises, which might indicate exposure to infectious diseases that cause hepatitis like Pacheco's disease virus or chlamydia.

Clinical Pathology

Bile Pigments

Green-colored urates are suggestive of liver disease. This discoloration is the result of increased excretion of biliverdin (biliverdinuria), which is the most important bile pigment in birds. Icterus or jaundice, which is caused by a hyperbilirubinemia, is seen very infrequently in birds.

Avian plasma may be colored yellow because of the presence of carotenoids, and this normal color should not be misinterpreted as icteric plasma.

Clinical Enzymology

Increases in plasma enzyme activities are usually related to leakage of enzymes from damaged cells, but sometimes there may be increased production in affected tissues.

Glutamate dehydrogenase (GLDH) is the most liver-specific enzyme in the racing pigeon. Since GLDH is localized within the mitochondria of the liver cells, elevated plasma GLDH activities are seen only after severe liver cell damage (necrosis). In the budgerigar, GLDH activity in liver tissue is relatively low when compared to man and most other birds tested. However, increased GLDH activities were observed in Amazon parrots with extensive liver necrosis due to Pacheco's disease virus, suggesting that this enzyme may be useful for the detection of liver necrosis in at least some psittacine species.

Aspartate aminotransferase (AST, formerly GOT) is the most sensitive indicator of liver disease in the pigeon. This variable, however, is not specific because elevated AST activities can also be seen with muscle damage.

Despite relatively low alanine aminotransferase (ALT, formerly GPT) activities in liver tissue of racing pigeons, this enzyme is useful for detecting liver cell damage because the elimination half-life in plasma is relatively long.

Lactate dehydrogenase (LDH) disappears rapidly from plasma, making it a poor indicator of liver damage, despite relatively high concentrations of this enzyme in liver tissue. Neither ALT nor LDH is specific for the liver because these enzymes, like AST, also occur in muscle.

Alkaline phosphatase (AP) and creatine kinase (CK) are not elevated after liver cell damage, because levels of these enzymes in liver tissue are negligible.

It should be emphasized that elevated activities of "liver enzymes" in plasma may indicate recent damage to liver cells and does not give information on liver function.

Intramuscular injections given within one to five days before collection of a blood sample may cause an elevation of some plasma enzyme activities due to damage of muscle tissue. This can lead to an erroneous diagnosis of liver disease.

Bile Salts

Plasma bile acid concentrations (PBAC), including their salts and corresponding glycine and taurine conjugates, are a reflection of the clearing capacity for bile acids by the liver.

Circulatory levels of bile acids increase if the liver is damaged and cannot extract bile from the portal vein or if the enterohepatic cycle is blocked and blood from the portal vein does not reach the liver. PBAC should be considered a sensitive and specific variable for testing liver function in birds as it is in mammals. In experimentally induced liver disease, five- to ten-fold increases of PBAC over the upper limit of the reference interval are common.

Food consumption significantly increased PBAC. Although up to a 4.5-fold postprandial increase of PBAC was seen in individual birds, the concentrations were never elevated more than 1.65-fold over the upper limit of the reference range. In hepatobiliary disease, five- to ten-fold increases over the upper limit of the reference range were common. Experimental findings suggest that values >70 mmol/L in fasted racing pigeons and most psittacine species, and values >100 mmol/L postprandially should be considered elevated, and therefore suggestive for hepatobiliary disease. In Amazon parrots, PBAC values >145 mmol/L are considered elevated.

Hepatic Encephalopathy

A tentative diagnosis of hepatic encephalopathy is often made when neurologic signs are seen in birds with documented liver disease; however, this syndrome has not been well documented in avian species. It is believed that degradation products from protein catabolism act as false neurotransmitters. For this reason, protein-rich diets in patients with liver disease frequently trigger neurologic symptoms.

Fasting plasma ammonia concentrations in healthy psittacines have shown values ranging from 36-274 mmol/L, which are well above the fasting concentrations described in dogs. Further work is needed to properly diagnose and document the occurrence of hepatic encephalopathy in birds.

Avian Hemochromatosis

The iron status of an individual bird is determined by measuring three main areas of iron: storage iron, transport iron and erythrocyte iron. Storage iron can be semiquantitated by histologic examination of liver biopsies for stainable iron.

In pigeons normal plasma iron value is 11-33 mmol/L, and normal total iron-binding capacity (TIBC) is 30-45 mmol/L. In Ramphastidae, total serum iron concentrations should be below 63 mmol/L, while TIBC should fall below 100 mmol/L. Total serum iron in a mynah bird with confirmed hemochromatosis exceeded 360 mmol/L, while control birds had values that were about 36 mmol/L. (See update on need for biopsy in Chapter 47.)

Plasma Chemistry and Liver Disease

To facilitate interpretation of plasma chemistry, it is advisable to include specific and sensitive indicators of both liver and muscle disease in the plasma chemistry panel (eg, GLDH, AST, CPK, bile acids). It should be stressed that elevated plasma enzyme activities are a sign of recent cell damage and not necessarily of impaired organ function. In chronic conditions, extensive damage occurring in the past may have led to major dysfunction of an organ while enzyme activities may have returned to normal. This is a common finding in birds with liver fibrosis (normal AST, but elevated bile acids and extremely low protein and albumin).

Radiology

Both hepatomegaly and ascites due to liver disease may be diagnosed radiographically. Hepatomegaly and microhepatia are common findings in birds (see Chapter 12). It is important to differentiate between hepatomegaly and cardio-hepatomegaly, because the latter indicates the presence of cardiac failure and secondary congestion of the liver. Caudal displacement of the ventriculus on a lateral radiograph is often caused by enlargement of the liver or associated structures (eg, bile duct or gallbladder in those species that possess one). Loss of the hourglass appearance between the heart and the liver on a ventrodorsal radiograph and widening of the liver beyond a line between the scapula and the acetabulum indicate hepatomegaly. Caudodorsal displacement of the ventriculus is also possible with hepatomegaly. Ascites and peritonitis may complicate radiographic interpretation and obscure hepatic enlargement by overshadowing the liver. Repeat radiography of the abdomen after removal of peritoneal effusion fluid by paracentesis or diuretic treatment may be needed to visualize an enlarged liver and heart.

Liver Biopsy

In order for the clinician to establish a definitive diagnosis of liver disease, it is essential to take biopsies for histologic examination. Indications for liver biopsy include biochemical and radiographic changes suggestive of liver disease. Laparoscopic examination and biopsy of the liver through a midline ventral approach just caudal to the sternum is the method of choice to confirm a diagnosis of liver disease (see Chapter 13). Alternatively, the liver can be exposed through a ventral laparotomy incision and a small wedge of liver tissue can be excised with small surgical scissors. The possibility of severe, life-threatening hemorrhage secondary to liver congestion should be considered prior to biopsy in cases showing radiographic signs of congestive heart failure or electrocardiographic abnormalities indicative of cardiac disease. A liver biopsy site will usually clot without complication, but caution should be exercised when performing biopsies in birds that have prolonged bleeding times after blood collection. Routine tests to determine the efficiency of the avian clotting mechanism are presently not available. In birds with ascites, it is important to perform a biopsy by entering just caudal to the carina to avoid damaging the air sacs and asphyxiating the bird with its own ascitic fluid. Liver biopsies should be examined histologically and cultured for bacteria. Acid-fast staining is of importance for the detection of mycobacteria.

Liver Diseases

Infectious Diseases

Bacteria

A diagnosis can be made by culturing the organisms from a biopsy specimen. If bacteremia occurs, the same organisms can be isolated by blood culture. Elevated white blood cell counts and monocytosis are common with hepatitis caused by *Mycobacterium avium*.

Chlamydiosis

Chlamydia psittaci is an extremely common cause of hepatitis in psittacine birds. Hepatosplenomegaly on radiographs of a bird that has been in recent contact with infected birds is a characteristic clinical presentation. A tentative diagnosis can be made by using an ELISA-type antigen capture test for the detection of chlamydial organisms in a fecal swab. Liver biopsies can be screened for chlamydiosis with a Stamp, Giemsa or Macchiavello's stain, or by fluorescent antibody IFA or ELISA.

Viruses

Pacheco's disease virus, adenovirus, polyomavirus, reovirus, coronavirus and avian serositis virus have all been associated with hepatitis in companion birds.

Duck virus hepatitis is a highly fatal, rapidly spreading viral disease of young ducklings that can be caused by either of one of the three known duck hepatitis viruses. The sudden onset, rapid spread and acute course of this disease, in combination with hemorrhagic lesions in livers of ducklings up to three weeks of age, are practically pathognomonic.

Turkey viral hepatitis is a highly contagious, often subclinical disease of turkeys that produces lesions only in the liver and pancreas (hence the suggested name hepatopancreatitis).

Helminths

Trematode infections have been reported in the liver and bile ducts of cockatoos (*Platynosomum proxillicens*), penguins (*Renicola* sp.), cormorants (*Amphimerus elongatus*), ducks and turkeys. A diagnosis can be made by examination of the feces for trematode eggs. It should be noted that in birds, trematode eggs in the feces do not always originate from parasites in the liver.

Protozoa

A variety of protozoa can cause hepatopathies. *Trichomonas gallinae*-induced hepatic necrosis has been reported in Columbiformes, Falconiformes and Passeriformes.

Histomonas meleagridis is a common cause of hepatitis in captive Galliformes.

Leucocytozoon simondi is a well known cause of mortality in ducks and geese; however, the infection can also occur in other species. Hepatosplenomegaly is common, and parasites can often be detected in a peripheral blood smear.

Atoxoplasma (*Lancesterella* sp.) and toxoplasma infections are common in Passeriformes, but the latter also occurs in Psittaciformes. An enlarged liver can often be seen through the transparent abdominal wall in Passeriformes with atoxoplasmosis. Sporozoites may be seen in small lymphocytes in a peripheral blood smear.

Microsporidian infections have been associated with hepatitis in lovebirds.

Noninfectious Diseases

Metabolic Disorders

In zoological collections, Psittaciformes show a high prevalence of fatty infiltration of the liver. Hepatic steatosis, hepatic lipidosis and fatty degeneration have all been used to describe the condition. It has been well established that an unbalanced diet (biotin, choline and methionine deficiencies) or excessive consumption of high-energy diets with restricted exercise may lead to fatty degeneration. It should be stressed that many companion psittacine birds are fed high-energy, multinutrient-deficient, all-seed diets that predispose them to fatty liver degeneration.

Fatty liver hemorrhagic syndrome in laying hens has been associated with high-energy diets fed to birds with restricted exercise. The dramatic estrogen-induced increase in liver lipogenesis to supply the developing ova has been suggested as the etiology of this condition.

Iron Storage Disease

Hemosiderosis has been defined as an accumulation of an increased amount of hemosiderin in tissues without alteration of tissue morphology, while hemochromatosis is associated with pathologic lesions in hemosiderin-containing tissues. The abnormal storage of iron is most frequently seen in the liver, but other organs may be involved.

Hemochromatosis is most frequently described in Ramphastidae (see Chapter 47), Sturnidae (birds of paradise), mynahs and quetzals, but has also been reported in Psittaciformes. Ramphastidae are generally clinically normal prior to death, but occasionally affected birds are listless 24 hours prior to dying. Cardiac disease has been reported in mynahs due to iron storage in the myocardium. Electrocardiographic changes are possible due to cardiomegaly. In mynahs, generalized weakness, dyspnea and ascites are common. Radiography may reveal (cardio)hepatomegaly and ascites, and blood chemistry may indicate a liver function disorder. A specific diagnosis can be made by histologic examination of a liver biopsy after specific staining for iron. Total serum or plasma iron and TIBC may not be helpful in evaluating the iron status of the animal.

Circulatory Disorders

Portal hypertension can occur as the result of right atrioventricular valvular insufficiency. Portal hypertension may cause hepatic congestion. In the acute stage, the liver is swollen; as the disease progresses, the organ may be fibrotic and have a shrunken appearance. When liver enlargement is caused by congestion, a liver biopsy may result in fatal hemorrhage. The use of an artificial substrate (eg, Gelfoam) at the biopsy site to facilitate clotting may help control bleeding.

Anemic infarctions of the liver, especially of the caudal margins, can be seen as a result of bacterial endocarditis.

Hepatotoxins

Many plants are known to be hepatotoxic in some birds including: rapeseed (*Brassica napus*), ragwort (*Senecio jacobea*), castor bean (*Ricinus communis*), hemlock (*Conium maculatum*), oleander (*Nerium oleander*), *Oxalis* spp., *Grantia* spp., *Crotalaria* spp., *Daubentonia* seed and cotton seed (*Gossypium* spp.). Interestingly, canaries are routinely fed rapeseed and do not appear to be affected by its toxins.

The following substances are hepatotoxic: arsenic, phosphorus, carbon tetrachloride, toxins from certain blue-green algae, halothane, methoxyflurane and mycotoxins (especially aflatoxin from *Aspergillus flavus, A. parasiticus* and *Penicillium puberulum*). Degeneration and necrosis of hepatocytes are typical with aflatoxicosis. Bile duct proliferation and fibrosis leaving only islands of hepatocytes are common in chronic cases.

Peanuts and Brazil nuts are notorious sources of aflatoxins, but many other seed mixtures can be contaminated. Chemical analysis of food for aflatoxin is possible.

Neoplasia

Liver tumors can be classed as primary and multicentric (metastatic). It has been suggested that there is an association between cholangiocarcinoma and the presence of cloacal papillomatosis in Amazon parrots (see Chapter 19). Likewise, it has been suggested that hemochromatosis in mynah birds and aflatoxicosis in ducks are associated with hepatomas.

Amyloidosis

Amyloidosis is commonly seen in Anseriformes, gulls and shorebirds. Amyloid A is a degradation product of an acute phase, reactant protein. Amyloidosis is often seen in birds with chronic infections (bumblefoot, tuberculosis and aspergillosis). Severe hypoalbuminemia caused by glomerular and hepatic damage can cause ascites and peripheral edema of the feet and legs.

Traumatic Rupture

Rupture of the liver is most likely to occur secondary to liver diseases, such as fatty degeneration, amyloidosis, mycobacteriosis and neoplasia, but can also occur as a result of trauma. When the bleeding is limited or confined to a subcapsular hematoma, survival is possible. Birds can also survive liver hemorrhage confined to one of the hepatic peritoneal cavities.

Treatment of Liver Disorders

The single most important treatment seems to be the administration of a well balanced diet free of hepatotoxins. The use of lactulose, hemicellulose and supportive care including IV fluids and assisted feeding are indicated in many cases of hepatitis. A multivitamin injection is indicated when malnutrition is suspected.

In birds with hemochromatosis, the iron content of the diet should be drastically reduced (<100 ppm), although high iron content of the diet may not be the only cause of excessive iron storage in the body. A few birds with hemochromatosis have responded to phlebotomy therapy (see Chapter 47).

When a microbiologic cause of liver disease can be diagnosed, a specific treatment against the causative organism is possible. Doxycycline is the treatment of choice for chlamydiosis (see Chapter 34). Pacheco's disease virus infections can be treated with acyclovir. Liver flukes may be susceptible to praziquantel.

Outbreaks of duck hepatitis virus can be controlled by IM injection of DHV antiserum into each duckling at the time the first deaths are noted.

Ascitic fluid should not be removed from birds with liver disease. Removal of this fluid will further deplete body stores of protein in a bird with an already compromised liver function. The author's preference for treating ascites is to use a potent diuretic, such as furosemide, to effect, and to take only a small amount of ascitic fluid for diagnostic purposes.

Limited experience with prednisolone in cases of chronic active hepatitis of unknown etiology in African Grey Parrots suggests that this drug may be beneficial for treating some avian liver disorders. The use of corticosteroids in mycotoxicosis may limit the formation of fibrosis; however, corticosteroids may exacerbate an underlying infection and may be contraindicated in cases of infectious hepatitis. Colchicine has been used to prevent the progression of hepatic fibrosis in a conure.

NEPHROLOGY

J. T. Lumeij

Confirming a diagnosis of renal disease in birds is often difficult because clinical signs are generally nonspecific and are frequently complicated by secondary changes caused by renal dysfunction. Lethargy, with a diminished appetite leading to emaciation, is typical of renal disease. Birds may appear unable to fly, while in reality they are too weak to fly. A distended abdomen with or without ascites may be seen with renal tumors.

Urinary output may vary from anuria to polyuria. In oliguric patients, the possibility of acute nephrotoxic renal failure should be considered, and the client should be carefully questioned concerning the administration of nephrotoxic drugs (eg, allopurinol, aminoglycosides, polypeptide antibiotics, sulfonamides), exposure to sodium chloride (eg, saline drinking water, sand for bedding, heavily salted foods) or other nephrotoxic substances (eg, heavy metals, ethylene glycol, carbon tetrachloride).

Etiology of Gout

Uric acid is synthesized in the liver. Ninety percent of its excretion is via tubular secretion from reptilian-type nephrons and therefore largely independent of urine flow rate. The clearance of uric acid surpasses the glomerular filtration rate by a factor of eight to sixteen and is occasionally even higher. The rate of secretion is largely independent of the state of hydration because UA excretion is independent of tubular water reabsorption. Very high concentrations of uric acid can be found in ureteral urine in dehydrated birds. Renal function disorders can eventually lead to elevated uric acid concentrations. However, nonprotein nitrogen substances in plasma, such as uric acid, creatinine and urea will be elevated only when renal function is below 30% of its original capacity.

Hyperuricemia is defined as any plasma uric acid concentration higher than the calculated limit of solubility of sodium urate in plasma and is an indication of nephrosis or impaired renal function. It is generally accepted that the upper limit of solubility of urate in human plasma, is 420 mmol/L. Urate solubility increases with higher sodium concentrations and higher temperatures. When the higher body temperature of birds (up to 43°C) is taken into account, the theoretical limit of solubility would be about 600 mmol/L. Because avian species have a higher plasma sodium concentration than humans (136-145 mmol/L), the theoretical limit of urate solubility is even higher. Hyperuricemia can result in urate precipitation in joints (articular gout) and in visceral organs or other extra-visceral sites (visceral gout). Gout should not be regarded as a disease entity, but as a clinical sign of any severe renal dysfunction that causes a chronic, moderate hyperuricemia.

When birds are provided with dietary protein in excess of their requirements, the surplus protein is catabolized and the nitrogen released is converted to uric acid. The use of high-protein poultry pellets as the bulk food in psittacine aviaries may result in an increased incidence of gout (See Chapter 3).

Articular and Visceral Gout: A plasma uric acid concentration that is slightly above the solubility of sodium urate will lead to uric acid precipitates in the body. The joints and synovial sheaths may be predilection sites because of a lower temperature than the rest of the body. Once uric acid deposits have occurred in a specific area, these deposits will grow with time, forming tophi (accumulations of uric acid). If, for whatever reason, uric acid crystals precipitate in the tubules or collecting ducts of the kidney (eg, severe dehydration of long duration, hypovitaminosis A) or the ureters, an acute obstructive uropathy (postrenal obstruction) will occur. These birds develop anuria or gross oliguria, and tubular secretion of uric acid is severely compromised or stops. This results in a rapid and severe elevation of plasma uric acid concentration with precipitation of urates on many visceral surfaces, including those predilection sites for articular gout. Visceral gout will rapidly lead to death of the affected animal. This hypothesis is supported by the fact that inflammation and tophi formation are rare with visceral gout, because the condition has a rapidly fatal course.

Acute, renal tubular failure, which would lead to acute abolishment of uric acid secretion, would result in a similar course of events. In this situation, visceral gout could develop without uric acid deposits forming in the tubules, collecting ducts and ureters.

The acute mortality seen in birds with visceral gout is probably not due to the effects of hyperuricemia, because uric acid is generally a nontoxic, insoluble substance. It is likely that these birds die from cardiac arrest caused by hyperkalemia, although this hypothesis needs confirmation.

Acute and Chronic Renal Failure

Renal dysfunction may result from any progressive destructive condition affecting both kidneys (chronic renal failure), but can also occur in conditions wherein the function of the kidneys is rapidly and severely, but often reversibly, compromised (acute renal failure). In the latter condition, oliguria usually occurs, while in the former situation, polyuria is normally seen. Dehydration and shock (prerenal renal failure), urolithiasis (postrenal renal failure) and urinary tract infections and the administration of nephrotoxic drugs can all cause changes that mimic irreversible chronic renal failure.

Prerenal Azotemia

Prerenal azotemia can be defined as the clinical condition associated with reduced renal arterial pressure or perfusion leading to oliguria and retention of nitrogenous urinary waste products in the blood. It is often seen during shock or severe dehydration. In recent experimental studies, elevated plasma uric acid concentrations were not observed in racing pigeons that were deprived of water for four days, while plasma urea concentration showed a significant 6.5- to 15.3-fold increase above reference values. Urea is normally present in low concentration in avian plasma and determination of this has traditionally been considered of little value in evaluating renal function in birds; however, plasma urea appears to be the single most useful variable for early detection of prerenal causes of renal failure (dehydration).

Postprandial Effects

It has been demonstrated that a significant postprandial increase in plasma uric acid (UA) and urea concentration occurs in Peregrine Falcons and Red-tailed Hawks.

It is not clear why at least twelve hours of postprandial hyperuricemia does not result in uric acid deposition in the tissues. In order to prevent misinterpretation of high plasma UA levels caused by the ingestion of food, it is recommended that repeat samples be evaluated following a fasting period in any bird that initially has a high plasma UA or urea concentration.

Evaluation of Urate Tophi

Macroscopically, the aspirated material from articular gout looks like toothpaste. The presence of urate can be confirmed by performing the murexide test or by microscopic examination of aspirates from suspected tophi. The murexide test is performed by mixing a drop of nitric acid with a small amount of the suspected material on a slide. The material is dried by evaporation in a flame and allowed to cool. One drop of concentrated ammonia is added, and if urates are present, a mauve color will develop. Microscopically, sharp, needle-shaped crystals can be seen in smears. A polarizing microscope is helpful in identifying the typical crystals.

Blood Changes

Apart from elevated concentrations of nonprotein nitrogen substances, a number of other variables are known to change in mammals as a result of acute or chronic renal failure. Hyperkalemia, which may lead to severe electrocardiographic changes and cardiac arrest, is a particular problem in acute renal failure. Hyperkalemia (5.2 mmol/L) was described in a Red-tailed Hawk with acute renal failure. Infusion of 10% calcium gluconate solution may reverse the cardiotoxic effects of severe hyperkalemia without affecting plasma potassium concentration. Hypocalcemia and hyperphosphatemia are common in mammals with renal failure. The former may lead to hypocalcemic tetany, especially with rapid correction of acidosis. Because these variables have significant therapeutic implications, documentation of their occurrence in avian renal disease is necessary. Anemia has also been documented in birds with chronic renal failure.

Clinicopathologic Diagnosis of Renal Dysfunction

Urinalysis

Despite its high diagnostic value, urinalysis is not routinely performed in avian medicine, perhaps because it seems difficult to separate urine from feces. The identification of casts in urinary sediment is strongly suggestive of renal disease. In polyuric cases, collection of a urine sample is relatively simple and can be performed by aspirating the fluid part of the excreta into a syringe from a clean enclosure floor covered by wax paper. It is important that the urine sample be relatively free of urates to ensure the diagnostic value of microscopic examination of the sediment.

Urate-free urine samples should be examined for specific gravity or osmolality, color, clearness, pH, protein, glucose and hemoglobin, and the sediment should be examined microscopically.

Osmolality and Specific Gravity

High urine osmolalities are common in avian species that are adapted to desert situations (Zebra Finch and budgerigar). Maximum urine osmolalities in birds vary from 500-1000 mOsmol/kg. The emu is adapted to the Australian semidesert and has a low turnover rate of water, but has a limited renal concentrating ability with a maximal urine:plasma osmotic ratio of only 1.4:1.5. In this species, the large intestine has been adapted to preserve water.

In polyuric birds without a diminished concentrating capacity, one day of water deprivation should be sufficient to cause a demonstrable rise in urine osmolality.

Because the specific gravity of urine has a positive correlation with the osmolality, it should be possible to determine specific gravity of avian urine with a refractometer. Further work is needed to establish the correlation between refractometric readings and osmometric values before refractometry can be recommended. Some practitioners believe that they can make an empirical prognostic determination based on the specific gravity of the urine in a patient.

Polyuria is confirmed by demonstrating hypotonic urine (osmolality, mOsmol/L or specific gravity).

Protein

In healthy pigeons, protein concentrations in urine collected with the cloacal cannula method can be as high as 2 g/L. The excretion of mucoproteins and glycoproteins in the distal portion of the nephrons and the ureters is responsible for this low level proteinuria. Severe, persistent proteinuria is a sign of increased glomerular permeability (eg, glomerulonephritis). Proteinuria is usually minimal or absent in diseases that primarily involve the tubules or interstitial tissue. Extreme protein loss through the kidneys can lead to severe hypoproteinemia.

Most urine dipsticks are too insensitive to distinguish between moderate and severe proteinuria and may not properly detect proteinuria in polyuric patients. A false-positive protein result is common in psittacine birds that have had an alkaline urine. The use of the Ponceau S method for determination of urine protein concentration is recommended.

Glucose

Glucose is normally absent from chicken urine, though small quantities (1.6 mmol/L) of monosaccharides have been described in ureteral urine samples collected from birds.

Polyuria and polydipsia accompanied by glucosuria do not always indicate diabetes mellitus. Diabetes mellitus can be diagnosed only if elevated plasma glucose concentrations have been demonstrated. In mammals, Fanconi's syndrome is characterized by renal glucosuria, hyperaminoaciduria and hyperphosphaturia, as well as renal loss of potassium, bicarbonate, water and other substances conserved by the proximal tubule. A case of renal glucosuria and proteinuria in an African Grey Parrot with severe renal damage was considered to be similar to the Fanconi's syndrome. Glucosuria is frequently seen in psittacine hens with egg-related peritonitis. The problem is transitory if the peritonitis can be successfully managed.

Ketonuria

It has been stated that ketonuria is a poor prognostic sign in birds, suggesting that catabolic processes lead to mobilization of fat and ketoacidosis. This statement is probably incorrect for migratory birds. The primary energy source during migration is fat. Diabetes mellitus has been mentioned as a cause of ketonuria in birds; however, in the author's opinion, the clinical importance of ketonuria needs further clarification.

Color

The color of urine varies but is generally white or off-white, pale yellow or light beige. Pigmented food items and medications may alter urinary color. B-complex vitamins can cause a yellow or brownish discoloration of the urine that can be misinterpreted as bilirubinuria. Berries in the diet can cause a blue-red discoloration of the urine. In liver diseases, biliverdinuria may result in a green-tinged urine.

Microscopic Examination of Urinary Sediment

Microscopic examination of urine sediment is diagnostic only when evaluating urine that contains relatively little uric acid. Furthermore, contamination of the urine with nonrenal components, such as feces or blood originating from the cloaca, must be considered. Various cast types and cellular elements can be encountered in urinary sediment. Cellular casts can contain epithelial cells, erythrocytes, leukocytes, bacteria and fungi. Granular casts are composed of degraded cellular components. Casts that have no cellular elements but have a yellow-orange color are suggestive of hemoglobin casts. Clinical experience suggests that the transition from cellular or granular casts to hemoglobin casts is a favorable prognostic sign and indicates resolution of the inflammatory process.

Microorganisms found in urine sediments are usually from fecal contamination; however, high bacterial counts in a relatively clean sample, together with urinary cast formation, is indicative of urinary tract infection. In male birds, sperm cells may be seen on routine microscopic examination of urinary sediment. Avian urine contains many amorphous urates, but other crystals may sometimes be noted.

Abnormal Urine Coloration

Hematuria is macroscopically visible when 0.1% of the urine contains blood. Chemical test strips, like Hemastix, will show a positive reaction when 0.002-0.001% of the urine contains blood. The combination of microscopic examination of the sediment and the use of a test strip is more sensitive for the detection of hematuria than when either test is used alone. In birds, hematuria is possible when blood cells from the gastrointestinal and genital tract or cloaca are mixed with the urine sample. In carnivorous birds, the meat diet frequently results in a positive reaction.

Myoglobinuria can also cause a red coloration of urine, which cannot be distinguished from hemoglobinuria on routine chemical urinalysis. Myoglobinuria can induce a severe toxic nephropathy.

Porphyrinuria is another cause of red coloration of the urine. In birds, the most common cause of porphyrinuria is lead poisoning. Amazon parrots with lead poisoning often produce a red or brown urine, which is assumed to be hemoglobinuria. It is possible that the red or brown urine seen in Amazon parrots with lead poisoning is caused by porphyrins mixed with urates rather than hemoglobinuria. Porphyrins in urine will show a red fluorescence in ultraviolet light. When the test is negative, a blue fluorescence will be seen.

Radiology of the Urinary Tract

Survey radiographs provide information about the size, location and radiopacity of the kidneys. The kidneys are surrounded by the abdominal air sacs, which extend as diverticuli between the kidneys and the pelvis. This finding explains why, at least in Psittaciformes, a rim of air can be seen dorsal to the kidneys. The loss of this dorsal rim of air is seen during pathologic swelling of the kidneys. Abnormalities that can be detected on survey radiographs include swelling and crystalline inclusions indicative of urate deposits. Nephrocalcinosis or concrements in the kidney, ureters or cloaca can also be detected. Barium sulphate contrast of the gastrointestinal tract may be helpful in localizing intra-abdominal space-occupying lesions such as renal tumors. Occasionally, urate tophi of articular gout are visible on radiographs.

Endoscopy and Biopsy

Endoscopy allows direct visualization of the complete urinary system (kidneys, ureters and cloaca). The endoscopic approach of choice is through a puncture site dorsal to the pubic bone and caudal to the ischium on the left side of the bird (see Chapter 13). Although it is feasible to take renal biopsies in healthy birds, there is considerable risk of fatal hemorrhage from this procedure, and it should always be performed with the appropriate equipment and ample experience.

In visceral gout, urate deposits can be seen on visceral organs, especially the pericardium and cranial border of the liver capsule. A ventral midline approach just caudal to the sternum is preferred to endoscopically evaluate these structures.

Diseases of the Kidney

Infectious Diseases

Bacterial Infections

Bacterial infections of the kidney often occur secondary to septicemia but may also result from bacteria that ascend from the cloaca. Diagnostically, WBC evaluation, total protein and protein electrophoresis provide useful information on the systemic inflammatory reaction. Bacterial cultures of blood and urine may reveal the causative organism. Mycobacterial infections often cause monocytosis that can be demonstrated on a peripheral blood smear.

Viral Infections

Viral infections are usually multisystemic, although some viruses like avian polyomavirus and infectious bronchitis virus in chickens demonstrate a trophism for the kidney. Other viruses that have been associated with renal lesions include Newcastle disease virus, paramyxovirus of pigeons, reoviruses, viruses belonging to the leukosis/sarcoma group and herpesviruses (eg, Pacheco's disease virus and pigeon herpesvirus).

Mycotic Infections

Renal infarction as a complication of mycelium invasion of blood vessels secondary to pulmonary mycotic disease is common. Abdominal air sac aspergillosis with renal involvement *per continuitatem* has also been reported. In the latter case, ischiatic nerve involvement resulted in unilateral paralysis.

Parasitic Infections

Granulomatous nephritis due to *Isospora, Cryptosporidium, Microsporidium* and *Encephalitozoon* spp. has been reported in a variety of avian species. *Eimeria truncata* is a well known cause of renal coccidiosis in geese. Adult trematodes of *Tanaisia bragai* can be found in collecting ducts of chickens, turkeys and pigeons.

Noninfectious Diseases

Congenital Defects

Agenesis and hypoplasia of part of the kidneys have been described in birds. Compensatory hypertrophy of the intact poles is common. Renal cysts have also been described and may be congenital in origin. Diagnosis can be made with urography and laparoscopy.

Metabolic Disorders

Hypervitaminosis D and elevated dietary calcium can both cause hypercalcemia and lead to deposition of calcium salts in the renal parenchyma (nephrocalcinosis). Calcinosis of other organs may also be noted. This condition can be detected radiographically, and the history may indicate oversupplementation of calcium or vitamin D in the diet.

Hypovitaminosis A can cause metaplasia of the epithelium of the ureters and collecting ducts and decreased secretions of mucus in these structures. This may lead to precipitation of urates and ureteral impaction.

Amyloidosis

Renal amyloidosis often occurs in Anseriformes in conjunction with amyloidosis of other organs (eg, liver) secondary to chronic inflammation.

Toxic Nephropathies

Many nephrotoxins cause renal tubular necrosis including aminoglycosides, heavy metals, and mycotoxins such as aflatoxin (*A. flavus* and *A. parasiticus*), ochratoxin (*A. ochraceus* and *Penicillium viridicatum*), oosporein (*Chaetomium trilaterale*) and citrinin (*P. citrinum*).

Salt (NaCl) poisoning has been documented in various species. Salt poisoning via drinking water can lead to right ventricular failure and ascites. Salt poisoning via food leads to acute renal failure with urate impaction of the ureters. Clinical signs include polydipsia and polyuria, or anuria if urate impaction of the ureters occurs.

Neoplasia

Budgerigars have a high incidence of primary renal tumors, especially adenocarcinoma and nephroblastoma (younger birds). A viral origin has been suggested. The kidney is a potential metastatic site for tumors of nonrenal origin, especially lymphoproliferative diseases (leukosis). Unilateral or bilateral paralysis caused by compression of the ischiatic nerve is a common clinical sign associated with renal malignancies in birds. Abdominal enlargement is common when a renal mass causes caudoventral displacement of the ventriculus or ascites. A renal tumor may be radiographically detectable with or without the use of barium sulphate to differentiate the margins of the gastrointestinal tract.

Ureteral Obstruction

Displacement or obstruction of ureteral orifices can occur due to intestinal or cloacal prolapse or cloacal obstruction caused by fecaliths, uroliths, foreign bodies, tumors or inflammatory processes. A bilateral obstruction will rapidly lead to visceral gout. Unilateral obstructions will lead to atrophy and compensatory hypertrophy of the contralateral kidney.

Therapeutic Considerations

Prerenal Renal Failure

Treatment of prerenal renal failure caused by dehydration or shock is usually successful; however, the challenge is diagnosing and treating the initial cause of dehydration. Rapidly expanding the circulatory volume with intravenous fluids will usually restore normal renal function within hours (see Chapter 15).

Postrenal Renal Failure

The treatment of postrenal renal failure caused by urolithiasis requires removal of the uroliths. This is a substantial surgical challenge. Successful extracorporeal shock wave lithotripsy for removal of uric acid concrements in the urinary tract has been reported in a Magellanic Penguin and may be attempted in other affected birds.

Acute Renal Failure

Once a diagnosis of acute (reversible) renal failure is made, immediate and aggressive therapy is indicated to prevent further damage. Treatment includes maintaining a high alkaline urine flow by infusing mannitol 20% (1000 mg/kg) every 15-20 min and sodium bicarbonate supplemented with intravenous furosemide. The prognosis for recovery of renal function is good if diuresis can be achieved.

In anuric/oliguric renal failure, fluid intake in the patient should be restricted to fluid loss (renal loss, loss from the gastrointestinal tract and insensible loss of about 20 ml/kg/day). Assessment of fluid requirements can be based on this general outline but must be monitored by daily weight determination and observation for clinical signs that would indicate overhydration or dehydration. In patients that are anorectic and not receiving assisted feedings, some allowance should be made to account for tissue catabolism. Losses of 2.5% body weight per day are possible in totally anorectic parrots. Sodium, potassium and protein intake should be discontinued and calories should be given in the form of fat and carbohydrates. Alternatively, a low-protein diet containing all essential amino acids can be given. Furosemide should be used in an attempt to restore or increase urine flow and potassium excretion.

In the polyuric phase that follows the anuric phase, fluid and electrolyte balance should be carefully monitored to prevent dehydration, hyponatremia and hypokalemia. Intravenous and subcutaneous infusions with lactated Ringer's solution should be continued on a daily basis. Because bacteria are often incriminated as the cause of renal failure, use of non-nephrotoxic bactericidal antibiotics that are effective against the most commonly encountered bacteria are indicated. A combination of piperacillin and claforan has been suggested, although these drugs have a similar mode of action. Vitamin A supplementation is always indicated in hyperuricemia, because hypovitaminosis A is a common cause of renal failure.

Effects of Drugs

Allopurinol

Contrary to expected findings, administration of allopurinol caused a severe hyperuricemia and induced gout in three out of six, clinically normal Red-tailed Hawks. Further work is needed in carnivorous and granivorous birds to establish fasting and postprandial reference intervals of plasma UA concentrations and the possible effects of allopurinol in birds.

Corticosteroids

Corticosteroids are known to be uricosuric in man and may be contraindicated in avian hyperuricemic conditions. Prednisolone has been used in budgerigars with renal tumors. The author states that although she does not know whether the prednisolone prolongs life, it may improve the quality of life by diminishing the pressure on the ischiatic nerve and stimulating appetite.

Pneumonology

Thomas N. Tully, Jr.
Greg J. Harrison

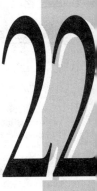

The rapid progression of many avian respiratory diseases makes early recognition by the client and rapid diagnosis and effective treatment by the practitioner critical. Conversely, chronic rhinitis and air sacculitis can fulminate for many years with subtle clinical changes. The difficulty in distinguishing between clinical signs originating from the upper versus the lower respiratory system makes the diagnosis of these problems challenging.

Normal respiratory effort in the bird should not be noticeable, and the mouth should remain closed. An increase in abdominal effort or head movement may be recognized in association with increased respiration following exercise, but should return to normal within minutes of ceasing exertional activity.

Mild upper respiratory or lung-induced dyspnea is frequently accompanied by open-mouthed breathing with a dilated glottis. Lung and lower respiratory tract problems are usually associated with a rhythmic jerking of the tail (tail-bob). A bird in severe respiratory distress may also move its head forward in an effort to increase air intake. If the respiratory problem is associated with excessive fluid production, bubbling and gurgling sounds are common on both inspiration and expiration.

Overt signs of respiratory disease are easy to identify and include oculonasal discharge, stained or matted feathers around the nares, sneezing, coughing, dyspnea or audible inspirations or expirations. Changes in pitch or vocalization of the patient may indicate problems in the glottis, trachea or syrinx. Shallow, labored breathing in a bird with weak, altered or absent voice is common with acute zinc toxicosis. Many psittacine birds may mimic the sneeze or cough of household members, which should not be misinterpreted as a sign of respiratory disease.

When dyspnea is induced by protracted respiratory disease, it is usually associated with other clinical signs including weight loss, depression, ocular or nasal discharge, sneezing or wheezing. Acute dyspnea in an apparently healthy bird usually results from exposure to aerosolized toxins, dislocation and movement

TABLE 22.1   Clinical Considerations of Respiratory Disease

UPPER RESPIRATORY DISEASE

Clinical Signs
- Open-mouthed breathing
- Sneezing
- Rhinorrhea
- Exercise intolerance
- Head-shaking
- Inflamed swollen cere
- Yawning
- Periophthalmic swellings
- Change in voice
- Sinus swelling
- Nasal granulomas
- Dyspnea
- Mucopurulent nasal discharge
- Stretching the neck
- Epiphora
- Plugged nares

Diagnostic Protocol
- Thorough review of nutritional status
- Thorough history (exposure to smoke, PTFE)
- Gram's stain of feces; direct fecal smear for parasites; special pathology stains
- Sinus flush
- Cytology of affected area (sinus aspirate, flush, scraping for parasites); Gram's stain
- Radiographs (whole body, sinus views)
- Rhinoscopy (foreign body examination)
- Culture and sensitivity
- Special bacterial & viral diagnostic testing (also chlamydia, mollicutes)
- Biopsy of lesion
- CBC, biochemistry panels

Normal Flora
- Gram-positive bacteria (eg, *Lactobacillus* spp., *Streptococcus* spp. and *Micrococcus* spp.)
- Small numbers of gram-negative organisms (eg, *E. coli, Bordetella*)
- Occasional non-budding yeast

Abnormal Flora
- Large numbers of gram-negative bacteria (over 5%)
- 10 budding yeast per oil immersion field examined

LOWER RESPIRATORY DISEASE

Clinical Signs
- Tail-bobbing
- Change in vocalization
- Exercise intolerance
- Sounds on auscultation
- Loss of voice
- Labored respiration
- Coughing

Diagnostic Protocol
- Radiographs of lungs, air sacs
- Laparoscopy; tracheoscopy
- Biopsy of lungs, air sacs
- Culture of trachea, lungs, air sacs
- Compression reduction of air sacs
- Transtracheal lavage (cytology of sample)
- Suction and cytology
- Surgical intervention (air sac granuloma, tumor, tracheal foreign body)

Fluid Obtained by Tracheal and Air Sac Lavage
- Normal: Low cellularity and very few pulmonary macrophages or inflammatory cells
- Abnormal: Large numbers of heterophils, pulmonary macrophages and other inflammatory cells, bacteria or yeast

of plaques in the trachea (from malnutrition or infectious agents) or aspiration of foreign bodies (especially seed husks or cage litter).

Nares

The first areas to examine for respiratory disease are the nares and surrounding tissues. Unilateral or bilateral diseases of the upper respiratory tract are indicated by matted or mildly stained feathers around the nostrils, occluded nares, nasal discharge or a growth or change in size of the nasal opening. Bacterial, fungal, chlamydial and viral infections, neoplasia and trauma are common etiologic agents of upper respiratory disease. Chronic inflammation may lead to disfiguring lesions of the nares, beak and cere. Severe *Knemidokoptes* spp. infection may cause proliferation of the cere that blocks the external nares and causes respiratory difficulties.

The sinuses have simple mucous glands and are lined by stratified squamous and ciliated columnar epithelium. Hypovitaminosis A commonly causes squamous metaplasia and hyperkeratosis of the sinuses and nasal passages, leading to granuloma formation.

Sinuses

The infraorbital sinus is the only paranasal sinus in birds and is located lateral to the nasal cavity and surrounding the eyes ventrally. In some birds (insectivorous Passeriformes, Anseriformes and Psittaciformes), the right and left infraorbital sinuses communicate, while in other species (non-insectivorous Passeriformes), the right and left infraorbital sinuses are independent.

The numerous pockets and extensions of the nasal system make sinus infections difficult to treat. With severe chronic sinusitis, the accumulation of caseous necrotic debris can cause destruction of the nares, nasal cavity, operculum and nasal conchae. This degree of destruction is particularly common in Amazon parrots and African Grey Parrots with aspergillosis sinusitis. Inflammation or accumulation of debris in the infraorbital sinus can lead to periorbital swellings.

Birds do not have a soft palate. Instead, air moves from the nasal cavity through the choana via the choanal slit (oropharynx) and then into the rima glottis of the trachea. The configuration of the choanal slit varies with the species, but in all cases the slit should be slightly moist. On the ventral surface of the palate and along the choana are numerous caudally directed choanal papillae.

Swollen, inflamed choanal tissues, with a sloughing of the protruding papillae, are common with upper respiratory tract infections (particularly chlamydiosis), and secondarily infected with candidiasis in immunosuppressed states following prolonged illness, malnutrition or improper antibiotic administration. The presence or absence of papillae is not a diagnostic indicator of current respiratory disease, as they seldom regrow after sloughing. Laryngeal lesions may occur from viral infections (poxvirus, herpesvirus), hyperkeratosis secondary to hypovitaminosis A, candidiasis, trichomoniasis, papillomatosis and neoplasia. Seeds may also become lodged in the choanal slit and cause respiratory signs or constant movement of the tongue in an effort to dislodge the seed.

Table 22.2   Clinical Presentations of Avian Respiratory Disease with Associated Differential Diagnosis

Clinical Presentation	Differential Diagnosis
Sunken eye	Chronic bacterial sinusitis
Enlarged cere	Chronic rhinitis; foreign body; trauma; allergy; airborne irritants (eg, cigarette smoke); malnutrition (chronic); avian poxvirus; Knemidocoptes mites; normal female budgerigar
Enlarged cere with or without granuloma formation	Bacterial, mycotic, mycoplasmal, chlamydial; nutritional rhinitis
Rhinorrhea or sneezing	Bacterial infection; mycotic infection; foreign body; toxic insult (smoke); allergy; virus; malnutrition; chlamydia
Serous sinusitis	Chlamydia or mycoplasma infection; nutritional rhinitis; foreign body; papillomatosis; occluded choana (atresia); uncomplicated viral infections
Mucopurulent sinusitis	Bacterial infection with predominantly gram-negative organisms; mycotic infection (often secondary to serous sinusitis)
Irritated swollen cere with sloughed papillae	Chronic mycotic, bacterial or viral sinusitis; chronic exposure to airborne irritants; chlamydiosis; malnutrition; hypovitaminosis A
Coughing (chronic)	Bacterial, viral, fungal, chlamydial, parasitic, yeast, mycobacterial; ascites; abscess or granuloma; malnutrition; air sac mites; mimicry of humans; airborne toxins (eg, cigarette smoke)
Coughing (acute)	Foreign body inhalation; trauma; upper respiratory infection; abscess or neoplasia in lungs or body cavity; air sac mites; infectious tracheitis; avian viral serositis; mimicry of humans; bleeding into body cavity; sarcocystosis; syringeal granuloma; airborne toxins - PTFE gas
Dyspnea (acute)	Aspergillosis syringeal granuloma; infectious disease; foreign body inhalation; internal bleeding; allergy; toxin inhalation; plugged nares; avian viral serositis; sarcocystosis; anemia
Dyspnea (chronic)	Infectious disease; liver disease; kidney disease; ascites; heart disease; neoplasia; air sacculitis; malnutrition; sarcocystosis (lung edema); proliferative tracheitis; Pacheco's disease virus; pericardial effusion; egg-related peritonitis (binding); hemo-chromatosis; anemia; obesity; thyroid enlargement, tumors, goiter
Subcutaneous swelling	Overinflation of cervicocephalic air sac; trauma (bite wound); normal (pelicans)
Neonatal sneezing, coughing, dyspnea	Inhalation pneumonia; respiratory foreign body; infections (eg, chlamydia); avian viral serositis; mycotic infection

Trachea

The opening of the larynx, or rima glottis, is not covered by an epiglottis as it is in mammals. The larynx does not function for sound production in birds. There are no vocal cords in the larynx.

Pathology involving the syrinx is best diagnosed and treated when signs of disease are first recognized. If a bird stops talking or has a voice change it should be evaluated immediately for lesions developing in the perisyringeal area (frequently aspergillosis). Progressive changes recognized clinically as dyspnea, coughing or tracheal discharge are more difficult to successfully resolve.

Lungs

The paired lungs lie dorsally in the thoracic cavity, extending from the first through the seventh ribs in Psittaciformes; however, the boundaries of the lungs vary, and they may extend to the ilia in some species.

There are frequent and inaccurate suggestions that the avian lung is fixed and not expandable. While changes in the size or position of the avian lung are limited, it is a dynamic organ that does undergo expansion and contraction during the respiratory cycle.

Air Sacs

Pulmonary

Most birds have four paired and one unpaired pulmonary air sacs that connect to the lung and create a large respiratory capacity. The cranial air sacs are composed of the cervical, clavicular and cranial thoracic air sacs; the caudal air sacs are composed of the caudal thoracic air sac and abdominal air sac.

Cervicocephalic

The cervicocephalic air sacs are not connected to the lung and are divided into cephalic and cervical portions; they connect to caudal aspects of the infraorbital sinus.

The air sacs of a normal bird are completely transparent (appear similar to clear plastic wrap). Any alteration in transparency should be considered abnormal. The presence of blood vessels in the air sacs may be an indication of early inflammation.

The poor vascular supply and lack of ciliary transport system within the air sacs hinder parenteral treatment of air sacculitis.

Depending on the species of bird, the humerus, clavicles, coracoids and cervical vertebrae are connected to the respiratory system through extrathoracic diverticula. The sternum and sternal ribs are pneumatized through the intrathoracic diverticula that lie between the coracoid bones. The lungs connect directly to the thoracic vertebrae and their associated ribs. The femur may be pneumatized through a connection with the air sac.

If a bird is unable to move its ribs, it will rapidly suffocate. This can occur with an overly aggressive restraint or by the surgeon resting his hands on the body cavity during surgery. Bandages that encompass the body cavity can also interfere with breathing, particularly if they are wrapped tightly around the caudal portion of the sternum or ribs.

It is frequently discussed in veterinary literature that inspired air flows through the parabronchi or primary bronchus and directly into the caudal air sacs, thus bypassing the gas exchange portion of the lungs. This statement is not completely accurate. On inspiration, one-half of the inspired air volume goes to the lung and the other half goes to the caudal air sacs. The air that is already in the lungs enters the cranial air sacs. On expiration, the ambient air that is in the caudal air sacs enters the lungs. Although not clearly stated in any physiology reference, the air that is in the lungs must exit through the trachea along with the air that is in the cranial air sac. For this system to function, the volume of the caudal air sacs, the lungs and the cranial air sacs must be equal (each contains one-half of a total volume of inspired air at any one time).

Gas Exchange

The air capillaries are present in all birds. In some species, the parabronchi are divided into two systems. In these birds, the paleopulmonic parabronchi are the major sites of gas exchange, and air flows unidirectionally through these passages on inspiration and expiration. In the neoplumonic parabronchi, air passes bidirectionally through both phases of the respiratory cycle. Gas exchange occurs in the air capillaries. These air tubes branch and anastomose with each other, creating an extensive network. They are richly entwined with blood vessels, which form a blood gas barrier.

The respiratory cycle is controlled principally by sensitive CO_2 pulmonary receptors. Interestingly, these receptors have been shown to be inhibited by halothane.

Diagnostic Techniques

Auscultation

The sinuses, trachea, lung, thoracic air sacs and abdominal air sacs can be auscultated using a pediatric stethoscope. Audible sounds on inspiration generally correlate with upper respiratory tract disease, while sounds on expiration are more commonly associated with lower respiratory tract diseases. Because air moves through the lungs continuously and the air capillaries do not collapse and expand to the same degree as alveoli, a "smacking" sound characteristic of pneumonia in mammals does not occur in birds. However, mild respiratory lesions may be associated with audible respiratory sounds, while auscultation may be normal in patients with severe air sac pathology. Placing a thin towel around the bird and ascultating through the towel will actually enhance the clinician's ability to detect respiratory sounds.

Air sac pathology is best detected by placing the stethoscope along the lateral and dorsal body wall. An increased respiratory rate, particularly with dyspnea, is indicative of respiratory tract pathology, and harsh sounds may indicate chronic air sac or parabronchi pathology. Use of a small amount of wing flapping (exercise) serves to increase respiratory rate and accentuate pathologic sounds. The amount of time for the bird to return to normal respiration (respiratory recovery time) is usually under two minutes even in obese birds. Prolonged respiratory recovery time is an indication that further diagnostic tests are necessary.

Imaging

Radiography and endoscopy (with biopsy and culture) are the most effective diagnostic techniques for avian respiratory disease. Radiographically, generalized air sacculitis may be recognized by the appearance of air sac lines on lateral radiographs. Radiographic interpretation of the avian respiratory tract is different from mammals. Interstitial patterns, air bronchograms and atelectasis do not occur in avian radiography. Radiographs are usually of little value in diagnosing acute sinus infections but may be of value, particularly with respect to documenting involvement of bones in the head, with chronic inflammatory processes. Rhinography and sinography are helpful in the diagnosis of upper respiratory tract problems (see Chapter 12).

The ventrodorsal view should be used to assess the subtle disorders of the lung and air sacs. Radiographically, soft tissue masses are commonly associated with upper respiratory signs, pneumonia and air sacculitis On a lateral radiograph, the trachea of normal toucans and mynah birds deviates ventrally, which should not be misinterpreted as a displacement caused by a soft tissue mass. In many ducks, the male has an enlargement on the left side of the syrinx (syringeal bulla) that is not found in the female.

Sample Collection

The minimum database for respiratory problems includes cytology of samples collected from the affected area, a CBC, biochemistries, radiographs and, when indicated, endoscopy.

A sinus aspirate is important in determining the cause of sinusitis (see Chapter 10). Aspiration of the right and left infraorbital sinuses is needed for diagnostic procedures in some passerines. Samples collected from the rostral portion of the choanal slit may provide some useful information on the organisms present in the respiratory passages. Samples collected from the caudal choanal slit are of little diagnostic value with respect to the sinuses or nasal passages.

Tracheal Lavage

Tracheal lavage is indicated when pathology of the trachea or lower respiratory system is suspected. The procedure is relatively simple but requires general anesthesia in most avian patients. A normal wash should be low in cellularity with a minimum of pulmonary macrophages or inflammatory cells.

Increased numbers of heterophils, pulmonary macrophages and other inflammatory cells in the lavage fluid are clinically important. In a severely dyspneic bird, a large-gauge hypodermic needle or a respiratory catheter placed in the abdominal air sacs will help the patient breathe while the procedure is performed.

An intratracheal wash is performed by placing the bird in dorsal recumbency and passing a sterile, soft plastic or rubber tube (eg, Robnel catheter) through the glottis into the trachea, ending near the syrinx (just caudal to the thoracic inlet). A sterile saline solution (0.5-1.0 ml/kg body weight) is infused into the trachea and reaspirated in the sterile syringe attached to the tube.

A sterile endotracheal tube may be placed within the trachea prior to inserting the lavage tube to prevent sample contamination as the lavage tube is passed through the oral cavity. Tracheal swab samples for microbiology evaluation may be taken by passing a small sterile cotton swab directly into the trachea.

Endoscopy

An endoscope may be used to diagnose respiratory problems associated with the trachea, air sacs or lungs.

Endoscopic evaluation of the air sacs can be performed on both the right and left side of the patient. The caudal surface of the lung, which normally appears pale pink and spongy, may also be observed during this procedure (see Chapter 13).

Diffuse air sacculitis, recognized endoscopically as vascularized, translucent, thickened air sacs, commonly occurs with chlamydiosis, some viral diseases, poor air quality, bacterial infections and localized fungal infections. Granulomatous air sacculitis is difficult to resolve without surgery.

Air Sac Diagnostics

Cultures or biopsies of the air sacs can best be obtained using endoscopically guided procedures. Specially designed brushes are commercially available that will traverse the length of a sterile channel in the endoscope. Feather picking over the air sacs may be an indication of irritation that requires further investigation. The lung can also be biopsied using an endoscope (see Chapter 13).

A cytologic sample can be collected from the air sacs by passing a tube through an endoscopic cannula, lavaging with sterile LRS and immediately reaspirating. Sterile cotton swabs may be used to obtain samples for bacterial or fungal cultures using the same technique.

Lung Biopsy

Lung biopsies may be diagnostic in some cases of toxin inhalation and microbial or parasitic infections. This procedure does create the potential for localized pulmonary hemorrhage and should be performed with minimal trauma to the lungs (see Chapter 13).

Aerosol Therapy

Humidification, vaporization and nebulization are three types of aerosol therapy that have been used successfully to treat avian respiratory problems.

In the clinical setting, humidification is used in conjunction with a therapeutic agent but can be prescribed without additives for home treatment. Any source of cool, moist air could be used.

Vaporization is a form of aerosol therapy that utilizes cool or warm mist to deliver topical medications to the mucous membranes. Vaporized particles are large and do not reach the lower respiratory system. Eucalyptus-based products, available as over-the-counter medications for human vaporizers, may cause mucosal irritation in birds and should not be used.

Nebulization can be used to augment systemic therapy of some respiratory tract diseases. Nebulization can help maintain proper hydration of the respiratory epithelium, break up necrotic debris and deliver antimicrobial agents to the upper respiratory tract and portions of the lower respiratory tract. Nebulization therapy is indicated in birds exhibiting sinusitis, rhinitis, pharyngitis and bronchitis. Depending on the agents delivered, nebulization can be used three to four times per day for 10-15 minutes for each session. Therapy should be continued for three days after all clinical signs have been resolved.

The equipment needed for nebulization therapy includes an air compressor or some source of O_2, an enclosed chamber and an infant (human) nebulizer. The most important piece of equipment is the air compressor. An inexpensive reliable unit is commercially available, which should satisfy most nebulization requirements. At least two sizes of nebulization chambers should be maintained, one for larger patients and one for small birds. It has been shown that nebulization can be used to deliver antimicrobial agents to the lungs and some portions of the air sacs if the particle size is less than 0.5 microns in diameter.

All medications delivered to birds by nebulization are used empirically and should be based at least on results obtained from culture and sensitivity (Table 22.5). Mucolytic agents should be used only with infections localized to the sinuses and trachea. Amphotericin B, gentamicin, polymyxin B and tylosin have been found to be poorly absorbed from the respiratory epithelium, and these agents are used principally for their local effects. However, penetration of nebulized antibiotic particles into avian lung parenchyma and onto air sac surfaces may be effective.

The addition of DMSO to the nebulization solution was found to increase the local and systemic concentration of nebulized tylosin. However, the systemic effects of inhaling DMSO have not been evaluated. Nebulized tylosin required one hour to reach therapeutic concentrations in the air sacs and lungs of pigeons and quail.

Table 22.5　Medications Commonly Used in Nebulization Therapy

Drug	Dosage
Amphotericin B	100 mg in 15 ml saline
Chloramphenicol succinate	200 mg in 15 ml saline
Erythromycin	200 mg in 10 ml saline
Gentamicin	50 mg in 10 ml saline
Polymyxin B	333,000 IU in 5 ml saline
Spectinomycin	200 mg in 15 ml saline
Sulfa dimethoxine	200 mg in 15 ml saline
Tylosin	100 mg in 10 ml saline 1 g in 50 ml DMSO
Amikacin	50 mg in 10 ml saline
Enrofloxacin	100 mg in 10 ml saline

Specific Respiratory Diseases

Nutritional Disorders

Hypovitaminosis A has been associated with hyperkeratosis, abscessation of the palatine salivary glands and other oral salivary glands and respiratory lesions in psittacine birds.

Infectious Organisms

Chlamydia psittaci and *Mycoplasma* spp. are obligate intracellular organisms with a predilection for respiratory epithelium and have been implicated in cases of rhinorrhea, infraorbital sinusitis and inflamed choanae. Both organisms may persist as low-grade upper respiratory tract infections. This is particularly common in birds that are treated with immunosuppressive, over-the-counter antibiotics.

Birds with suggestive clinical signs frequently respond to treatment with tetracyclines, tylosin or spectinomycin. These drugs are rarely effective against microbial organisms other than *Chlamydia* or *Mycoplasma* spp.

Bacteria

Gram-negative bacterial infections cause a mucopurulent or thick serous drainage in comparison to the rhinorrhea (clear nasal discharge) associated with uncomplicated *C. psittaci* infections (see Chapter 33).

Serous nasal discharges may result from foreign bodies, allergies, uncomplicated viral, bacterial, fungal or chlamydial infections and with developmental defects or injuries that block the normal drainage of the sinuses into the oral cavity. With most infectious agents, the discharge will turn rapidly from serous to mucopurulent.

Pathogenic gram-positive bacteria commonly associated with respiratory infections include strains of *Streptococcus* spp. and *Staphylococcus* spp. *Mycobacterium tuberculosis* was recovered from the nasal cavity and infraorbital sinuses of a Red-lored Amazon Parrot.

Under most circumstances, *Streptococcus* spp. and *Staphylococcus* spp. would be considered normal bacterial flora. However, pure isolates of *Staphylococcus* spp. and *Streptococcus* spp. have been associated with respiratory and intestinal tract infections. Common nonpathogenic bacteria isolated from the respiratory tract of psittacines include *Bacillus* spp., *Corynebacterium* spp. and *Lactobacillus* spp. (see Chapter 33). Upper respiratory infections caused by spirochetes have been seen in cockatiels. This organism can be demonstrated on wet mount smears (see Chapter 10).

Mycotic Organisms

Aspergillus spp. are ubiquitous fungal organisms and are common pathogens in the respiratory system of immune-incompetent birds. African Grey Parrots, cockatoos, Amazon parrots, raptors, penguins, turkeys, swans and other waterfowl (see Chapter 37) seem to be more susceptible than most psittacine species to this mycotic infection (see Chapter 35). Mycotic granulomas may be found in the nasal cavity, oropharynx, glottal opening, tracheal bifurcation (syrinx), lungs or air sacs.

Clinical signs with acute mycotic tracheitis include dyspnea (mild to severe) and a white discharge originating from the glottis. Fungal hyphae may be seen cytologically in specimens taken from the choana or trachea. Tail-bobbing and peracute severe respiratory distress are common with chronic lower respiratory tract involvement if the passages from the air sacs to the lungs is occluded. Secondary infections may occur on organs in contact with infected air sacs, which might include the liver, kidneys, intestinal serosa and gonads (see Chapter 35). *Candida* spp. infections originating in the oral pharyngeal cavity may extend into the proximal trachea and infraorbital sinuses resulting in varying degrees of dyspnea. Infected birds may temporarily respond to antibiotics (alleviation of secondary bacteria) but fail to recover. In these cases, samples from the affected area should be evaluated by cytology and culture for the presence of fungal pathogens.

Although not common in psittacine birds, a few cases of respiratory cryptococcosis have been described. Affected birds were depressed with severe dyspnea and were unresponsive to treatment. Necropsy findings indicated gelatinous myxomatous material in the nasal cavity, infraorbital sinus and air sacs.

Parasites

Disseminated cases of trichomoniasis may involve the upper respiratory system, trachea and air sacs causing dyspnea and respiratory distress. In the oropharynx and ventral choanal surface, lesions may appear as white or yellow caseous nodules or ulcers (see Chapter 36).

The tracheal mite, *Sternostoma tracheacolum* may cause severe respiratory signs in finches and canaries. Symptoms include vocalization changes, a characteristic clicking during respiration, tail-bobbing and dyspnea. Severe cases lead to weakness and death. The mite may be present in any location of the respiratory system. Transtracheal illumination may be helpful in diagnosing infections. The identification of eggs in mucus from the trachea is diagnostic (see Chapter 36).

Gapeworms (*Syngamus trachea*) inhabit the trachea and glottis area of an infected bird. Clinical signs include dyspnea and changes in vocalization. Visualization of large, bright-red helminths that are in a Y-configuration in the glottal opening are indicative of infection. The earthworm is the primary vector for *Syngamus trachea*, and infections occur following ingestion of the worm.

Sarcocystis falcatula is a coccidian parasite with an obligatory two-host life cycle. This parasite causes an acute, fulminating, hemorrhagic, interstitial pneumonia. The clinical presentation may range from respiratory distress and severe dyspnea to peracute death with no premonitory signs (see Chapter 36).

Systemic microfilaria, trematodes, nematodes and cryptosporidia are other parasites that have been documented in the respiratory system of companion birds. These parasites may be incidental findings on necropsy or may cause varying degrees of upper or lower respiratory distress.

Inhalation Toxicosis

The clinical changes following inhalation of household fumes may include irritation of mucous membranes, conjunctivitis, rhinitis, dyspnea or peracute death (see Chapter 37).

Cigarette Smoke

Passive exposure to cigarette smoke is a common cause of primary respiratory problems in birds as well as a common complicating factor in other respiratory illnesses. Exposure to cigarette smoke can cause a mixture of clinical problems including conjunctivitis, sinusitis, air sacculitis, rhinitis and dermatitis. Diagnosis and treatment of respiratory disease in birds that are exposed to cigarette smoke are difficult, if not impossible. In many cases, complete cessation of all respiratory signs occurs from several weeks to several months after the bird is removed from an environment contaminated with cigarette smoke.

Rhinitis and Sinusitis

Precipitating environmental factors may include cigarette smoke, excessive powder down, dust from organic debris (bedding, flooring substrate), nutritional deficiencies and inappropriate use of antibiotics, all of which may damage the mucosa of the upper respiratory tract allowing pathogens to colonize. South American Psittaciformes that are exposed to the dander of cockatoos and cockatiels may develop a severe allergic pneumonitis. Antibiotics should be used with caution in mild undiagnosed rhinitis. Prolonged or inappropriate use can predispose the patient to secondary bacterial or fungal infections.

A seasonal occurrence (primarily winter months) of serous nasal discharge, mild sneezing and erythromatous nostrils has been described in some Psittaciformes (particularly South American species) maintained in cold, dry northern environments. Similar lesions are seen when the heat or air conditioning systems are first turned on, which might suggest the accumulation of debris or respiratory irritants (stale gases) in the duct system. These birds can frequently be maintained with conservative therapy by increasing humidity, as long as the discharge remains serous and no pathogens are demonstrated. Birds are susceptible to influenza-A virus and could, theoretically, be infected through exposure to diseased members of the household (see Chapter 32).

Miscellaneous Conditions

Choanal Atresia

An African Grey Parrot chick with bilateral serous nasal discharge starting at four days of age was found to have choanal atresia. Endoscopy of the choanal slit and surrounding structures revealed an intact membrane covering the choana at the level of the palate.

Proliferative Nasal Granulomas (Rhinoliths)

Proliferative nasal granulomas have been documented in numerous psittacine species, but are particularly common in African Grey Parrots.

Upper respiratory disease, wheezing, sneezing and insufflation of the infraorbital air sacs on expiration can be early clinical changes associated with the accumulation of debris in the nares. Subtle lesions can best be detected by examining the area around the operculum using magnification. It is best to remove accumulating necrotic debris by probing and flushing before it accumulates and alters the architecture of the nares or sinus passages (see Chapter 41). Recurrence is common unless dietary and management changes are made in conjunction with aggressive parenteral, topical and nebulization therapy.

Sunken Eye Sinusitis

A syndrome characterized by periorbital depression (sunken sinus syndrome) has been described as a sequela to sinusitis in macaws, conures and emus. Progressive collapse of the epithelium into the infraorbital sinus around the eye is typical. Gram-negative organisms have been isolated from the infraorbital sinuses and choana of affected birds. The pathogenesis of this lesion is unclear.

Foreign Body Inhalation

The inhalation of foreign bodies (seeds, granulomatous plaques, splinters and toys) occasionally occurs in companion birds. The acute onset of mild to severe dyspnea in an otherwise healthy bird is a suggestive finding. A thorough endoscopically assisted examination of the nares, choana, glottis, trachea and syrinx is helpful in the diagnosis of foreign body inhalation. Tumors, granulomas, abscesses and papillomas (glottis and choana) may cause varying degrees of dyspnea.

The methods chosen to remove a foreign body will depend on the size of the patient. In birds weighing over 300 g, an endoscope can be used to suction or guide grasping forceps in the removal of some foreign bodies. Once the foreign body is localized, a 30 ga needle can be passed through the trachea distal to the mass to prevent it from moving further down the trachea. Some foreign bodies that cannot be removed by grasping may be flushed out of the trachea by holding the bird upside down and infusing fluids through a small tube placed in the trachea or through a transtracheal needle passed caudal to the mass. In some smaller birds, the distance to the syrinx can be estimated and marked on an appropriate-sized tube. The tube is then passed blindly to this predetermined level and suction is applied to remove accumulated debris. If all other methods of removal fail, a tracheotomy is necessary (see Chapter 41).

Proliferative Tracheitis

Dyspnea, rales, pseudomembranous tracheitis, conjunctivitis and sinusitis have been described as clinical signs associated with proliferative tracheitis in psittacine birds. A herpesvirus with group-serologic relations to the infectious laryngotracheitis virus (ILT) has been shown to cause this lesion in *Amazona* spp. Swabs of the glottis and proximal trachea for cytology culture and viral isolation are necessary for diagnosis. Antiviral therapy utilizing acyclovir may be helpful along with supportive therapy and antibiotics. This disease is rarely reported in the USA, and has been described only in smuggled or recently imported Amazon parrots (see Chapter 32).

Air Sacculitis

Air sac infections are best treated aggressively with therapeutic agents that are chosen based on culture and sensitivity. Surgical debridement may be necessary to resolve air sac infections that result in the formation of masses.

Subcutaneous Emphysema

Subcutaneous emphysema can occur following damage to any air sac system but is most common with damage to the cervicocephalic, abdominal or caudal thoracic air sacs. Trauma, malnutrition and infectious agents have been implicated as causes of subcutaneous emphysema (see Chapter 41). In addition, the cervicocephalic air sac may distend as a result of rhinitis, which causes occlusion of the nasal passage or damage to the outflow tracts. The resulting lesion looks clinically like subcutaneous emphysema as the air sacs progressively inflate with each successive expiration.

When the air is removed with a needle, the sac will deflate but will typically reinflate with subsequent respiratory cycles. Initially, these problems can be managed by wrapping the area with a loose, self-adherent bandage. If the problem persists, long-term management can be achieved by inserting a Teflon stent in the dorsal wall of the air sac that allows air to escape. In some cases, the damage to the sac will repair itself and the stent can be removed. In other cases, the stent must remain in place permanently (see Chapter 41).

ENDOCRINOLOGY

J. T. Lumeij

A lthough endocrinopathies in birds do occur, endocrinology is a subject that is frequently unfamiliar to the avian practitioner. Endocrine system abnormalities may be more frequently diagnosed as practitioners expand their working knowledge of normal avian endocrinology, and appropriate clinical diagnostic tests can be used to document endocrine abnormalities.

A clinical presentation that suggests an endocrine disorder must always be confirmed before treatment is begun. Confirmation of the diagnosis may be difficult once replacement therapy is initiated, and improper or inadequate endocrine therapy can be fatal. Obesity is a good example of a clinical sign that is often misdiagnosed as an endocrine disorder (hypothyroidism) in birds, but is nearly always caused by malnutrition and lack of exercise instead. Feather abnormalities have also been reported in association with endocrine disorders without supporting evidence for an etiology. Polydipsia and polyuria can be of endocrine origin, but may also be psychogenic in origin.

The Hypothalamus and Pituitary Gland

Neurohypophyseal Hormones

Avian neurohypophyseal hormones, arginine vasotocin (AVT) and mesotocin (MT), are similar to the mammalian antidiuretic (arginine vasopressin, AVP) and oxytocic (oxytocin) hormones, respectively. The major effect of AVT in birds is to reduce urine production. This is accomplished by decreasing the glomerular filtration rate through constriction of the afferent arterioles of reptilian-type nephrons, and by increasing the permeability of collecting ducts of mammalian-type nephrons. AVT is released in response to plasma osmolality changes, which are registered by peripheral and central osmolality receptors.

Injections of both AVT and oxytocin increase intrauterine pressure in birds, and a large increase in blood AVT concentration has been observed shortly before oviposition.

Adenohypophyseal Hormones

Adenohypophyseal hormones are either glycoproteins or polypeptides. The glycoprotein hormones are luteinizing hormone (LH), follicle stimulating hormone (FSH) and thyroid stimulating hormone (TSH; thyrotropin).

The adenohypophyseal polypeptide hormones are growth hormone (GH; somatotropin), prolactin- and proopiomelanocortin (POMC)-derived hormones such as adrenocorticotrophic hormone (ACTH) and β-melanocyte stimulating hormone (α- and β-MSH), β- and τ-lipoprotein (β- and τ-LPH), β-endorphin and encephalin.

Both LH and FSH stimulate ovarian steroid synthesis and are essential for ovarian function in birds. During the ovulatory cycle, plasma FSH concentration shows little change. However, approximately five hours before ovulation, a rise in plasma LH concentration can be observed. Plasma LH concentration is low during egg laying, incubation and care for the chicks. An increase in LH secretion occurs toward the end of the chick-rearing period to prepare the hen for the next laying cycle.

In males, LH stimulates Leydig cell differentiation and testosterone synthesis, while FSH promotes Sertoli cell differentiation and spermatogenesis.

TSH increases the number of colloid droplets in thyroid cells, stimulates the uptake of iodide by the thyroid and stimulates the release of thyroxine (T_4).

Avian GH has effects both on growth and on the short-term control of metabolism. GH mobilizes stored lipids and increases free fatty acids, which are then available as an energy source. Lipogenesis is decreased. Muscle glycogen is increased and glucose utilization is reduced. GH seems to spare carbohydrates from use as a precursor for lipid synthesis.

In birds, prolactin is known to affect reproduction and osmoregulation. Effects on growth and metabolism have been suggested. In pigeons and doves, prolactin stimulates the production of crop milk. Just before the eggs are to hatch, there is a prolactin-induced proliferation and sloughing of mucosal cells in the crop sac. These cells are then regurgitated to feed the young during the first eight to eleven days of life. In other avian species, prolactin induces broodiness and suppresses ovarian function directly and indirectly via the hypothalamus. Prolactin is released after infusion of hypertonic NaCl solutions, and reduced urine flow occurs following the administration of prolactin.

ACTH stimulates corticosterone and aldosterone production by the avian adrenal cortical (interrenal) cells.

Hypothalamic Releasing or Inhibiting Hormones or Factors

The hypothalamic-hypophysiotropic factors are released from the median eminence and are transported to the anterior pituitary gland via the portal blood vessels. If the chemical structure of these hypothalamic chemotransmitters is known they are called hormones, and when the chemical structure is unknown, they are called factors. These chemotransmitters can have a stimulating or an inhibiting action on the release of the trophic anterior pituitary hormones and hence are called releasing or inhibiting hormones or factors.

The secretion of gonadotropin (LH and FSH) is controlled by LH releasing hormone (LHRH) which differs slightly from its mammalian counterpart.

The secretion of TSH is under stimulatory hypothalamic control. The hypophysiotropic factors regulating pituitary TSH release are somatostatin and thyrotropin releasing hormone (TRH), which are also physiologic regulators of GH secretion in birds.

GH release from the adenohypophysis is under hypothalamic control by TRH, growth hormone releasing factor (GRF) and somatostatin (somatotropin release inhibiting factor; SRIF), which inhibits GH secretion. Somatostatin is also formed in the avian pancreas.

Contrary to the situation in mammals, prolactin is under stimulatory hypothalamic control. The identity of avian prolactin releasing factor (PRF) remains undetermined.

The secretion of ACTH in birds is presumably under control of corticotrophin releasing factor (CRF).

Diseases in Relation to the Hypothalamic-Hypophyseal Complex

Diseases may be caused by hypo- or hypersecretion of one or, more commonly, several of the hypothalamic or pituitary hormones. These alterations in secretion may be caused by tumors that are primary or metastatic, benign or malignant, pituitary or parapituitary, or by granulomatous lesions, congenital lesions or trauma. In addition to causing endocrine abnormalities, space-occupying lesions may cause neurologic signs due to pressure on surrounding nerve tissue.

When a diagnosis of hypothalamic disease is based on circulating concentrations of hypothalamic or hypophyseal hormones, it should be considered that primary hypofunction of a target organ will result in hypersecretion of the trophic hormone. This makes it possible to distinguish between a primary disorder of the gland or a disorder of the gland secondary to pituitary dysfunction or a hypothalamic disorder (tertiary dysfunction).

Dwarfism

Dwarfism has been reported in various avian species such as the fowl, pheasant, Black-headed Gull and Great Crested Flycatcher. Dwarfism is sex-linked recessive in the fowl. Sex-linked dwarf growing chicks have lower concentrations of somatomedin C (insulin-like growth factor, IGF - I) and T_3, whereas GH and T_4 are increased, probably due to a decreased negative feedback effect on GH secretion.

Diabetes Insipidus

Diabetes insipidus has been reported to occur in chickens and might also occur in other avian species. The principal clinical signs of this disease are polyuria and polydipsia (PU/PD).

For healthy racing pigeons, it has been established that a urine osmolality of at least 450 mOsm/kg can be expected after 24 hours of water deprivation, which typifies the normal concentrating capacity of the kidneys. In avian patients with PU/PD in which urine osmolality does not increase in response to water deprivation, administration of exogenous ADH or AVT can be used to differentiate between central diabetes insipidus and other causes of PU/PD.

Pituitary Tumors in Budgerigars and Cockatiels

Chromophobe adenomas and carcinomas of the pituitary are common in budgerigars (see Chapter 25). In a review of 497 tumors in budgerigars, 156 were either chromophobe adenomas or carcinomas; however, in other reports, the incidence of these tumors was considerably lower. Variations in the reported incidence of pituitary tumors might be caused by the fact that these tumors are easily overlooked during a routine gross necropsy. The pituitary gland is easy to isolate and should always be evaluated. The mandible is removed with the bird in dorsal recumbency. The medial ridge of the sphenoid bone can be broken away with forceps, after which the pituitary will be found lying in the sella turcica of the sphenoid, just posterior to the optic chiasm. The normal pituitary gland from a budgerigar is about 2 mm in diameter, while the diameter can be 7 mm if a pituitary tumor is present. Pituitary tumors have been associated with a ten-fold weight increase of the pituitary gland.

Recently, pituitary adenoma and pituitary adenocarcinoma with metastasis to the liver have been reported in cockatiels.

Reported clinical signs of pituitary tumors in budgerigars and cockatiels are related to hormonal imbalance (eg, polyuria, polydipsia, reproductive failure, obesity and feather structure and pigmentation abnormalities) and to compression of surrounding nervous tissue (eg, stupor, blindness, uni- or bilateral exophthalmus, convulsions). Although it has been suggested that the PU/PD is caused by hyposecretion of AVT (diabetes insipidus), hypersecretion of ACTH (Cushing's disease, secondary hyperadrenocorticism), TSH (hyperthyroidism) and GH have not been excluded.

Clinical Applications

Pituitary gland tumors should be suspected in clinical cases with:
- PU/PD
- Feather dystrophy
- Obesity
- Blindness
- Uni- & bilateral exophthalmos
- Reproductive failure
- Pigmentation abnormalities
- Stupor
- Convulsions
- Hyperglycemia

If these signs are present and a bird dies, the pituitary gland should be submitted for histopathology.

Hyperglycemia and obesity occurred in birds with subcutaneous transplants of pituitary tumors. The obesity was characterized by an accumulation of adipose tissue beneath the skin of the breast and abdomen as well as in the peritoneum and mesentery. The liver was often enlarged, and histologic sections revealed an accumulation of fat in hepatic cells.

Calcium Metabolism

Calcium metabolism in birds is under the control of three major hormones: parathyroid hormone (PTH), calcitonin (CT) and 1,25 dihydrocholecalciferol ($1,25(OH)_2D_3$), the active metabolite of vitamin D_3.

Parathyroid Hormone

In companion birds, the parathyroids are normally visible as light-colored areas at the caudal end of the thyroid glands. Currently, a sensitive radioimmunoassay for avian PTH is not available.

PTH is secreted in response to hypocalcemia. The primary target organs of PTH are the kidney and bone. Calcium excretion in the urine is decreased by increasing tubular reabsorption of calcium, while circumstantial evidence suggests that calcium resorption from bone is increased. Under the influence of PTH, renal tubular secretion of phosphate is increased, while decreased tubular reabsorption may occur. The net result is a phosphate diuresis and a decrease in plasma phosphate.

PTH regulates vitamin D by enhancing the production of the key calcium-regulating hormone $1,25(OH)_2D_3$.

Calcitonin (CT)

In contrast to its action in mammals, CT does not induce a hypocalcemia in normocalcemic birds. It appears, rather, to control hypercalcemia and to protect the skeleton from excessive calcium resorption.

Vitamin D_3

Vitamin D_3 (cholecalciferol) is converted from its precursor, 7-dehydrocholesterol, under the influence of ultraviolet (UV) light. The next step occurs mainly in microsomal fractions of liver cells and is the formation of 25-hydroxycholecalciferol. The second and more important step in the activation of D_3 occurs in mitochondria of cells in the renal cortex, and involves the conversion to 1,25-dihydroxyvitamin D_3.

The main role of the active metabolite of vitamin D_3 is to elevate plasma calcium and inorganic phosphorus by increasing small intestinal absorption.

Lack of vitamin D_3 in young birds leads to rickets.

Calcium in Reproductive Physiology

Two independent physiologic phenomena related to calcium metabolism are seen in hens during reproduction. These normal changes should not be misinterpreted as pathologic.

Estrogen-induced Hypercalcemia: About four days before female pigeons are due to ovulate, the blood calcium concentration rises from a normal value of about 2.2 mmol/L (9 mg/dL) to a value of over 5.0 mmol/L (20 mg/dL) at the time of ovulation.

Physiologic Marrow Ossification: During egg-laying, there is a large increase in the quantities of calcium and phosphorus that are retained from the diet and deposited in the medullary bone. This medullary bone may completely fill the marrow cavity of long bones. When the hen starts to secrete the eggshell, the medullary bone is resorbed by osteoclastic activity. Calcium is deposited in the eggshell as calcium carbonate, and the phosphorus is excreted from the body. Normal medullary bone deposits should not be mistaken for a pathologic condition radiographically.

Relation Between Total Calcium and Protein in Avian Plasma

The plasma calcium concentration is normally about 2.0-2.8 mmol/L (8-11.2 mg/dL), depending on the species. About one-third of plasma calcium is protein-bound and is biologically inactive. Total calcium concentration is markedly influenced by plasma protein concentrations. The ionized fraction is important with regard to deposition of calcium salts and excitability of nervous tissues. For technical reasons, most laboratories determine only total calcium. Hence, total plasma calcium should be evaluated in conjunction with plasma protein concentrations.

Recently, a significant correlation was found between total calcium and albumin concentration in the plasma of 70 healthy African Grey Parrots. Approximately 14% of the variability of calcium was attributable to the change in the concentration of plasma albumin. A correction formula was derived on the basis of the concentration of albumin:

Adjusted Ca (mmol/L) = Ca (mmol/L) - 0.015 albumin (g/L) + 0.4

A significant correlation was also found between total calcium and total protein concentration in 124 plasma samples of Peregrine Falcons. About 42% of the variability in calcium was attributable to the change in the plasma total protein concentration. The correlation between calcium and albumin was significant, but significantly smaller than the correlation between calcium and total protein. An adjustment formula for plasma calcium concentration in the Peregrine Falcon was derived on the basis of the total protein concentration.

Adj. Ca (mmol/L) = Ca (mmol/L) - 0.02 Total Protein (g/L) + 0.67

Application of a correction formula in African Grey Parrots and Peregrine Falcons is indicated when extremely low or extremely high plasma protein concentrations are detected.

Diseases in Relation to the Metabolism of Calcium and Phosphorus

Hyperparathyroidism

Contrary to the situation in man and domestic mammals, primary hyperparathyroidism and pseudohyperparathyroidism have not been documented in birds. Because adenoma and carcinoma of the avian parathyroid gland do occur, it is likely that primary hyperparathyroidism will be reported in the future.

Secondary nutritional hyperparathyroidism is commonly reported in birds secondary to a calcium-deficient diet (see Chapter 3).

Diets that contain only seeds or only meat are deficient in calcium. Fruits and most vegetables are also calcium deficient. Nonetheless, many pet food retailers continue to market so-called "complete parrot foods," which consist only of seeds (mainly sunflower seeds). Affected birds have a low or normal plasma calcium concentration, a normal plasma phosphate concentration and increased AP activity. In young birds, rickets or rachitis is seen as a result of calcium-deficient diets, while in adult birds osteomalacia will occur.

Secondary hyperparathyroidism due to a renal disorder is well known in mammals and possibly occurs also in birds. In chronic renal disease, failure of the conversion of 25-hydroxycholecalciferol to 1,25-dihydroxyvitamin D_3, the key calcium-regulating hormone, will result in reduced intestinal absorption of calcium. Under these circumstances, a high plasma phosphate concentration may be seen due to decreased tubular secretion of phosphate. Plasma AP activity will be increased.

Rickets

Rickets or rachitis is a metabolically induced bone disease in growing animals. The skeleton and the beak (rubber beak) become soft and pliable. Rickets can be caused by inadequate dietary intake of calcium, phosphorus or vitamin D_3 or by an improper calcium:phosphorus ratio. With calcium and vitamin D deficiencies, the resulting hypocalcemia induces enlargement of the parathyroid gland (nutritional secondary hyperparathyroidism). Consistent parathyroid gland changes are not typical with a phosphate deficiency or excessive calcium intake. Histologically, it is possible to differentiate between rickets caused by vitamin D deficiency, hypocalcemia and hypophosphatemia/calcium excess.

Tachypnea and polycythemia have been observed in birds with rickets, presumably because of poor rib strength and infolding of ribs. Affected birds died of right ventricular failure, often accompanied by ascites.

Osteomalacia (Osteodystrophy)

In mature birds, calcium deficiencies will result in parathyroid enlargement and PTH-induced activation of osteoclastic activity, which eventually can result in complete demineralization of medullary bone, followed by cortical bone. The resorbed osseous tissue can be replaced by fibrous tissue (osteodystrophia fibrosa). The cortical bone can become so thin that spontaneous fractures may occur, especially in the vertebrae, ribs, tibiotarsus, tarsometatarsus and femur. The beak becomes soft and pliable. Plasma calcium concentrations remain generally normal until the end stage of the disease, when tetanic convulsions may be observed. Although calcium deficiencies accompanied by pathologic fractures seem relatively common in psittacine birds, nutritional osteodystrophia fibrosa is rarely diagnosed.

Osteoporosis

To a certain degree, osteoporosis (cage layer fatigue) is physiologic during egg production. Osteoporosis is characterized by the progressive reduction of bone mass.

Affected birds are found paralyzed in their enclosures, and have skeletal deformities and enlarged parathyroid glands. Paralysis may be explained by spinal cord compression due to fractures in the thoracic spine and possibly by hypocalcemia, although the latter has not yet been demonstrated.

Hypervitaminosis D$_3$

Oversupplementation of the diet with vitamin D$_3$ (>4 million IU/kg diet) causes dystrophic calcification of kidney tubules. Calcium nephropathy can also occur when birds are raised on diets containing 3% calcium instead of the normal 0.6% (see Chapters 3, 31).

Hypocalcemia Syndrome in African Grey Parrots

Hypocalcemia characterized by seizures has been described in raptors and African Grey Parrots. A unique feature of this syndrome in African Grey Parrots is that demineralization of the skeleton to maintain normal calcium levels does not occur. Hypocalcemia is an important problem to consider in an African Grey Parrot that repeatedly falls off its perch. Administration of parenteral calcium and sufficient dietary uptake of calcium resolves clinical signs. A dietary calcium deficiency is suspected, but not confirmed as the etiologic agent. In a recent study it was shown that African Grey Parrots have significantly lower calcium, albumin and total protein concentrations compared to Amazon Parrots; however, the significantly lower mean and median values for plasma calcium in African Greys could be explained only partially by the difference in albumin-bound calcium. The higher incidence of hypocalcemia in African Grey Parrots might therefore be associated with lower plasma concentrations of free calcium.

Polyostotic Hyperostosis

In female budgerigars, polyostotic hyperostosis, which resembles physiologic marrow ossification is often seen in association with ovarian tumors. Physiologic marrow ossification and polyostotic hyperostosis may be related, and the latter may be a pathologic exacerbation of a physiologic phenomenon caused by hyperestrogenism. Hyperestrogenism has also been associated with abdominal hernias.

The Thyroid Glands

Compared to the thyroid gland in mammals, the avian thyroid produces more T$_4$ than T$_3$. It is T$_3$ that is the principally active hormone, produced mostly by extrathyroidal 5'-monodeiodination of T$_4$ in liver and kidney. The activity of the 5'-monodeiodination enzyme is hormonally controlled by hypothalamic hormones (TRH, GRF) and GH.

Thyroid Disorders

Diseases of the thyroid gland may be accompanied by thyroid enlargement (goiter), hyperfunction or hypofunction. Functional disorders may be primary, secondary or tertiary, depending on the location of the lesion (thyroid gland, pituitary gland or hypothalamus, respectively). Only goiter has been adequately documented in birds and may be caused by neoplastic disease or by iodine deficiency. Hypothyroidism has been documented in chickens, pigeons and one parrot, and it has been suggested that hyperthyroidism may be induced by exposure to iodide-containing disinfectants. Thyroiditis occurs frequently in birds, but clinical signs associated with this condition have not yet been reported.

Thyroid Tumors

Thyroid neoplasia is rare in birds. Adenomas and adenocarcinomas have been reported in budgerigars, a Scarlet Macaw and some other birds from zoological collections (see Chapter 25).

Clinical signs associated with thyroid enlargement include regurgitation and dyspnea. Like thyroid tumors in man and domestic mammals, it is to be expected that some avian thyroid tumors will have autonomous hormone production and will cause hyperthyroidism; however, no reports are available in birds.

Goiter in Budgerigars

The most frequent clinical disease of the thyroid gland in birds is goiter in budgerigars, caused by feeding an iodine-deficient diet (usually seed mixtures). Goiter has occasionally been seen in other avian species, but is a well known and distinct clinical entity in the domestic pigeon. In budgerigars with goiter, clinical changes are limited to regurgitation and dyspnea caused by gland pressure on the trachea and esophagus. Specific signs of hypothyroid function are absent. Circulatory problems may occur due to compression of the heart and great vessels. The size of the glands can exceed 10 mm compared to a normal size of about 2 mm. Radiographically, a dorsal or ventral displacement of the trachea may be visible.

Goiter can be prevented by placing a bird on a complete formulated diet. The dietary requirement of iodine is about 20 micromg per week for a 35 g budgerigar. Affected animals can be treated with a 0.3% Lugol's solution in the drinking water (1 drop per 20 ml water): first week, daily; second week, three times a week; then once weekly.

Goiter in Domestic Pigeons

Goiter can occur in domestic pigeons on an iodine-deficient diet. Certain breeds (eg, White Carneaux) are more susceptible than others. Soybeans and fat-rich corns (like maize) may increase the iodine demand and potentiate goiter. Clinical signs in adult pigeons are different from those in budgerigars and include lethargy, obesity and a palpable thyroid gland in the thoracic inlet. Tail and wing feathers that are too long and narrow or structural defects in the contour feathers may give the bird a ruffled appearance and an irregular or failing molt. Dyspnea accompanied by a respiratory stridor occurs only in severe cases.

Hypothyroidism

Primary hypothyroidism is a well recognized disorder in birds. In chickens, it occurs as a hereditary autoimmune disorder. Low levels of thyroid hormones have also been associated with a malabsorption syndrome. The measurement of T_4 would seem to be the most logical choice for evaluating birds; however, even plasma T_4 concentrations can be influenced by drugs, handling, bleeding, food intake, environmental temperature, increased plasma corticosterone concentration and infections with *Eimeria maxima*. Normal plasma T_4 concentrations in birds are about one-fifth to one-tenth those characteristic for mammals. In many birds, resting plasma thyroxine concentrations are below the detection limit of the assay. Documentation that a low plasma T_4 level is caused by primary hypothyroidism requires a TSH stimulation test to rule out other causes for a decreased T_4 concentration.

For evaluation of thyroid function in racing pigeons, blood samples should be collected before and between 4 and 24 hours after administration of 0.1 IU of TSH. If a dose of 1 IU per pigeon is used, samples can be collected up to 32 hours later. In healthy individuals, at least a 2.5-fold increase will be observed over basal T_4 concentrations using these doses and sampling times. The TSH stimulation test can also be used in other avian species using 1 IU/kg. A diagnosis of hypothyroidism should not be based on low baseline thyroxine concentrations or on a "favorable response to administration of thyroxin." A diagnosis is based on suggestive clinical signs, especially defective plumage development, in conjunction with failure to respond to TSH.

Thyroiditis

Thyroiditis was reported in a large variety of avian species, including an Amazon parrot. At necropsy, 36.9% of avian thyroid lesions were of an inflammatory nature.

In an obese strain (OS) of chickens, circulating thyroglobulin autoantibodies have been shown to be the cause of spontaneous thyroiditis accompanied by hypothyroidism.

The Use of Thyroid Hormone in Non-thyroidal Disorders

Thyroid hormone has been frequently recommended for the treatment of obesity in birds. However, no controlled studies have been performed to demonstrate the effectiveness of this treatment. Pharmacologic doses of thyroid hormone sufficient to raise the basal metabolic rate to a hypermetabolic state undoubtedly result in increased weight loss. If caloric intake is not carefully controlled, however, predominantly fat-free tissue may be lost during treatment. The weight loss may be readily and rapidly reversed after discontinuation of therapy.

The occurrence of toxic effects is unavoidable when pharmacologic doses of thyroid hormone are used. In obese birds without proven hypothyroidism, thyroid hormone therapy can be dangerous and should not be used in lieu of providing a well balanced diet and adequate exercise.

Thyroid hormone can induce molt in a number of species. The molt is more pronounced after administration of a single dose compared with daily administration of small doses equal to the sum of the single dose.

The Adrenal Glands

Anatomy and Physiology

The microanatomy of the avian adrenal gland differs from that of mammals in that the avian adrenal gland is not clearly divided into an outer cortex and inner medulla. In birds, cortical and chromaffin tissue are intermingled. Chromaffin tissue accounts for about 25% of adrenal tissue and can be divided by means of cytochemistry into two types of chromaffin cells: those releasing epinephrine and those releasing norepinephrine.

Cortical or interrenal cells are arranged in numerous cords composed of a double row of cells. The major function of the avian adrenal cortical cells is to produce glucocorticoid and mineralocorticoid hormones, of which corticosterone is the most important corticoid hormone in birds. Aldosterone production is considerably less.

Adrenocortical Disorders

Although adrenal lesions have been described on postmortem examinations in a high percentage of birds (27% in one study involving psittacine birds), a clinical diagnosis of spontaneous adrenal disease has never been documented. The use of the ACTH stimulation test, dexamethasone screening test and dexamethasone suppression test as reported for dogs should prove useful for the diagnosis of both hypoadrenocorticism and hyperadrenocorticism in birds. The optimal dose for ACTH and sampling times for determination of plasma corticosterone (not cortisol) concentrations have been established for a number of avian species.

Hyperadrenocorticism (Cushing's syndrome)

Spontaneous hyperadrenocorticism has not been reported in birds, but the effects of exogenous glucocorticoids have been well documented. Hyperadrenocorticism can occur as a result of a primary tumor of the adrenal gland, a pituitary tumor that hypersecretes ACTH, or ectopic ACTH secretion from a nonpituitary tumor. Both of the latter conditions induce bilateral adrenocortical hyperplasia due to continuous ACTH secretion.

Pituitary and adrenal tumors have been reported in birds, and it is not unlikely that a number of these patients were in fact suffering from hyperadrenocorticism. The following conditions have been reported: bilateral adrenal adenoma and adrenal cortical hyperplasia in budgerigar, unilateral adrenal adenoma in a budgerigar, unilateral adrenocortical carcinoma in a pigeon, adrenal carcinoma with metastasis in the liver, and adrenal gland neoplasia in a variety of avian species.

Hypoadrenocorticism

In all avian species studied, corticosterone, and not cortisol, is considered to be the major glucocorticoid; therefore, cortisol is not a valid parameter to evaluate adrenocortical function in birds.

It has been demonstrated that Mallard Ducks consuming petroleum-contaminated food (South Louisiana crude oil) developed structural damage to the mitochondria of the inner zone cells in the adrenal cortex and had decreased circulating corticosterone concentrations. Adrenocortical testing procedures using corticosterone have been reported in Psittaciformes, raptors and pigeons. In pigeons, ACTH testing was accomplished by taking blood samples before and at 60 or 90 minutes after stimulation with 50 mg of ACTH or at 30, 60, 90 or 120 minutes after stimulation with 125 mg of ACTH. In healthy individuals, a 10- to 100-fold increase over baseline corticosterone concentrations and absolute concentrations in the range of 2.2-15 mg/dL should be considered normal for post-stimulation samples.

The Use of Corticosteroids in Non-endocrine Disease

Glucocorticoids are widely used in human and veterinary medicine for their beneficial effects in a wide variety of diseases, especially those in which inflammation is severe or in which immunologic-induced disease is involved. The adverse effects of glucocorticoids should always be considered before they are administered. The clinician has to consider whether the disease is serious enough to warrant long-term glucocorticosteroid therapy.

Pharmacologic concentrations of corticosterone in birds can cause involution of the cloacal bursa, thymus and spleen, resulting in suppression of both humoral and cell-mediated immunity. A single intramuscular injection of dexamethasone or prednisolone in racing pigeons was found to cause lymphopenia. There is a proportional increase in granulocytes that occurs with the lymphopenia.

Aspergillosis has been observed in racing pigeons and budgerigars as a complication of long-term administration of glucocorticosteroids.

Aspergillosis in recently captured free-ranging birds may be related to stress-induced hypercorticosteronism with associated suppression of monocyte function.

Glucocorticoids (Corticosteroids)

Appropriate dosages for glucocorticoids in birds have not been fully established and are currently being investigated. Dosage guidelines are based on data in mammals.

The cortisol dosage for replacement therapy is about 0.5-1 mg/kg daily.

Prednisolone is the agent of choice for anti-inflammatory immunosuppression and antineoplastic therapy to reduce the severity of negative feedback at the hypothalamus-hypophyseal level. Anti-inflammatory doses of prednisolone are 0.5-1.0 mg/kg. Immunosuppressive and chemotherapeutic doses are 2-4 mg/kg prednisolone daily. Corticosteroids are used as chemotherapy for lymphoreticular neoplasia because of their antimitotic effects on lymphoid tissue.

Dexamethasone is the steroid of choice for reducing cerebrospinal edema. Dosages used in mammals are 2 mg/kg q8h until improvement occurs.

In clinical situations where long-term glucocorticosteroid therapy is indicated, appropriate consideration should be given to exacerbations of subclinical infections (eg, viral, bacterial, mycotic or parasitic) or induction of iatrogenic secondary hypoadrenocorticism or iatrogenic hyperadrenocorticism-like disease. Local corticosteroid therapy should be considered in ophthalmic and dermatologic conditions, and alternate-day therapy should be considered in long-term systemic corticosteroid therapy to reduce these side-effects. However, the clinician should be aware that high or even toxic blood levels of steroids can occur following topical application.

Corticosteroid therapy in severe inflammatory diseases is best divided into several doses through the day. Once the desired effects are reached, the regimen should be tapered down to the least toxic dose. The divided daily dose is given in a single daily dose in the morning and gradually decreased to the minimal effective dose. Whenever glucocorticosteroid therapy has to be given for periods over two weeks, alternate-day therapy should be considered. The daily dose is doubled and given every other day, while the dose on the "off" day is gradually decreased to zero.

Iatrogenic Hyperadrenocorticism-like Disease

Exogenous glucocorticoids cause hyperphagia while reducing growth and body weight in birds. There is a marked increase in fat deposition (lipogenesis) and a concomitant increase in protein catabolism. Cholesterol levels increase, and true lipemic conditions may develop as a result of glucocorticoid injections. Furthermore, gluconeogenesis is increased (production of blood glucose at the expense of muscle and adipose tissue) and hence plasma glucose concentrations are elevated. Steroid diabetes may be induced with accompanying glucosuria. Hepatic glycogen is increased. Calcium absorption from the intestinal tract is reduced after administration of betamethasone and cortisol. Corticosterone increases the glomerular filtration rate which, together with glucosuria, may be recognized as polyuria and polydipsia.

Iatrogenic Secondary Hypoadrenocorticism

Glucocorticoids exert a negative feedback influence at the hypothalamo-hypophyseal level and suppress basal and stress-induced corticosterone release. Failure of the adrenal gland to respond to stress factors may result in adrenocortical insufficiency. It has been shown in pigeons that short-term, high-dose glucocorticoid therapy produces only transient suppression of the HPA axis. An ACTH stimulation test can be performed to evaluate the integrity of the HPA axis. Replacement therapy is indicated in stressed birds with hypoadrenocorticism.

Stress Marks

A common disorder of developing feathers is the symmetrical development of stress marks or hunger traces. These represent a segmental dysplasia in the barbs and barbules. Stress lines can be easily identified by holding the spread wing or tail feathers against a light and looking for bilateral symmetrical lines perpendicular to the feather shaft. These lesions represent a period of malnutrition or stress while the feathers were developing. They can also be induced by a single injection of a glucocorticoid. Administration of glucocorticoids strongly suppresses growth and increases protein catabolism, and these lesions probably reflect a short period of decreased amino acid available to the developing feather. Chronic malnutrition and chronic stress in birds with developing feathers will result in more severely affected feathers.

Adrenomedullary Disorders

Pheochromocytoma (Chromaffinoma)

A pheochromocytoma of the adrenal gland in a 14-week-old broiler pullet has been reported. The bird died suddenly. The only obvious abnormality was an enlarged left adrenal gland measuring 15 mm in diameter.

Diabetes Mellitus

Spontaneous diabetes mellitus has been reported in a variety of granivorous avian species, including the domestic pigeon. One case of spontaneous diabetes mellitus has been reported in a raptor. Budgerigars and cockatiels frequently develop diabetes mellitus. The most striking clinical signs are PU/PD and loss of weight despite a good appetite. A tentative diagnosis can be made by demonstrating glucosuria while a definitive diagnosis can be made by finding persistent hyperglycemia.

It is generally accepted that glucagon is more effective in granivorous birds, which exhibit a marked insulin insensitivity. The limited data available on spontaneous diabetes mellitus in granivorous birds suggest that in these species diabetes mellitus is not caused by an insulin deficiency. Birds of prey may be more insulin dependent than granivorous birds.

There are several case reports of successful treatment of spontaneous diabetes mellitus in birds with daily injections of insulin using dosages comparable to those used in dogs. These reported "successful treatments" of diabetic birds (disappearance of clinical signs) are surprising, considering the relative insulin insensitivity that has been reported to occur in a variety of avian species.

Plasma insulin and glucagon concentrations have been established in three birds with hyperglycemia. It is not clear whether these determinations were accurate. In all cases, insulin concentrations were similar to controls. Glucagon concentrations on the other hand were extremely high or extremely low. This suggests that the hyperglycemia may have been from varying etiologies.

An islet cell carcinoma has been diagnosed in one case of diabetes mellitus in a parakeet. The cellular origin of the tumor was not identified, but it was suggested that it could be an alpha-cell tumor.

The pathogenesis of diabetes mellitus in birds remains unclear.

Polyuria/Polydipsia (PU/PD)

The minimal data-base for an avian patient with PU/PD should include dietary history, social and behavioral history, vaccination status (paramyxovirus in pigeons) and recent medications (eg, corticosteroid therapy), urine glucose, plasma glucose, urea, uric acid, AST, bile acids, total calcium, total protein, protein electrophoresis and HAI-titer for paramyxovirus in pigeons.

Determining the reproductive history is important in hens with PU/PD. Birds with egg-related peritonitis may have previously laid eggs and then stopped because of the egg-related peritonitis. These birds may have a swollen abdomen in association with PU/PD.

Polyuria/Polydipsia Syndrome in Pigeons Feeding Squabs

Pigeons feed their young crop milk during the first 7-11 days after hatching, at which time the squabs are fed regurgitated grains. The parent birds and the squabs often develop PU/PD for a couple of days during the transition period.

The observed PU/PD in the parent birds may be caused by a decrease in the circulating concentrations of prolactin. It has been shown that prolactin has an influence on water and electrolyte regulation in birds.

Renal Glucosuria

Glucosuria is not always associated with hyperglycemia, and the two should occur together to warrant a diagnosis of diabetes mellitus. Glucosuria without hyperglycemia in man is associated with the Fanconi syndrome, which is caused by inherited or acquired damage to the proximal convoluted tubules of the kidney. Glucosuria without hyperglycemia has been observed in an African Grey Parrot.

Apparent Psychogenic Polydipsia

Some avian patients may develop psychogenic polydipsia that results in polyuria. A water deprivation test may be useful in documenting a primary polydipsia or compulsive water drinking. In these patients, water restriction results in disappearance of the clinical signs. It seems that psychogenic polydipsia should be added to the list of behavioral problems that can be encountered in companion birds.

Paramyxovirus Infection in Racing Pigeons

When a pigeon strain of paramyxovirus serotype-1 infects an unvaccinated flock of pigeons, about 80% of the birds will develop severe PU/PD, which can last for several months and then gradually resolve. The pathophysiologic mechanism for these clinical changes has not been defined.

Table 23.3 Some Conditions Associated with Polyuria/Polydipsia	
• Dietary-induced polyuria	• Pigeons feeding squabs
• Excitement or nervousness	• Paramyxovirus (racing pigeons)
• Apparent psychogenic polydipsia	• Liver disease
• Medications (corticosteroids, diuretics, progesterones)	• Renal disease
• Toxins (eg, gentamicin)	• (Hypercalcemia?)
• Nephrogenic diabetes insipidus	• (Hyperadrenocorticism?)
• Diabetes insipidus	• (Hyperthyroidism?)
• Diabetes mellitus	• Hypervitaminosis D_3
• Renal glucosuria	• Elevated dietary sodium
• Excessive fruit consumption	• Excess dietary protein

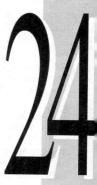

Dermatology

John E. Cooper
Greg J. Harrison

Cere

The cere is affected by a number of conditions, and its appearance can change with the health of the bird. In raptors, the cere may change from bright yellow to pale yellow based on the quantity of carotenoids in the diet.

Brown hypertrophy of the cere may occur in male budgerigars, presumably due to changes in the ratio of sex hormones, and is frequently associated with testicular tumors. The discolored hyperkeratotic material can be moistened and gently peeled away or removed by scraping or rasping.

Hyperkeratosis and flaking of the skin around the cere may be pronounced in malnourished birds. Some hypertrophy is normal in reproductively active hens.

Beak

The beak should remain in proper condition without trimming in birds that are maintained on a formulated diet supplemented with fresh fruits and vegetables, exposed to adequate sunlight, allowed to bathe regularly and provided with hard woods to chew.

Any companion bird that requires repeated beak trimming should receive a thorough diagnostic evaluation to detect the underlying management, nutritional or systemic abnormality that is causing excessive growth or improper wear. Overgrowth of the lower beak may lead to occlusion of the openings to the bill tip organ and a loss of function. To improve the sensory capacity of the bill tip organ, the lower beak should be included in routine grooming if it is overgrown.

Abnormalities of the beak are caused by:
- Malformation (often due to nutritional disorders)
- Primary viral infection
- Overgrowth (associated with a high-protein diet in some frugivorous birds, believed to be secondary to malnutrition or organopathy [liver] in many species)
- Fracture or puncture (usually traumatic).

Color changes in the beak of some species (toucans, lorikeets) may be associated with malnutrition or systemic disease. Bacterial or fungal infections are usually secondary to injuries that result in damage to the horny layer of the beak (see Chapter 42). Bragnathism and scissors beak occur commonly in some neonatal psittacines (see Chapters 30 and 42). A discussion of the diseases of the beak is provided in Chapter 19.

Skin

Although avian skin is noted for its paucity of glands, it has been suggested that the lipid production by the keratinocytes (a function unique to birds) makes the entire skin an oil-producing holocrine gland. The lipids produced by the keratinocytes are combined with oils secreted by the uropygial gland to form a thin film that is deposited over the feathers.

It can be theorized that the severe and generalized feather pathology associated with systemic diseases (eg, organopathy, malnutrition) is a result of improperly functioning keratinocytes.

Patagia

Skin may be reflected into flat, membrane-like structures (patagia) in areas where the wings, legs, neck and tail join the body.

Patagia and webs represent sites of major skin flexion and can be used clinically for subcutaneous injections or tattooing. These anatomic areas as well as the ventral tail region appear to be frequent sites for the occurrence of ulcerative dermatitis.

Uropygial Gland

The uropygial gland is a bilobed gland located at the base of the tail dorsal to the pygostyle. The gland is absent in many Columbiformes, Amazon parrots and other Psittaciformes. This holocrine gland opens to the outside through a caudally directed nipple that is frequently surrounded by a tuft of feathers.

Abnormalities associated with the uropygial gland include neoplasm (primarily squamous cell or adenocarcinoma), abscessation and impactions. A presumptive diagnosis of uropygial gland abnormalities can be based on microbiological culture and cytologic examination of exudate, an aspirate or a biopsy.

Impacted glands are frequently discussed in the literature but appear to be uncommon clinically. The gland is normally swollen and appears as though it may need expressing. In some birds, hyperkeratotic plugs may form in the gland. These cases will generally respond to removal of the plug and improving the bird's diet. An African Grey Parrot with widespread feather loss and a cystic uropygial gland failed to respond to extensive treatment that included laser therapy, but recovered three months later after a deficient diet was corrected.

Surgical extirpation of the gland may be necessary if neoplasia occurs. In ducks, removing the gland will cause the birds to lose the ability to waterproof their feathers. In other birds, removal of the gland seems to have few clinically detectable effects.

Feathers

The three principal functions of the feathers are flight, insulation and waterproofing.

The feathers can be characterized based on the structure of the rachis, barbs and barbules, and are divided into ten feather types:

Contour feathers represent the predominant feathers that cover a bird's body. They are the largest feathers and have a well developed shaft, pennaceous and plumulaceous components of the vane and an afterfeather.

Coverts are the small contour feathers that are found in rows on the wing and tail.

Remiges are large, stiff, well developed feathers found in the wing and are principally responsible for flight. These feathers are generally asymmetric in form and have an entirely pennaceous vane. The remiges that arise from the periosteum of the metacarpus are called primaries, and those that arise from the periosteum of the ulna are called secondaries. The primaries are counted from proximal to distal (digits), while the secondaries are counted from distal (carpus) to proximal (elbow). The number of primary and secondary feathers varies among species.

Rectrices are large flight feathers found in the tail. They are structurally similar to the remiges. Tail feathers are counted from the center laterally.

Downs (juvenile and definitive) are small, fluffy, wholly plumulaceous feathers with a short or absent rachis.

Powder down are specialized down feathers that disintegrate and produce a powder (keratin) that is spread through the feathers during preening. African Grey Parrots, cockatiels and cockatoos have the most abundant powder down feathers. Birds with damaged powder down feathers frequently have soiled-appearing feathers, suggesting their involvement in the maintenance of normal feather condition.

Semiplumes have a long rachis and entirely plumulaceous vane.

Hypopnea (afterfeathers) are structures attached to the underside of a feather at the superior umbilicus. They may consist only of barbs or have a shaft and plumulaceous barbs.

Filoplumes are fine, hair-like feathers with a long rachis and a tuft or barb on the tip. They generally accompany contour feathers in most species. They are believed to serve a proprioceptive function.

Bristles are characterized by a stiff, tapered rachis with no barbs except at the proximal end. They are usually found around the mouth, nostrils and eyes and are believed to serve a sensory function.

Feather Color

The color of feathers is determined by two factors: the pigments that are deposited at the time of development, and structural features of the feather that alter the absorption or reflection of light. These structural features of the feather can be inherent in the development of the feather or can be induced by materials that are placed on the feathers after development.

The normal iridescent glow of the feathers may be induced in part by lipids derived from the keratinocytes. This "glow" is frequently absent in birds with clinical abnormalities and returns as a bird responds to therapy.

It is interesting to note that abnormally colored feathers may return to normal without a molt. This is particularly common in cockatiels with feathers that are stained yellow secondary to chronic biliverdinuria (liver disease). As birds respond to therapy for hepatitis, these feathers will return to a normal white coloration, presumably because biliverdin-laden, keratinocyte-produced lipids are replaced with lipids that do not contain biliverdin.

Yellow or red pigments derived from the uropygial gland can be spread on the feathers where the pigment remains bright until it fades due to oxidation from exposure to air and light. In a healthy bird, feathers maintain their bright pigmentation through the addition of newly synthesized oils during preening. These mechanisms for imparting color to a feather would allow changes in feather pigmentation to occur without a bird undergoing a molt. Birds receiving higher fat diets would be expected to produce a lipid-rich, keratinocyte-derived uropygial gland secretion that may enhance the color and sheen of the feathers.

Peach-faced Lovebirds may develop red patches on their normally green plumage, and both diet and blood parasites have been suggested as a cause of this condition. Abnormal yellow, red and pink feathers may be noted in Amazon parrots and African Grey Parrots, and it has been suggested that these are associated with hepatopathies, renal dysfunction or systemic disease. Psittacine beak and feather disease has been implicated in some cases of the abnormal occurrence of red feathers in African Grey Parrots. Excess dietary levels of beta carotene can cause a similar feather change.

Molt

Soft keratin structures (skin, comb, wattles, cere) undergo constant replacement through the sloughing of the outer cornified layer. Old or damaged outer layers of hard keratin structures (rhamphotheca and metatarsal spurs) are replaced through normal wear. The thick, horny heel pads on the back joints of woodpecker, toucan and barbet neonates are molted at fledging. In cases of malnutrition or systemic disease, hyperkeratotic layers of the rhamphotheca can accumulate and be peeled off with a blunt instrument.

Molting is the process whereby the growth of a new feather causes the shedding of an old feather. The single generation of feathers that occurs as a result of a molt is collectively known as plumage. At any one time, a bird may have feathers derived from more than one molt. This is because some molts involve all of the feather tracts, while others involve only certain tracts or specific feathers. Collectively, the feathers present on the body at one time, regardless of when they first appeared, are called the feather coat.

A new feather that is still enclosed in a feather sheath is called a pin feather. Any infectious agent or systemic abnormality that alters the nutrients or blood supply available to the developing feather will alter its appearance. Additionally, damage to the epidermal collar will be manifested clinically as an abnormal feather.

The molting process in adult birds occurs on a cyclic basis. A molt cycle is defined as the period that runs from the appearance of a plumage to the appearance of its replacement. The cycle length for most birds is one year; however, some species will molt throughout the year, while others will molt annually or several times a year during distinct periods. Large Psittaciformes may have a two-year molt cycle. Powder down feathers are shed continuously.

General Diagnosis and Therapy

Investigation of Dermatologic Disease

Integumentary diseases can be broadly classified as being caused by infectious or noninfectious agents (Table 24.3). In many cases, dermatologic lesions are secondarily infected with bacterial or fungal agents, and the identification of microbial agents from cultures of the skin does not necessarily implicate these organisms as the precipitating cause of the lesions.

Table 24.3   An Etiologic Approach to Integumentary Diseases

Infectious	Non-infectious
Viral	Traumatic
Mycoplasmal	Chemical/toxic
Chlamydial	Nutritional
Bacterial	Hormonal
Fungal	Developmental/genetic
Protozoal	Irradiation
Metazoal (parasitic)	Neoplastic
	Immune-mediated
	Behavioral
	Allergic

Using a dermatology examination form is a concise way to consistently evaluate and record integumentary lesions. The evaluation of feather and skin lesions, particularly in small birds, can be facilitated by the use of a magnifying loupe. Inflammation of the skin can occur as a result of trauma, chemical irritation, bacterial, fungal, viral or parasitic agents. Pericloacal inflammation may be associated with the accumulation of excrement.

Cytology, culture and biopsy are indicated in cases of dermatitis. Cultures should be obtained by removing any scabs, moistening the culturette in the sterile transport media and rolling the tip over the lesion. Moistened swabs will yield better results than dry ones, and it is important that the swab be plated as soon as possible after collection. A quick and inexpensive diagnostic technique in practice is to apply a microscope slide to the affected area and to examine it cytologically (see Chapter 10). Skin biopsies are most diagnostic if collected from the center and the periphery of the lesion.

Table 24.5   Dermatology Database

Systemic
  Physical examination
  CBC, AST, LDH, UA, bile acids, CPK
  DNA probe for PBFD virus
  DNA probe for polyomavirus
  Gram's stain of feces

Fecal examination for parasites
Radiographs
Thyroid levels - TSH test
Specific Integumentary Examination
Microscopic (operating or dissecting) examination of feather for
parasites
Cytology of pulp cavity (bacterial and fungal)
Bacterial and fungal cultures of feather pulp
Histopathology of biopsy specimens (skin and follicle)
Electron microscopy of feather sections

General Therapy for Integumentary Lesions

General therapeutic considerations include:

- Correcting any nutritional deficiencies by administering parenteral multivitamins, minerals (trace minerals) and placing
the bird on a formulated diet supplemented with some fruits
and vegetables.
- Removing the bird from all exposure to aerosolized toxins that
may accumulate on the feathers and skin and cause irritation
(eg, cigarette smoke, kerosene fumes, cooking oils).
- Ensuring that the bird has frequent exposure to sunlight, and
that a regular bathing program is instigated.
- Identifying and correcting any behavioral abnormalities that
are causing over-grooming (feather picking).

Aloe vera gel, human skin softeners with a vanishing cream
base, nystatin-neomycin sulfate ointment (for pruritic lesions and
moist dermatitis) and silver sulfadiazine cream (for moist dermatitis and burns) are particularly effective topical medications.
A mixture of Penetran and aloe vera may relieve severe pruritus
in some cases (see Chapter 18). This therapy should be discontinued or the solution should be diluted further if a bird becomes depressed or lethargic. If a bird does not improve within 48 hours of
initiating therapy, the preparation should be considered ineffective and discontinued.

If an infectious agent is identified, specific antimicrobial therapy should be initiated. In some cases of severe ulcerative dermatitis, surgical debridement and primary wound management
may be necessary; however, surgery should not be considered until all other therapeutic modalities have failed to resolve the lesions over a six-month treatment period. Peeling, flaking skin and
heavy molts are common for prolonged periods (up to a year) when
a diet change is initiated in a malnourished bird.

Lesions should be evaluated regularly (generally on a weekly
basis) to determine if prescribed therapy is effective. Trimming
the tip of the beak to prevent a bird from self-mutilating or applying a neck brace is justified only as a last resort.

Dystrophic feathers may occur in birds infected with PBFD
virus, polyomavirus, adenovirus and a parvo-like virus (waterfowl). Dermatologic lesions may occur with poxvirus, papillomavirus and herpesvirus infections (see Chapter 32).

Young birds are most susceptible to PBFD virus, which is characterized by the progressive appearance of dystrophic feathers after a molt. The disease progression can be acute or chronic de-

pending on the age and species of bird. A diagnosis of PBFD is made by demonstrating viral antigens or nucleic acid in affected tissues. DNA probes are available that can be used to detect the virus in circulating white blood cells (see Chapter 32).

Avian polyomavirus (budgerigar fledgling disease) causes feather pathology in some affected budgerigars and occasionally in large Psittaciformes (see Chapter 32).

"French moult" is a descriptive term used to describe feather dystrophy in young psittacine birds, primarily budgerigars. The classic clinical changes include premature molting of the wing and tail feathers and associated hemorrhage and poor plumage. Affected young birds are termed "runners" because they are usually incapable of flying. Feather changes characteristic of "French moult" can be caused by PBFD virus, polyomavirus or both. It should be noted that any factor (infectious or noninfectious) that damages the epidermal collar can result in a gross lesion resembling that induced by PBFD virus or polyomavirus. There is no specific treatment for French moult.

Poxvirus can cause skin lesions in most avian species and may retard wound healing. Uncomplicated lesions are characterized by the formation of nodules on the unfeathered skin. Skin lesions should be kept clean and dry to prevent secondary bacterial or fungal infections (see Chapter 32).

Cutaneous papillomas may occur on the head, neck, beak commissure, feet or uropygial glands. Some of these lesions have been associated with papillomavirus or herpesvirus while others are of undetermined etiology. Therapy is generally limited to removal of the masses in birds in which they cause problems. A herpesvirus has been associated with "feather dusters," and adenoviral folliculitis has been reported in lovebirds (see Chapter 32).

Parasites

Wasps, bees or other stinging insects will occasionally attack birds causing characteristic hyperemic swellings. Most affected birds heal with no therapy; however, in severe cases steroids may be indicated to reduce inflammation. The likelihood of a bird being stung can be reduced by removing uneaten soft foods (particularly fruits) from the enclosure and destroying wasp nests found near the aviary.

Flies, mosquitoes and gnats can cause severe dermatitis on the face, feet and legs, particularly in birds raised in warm coastal areas. Lesions are most common in Amazon parrots and macaws, but can occur in any species. The flies that commonly parasitize cattle and deer can induce small bleeding ulcers on the unfeathered areas of the body.

Ants (especially fire ants) can be a nuisance to nesting birds. If necessary, five per cent Sevin dust can be used in the nest box to prevent chicks from being eaten alive. Many affected chicks die, and those that survive may have localized necrotic areas that are secondarily infected with *Staphylococcus* spp. Topical application of antibiotic and steroid lotions or creams can be used to reduce swollen or hyperemic lesions. Ant bites also may cause localized necrosis that results in defects in the webs of the feet in waterfowl. Some helminths and mites can cause dermatitis (see Chapter 36).

A sarcoptid mite infection was described in a Grey-cheeked Parakeet with feather loss and flaking skin on the head and trunk. Severe pyogranulomatous dermatitis was associated with a sarcoptic mite infection in a Green-winged Macaw. The bird did not respond to ivermectin therapy. Generalized alopecia and thickening of the calamus occurred in a Red-fronted Parakeet infected with *Knemidokoptes* spp. (see Chapter 36). Mites are more likely to be a primary cause of dermatitis on the head than are lice. Control of ectoparasites, whether on the head or elsewhere, must be undertaken with caution. Only those parasiticidal agents that are licensed or recommended for use in birds should be applied, and such therapy must be accompanied by other measures to exclude the parasites.

In subtropical and tropical areas, the sticktight flea (*Echidnophaga gallinacea*) can be a problem on many species of birds. This is a sessile flea, and large numbers may attach to the skin of the head, especially around the eyes, and cause anemia. This parasite can be controlled with the topical application of a pyrethrin-based product.

Bacterial and Fungal Diseases

Many authors have suggested theories to explain the apparent paucity of primary skin infections in birds, including a high body temperature, which might inhibit the growth of some organisms, and keratinocyte-derived lipids that may inhibit certain pathogenic bacteria or may provide appropriate nutrients for competitive autochthonous flora. Bacterial and fungal infections of facial skin are usually secondary to trauma or possibly a contact dermatitis. Avian skin abscesses are rare but can be found following wounds or in association with feather cysts. Treatment is routine with surgical drainage or removal.

Although frequently discussed, documented cases of bacterial folliculitis in birds are rare. The pulp can be examined for the presence of bacteria by making impression smears or by culturing the pulp cavity. Secondary fungal agents may also be recovered from these lesions.

Nutritional Factors

The ability of avian skin to resist infections and to heal properly is related to many factors, the most important of which is the nutritional status of the bird. Malnutrition, particularly hypovitaminosis A, is suggested by the smoothing of the normally papillary surface of the plantar surface of the feet.

Hyperkeratosis of the feather sheath may occur as a result of malnutrition or in association with some infectious agents that affect the developing feather (eg, PBFD virus, polyomavirus). In affected feathers, the sheath on the developing feather is retained, resulting in a bird that appears to have an excess number of pin feathers.

A malnutrition-induced loss of feathers on the back of the head and neck is believed to occur in canaries. Affected birds are usually egg-laying females and also may show decreased fertility and produce weak chicks. Dietary changes will usually resolve the lesions.

Nonspecific Dermatopathies

Many minor scratches and cuts (that are not caused by animal bites) require no medical attention, especially if they are in the non-feathered areas of a healthy bird. If a severe wound occurs, the feathers can be trimmed or pulled from the periphery of a lesion to prevent the accumulation of necrotic debris. Most companion and aviary birds do not pick at skin injuries (see Chapter 16).

Chronic ulcerative dermatitis (CUD) is characterized by septic, edematous and hyperemic ulceration and exudation of the skin. Chronic ulcerative dermatitis has been associated with tumors (lipomas, squamous cell carcinomas and papillomas), abscesses, unhealed wounds, hernias, mycobacteriosis, diabetes, nephritis, hepatitis and giardiasis. Biopsies should always be performed on proliferative, chronic skin lesions to determine if they are neoplastic in origin.

Giardiasis and hypovitaminosis E seem to be associated with ulcerative dermatitis in lovebirds and cockatiels. The precise nutrients that may be missing in the diet have not been defined, but these birds are frequently fed seed-based diets with or without the addition of fruits and vegetables. Many cases of CUD will improve when a bird is placed on a balanced, formulated diet and provided with adequate exposure to sunlight. Complete resolution may not occur for several months after these management changes are initiated.

Propatagial CUD

Lovebirds, cockatiels, Grey-cheeked Parakeets and occasionally Amazon parrots and cockatoos may develop chronic ulcerative dermatitis involving the metapatagium or propatagium. Lesions may also be noted in the proventer and in the interscapular regions of the body. The lesions appear to be extremely pruritic. Outbreaks of ulcerative dermatitis affecting patagial membranes have been described. In one outbreak, 60% of the lovebirds in a flock were affected, and the progression of the disease suggested an infectious agent.

Treatment for propatagial CUD should include metronidazole for giardiasis (if identified), administration of parenteral vitamin E, removing the feathers from the periphery of the lesion and placement of a figure-of-eight bandage to prevent mutilation. Secondary bacterial or fungal infections should be treated with appropriate topical medications.

Surgical debridement and primary wound closure may be necessary if the lesions do not heal in five to six weeks. Radiosurgery should not be used to debride or control hemorrhage associated with these lesions. Birds with long-term or severe lesions will replace the normally elastic patagial tissue with scar tissue, which may make the bird more susceptible to future lesions.

CUD in Other Regions of the Body

Ulcerative dermatitis of the proventer region may occur in heavy-bodied birds (African Grey and Mealy Amazon Parrots) that have had improper wing trims. A bird that attempts to fly from a high perch and has no lift may land on its sternum, resulting in a bruise or open wound over the cranial portion of the keel. These damaged tissues seldom become infected although cellulitis of the area is common.

The skin wounds should be treated as discussed under general therapy for integumentary lesions, and several of the clipped primary and secondary feathers from each wing should be removed to stimulate replacement of the feathers. These new feathers will provide the bird with the necessary lift to prevent further injury. In severe cases, necrotic portions of the keel must be surgically removed. Supportive care is successful in most minor cases and the lesions generally resolve in six to nine weeks.

Birds with chronic ulcerative dermatitis in the caudal aspect of the postventer region may be presented with a history of blood-tinged excrement. Feathers adjacent to and covering the skin lesion may be stained with blood. This lesion is common in malnourished birds and may begin when a bird with an improper wing clip lands on a hard surface. The impact of the tail with the ground causes a hyperextension of the rectrices and places excessive pressure on the tight skin of the proventer region.

Disorders Affecting the Feet and Legs

Skin on the legs may be damaged by bands or, in the case of falconers' birds, by badly fitted leather jesses. Secondary bacterial infections of skin wounds can occur and impair healing, particularly when a foreign object is constantly in contact with the wound. The application of a self-adherent wound dressing (see Chapter 16) will keep the wound clean and moist and permit regular visual inspection.

Pox lesions on the feet and legs are characterized by dry, brown plaques. Other viral infections appear to be rare, but a herpesvirus has been implicated in skin lesions in Mallard Ducks and cockatoos (see Chapter 32). Proliferative, hyperplastic lesions on the feet of canaries and mynahs have been associated with abrasions, aging and malnutrition. A condition involving cracking of the feet that is responsive to high doses of biotin has been documented in flamingos, ratites and waders.

Keratomas that appear clinically as digit-like projections composed of hyperkeratotic scales have been described in some species. These callus-like growths may predispose a bird to bumblefoot (see Chapter 43). Virus-induced papillomas are common on the feet of finches in Europe.

A "constricted toe syndrome" has been described in a number of Psittaciforme neonates. The fibrous band can be surgically excised to correct the problem (see Chapter 41). Other causes of ischemic necrosis of the feet or legs may include entangled fibers, hairs, bedding material, leg bands, strings, jesses, dried skin, frostbite or ergot poisoning.

Pruritic, ulcerative lesions have been described on the feet and legs of Amazon parrots (particularly Yellow-naped and Double Yellow-headed Amazon Parrots). The lesions start with a bird chewing at the feet and legs followed by the formation of hyperemic lesions, sometimes within minutes of the initial pruritic episode. The role that the bacteria or fungi play in the pathogenesis of this syndrome is undetermined. Immune-mediated and allergic reactions with secondary involvement of autochthonous skin flora have been proposed as etiologies for these lesions (see Chapter 33).

Staphylococcus spp. are frequently isolated from the lesions, but the birds will usually not respond to antibiotic therapy alone. The syndrome appears to be more common in the spring (suggesting a seasonal allergen), and many affected birds belong to cigarette smokers. In these latter birds, the lesions may spontaneously resolve when the clients stop smoking or wash their hands before handling the birds. Other cases will respond to a change in diet, frequent exposure to sunlight and a topical antimicrobial cream containing steroids. Topical steroids should be applied with caution to prevent toxicity.

Atarax and oral antibiotics were found to be effective in some cases. Seasonal recurrence of the lesions may be prevented by the oral administration of prednisolone about one month prior to the time that lesions typically occur.

A hydroactive dressing can be used to facilitate healing of these wounds. Initially, the bandage may require daily changing. The frequency of bandage changes can be reduced as the wound becomes less exudative. Once granulation tissue forms at the edge of the ulcers, scabs should be removed and the lesions should be kept clean to facilitate healing (see Chapters 15, 16).

Some reports detail the use of thyroid supplementation as a therapeutic regimen for foot necrosis syndrome; however, thyroid levels were not determined in the treated birds, and the indiscriminate administration of thyroxine can cause fatal toxicity (see Chapter 23).

Diseases of the Feathers

Feather conditions can be divided into two main groups: those affecting normal feathers and those in which abnormality of the feather is the primary feature. A simple method to determine if a feather problem occurs during or after development is to remove an affected feather (it should be examined cytologically, microscopically and possibly histologically) and evaluate the growth of the new feather over the next one to three weeks. There are three possibilities with respect to the new feather:

- The feather does not regrow (suggests a systemic or follicular abnormality)
- The feather regrows but is not normal (suggests a problem in the feather follicle or organopathy)
- The feather regrows normally (suggests that the feathers are being damaged after development, eg, feather chewing, enclosure trauma).

Biopsy and histopathology are indispensable for diagnosing the cause of feather lesions.

Stress Marks

Translucent lines across the vane of a feather are frequently referred to as stress marks. These abnormalities represent segmental dysplasia that occurred in the developing barbs and barbules and represent a brief period of dysfunction in the epidermal collar. These marks can be induced by the administration of exogenous corticosteroids, suggesting that they are truly "stress" marks. Restraint, illness, a brief period of food deprivation or exposure to environmental extremes should be expected to induce these lesions. Deficiencies of arginine (curled wing feathers), riboflavin (clubbed down feathers) and pantothenic acid, niacin and selenium (poor feathering) are nutritional causes of poor feather structure in poultry.

Preening

Much of a bird's day is spent in feather preening, a natural process for maintaining feather condition. Feather preening appears to be innate, but occasionally a hand-raised neonate will have poor quality feathers or an excess number of pin feathers because of an improper preening response. These birds should be taught to preen the feathers by gently breaking the sheaths while encouraging the bird to pick at an area with its beak.

Damage to the feathers of the breast, abdomen and legs during the breeding season may indicate reproductive frustration. Seasonal feather picking associated with breeding activity is usually temporary and no specific therapy is necessary or warranted unless the feather loss is persistent or involves areas other than the lower abdomen.

Feather Picking

Feather picking occurs when a bird damages its feathers or skin (or the feather and skin of a companion). Feather picking is a condition of captivity. With the importance of the feathers for thermal regulation and flight, severe, self-induced feather damage would be life-threatening to a free-ranging bird.

Many feather-picking or self-mutilating birds are considered to be pruritic, which is difficult to document. Over-preening and scratching an area with the nails is suggestive. Inflammation or irritation associated with internal pathology, including that caused by infectious agents, has been suggested as a precipitating factor for feather picking. Organopathy, toxins, malnutrition, bacteria, viruses, fungi, parasites (blood or intestinal), boredom, anxiety, lack of sleep, psychosis and undesired contact with strangers or family pets (dogs or cats) have all been implicated in cases of self-mutilation. Feather loss on the neck of lories and Hyacinth Macaws has been attributed to contact with conifers.

Some birds may be mutilated by other birds (canaries, finches, conures, cockatoos). In colony-breeding flocks, reducing the number of birds in the enclosure, increasing the number of hiding places and nest boxes or removing the offending birds may be necessary for control. Cockatoos may occasionally over-preen a mate, but more commonly a male bird will kill its mate with no previous indication of aggressive behavior (see Chapter 2).

Examination of the Feather-picking Bird

Feather-picking birds should be approached in a systematic fashion. A diagnosis of psychologically induced self-mutilation should be reserved for patients in which no cause for the problem can be identified by physical examination, complete blood count (CBC), serum chemistries, feather pulp culture and cytology, skin lesion culture and cytology, radiographs, endoscopy and direct microscopic examination and biopsies of affected feathers. If no etiology can be determined for the over-preening, then behavioral abnormalities should be considered.

There is an apparent species' predilection to feather-picking behavior. African Grey Parrots appear to be particularly prone to feather picking, perhaps as a result of their sensitive natures or need for a highly stimulated environment. Spoiled, improperly socialized, hand-raised birds of any species may also be prone to self-mutilation. Cockatoos and conures frequently develop feather-picking behavior for which an etiology cannot be conclusively identified, necessitating a diagnosis of psychologic feather picking. By comparison, idiopathic feather picking in budgerigars and cockatiels is rare. In these species, feather picking associated with ulcerative dermatitis of the patagial membranes is most common.

Treatment of Feather Picking

Once initiated, feather picking can become habitual and continue even though the precipitating cause is no longer present. Chronic feather picking can result in sufficient damage to the follicles to prevent any future feather growth. Therapy for self-mutilation of undetermined etiology should be considered effective if the destructive behavior can be reduced. Complete cessation of self-mutilation is rare.

Occasionally, a bird will self-mutilate as a result of sexual frustration. Some of these birds will stop mutilating when placed in a breeding situation; however, others will continue self-mutilation activities and may also over-preen a mate. Assuming that idiopathic self-mutilation is a result of some undetectable neurosis, it would be considered unwise for these birds to be added to a breeding collection where they may pass on genes that will predispose their progeny to the same problem.

Treatment for feather picking should include the correction of organopathies, specific therapies for folliculitis (bacterial or fungal), improving the diet, removing exposure to cigarette smoke, providing frequent exposure to fresh air and sunlight, providing an 8- to 14-hour photoperiod that varies naturally with the seasons, and behavioral modification (see Chapter 4). If these therapies are determined to be ineffective over a two-month period, then mood-altering drugs may be necessary.

Where feather picking is determined to be psychological (a failure in the ability to diagnose a cause for the problem), a video recorder may be helpful in documenting a bird's behavior in its normal environment. Identifying the specific factors that induce the feather-picking behavior (separation anxiety, a tormenting pet, an unliked child, an abusive adult) can guide the clinician in making specific recommendations to correct the behavior and resolve the problem (see Chapter 4). Striving to improve the human-animal bond may be the most effective therapy in these cases.

Some problems with separation anxiety can be corrected by leaving tape recordings of family activities or a radio or TV playing in the family's absence. With some birds, the addition of new toys or moving an enclosure to a different location will be a stress factor that induces feather-picking, while with other birds these moves are positive and help to keep a bird mentally stimulated. A bird that is properly socialized and adapted early in life to changes in daily routine is less likely to develop emotional problems due to separation anxiety when changes occur later in life.

If psychological feather picking cannot be stopped with behavior modification, drugs may be necessary. Mood-altering drugs that have been suggested for use in feather-picking birds include tricyclic antidepressants and antihistamines (hydroxyzine hydrochloride, 2 mg/kg oral). These therapeutic agents are frequently discussed but are rarely effective. Hormonal therapies including thyroxine, testosterone and medroxyprogesterone have also been suggested for some cases of feather picking; however, all of these agents have undesirable side-effects and should be used only to treat specifically identified problems.

Medroxyprogesterone acetate may be effective in stopping some sexually related behavioral disorders including feather picking, aggressiveness and masturbation; however, the drug can have severe side-effects including obesity, polydipsia, polyuria, glucosuria and liver disease.

Haloperidol has been used in some feather-picking cases. This drug is used to control hyperactive and impulsive behavior in humans. The dose used in cockatoos is 0.08 mg/kg orally q24h. It takes two days to stabilize the dose. Side-effects include loss of appetite, incoordination and vomiting. If there are no side-effects and a bird is still picking, the dose can be increased in 0.01 ml increments every two days. The maximum dose should not exceed two times the initial dose.

If the treatment is successful the bird stops over-preening or self-mutilating and begins to play, sing and interact with the client. There is also a haloperidol decanoate (50; 100 mg/ml) injectable repositol for IM administration. Dosed at 1-2 mg/kg, the patients respond for up to 14-21 days. Both administration forms have to be used continually unless the initiating cause of the feather picking can be corrected. Clinical experience suggests that Moluccan and Umbrella Cockatoos, Quaker Parakeets and African Grey Parrots may respond to a lower dose (half that used for other birds).

Endocrine-related Feather Disorders

Documented cases of hypothyroidism in companion birds are rare. It should be noted that some species of birds that are deficient in iodine will have a TSH response test that suggests hypothyroidism (see Chapter 23).

There are no documented cases of feather abnormalities resulting from hyperadrenocorticism or hypoadrenocorticism in birds although both conditions would be expected to occur.

Hyperestrogenism has been associated with proliferation of endosteal bone in birds, but has not been associated with feather lesions (see Chapter 23).

Inactive Feather Follicles

A feather follicle is normally inactive between molts. Persistent generalized inactivity of the feather follicles should be considered abnormal. In one study, many birds with inactive follicles had abnormal bacterial populations, elevated CPK activity and toxic heterophils. Some birds had a leukocytosis and elevated calcium levels; a few of these cases responded to antibacterial therapy. Epidermal atrophy accompanied chronic inactive feather follicles, hyperkeratosis and follicular atrophy in some birds.

Cysts

Cutaneous cysts are characterized by an epithelial wall surrounding keratinaceous contents. If the orifice of the feather follicle is occluded from a traumatic or infectious episode, keratinaceous debris will accumulate in the follicle resulting in a follicular cyst. These lesions are particularly common in canaries. Therapy is excisional (see Chapters 41 and 43).

Polyfolliculitis

Pruritic polyfolliculitis and dermatitis that may be caused by a virus have been described in lovebirds and budgerigars. Lesions appear to be particularly common in the feather tracts of the tail and dorsal region of the neck. The newly emerging feathers have short, stout quills with retained sheaths. Some of these birds have been histologically diagnosed with PBFD virus infections, whereas others have not been shown to be infected.

Other Feather Abnormalities

Bleeding occurs if the protective keratin sheath of a developing feather (pin or blood feather) is injured or the feather is dislodged from the follicle. In the clinical setting, it is best to remove damaged pin feathers (see Chapter 15).

Neonates kept in areas with low humidity may have dystrophic feather growth characterized by failure of the developing feather to exsheath. The lesions will usually resolve when the humidity is increased (and the affected feathers are removed).

ONCOLOGY

Kenneth S. Latimer

Integumentary System

Adipose Neoplasms and Masses

Lipoma: Lipomas are benign proliferations of well differentiated adipocytes (lipocytes) that may exhibit slow-to-rapid, progressive growth over time. Lipomas are the most frequently observed neoplasm of companion birds, with a reported incidence of 10-40% in budgerigars. Besides budgerigars, lipomas may be observed frequently in Rose-breasted Cockatoos (galahs) and Amazon parrots.

Lipomas usually arise in the subcutis of the sternal or abdominal skin, but may also be observed on the wings, back, neck, legs or near the uropygial gland. In addition, lipomas may occur in the thoracoabdominal cavity (arising from thoracic or mesenteric fat, ovary, ventriculus and liver) or in association with skeletal muscle.

Dietary changes and increased exercise are frequently curative in early cases and should be implemented prior to surgery to reduce the size of the mass. Because lipomas are often accompanied by body fat that may interfere with caudal air sac volume, exercise programs should be initiated with care, especially in tachypneic patients. Surgical excision is necessary if the tumor is causing clinical problems that are not resolved with diet change and increased exercise. Lipomas may be vascular; therefore, attention to hemostasis through the use of bipolar radiosurgery is important. Feeding formulated diets should prevent goiter and may also reduce the likelihood of a bird developing lipomas. Nonspecific use of thyroxine should be avoided, and treatment of lipomas in the absence of hypothyroidism is not an indication for thyroxine administration.

Myelolipoma: Myelolipomas are composed of adipose and hematopoietic tissues that may arise in the subcutis of the trunk, wings and legs. Occasionally they may occur in the liver or spleen. The outward appearance is similar to a lipoma.

Liposarcoma: Liposarcomas are malignant, fatty neoplasms composed of lipoblasts and immature adipocytes. These neoplasms are firm on palpation, poorly encapsulated, highly vascularized and usually arise in the subcutis of the sternum or uropygial gland area. Infrequently, liposarcomas may present as poorly demarcated nodules in the thoracoabdominal cavity, liver or skeletal muscles. Liposarcomas are locally invasive, have the potential to metastasize and may arise in a multicentric pattern. Multicentric origin or widespread metastasis is typical.

Hibernoma is a rare benign tumor of brown fat origin.

Xanthoma/Xanthomatosis: An xanthoma is not a true neoplasm, but an inflammatory intumescence resulting from the accumulation of lipid-laden macrophages, giant cells, free cholesterol and variable degrees of fibrosis.

Unresectable or multiple skin xanthomas may respond to irradiation (low-energy X-rays; 20-30 Gy) or hyperthermia. Dietary restriction of oily seeds may be beneficial in the medical management of xanthomatosis.

Connective Tissue Neoplasms and Masses

Fibrosarcoma: Fibrosarcoma is a malignant neoplasm of fibroblast or mesenchymal cells, which possess the ability to produce collagen fibers. Fibrosarcomas occur commonly in budgerigars, cockatiels, macaws and parrots.

Superficial fibrosarcomas may be covered by an intact-to-ulcerated epidermis accompanied by hemorrhage and secondary bacterial infections. Fibrosarcomas commonly arise from the soft tissues of the wing, leg, head, beak, cere and trunk. They also may arise in the viscera and deep tissues including thoracoabdominal cavity, spleen, liver, mouth, tongue, syrinx, lung, small intestine, proventricular wall, testes and ovary.

Fibroma is an uncommon benign neoplasm composed of well differentiated fibroblasts distributed within a collagenous matrix.

Myxoma and Myxosarcoma: These neoplasms are of fibroblast or mesenchymal cell origin, but possess abundant mucinous stroma. These rare neoplasms may arise wherever connective tissue exists. Clinically, these masses may appear soft on palpation and gelatinous on cut surface.

Epithelial Neoplasms and Cysts

Papillomas and Papilloma-like Lesions: Cutaneous papillomas are observed occasionally in domestic, captive and free ranging birds. Multiple papillomas most frequently originate from the skin of the eyelids, at the junction of the beak and face, and on the feet and legs. Cutaneous papillomas are viral-induced, at least in African Grey Parrots, Chaffinches and Bramblings (see Chapter 32).

Squamous Cell Carcinoma: Squamous cell carcinoma is observed most frequently in chickens but has also been described in captive and free-ranging birds in the skin of the head, eyelids, neck, chest, wings or around the beak.

Uropygial Gland Adenoma and Adenocarcinoma: Uropygial gland neoplasms occur sporadically in captive birds, especially budgerigars and canaries. On physical examination, the uropygial gland may appear enlarged, ulcerated and hemorrhagic. Neoplasia must be distinguished from adenitis, which usually requires histologic examination. Partial or complete removal of the affected gland is recommended.

Feather Folliculoma: Feather folliculomas occur primarily in canaries and budgerigars. These neoplasms may appear as discrete, mobile, single or multiple dermal nodules that may ulcerate or hemorrhage.

Miscellaneous Basal Cell Tumors and Cutaneous Cysts: All of these neoplasms present as discrete skin nodules. Basal cell tumors are composed of sheets, nests or cords of basaloid epithelial cells.

Intradermal cystic lesions occasionally are observed in captive and free-ranging birds. Those benign neoplasms that exhibit glandular differentiation are cystadenomas. Cystic lesions with keratin production are classified on the basis of gradual or abrupt keratinization. Gradual keratinization is observed with epidermal inclusion cysts, follicular cysts and intracutaneous cornifying epitheliomas. Those cystic lesions with abrupt keratinization include trichoepithelioma and pilomatrixoma.

Miscellaneous Neoplasms

Cutaneous Lymphosarcoma: Cutaneous lymphosarcoma is observed in chickens as a manifestation of Marek's disease and may occasionally occur in captive and free-ranging birds.

Mast Cell Tumor: Mast cell tumors have been reported in three owls and a chicken. Generally, animal species with a higher circulating basophil count have fewer tissue mast cells, which may explain the rarity of mast cell tumors in avian species. Mast cell tumors appear grossly as raised-to-spherical, pink-to-red, dermal or submucosal masses.

Respiratory System

The avian lung serves as a metastatic site for many neoplasms including fibrosarcoma, adenocarcinoma, hemangiosarcoma, malignant melanoma, mesothelioma and osteosarcoma. In contrast, primary neoplasms of the avian respiratory system are rare in species other than chickens.

Papilloma: Laryngeal papillomas are observed occasionally in psittacine birds, especially Amazon parrots and macaws. Papillomas also may occur within the nares and choanal area. Clinically, laryngeal papillomas may cause dyspnea. These lesions may be surgically excised, but will recur if excision is incomplete.

Bronchiolar Adenoma and Adenocarcinoma: A bronchiolar adenoma has been reported in a parrot. A bronchiogenic adenocarcinoma has been reported in a quail.

Fibrosarcoma: A solitary pulmonary fibrosarcoma has been described in a cockatiel.

Ectopic Pulmonary Ossification: Ectopic pulmonary ossification may be confused radiographically with pulmonary metastasis.

Ultimobranchial Cyst: Ultimobranchial cysts develop from branchial pouch remnants following embryogenesis. A large ultimobranchial cyst has been observed in the lower neck of a lorikeet. The thyroid gland was displaced by this mass.

Circulatory System

Vasoformative neoplasms originate from endothelial cell proliferation with subsequent formation of irregular vascular channels and spaces filled with blood (or rarely with lymph). Vasoformative neoplasms are classified as benign (hemangioma, lymphangioma) or malignant (hemangiosarcoma, lymphangiosarcoma).

Hemangioma: Cutaneous hemangiomas often arise within subcutaneous tissues of the dorsum of the neck, wing or legs. Feather follicles also may be involved. Abdominal hemangiomas may arise in the spleen, liver, kidney or testicular capsule. These latter neoplasms may cause abdominal distention by tumor mass or hemorrhage hemoperitoneum). External hemangiomas, particularly on the wing tips, are subject to trauma and may bleed profusely.

Cytologic aspirates of hemangiomas are of limited diagnostic value and generally consist of blood. Endothelial cells are rarely observed. Hematoma, hemangioma and hemangiosarcoma may be difficult or impossible to distinguish cytologically.

Hemangiosarcoma: Hemangiosarcomas may arise singly or in a multicentric pattern. These neoplasms often arise in the skin, liver, lungs, spleen, muscle, mesentery, kidney, heart, oviduct, bone or synovium. Hemangiosarcomas that develop in the distal diaphysis of long bones may exhibit aggressive osteolysis and surface hemorrhage.

Lymphangioma: Birds possess lymphatic channels but they appear less well developed than corresponding structures in mammals. Lymphangiomas are benign neoplasms wherein endothelial cells form lymphatic channels. These neoplasms are extremely rare in all species, especially birds.

Musculoskeletal System

Neoplasms of Smooth and Striated Muscle

Generally, smooth muscle neoplasms are reported about twice as frequently as striated muscle tumors. Furthermore, malignant neoplasms are reported twice as frequently as their benign counterparts.

Leiomyoma: Leiomyomas are benign neoplasms that generally are nodular and may arise from smooth muscle of the gastrointestinal or female reproductive tract, especially the oviduct. Other sites of origin include smooth muscle trabeculae within the spleen or smooth muscle associated with vessels or ducts in the pancreas.

Cytologic aspirates and imprints are sparsely cellular, containing only scattered free nuclei or a few spindle cells with elongate nuclei.

Leiomyosarcoma: Leiomyosarcomas are the most common muscle neoplasm reported in captive and free-ranging birds. They may arise from smooth muscle in any location, but usually arise from splenic smooth muscle trabeculae. Other sites of origin include crop, intestinal tract, trachea, pancreas, oviduct, ventral ligament of the oviduct, vas deferens and testicular capsule. Cytologic imprints of leiomyosarcomas may contain free nuclei and a pleomorphic but sparse population of spindle cells. Distinguishing leiomyosarcomas from fibrosarcomas may be difficult cytologically.

Rhabdomyoma: Rhabdomyomas are benign neoplasms of striated muscle and are the rarest muscle neoplasm reported in captive birds. Reported sites of origin include the wing, tongue and eyelid.

Cytologic aspirates are unrewarding except for possible fragments of striated muscle cells.

Rhabdomyosarcoma: Rhabdomyosarcomas are of skeletal muscle origin and frequently present as irregular, elevated, lobulated, relatively firm subcutaneous swellings of the wing or shoulder that limit the use of the wing. Because these neoplasms blend with surrounding skeletal muscle, they are immobile or firmly attached on palpation.

Neoplasms of Cartilage and Bone

Neoplasms arising from cartilage and bone are observed occasionally. Osseous neoplasms usually arise from the long bones, while cartilaginous neoplasms often arise on the foot. Cytology may suggest the presence of mesenchymal neoplasia by demonstrating a pleomorphic population of spindle-to-polyhedral cells and possible matrix material.

Chondroma: Chondromas are reported occasionally in captive and free-ranging birds, especially of the order Anseriformes. Grossly, these neoplasms may be single or multiple. They often arise on the plantar surface of the foot pad where they may be subjected to trauma with subsequent hemorrhage and ulceration of the overlying epidermis. Other sites of origin of chondromas include the cranium (especially in canaries) and proximal humerus.

Chondrosarcoma: Chondrosarcomas are very rare in comparison to chondromas.

Osteoma: Osteomas are observed infrequently in birds compared to osteosarcomas. Osteomas may originate from the cranium, scapula, tarsometatarsus, plantar foot pad and elbow joint. Histologically, osteomas are small, well encapsulated nodules composed of disorganized bony trabeculae and are attached to adjacent bone. Surgical excision is the treatment of choice.

Osteosarcoma: Osteosarcomas occur 3.5 times more frequently than osteomas and usually originate from the proximal or distal portion of long bones including the radius, humerus, femur, tibiotarsus and tarsometatarsus Osteosarcomas may metastasize widely.

Bone Proliferation Resembling Neoplasia

Radiographically, skeletal hyperostosis is recognized by increased medullary bone density, increased bone thickness and deformities involving one or multiple long bones. The differential diagnosis for increased medullary opacity of long bones includes osteopetrosis, polyostotic hyperostosis, metastatic neoplasia, hypertrophic osteopathy and metabolic bone disease.

Osteopetrosis: Osteopetrosis is defined as marked subperiosteal proliferation of bone resulting in loss of medullary space, increased bone thickness and deformity.

Ovarian and Oviductal Neoplasms and Cysts: Cystic ovaries, oviductal carcinoma and ovarian neoplasms may induce generalized or localized bone formation in companion birds. Increased medullary bone density is apparent on survey radiographs.

Ectopic Pulmonary Cartilage and Bone: Ectopic pulmonary ossification has been observed in an Orange-winged Amazon Parrot and a Senegal Parrot. Survey radiographs in both birds detected multifocal opacities throughout the lung fields, suggesting deep mycosis or metastatic neoplasia. Lung biopsy specimens, however, contained only small foci of osseous tissue within the parenchyma.

Urogenital System

Neoplasms of the urogenital system are reported frequently, especially in budgerigars. Testicular neoplasms of captive and free-ranging birds are approximately three times as common as ovarian and oviductal neoplasms.

Larger neoplasms may cause abdominal distention or respiratory embarrassment. Some renal, testicular, ovarian and oviductal neoplasms may cause unilateral or bilateral leg paresis or paralysis with difficulty or inability to perch. This occurs because the nerves of the sacral plexus pass through the mid-portion of the kidney where they are subject to compression or infiltration by neoplastic cells. Lastly, gonadal neoplasms may be associated with various paraneoplastic syndromes such as feminization or masculinization and localized or polyostotic hyperostosis. Feminization or masculinization is most apparent in budgerigars where the male's cere may change from blue to brown, or the female's cere may turn from brown to blue.

Renal Neoplasms

Renal neoplasms are observed occasionally in free-ranging and captive birds, especially budgerigars. Renal neoplasms usually occur unilaterally, but may occur bilaterally, and presenting complaints generally include an inability to perch or ambulate. Abdominal enlargement and articular gout also may occur.

Renal neoplasms are difficult to manage surgically. Renal carcinomas may aggressively invade adjacent muscle and bone. Because the kidneys are located in the renal fossae, neoplasms are difficult to isolate and excise. The sacral plexus passes through the mid-portion of the kidney and is subject to trauma. Finally, the kidneys are highly vascular and marked hemorrhage is expected. Treatment of renal neoplasms using radioisotope implants appears promising, but will require further evaluation.

Renal Carcinoma: Renal carcinoma is the most frequently observed renal neoplasm in captive and free-ranging birds. Renal adenocarcinomas may infiltrate adjacent muscle and bone with extension into the spinal canal. Distant metastasis to the liver and oviduct may occur, but is unusual.

Renal Adenoma: Renal adenomas are benign neoplasms that are observed infrequently compared to renal adenocarcinomas.

Embryonal Nephroma: Embryonal nephroma (nephroblastoma, Wilms's tumor) has been observed most commonly in chickens infected with leukosis (sarcoma) virus. In captive and free-ranging birds, these neoplasms are observed occasionally, especially in budgerigars. The literature suggests they are more frequent than adenomas but less common than adenocarcinomas.

Testicular Neoplasms

Testicular neoplasms are usually unilateral, but may occur bilaterally. With unilateral neoplasms, atrophy of the contralateral testis may be observed. In rare instances, a collision tumor may be observed in which two or more cell lines are involved in the neoplastic process.

Sertoli Cell Tumor: Sertoli cell tumor is one of the most frequent testicular neoplasms encountered in captive and free-ranging birds. If neoplastic Sertoli cells are synthesizing estrogen, feminization may be present. This phenomenon is most noticeable in male budgerigars in which the cere color changes from blue to brown.

Seminoma: Seminomas are neoplasms of germ cell origin. These tumors also occur frequently in captive and free-ranging birds. The most common clinical signs include dyspnea, lethargy, anorexia, ascites and abdominal enlargement (occasionally with a palpable intraabdominal mass). Seminomas infrequently may be associated with signs of feminization in budgerigars.

Interstitial Cell Tumor: Interstitial (Leydig) cell tumor is the least frequently reported gonadal stromal testicular neoplasm of birds.

Miscellaneous Testicular Neoplasms: Lymphosarcoma (Marek's disease, Marek's lymphoma) is the most frequent testicular neoplasm of chickens. This neoplasm is herpesvirus-induced.

Ovarian and Oviductal Neoplasms

Ovarian neoplasms are reported more frequently than neoplasms arising from the oviduct. Clinical signs may include abdominal distention, ascites, dyspnea, intra-abdominal mass and leg paresis or paralysis. Usually the left leg exhibits paresis or paralysis initially, but both limbs ultimately may be affected. Paraneoplastic syndromes that may be observed in conjunction with ovarian and oviductal neoplasms include localized exostosis or polyostotic hyperostosis.

Oviductal neoplasms are also described, and most of these tumors are of epithelial cell origin. Ovariectomy or salpingectomy is the treatment of choice.

Granulosa Cell Tumor: Granulosa cell tumors are the most frequently reported ovarian neoplasm in captive and free-ranging birds.

Ovarian Carcinoma: Ovarian carcinomas or adenocarcinomas are the second most frequently reported neoplasm originating in the ovary. Ovarian carcinomas may metastasize to the mesentery, intestinal serosa, liver, lung, pancreas, muscle and bone.

Miscellaneous Ovarian/Oviductal Neoplasms: Stromal tissues of the ovary are infrequent sites of origin for lipomas and fibrosarcomas. Teratomas also may originate in the ovary and are discussed under neoplasms of the nervous system.

The oviduct and ventral ligament of the oviduct occasionally are the sites of origin of leiomyomas and leiomyosarcomas.

Carcinomatosis: Carcinomatosis is the seeding of the thoracoabdominal cavity with neoplastic cells that subsequently proliferate, forming variably sized white nodules. Carcinomatosis may be observed with ovarian and oviductal adenocarcinomas, intestinal adenocarcinoma, pancreatic adenocarcinoma, mesothelioma and undifferentiated adenocarcinoma. Both disseminated mycobacteriosis and egg-related peritonitis of hens may mimic neoplasia clinically and at necropsy. Both cytology and histopathology can confirm the presence of carcinomatosis.

Digestive System

Oral Cavity

Papilloma: Papillomas are composed of proliferative squamous epithelium with a fibrovascular stroma. Oral papillomas are occasionally encountered, especially in psittacine birds, and may involve the oropharyngeal, choanal or laryngeal regions of the pharynx. Papillomas may undergo malignant transformation to squamous cell carcinoma.

Squamous Cell Carcinoma: Squamous cell carcinomas are second to papillomas in frequency and may involve the oral cavity and tongue. These carcinomas appear as ulcerative-to-cauliflower-like, painful lesions or masses that are associated with inappetence, dysphagia, regurgitation, halitosis and frequent head shaking. The differential diagnosis for this lesion should include oral neoplasia, hypovitaminosis A, trauma, candidiasis or protozoal infection (trichomoniasis).

Cytologic examination may demonstrate a pleomorphic population of epithelial cells, but squamous cell hyperplasia and squamous cell carcinoma may be difficult or impossible to distinguish.

Miscellaneous Neoplasms: Miscellaneous oral neoplasms include a mast cell tumor in an owl and a fibrosarcoma in a budgerigar. Mucinous adenocarcinoma of the tongue also has been described in an owl.

Esophagus and Crop

Squamous Plaque: Squamous plaques are focal or multifocal thickening of stratified squamous epithelium that may be accompanied by dysplastic change. This lesion has been described as an "epithelioma" in the crop of a pigeon. Squamous plaques are caused by chronic irritation and may undergo neoplastic transformation.

Papilloma: Papillomas account for the vast majority of neoplasms observed on the mucosal surfaces of the esophagus and crop, especially in psittacine species. Papillomas may undergo malignant transformation.

Squamous Cell Carcinoma: Squamous cell carcinoma of the crop has been observed in a budgerigar and an Amazon parrot.

Leiomyosarcoma: A multifocal leiomyosarcoma has been reported to originate in the crop wall of a budgerigar. The only clinical sign attributed to this neoplasm was difficulty in swallowing.

Proventriculus and Ventriculus

Neoplasms of the proventriculus are approximately twice as common compared to neoplasms of the ventriculus. Adenocarcinomas are most commonly observed and often arise from the junction of these two organs.

Proventricular Carcinoma: Proventricular carcinoma is the most frequent neoplasm observed in this organ. These neoplasms are more common in psittacine species, especially Grey-cheeked Parakeets.

Clinically, gastrointestinal bleeding, as determined by observation of melena, anemia or a positive fecal occult blood test, should alert the clinician to the possibility of gastrointestinal neoplasia. Severe bleeding, hypovolemic shock or exsanguination may occur.

Ventricular Carcinoma: Ventricular carcinomas are infrequent in comparison to proventricular carcinomas but the clinical signs are similar.

Papillomas: Papillomas are reported to occur within the proventriculus and ventriculus. They are apparently more common in the ventriculus.

Proventricular Adenoma: A proventricular adenoma has been observed in a teal.

Intestine

Although rare, some neoplasms originating in the small intestine have been reported. Intestinal neoplasms can best be managed by surgical excision and intestinal anastomosis if the lesions are diagnosed early, if metastasis has not occurred and if the site can be adequately exposed.

Leiomyosarcoma: Primary intestinal leiomyosarcomas have been observed in budgerigars.

Intestinal Carcinoma: Intestinal carcinoma has been reported in a budgerigar, duck and gull.

Cloaca

Cloacal neoplasms and masses, including papillomas, adenocarcinomas, and adenomatous polyps and hyperplasia are observed most commonly in psittacine birds, especially Amazon parrots.

Cloacal Papilloma: Cloacal papillomas are recognized frequently in psittacine birds. Cloacal papillomas and bile duct carcinoma may show concurrent development, especially in Amazon parrots. Grossly, cloacal papillomas appear as broad-based, pink-to-red, proliferative-to-ulcerative masses. They may closely resemble granulation tissue. Major clinical signs associated with cloacal papillomas are straining, bleeding from the vent and cloacal prolapse. A viral etiology has been suggested for these neoplasms, but has yet to be confirmed.

Cloacal Carcinoma: Cloacal carcinomas are observed infrequently compared to papillomas.

Cloacal Adenomatous Polyp or Hyperplasia: Histologically, these lesions are characterized by epithelial cell hyperplasia resulting in a visible mass.

Hepatic Neoplasms

Both primary and metastatic neoplasia occur in the liver. The most frequent primary hepatic neoplasms are hepatocellular carcinoma and bile duct carcinoma.

Cholangiocarcinoma: Cholangiocarcinoma (cholangiocellular carcinoma, bile duct carcinoma) originates from bile duct epithelium. This is the most frequent hepatic neoplasm reported in captive and free-ranging birds (lymphoid neoplasms are most common in gallinaceous birds). Specific clinical signs are infrequent, although emaciation, weakness, hepatomegaly, ataxia, trembling and seizures have been observed. Some neurologic signs are suggestive of hepatoencephalopathy.

Cholangioma: Cholangiomas are of bile duct epithelial origin and are rare in comparison to cholangiocarcinoma. Cholangiomas may occur as single or multiple, firm nodules.

Bile Duct Hyperplasia: Bile duct hyperplasia is observed with some frequency in psittacine birds with liver disease. Bile duct hyperplasia is often seen concurrently with hepatic fibrosis and hepatocellular lipidosis. The etiology of bile duct hyperplasia is often undetermined; however, ingestion of mycotoxin-contaminated feed should be considered in the differential diagnosis (see Chapter 20).

Biliary Cyst: Biliary cysts are reported infrequently in birds. Such cysts are generally congenital and may be intra- or extrahepatic. Biliary cysts may be observed in conjunction with polycystic kidneys.

Hepatocellular Carcinoma: In captive and free-ranging birds, the incidence of hepatocellular carcinoma is superseded only by cholangiocarcinoma. Birds with hepatocellular carcinoma frequently present in a debilitated state with enlargement of one liver lobe. Abdominal enlargement may be apparent on physical examination.

Antemortem liver lobe enlargement may be confirmed by radiography, ultrasound, endoscopy or laparotomy.

Hepatocellular Adenoma: Hepatocellular adenoma (hepatoma) is poorly documented in birds, having been reported in a cissa, guineafowl, hornbill and mynah bird.

Nodular Hyperplasia: Nodular hyperplasia of the liver may be viewed as attempted parenchymal regeneration following injury. Nodular hyperplasia is usually an incidental finding at necropsy in birds with evidence of chronic liver disease. The most common associations with nodular hyperplasia are mycotoxin exposure and iron-accumulating hepatopathy.

Pancreatic Neoplasms

Most pancreatic neoplasms reported in birds arise from the exocrine pancreas, especially ductular structures.

Pancreatic Adenoma: Pancreatic adenomas occur in psittacine birds, especially Amazon parrots, macaws and budgerigars. In Amazon parrots, pancreatic adenomas may be associated with internal papillomas or may be observed as incidental findings at necropsy.

Pancreatic Adenocarcinoma: Pancreatic adenocarcinoma may be observed in various species of birds including psittacines, doves, Anseriformes and ratites. These neoplasms occasionally may be quite large, envelop bowel loops and result in abdominal effusion. They are not amenable to treatment.

Endocrine System

Pituitary Gland

Pituitary neoplasms are the most frequently reported endocrine neoplasm in birds and there is no effective treatment for them.

Pituitary Adenoma: Pituitary adenoma is the most frequently reported endocrine neoplasm of birds, especially budgerigars. These neoplasms often originate from proliferation of chromophobe cells in the anterior lobe. Because of the anatomic location of the pituitary gland, expansive neoplasms follow the path of least resistance, compressing the hypothalamus and optic chiasm. Neurologic signs resulting from compression include incoordination, poor perching or posture, somnolence, seizures and convulsions, and visual impairment including blindness associated with dilated, fixed pupils. Unilateral or bilateral exophthalmos may result from neoplastic cell infiltration along the optic nerve(s).

Pituitary adenomas also may be associated with polydipsia and polyuria. The mechanisms of polydipsia and polyuria have not been investigated in birds, but may be caused by decreased antidiuretic hormone (ADH) concentrations or by overproduction of adrenocorticotrophic hormone (ACTH).

Necropsy usually reveals a mass in the location of the pituitary that compresses the overlying hypothalamus.

Pituitary Carcinoma: Pituitary carcinomas are rare neoplasms in birds, but have been reported and characterized in two budgerigars.

Pineal Gland

Neoplasms of the pineal gland are rare. These expansive neoplasms may displace or compress adjacent neural tissue resulting in neurologic deficits. Because of their anatomic location, surgical excision of pineal gland neoplasms is virtually impossible.

Pineoblastoma: A pineoblastoma has been described in a cockatiel. Clinical signs included polydipsia, depression, right-sided head tilt and inability to grasp objects with the right foot.

Pinealoma: Pinealoma has been reported in two chickens and a dove.

Thyroid Gland

Enlargement of the thyroid glands may be observed with hyperplasia or neoplasia. Signs of thyroid gland enlargement may include dyspnea and a distinctive squawk on vocalization. Their anatomic location near the thoracic inlet precludes palpation of masses unless glandular enlargements are extreme. Thyroid hyperplasia can be managed medically. Theoretically, thyroid neoplasia can be managed surgically, but diagnosis and extirpation of intrathoracic lesions are difficult.

Thyroid Hyperplasia: Thyroid hyperplasia (goiter) may be associated with iodine-deficient diets, ingestion of goitrogenic plants such as *Brassica* species, exposure to iodine-containing disinfectants or excessive dietary iodine. Thyroid hyperplasia is manifested by bilateral glandular enlargement. Colloid-distended follicles may result in glandular enlargements reaching 20 mm in diameter. Because of improved diets for companion birds, thyroid hyperplasia is reported less frequently than three decades ago.

Thyroid Adenoma: Thyroid adenomas are usually unilateral but may occasionally cause bilateral glandular enlargement. These neoplasms usually represent incidental necropsy findings in birds.

Thyroid Carcinoma: Thyroid carcinomas are rare and poorly characterized in birds. Thyroid gland enlargement may be unilateral or bilateral. Dyspnea may be a presenting complaint.

Adrenal Gland

In contrast to mammals, avian adrenal glands have no distinct cortex or medulla. Both interrenal (cortical) and enterochromaffin (medullary) cells are intermingled throughout the gland. Adrenal neoplasms are rare in captive and free-ranging birds and have not been studied in detail. When enlargement of the adrenal glands is observed at necropsy, a primary consideration is adrenal gland hyperplasia.

Adrenal Adenoma: Adrenal adenomas arise from interrenal (cortical) cells and have rarely been reported in birds and generally are not associated with clinical signs of disease.

Adrenal Carcinoma: Adrenal carcinoma was described in a Mountain Duck that was depressed and had leg paralysis.

Pheochromocytoma: A single pheochromocytoma has been reported in a Mouflon, but clinical, necropsy and histologic findings were not discussed.

Endocrine Pancreas

Islet Cell Carcinoma: The islets of Langerhans constitute the endocrine portion of the pancreas. These scattered islets are composed of a diverse aggregation of alpha, beta and delta cells that secrete glucagon, insulin and gastrin, respectively. Islet cell neoplasms may be secretory or non-secretory. Secretory islet cell neoplasms may have diverse clinical presentations.

Chemoreceptor Neoplasms

Chemoreceptors, in concert with the parasympathetic and sympathetic nervous systems, regulate blood pH, pCO_2 and pO_2. These neoplasms are very rare in birds. A carotid body tumor has been reported in a parakeet, but no details of the neoplasm were presented.

Nervous System and Eye

Central Nervous System

Neoplasms of the central nervous system may represent an interesting incidental finding at necropsy or may be related to profound neurologic deficits from compression and infiltration of neural tissue, obstruction of cerebrospinal flow, or secondary edema, hemorrhage or necrosis. These neoplasms have a poor prognosis, and effective treatment regimens have yet to be developed. The discussion below is confined to those neoplasms recently reported in birds.

Astrocytoma: An astrocytoma is a differentiated neoplasm of astrocytes that exhibits slow but progressive growth. These neoplasms usually arise in the cerebral hemispheres, thalamus, brainstem, cerebellum or spinal cord. A single astrocytoma has been reported in a duck with neurologic signs.

Glioblastoma: A glioblastoma is an undifferentiated neoplasm of astrocyte origin. These neoplasms grow rapidly, infiltrate surrounding neural tissue, and are very destructive. A glioblastoma has been described in a budgerigar with weakness, incoordination, inability to perch properly, tremors of the wings and rigidity of the legs.

Oligodendroglioma: This neoplasm originates from oligodendroglial cells. These neoplasms usually arise in the cerebral hemispheres. A single "glioma" has been reported in the left cerebral hemisphere of a budgerigar, but microscopic characteristics of the neoplasm were not reported.

Choroid Plexus Papilloma: These benign neoplasms originate from the choroid plexus epithelium, usually in the fourth ventricle at the cerebropontine angle. A choroid plexus papilloma has been observed in a budgerigar with blindness, exophthalmos and seizures.

Neuroblastoma and Ganglioneuroma: These neoplasms are derived from primitive neuroepithelial cells that differentiate toward neuroblasts (neuroblastoma) or neurons (ganglioneuroma).

Ganglioneuromas have been reported in chickens where they may arise in the nervous system, gastrointestinal tract, ovary, muscle or heart.

Vascular Neoplasms: The most common vascular neoplasms observed in the central nervous system are hemangiosarcoma and hamartoma. A hamartoma is a benign tumor-like nodule composed of an overgrowth of mature cells. A hamartoma-like lesion has been reported in the brain of an 11-week-old budgerigar.

Teratoma: Grossly, these primordial germ cell neoplasms, which may be large and cystic, have been observed in chickens and ducks. Teratomas have diverse sites of origin including the brain, pineal gland, testis, ovary, kidney, orbit, cranium, thoracoabdominal cavity and retroperitoneal space. Teratomas arising within the cranial vault may cause neurologic deficits such as head tilt, circling and facial nerve paralysis.

Lymphosarcoma: Lymphosarcoma of the central nervous system may be classified as a primary or secondary disease. Primary lymphosarcoma originates in the CNS, while secondary lymphosarcoma represents a metastatic event. Evidence exists for both of these presentations of lymphoid neoplasia in birds, although metastatic neoplasia is more common. Most instances of CNS lymphosarcoma occur in poultry and are viral-induced. Lymphosarcoma is discussed in detail under the hemolymphatic system.

Meningioma: Meningiomas originate from neural crest cells or mesenchymal cells in contact with neural crest cells.

Peripheral Nervous System

Localized neoplasms may be amenable to surgical excision based upon their location, size and proximity to vital structures.

Schwannoma: These neoplasms previously have been reported as neurolemmomas or neurofibroma, the latter term being a misnomer. Schwannomas may arise from Schwann cells or perineural cells of the peripheral nerve sheaths in any location including unspecified peripheral nerves, cranial nerves, sciatic plexus, gastrointestinal tract, testis, pineal gland, kidney, skin, muscle and spleen.

Malignant Schwannoma: Malignant schwannomas (neurofibrosarcoma is a misnomer) also originate from Schwann cells or perineural cells.

Lymphoid Neoplasia (Lymphosarcoma): Marek's disease in chickens is often associated with leg paralysis secondary to ischiatic nerve infiltration by neoplastic lymphocytes. Affected nerves appear thickened.

Ocular Neoplasms

Intraocular neoplasms in birds may be associated with blindness, hyphema or aqueous flare. Some neoplasms, such as malignant lymphoma, may be visualized occasionally by ophthalmoscopy. Because the avian eye is reinforced by scleral ossicles, buphthalmos is not expected. In contrast, exophthalmos occurs with some frequency and usually indicates a retrobulbar space-occupying lesion or extension of malignant ocular neoplasia into the retrobulbar area. In birds, exophthalmos has been associated with various retrobulbar neoplasms including malignant lymphoma, pituitary adenoma and adenocarcinoma, malignant intraocular medulloepithelioma, intraocular rhabdomyosarcoma, undifferentiated carcinoma, teratoma, and glioma.

Lymphosarcoma: Lymphosarcoma (malignant lymphoma) involving the iris, ciliary body and choroid is observed most frequently in chickens with Marek's disease. When visualized, these neoplasms may appear as yellow-to-white proliferative masses. Most occurrences of ocular lymphoid neoplasia represent metastatic lesions.

Rhabdomyosarcoma: Intraocular rhabdomyosarcomas have been reported in two chickens. These neoplasms may have arisen from the ciliary muscles, which are striated in birds. One neoplasm extended into the retrobulbar space. The other neoplasm replaced the iris, ciliary body and choroid.

Malignant Medulloepithelioma: Intraocular medulloepitheliomas are primitive neoplasms that originate from the optic cup epithelium and have been described in two cockatiels.

Malignant Melanoma: Metastatic ocular malignant melanoma has been reported in a Pintail Duck in association with multiple neoplasms involving adrenal gland, skin, liver, skeletal muscle, heart, lung, kidney, brain and bone.

Hemolymphatic System

Clinical signs related to hemolymphatic neoplasia are variable and vague including lethargy, anorexia, weight loss, lameness, swellings, dyspnea, loose droppings and petechial-to-ecchymotic hemorrhages. Death often occurs from organ dysfunction secondary to infiltrative disease.

Lymphoid Neoplasia

Lymphoid neoplasia is the most common form of hemolymphatic neoplasia occurring in domestic, captive, and free-ranging birds. This form of neoplasia may originate from the peripheral lymphoid tissues as lymphosarcoma (malignant lymphoma) or in the bone marrow as leukemia.

In chickens, lymphoid neoplasms may be induced by herpesvirus or retrovirus infections. Herpesvirus infection causes Marek's disease. Following neoplastic transformation, lymphoid neoplasms appear more progressive and are composed of lymphoblasts. In contrast, lymphoid leukosis is caused by retroviral-induced neoplastic transformation of B-lymphocytes.

Lymphoid neoplasia of free-ranging and captive birds has not been studied in detail. A recent pathologic survey subclassified avian lymphoid neoplasia as plasmacytoma or fibrifying, lymphoblastic, lymphocytic or mixed-cell lymphosarcoma. However, the prognostic importance of these subclassifications has not been demonstrated and requires further clinico-pathologic study.

Currently, there is no effective treatment for avian lymphoid neoplasia. Radiation therapy may be palliative. Combination chemotherapy with vincristine sulfate, prednisone and chlorambucil appears promising but requires more clinical research.

Lymphosarcoma: Lymphosarcoma (malignant lymphoma) is defined as any lymphoid neoplasm that originates in the peripheral lymphoid tissues. This form of lymphoid neoplasia is commonly observed in birds and is characterized by the formation of white-to-yellow tissue discolorations or sarcomatous masses.

Lymphosarcoma usually presents as a disseminated multisystemic disease that can involve all tissues of the body, including bone marrow. The abdominal viscera often are involved (visceral leukosis), especially the liver, spleen and kidney. Occasionally, lymphosarcoma may show tissue tropism with multiple neoplasms being observed in one tissue such as skin. The rarest presentation of lymphosarcoma is the presence of a single, localized neoplasm. This presentation was documented as a single neoplasm at the optic chiasm of a cockatiel.

Lymphoid Leukemia: Lymphoid leukemia originates in the bone marrow and disseminates to various body tissues. This presentation of lymphoid neoplasia is rare compared to lymphosarcoma. Birds with lymphocytic leukemia may have anemia, thrombocytopenia and marked lymphocytosis. Lymphocytes in blood smears may be well differentiated or blastic. Bone marrow aspirates contain innumerable lymphocytes. Sarcomatous masses are not observed in tissues at necropsy; however, hepatosplenomegaly may be prominent. Infiltration of various tissues by neoplastic lymphocytes is observed microscopically.

Thymoma: Thymoma is a localized form of lymphoid neoplasia that is confined to one or more thymic lobes.

Nonlymphoid Neoplasia

Granulocytic Leukemia: Granulocytic leukemia is the unregulated proliferation of granulocytes. In chickens, this disease (myeloblastosis) is caused by retrovirus infection; the etiology in captive and free-ranging birds has not been identified.

Erythremic Myelosis: Erythremic myelosis is the unregulated production of erythrocyte precursors. This form of leukemia is caused by retrovirus infection in chickens and has been called erythroblastosis.

An erythremic myelosis-like syndrome has been described in conures. Most of these birds appear weak and have a history of spontaneous hemorrhage. Although the evidence occasionally appears supportive of erythremic myelosis, marked extramedullary erythropoiesis cannot be excluded. In comparison to mammalian erythrocytes, avian erythrocytes have a very short life span (20-25 days). Following acute and ongoing hemorrhage, intense extramedullary erythropoiesis could occur, especially with concurrent recycling of iron from internal hemorrhage. Therefore, the conure bleeding syndrome will require further hematologic characterization before it can be classified absolutely as erythremic myelosis.

OPHTHALMOLOGY

David Williams

The detailed ophthalmic examination requires adequate restraint, and a darkened room will calm the bird and improve the illumination provided by a focal light source.

Some larger Psittaciformes may inflate a portion of their periorbital sinus as an aggressive gesture, creating a transient swelling in the periorbital region. This swelling should not be mistaken for periorbital disease. Collapse of the anterior chamber may occur in an otherwise normal eye following a period of head restraint or lateral recumbency during anesthesia. Normal anterior chamber depth is rapidly regained.

Examination of the anterior segment can be performed with a bright pen light, a binocular loupe, an operating microscope, an ophthalmoscope set on +20 diopters or, ideally, a slit lamp. Key features to evaluate are the clarity of the cornea, the aqueous, the lens and the color and vascularization of the iris. Aqueous flare, as seen in uveitis, can be detected by looking for scattering of a slit light beam that is passing through the anterior chamber.

Retinal examination is difficult in many birds because of the small size of the eye and the lack of response of the avian iris to conventional parasympathomimetic mydriatics. Mydriasis can be accomplished by intracemeral injection of d-tubocurarine or by the frequent use of a freshly prepared topical 3 mg/ml solution of crystalline d-tubocurarine in 0.025% benzilonium chloride over a fifteen-minute period. A more practical approach may be the topical use of commercially available neuromuscular blocking agents commonly used for intravenous injections (eg, vecuronium bromide solution 4 mg/ml q 5 min x 3 in raptors, see Chapter 18).

With or without mydriasis, the easiest way to view the fundus is to start with the direct ophthalmoscope at the +20 dioptre setting, and with the instrument close to the bird's eye, change the dioptre setting gradually back to zero. This will bring the pleated pecten into view. It is then possible to focus on the avascular retina at the posterior of the eye.

Ancillary Tests for Evaluation of the Eye

Corneal ulcerations can be detected by staining with fluorescein dye. The Schirmer Tear Tests can be used on birds, although normal data for psittacine birds have not been published. Conventional 6 mm-wide Schirmer tear test filter paper strips have been found to be difficult to insert in the lower conjunctival sac of the smaller Psittaciformes; thus trimming these to 4 mm is more useful. To date, Schirmer tear test readings have been found to be 8 ± 1.5 mm in the larger Psittaciformes such as the African Grey Parrot, and 4.5 ± 1 mm in smaller species such as lories and conures.

Tonometry is possible in birds, but little normal data has been published. The portable Tonopen applanation tonometer is ideal for use in birds. A tonometric examination of 275 birds (39 species) showed intraocular pressures in normal eyes of between 9.2 and 16.3 mmHg. Among 14 species of psittacine birds, values were found to be 14.4 ± 4.2 mmHg with a sample size of 74 birds.

Avian periorbital and external eye disease is frequently associated with infectious agents. The best diagnostic bacteriologic samples can be obtained by inserting a sterile swab moistened in transport medium into the upper conjunctival fornix and rubbing it from side to side two or three times.

As an overview, the avian eyelids are mobile, the lower more so than the upper. The meibomian glands are absent, but a lacrimal gland (varying in size between species) is present, inferior and lateral to the globe. The Harderian gland acts as a second lacrimal gland at the base of the nictitating membrane. Inferior and superior nasolacrimal puncta at the medial canthus drain lacrimal secretions into the nasal cavity.

A key point in the anatomy of the avian orbit is the close proximity of the tightly packed orbit with the infraorbital diverticulum of the infraorbital sinus. Sinusitis and enlargement of this diverticulum will therefore lead to periorbital or orbital compression and signs of periorbital swelling, conjunctivitis and sometimes intraocular disease.

Ophthalmic Disorders

Lids and Periorbita

One of the most common ocular presentations in large psittacine birds is periorbital disease secondary to upper respiratory infection, particularly chronic rhinitis and sinusitis. As stated above, the close proximity of the infraorbital sinus to the orbit predisposes it to physical displacement when the sinus diverticulum is enlarged. In some cases, cellulitis or abscessation occur from spread of organisms from the sinus cavity. Antibiotics alone are rarely efficacious in these cases; flushing the sinus and, in some cases, more aggressive surgical debridement is required (see Chapter 41).

Poxvirus

The initial changes include a mild, predominantly unilateral blepharitis with eyelid edema and serous discharge starting about 10-14 days post-infection. As the disease progresses, ulcerative lesions on the lid margins and at the medial or lateral canthus develop; these can become secondarily infected, giving rise to a mucopurulent discharge and transient ankyloblepharon. The lids become sealed shut with a caseous plug or with dry crusty scabs, which fall off within two weeks.

Clinical lesions provide a tentative diagnosis. An infection can be confirmed through histopathologic identification of eosinophilic intracytoplasmic inclusion bodies (Bollinger bodies) in scabs or scrapings of periocular ulcers.

Poxvirus infections may cause keratitis and, less commonly, anterior uveitis. The keratitis can be mild with corneal clouding or severe with ulceration that progresses to panophthalmitis and rupture of the globe. Keratitis may lead to permanent corneal scarring. Cicatricial changes in the lid margins can lead to entropion, ankyloblepharon or deformities of the lid edge, resulting in keratitis from corneal abrasion or environmental exposure. These patients may need corrective surgery (lid retraction) or can be placed on lifelong therapy with ocular lubricants.

Eyelid and corneal lesions are most severe if poxvirus lesions are secondarily infected with bacteria or fungus. Treatment of poxvirus lesions should include topical antibiotic ophthalmic ointments to reduce the incidence of these sequelae. Systemic antibiotics may also be required in severely affected birds. Early eye lesions should be flushed with dilute antiseptic solutions. Once scabs have formed they should not be removed. It may be beneficial to soften scabs with hot or cold compresses soaked in nonirritating baby shampoo. It has been reported that prophylactic vitamin A supplementation of exposed birds decreases the severity of infection.

Hypovitaminosis A

Xerophthalmia is said to be the classic sign of hypovitaminosis A in many avian species, but the most common ocular change in psittacine birds is mild periorbital and conjunctival swelling with some discharge. These signs can be subtle. Hypovitaminosis A should be considered in cases of unexplained ocular discharge or swelling.

Nasal discharge, sneezing, crusted nares, dry oral membranes and palatine and choanal abscesses are highly suggestive of primary hypovitaminosis A, particularly in Amazon parrots. Response to injectable vitamin A or oral beta carotene supplementation suggests the involvement of a deficiency in the disease process.

Lovebird Eye Disease

A severe and often fatal systemic disease with periocular lesions as the presenting sign has been reported in lovebirds. Generalized depression is accompanied by blepharitis and serous ocular discharge, followed by hyperemia and edema of the periorbita with a mucopurulent ocular discharge. Affected birds are often attacked by enclosure mates and usually die within a few days of the onset of ocular signs. The disease is most commonly seen in the Peach-faced mutations, and it is in these birds that the lesions are most severe.

No definitive isolation of an infectious agent has been achieved, but an adenovirus-like particle has been demonstrated in renal tissue by electron microscopy. Conjunctival inclusions have been found in some affected birds. The disease occurs most frequently immediately after shipping or introduction into a new aviary, suggesting that stress may be involved in initiating pathologic changes. Symptomatic therapy that includes isolation of affected birds in a stress-free environment and administration of antibiotics has been suggested.

Pasteurella spp. septicemia and gram-positive cocci have been associated with conjunctivitis in lovebirds. A poxvirus has been described in Masked and Peach-faced Lovebirds.

Periorbital and Orbital Abscesses

Periorbital disease with exophthalmos or strabismus is most likely to be caused by an abscess of the orbit or lacrimal gland. In some cases, periorbital neoplasia, either primary or secondary, can cause similar clinical changes. Periorbital abscesses generally result from chronic upper respiratory tract infection and sinusitis. They are most often seen in cockatiels, and can occur in any position in the orbit. Early treatment of sinusitis reduces the incidence of these lesions. Surgical debridement of the abscesses with concomitant systemic antibiotics is the only effective treatment. Lacrimal sac abscesses must be differentiated from periorbital abscesses. The lacrimal sac masses present as mobile swellings at, or immediately anteroventral to, the medial canthus. Early dacryocystitis can sometimes be treated by expressing the inflammatory debris through the lacrimal punctum. More severe cases with firm, necrotic debris require cannulation and regular flushing with antibiotic solutions as dictated by bacteriologic culture and sensitivity. Surgical removal is not recommended because of the potential for scarring and long-term nasolacrimal drainage problems.

Periorbital Swelling of Neoplastic Origin

Any primary tumor arising in the periorbital or retrobulbar area can cause swelling with or without globe displacement. Exophthalmia or posteriorly directed strabismus may be noted.

Other less common causes of retrobulbar masses include *Mycobacterium* spp., *Aspergillus* spp. granulomas and disseminated cryptococcosis.

Hyperplastic Periocular Lesions

Proliferative and hyperplastic periorbital lesions are most commonly seen in budgerigars and canaries in response to *Knemidokoptes* spp. infections. Pitted or honeycombed, scaly and crusting lesions are easily noted in the periorbital area as well as on the beak, vent and legs. The periorbital lesions seldom cause problems even though they may be quite severe. Ivermectin can be used topically.

A potential differential diagnosis would include vitamin A deficiency, which can lead to periorbital epithelial hyperplasia and hyperkeratosis, but hypovitaminosis A lesions rarely achieve the size or proliferative extent seen with knemidokoptes. Periorbital papilloma-like virus infection in an African Grey Parrot resulted in hyperplastic parakeratotic epithelial proliferations. Other periorbital papillomas have been described without viral isolation.

Congenital Deformities

Partial agenesis of the upper eyelid, which was surgically corrected by creating a new lateral canthus at the point at which normal upper eyelid would be found, has been reported in a raptor.

Cryptophthalmos (fusion of the eyelid margins) has been reported in four cockatiels in which dramatically reduced or absent palpebral fissures were described without other ocular abnormalities. Reconstructive surgery was uniformly unsuccessful. Corneal dermoids have been reported in one goose, in which feathers grew out of the aberrant dermal tissue on the lateral aspect of the globe.

The lacrimal ducts did not drain properly in an Umbrella Cockatoo with choanal atresia, resulting in a chronic ocular discharge.

Conjunctivitis

Conjunctivitis can be classified clinically into three groups. The first are those caused by strictly local factors, such as localized conjunctival infection or foreign bodies. The second are those in which conjunctivitis is a manifestation of periorbital or orbital disease. These are mainly related to sinusitis (see Chapter 22). The third group are those in which conjunctival hyperemia is caused by a septicemia. Almost any organism causing systemic infection can result in conjunctivitis. A careful examination of the bird for upper respiratory disease is mandatory in determining the cause of ocular discharge or conjunctival hyperemia. Exposure to cigarette smoke, chemical fumes and other aerosolized environmental toxins should always be considered in the differential diagnosis of conjunctivitis, with or without signs of upper respiratory disease.

Various infectious agents have been implicated in conjunctivitis, but mere isolation of a bacteria or protozoan does not imply that it is the cause of the disease.

Chlamydia psittaci is a frequent cause of keratoconjunctivitis in Australian parakeets and of conjunctivitis without other signs in pigeons and finches. In these cases, treatment with topical oxytetracycline is effective. Clinical chlamydiosis in Psittaciformes is generally associated with conjunctivitis, diarrhea and polyuria.

Mycoplasma spp. are important causes of conjunctivitis in pigeons and are suspected in many cases of conjunctivitis in cockatiels. Ocular discharge and conjunctivitis may be the only presenting signs. Other affected birds may develop rales, nasal discharge and sneezing. Unilateral conjunctivitis (one-eyed cold) in pigeons is frequently associated with mycoplasma but can also be caused by chlamydia or salmonella.

The presence of foreign bodies in the fornix, or behind the third eyelid, may be a cause of conjunctival irritation and should be suspected in cases of unilateral conjunctivitis that are not responsive to antibiotics.

Cockatiel Conjunctivitis

Cockatiels are frequently presented with a conjunctivitis from which no infectious agent can be isolated. Clinical signs involve blepharitis and serous ocular discharge, progressing to conjunctival chemosis and inflammation with hyperemic conjunctiva protruding in front of the eye. These signs are seen much more frequently in white or albino mutations than in birds of normal gray color.

The lesions are often associated with upper respiratory tract infection, and *Mycoplasma* spp. and *Chlamydia* spp. have been suggested as agents. Isolating mycoplasma requires specialized techniques, and diagnostic samples should be sent in specific media to qualified laboratories. Many cockatiels with conjunctivitis are not systemically positive for *Chlamydia* spp., shedding some doubt on the importance of this organism in the cockatiel syndrome.

Treatment with topical antibiotics often ameliorates the signs but recurrences are common. Systemic tetracycline is often curative but should be combined with symptomatic treatment of the inflamed periorbita. Antibiotic ophthalmic ointments may be used or the eyes can be sprayed with tylosin (1:10 dilution in sterile water) or lincomycin and spectinomycin. The problem seems to follow familial lines, suggesting that affected birds should not be used in breeding programs. In some cockatiels, the conjunctivitis is associated with partial lid paresis and reduced jaw tone. Many of these birds have giardiasis and respond to treatment with metronidazole and vitamin E. A similar condition has been noted in budgerigars, and again, the etiologic agent has yet to be identified.

Parasitic Conjunctivitis

A number of nematode and trematode parasites can occasionally cause conjunctival irritation in a wide variety of avian species (see Chapter 36). *Oxyspirura mansoni* is a nematode that has been associated with conjunctival irritation and pruritus in cockatoos, mynahs and other avian species. Nematode eggs are passed through the nasolacrimal duct, swallowed and passed in the feces, where they are consumed by cockroaches (*Pycnoscellus* spp.). When a bird eats the cockroach, the mature nematode larvae escape into the crop, move up the esophagus and enter the nasolacrimal duct to reach the eye. Companion birds maintained in indoor environments are less likely to be infected. *Thelazia* spp. are reported to cause conjunctivitis in birds.

Trematode flukes of the genus *Philophthalmus* have been reported as a cause of conjunctivitis in many avian species. Repeated applications of topical carbamate powder eliminated the flukes.

Cornea

Treating Corneal Ulcers and Keratitis

Most corneal problems seen in Psittaciformes are epithelial erosions secondary to trauma or keratitis secondary to lid abnormalities. Fluorescein dye will stain denuded stroma indicating the presence of an ulcer. In subtle lesions such as Amazon punctate keratitis, an ultraviolet Wood's lamp can be used to augment the detection of fluorescein retention. Keratitis can be difficult to resolve, but, as a rule, topical antibiotics and corneal bandaging techniques provide a sterile environment and time for corneal epithelium to heal. By extrapolation from other species, anticollagenases should be used in deep ulcers, especially in hotter climates, where corneal melting may be a cause of rupture of the globe. Acetylcysteine can be applied by spray every few hours without having to restrain the bird. A temporary tarsorrhaphy created by placing one or two horizontal mattress sutures of 4-0 or 6-0 nylon provides a corneal "bandage." This is preferable to a third eyelid flap because the muscular action moving the third eyelid can cause the suture to pull through. The use of a hydrated collagen shield to provide a medicated corneal bandage has not been reported in birds but may be useful in selected cases. Chronic corneal erosions may occur in older birds. To provide a suitable surface for reattachment of the epithelium, devitalized epithelium can be removed with a dry cotton-tipped applicator or by using a punctate or grid keratotomy.

Mynah Bird Keratitis

Corneal erosions may be noted secondary to capture and transport in many imported companion birds. Mynahs appear to be especially prone to handling-related keratitis. In one study, 96% of birds examined immediately after shipping were found to have corneal scratches. Blepharospasm or some degree of conjunctival hyperemia is a characteristic finding. Many of these lesions regress spontaneously in a few weeks, but some may lead to corneal scarring and permanent opacity. Some birds develop a chronic keratoconjunctivitis with conjunctival masses, severe geographic corneal ulceration and corneal vascularization. Systemic aspergillosis is found in many chronically affected birds, suggesting an immunosuppressed condition. Acyclovir-responsive herpesvirus lesions have been suggested as complicating factors in some affected birds.

Amazon Punctate Keratitis

A transient keratitis with a characteristic subtle punctate appearance has been reported in Central American Amazon parrots. Lesions are bilateral, and the presenting signs are normally blepharospasm and a clear ocular discharge. The keratitis normally starts in the medial cornea. In 50% of the birds, lesions progress to cover the cornea but resolve generally within one to two weeks. The lesions are transiently fluorescein-positive. A small minority of birds develops more serious lesions with deep corneal ulceration and anterior uveitis, manifesting either as a flare and "muddiness" of the iris or as a more severe inflammation with fibrin clots and synechiae. Some birds develop concomitant sinusitis. The use of topical antibiotics or antivirals has not been found to significantly alter the outcome of the disease.

Amazon parrots from northern South America have also been reported with a chronic keratitis. There are fewer cases reported in this group of birds, but the incidence of long-term corneal scarring is higher.

Treatment of more severely affected birds, such as those with intraocular lesions, includes topical and systemic antibiotics.

Topical corticosteroid to control intraocular inflammation can reduce the healing of concurrent corneal ulceration; topical nonsteroidal anti-inflammatories such as indomethacin or flubruprofen may be more appropriate in these cases.

Uvea

Uveitis in raptors is most commonly seen as a sequela to intraocular trauma and is characterized by aqueous flare, hypopyon and fibrin clots in the anterior chamber, iridal hemorrhages or gross hyphema. Uveitis can occur following rupture of the crystalline lens or secondary to severe extraocular disease in conditions such as poxvirus infection. Uveitis has been reported in psittacine birds with reovirus infection in which histopathologic changes suggested disseminated intravascular coagulopathy. Hypopyon and hemorrhage, sometimes with fixed dilated pupils (atypical for uveitis where miosis is more common), are characteristic ocular signs. Birds that recover may have synechiae.

Active inflammation may be mild, with increased levels of aqueous proteins causing a flare that reduces the clarity of iris detail and pupil margin. More severe cases may be characterized by accumulation of pus or hemorrhage in the anterior chamber. Glaucoma is seen secondary to traumatic uveitis in raptors, and has been diagnosed without concurrent ocular disease in a canary. If the eye appears painful, enucleation or evisceration is the only treatment.

Lens

Cataract and lens luxation can occur in birds. Both conditions can be treated surgically in suitable cases. Senile cataracts have been described in macaws.

There is clear evidence for familial cataracts in Yorkshire and Norwich Canaries. In affected canaries, the cataracts were mature with lens-induced uveitis and posterior synechiae formation. Lens removal by the irrigation-aspiration technique was unsuccessful in these birds. Patients requiring cataract removal should be referred to a veterinary ophthalmologist.

Because of the small size of the avian eye, conventional extracapsular cataract extraction techniques are generally difficult. In small birds, soft lenses can be removed through a 26 ga needle. Phacoemulsification is the technique of choice for avian cataract removal in patients with eyes large enough to accommodate the phacoemulsification probe. The extra-capsular technique can be used in intumescent or resorbing cataracts where the lens material can be aspirated or flushed from the anterior chamber. An intracapsular technique has been used for removal of an anteriorly luxated lens in an owl. In eight aging macaws with senile cataracts, the lens was disrupted and removed with an irrigation aspiration technique, resulting in vision in 77% of the eyes. Post-operative treatment with 17% maxitrol was considered an indispensable part of the therapy. Topical medications, particularly steroids, must be applied cautiously to small birds to prevent intoxication.

Miscellaneous Eye Conditions

Retinal Diseases

Some reports of retinal disease in birds have found their way into the literature. Lesions include pigmentary deposits on the otherwise unpigmented peripheral retina, focal scarring, pre-retinal membranes, vitreal opacities and gross inflammatory disease of the entire posterior segment. Many of these lesions in free-ranging birds may be caused by trauma with hemorrhage that causes vitreal scarring and contraction.

Toxoplasmosis has been suggested as a cause of retinal lesions in raptors. Toxoplasmosis was confirmed as a cause of retinitis and blindness in canaries. Several of the infected birds had neurologic signs characterized by circling and head tremors. High latex agglutination antibody titers to *T. gondii* were seen in five of the seven affected birds.

Intraocular Tumors

Intraocular tumors are rare in birds. Malignant intraocular medulloepithelioma has been reported in two-year-old cockatiels. An intraocular adenocarcinoma has been reported in a budgerigar.

Neurophthalmology and Central Blindness

In cases where no obvious ocular cause of blindness can be observed, an electroretinogram can be used to differentiate between retinal or central lesions.

Causes of central blindness may include cataracts, neoplasia or encephalitis that may be localized or related to systemic disease. Heavy metal toxicities can result in blindness, but the visual changes are only one of a number of multifocal nervous signs. One large survey of 50 chromophobe pituitary tumors reported central blindness in a number of birds with associated neurologic and endocrine signs.

Evaluating the Blind Bird: Determining if visually defective birds are sound for release can be difficult. Some birds such as owls perform well with one eye, while releasing a one-eyed diurnal falcon to the wild might be considered unwise. Many companion birds can survive remarkably well with little or no vision.

Enucleation

Enucleation is frequently necessary in birds because of trauma, nonresponsive inflammation or tumors. Enucleation is difficult because of the large size of the avian eye and the tight fit of the globe into the orbit. For further information on enucleation and other ophthalmic surgeries, see Chapter 41.

CARDIOLOGY

J. T. Lumeij
Branson W. Ritchie

The avian heart is divided into four complete chambers and is located midway in the thoracic cavity in an indention in the sternum parallel to the long axis of the body. The right atrioventricular (AV) valve is a simple muscular flap devoid of chordae tendineae, while the left bicuspid AV valve is thin and membranous. Both the aortic and pulmonary valves are membranous and tricuspid as in mammals. The left ventricle is heavily walled and is about two to three times thicker than the right. Rigor mortis in a normal heart always results in complete emptying of the left ventricle. Rigor mortis may not occur if severe degenerative disease of the myocardium is present.

The apex of the avian heart is covered ventrally by the cranial portion of the right and left liver lobes. The normal pericardial sac is clear and in contact with the epicardium circumferentially and the mediastinal pleura dorsally. A normal bird should have a small quantity of clear to slightly yellow fluid in the pericardial sac. The heart is normally even in color and is deep reddish-tan. In neonates, the heart is normally a lighter pink color and may appear pale.

On a body weight basis, smaller birds, in general, have a bigger heart than larger birds. Systolic blood pressure ranges from 108-220 mmHg depending on the species.

Evaluating the Avian Heart

Diagnostic Methods

Primary heart diseases should be included in the differential diagnosis when patients are presented with lethargy, periodic weakness, dyspnea, coughing and abdominal swelling (ascites). Drugs taken, potential exposure to toxins and concurrent diseases should always be evaluated when determining if the heart is abnormal. Cardiac-induced ascites appears to be less common in Psittaciformes than in Galliformes and Anseriformes.

Auscultation of the avian heart is difficult and the information that can be gained is limited. Subtle murmurs are easiest to detect when birds are under isoflurane anesthesia and the heart rate is decreased. Auscultation of the heart can best be performed on the left and right ventral thorax. Pleural or pulmonary fluid accumulation may cause muffled lung sounds or rales when a bird is auscultated over the back between the shoulder blades.

Diagnostic aids that have proven to be effective in evaluating cardiac diseases include CBC, plasma chemistries (eg, AST, LDH, CPK), cytologic examination of pericardial or peritoneal effusions, plasma electrolytes, blood culture, radiographs (including contrast studies such as nonselective angiocardiography), electrocardiography, cardiac ultrasonography (echocardiography) and color flow doppler. CPK activity from cardiac muscle origin (CPK-MB isoenzyme) was significantly higher in ducklings with furazolidone-induced cardiotoxicosis when compared to controls.

Imaging

Radiographic detection of cardiovascular abnormalities may be difficult, although an enlarged cardiac silhouette or microcardia can often be visualized. Radiographic detection of an enlarged cardiac silhouette with muffled heart sounds is suggestive of pericardial effusion. An enlarged cardiac silhouette with normal heart sounds is suggestive of dilative heart disease.

Electrocardiography (low voltage in pericardial effusion) and ultrasonography may demonstrate free pericardial fluid. Microcardia is indicative of severe dehydration or blood loss that has resulted in hypovolemia. Other radiographic changes that suggest cardiac disease include congestion of pulmonary vessels, pulmonary edema, pleural effusion, hepatomegaly and ascites.

Non-selective angiocardiography with rapid sequence serial radiographs has been used to confirm impaired cardiac function in a racing pigeon. This technique has also been used to rule out cardiovascular shunt as the cause of severe dyspnea and hypoxia in a Blue and Gold Macaw. The procedure is performed by injecting a bolus dose of contrast medium into the catheterized basilic vein.

Of the imaging techniques, echocardiograms generally provide the most diagnostic information. In small birds, the echocardiographic image of the heart is best obtained by sweeping through the liver. Color flow doppler was used to demonstrate mitral regurgitation and right-sided heart failure in a mynah.

Electrocardiology

It was demonstrated in 1949 that the negative mean electrical axis of ventricular depolarization in birds occurs because the depolarization wave begins subepicardial and then spreads through the myocardium towards the endocardium.

Electrocardiography may be useful for detecting cardiac enlargement from hypertrophy of any of the four cardiac chambers. Electrocardiography is indispensable for the diagnosis and treatment of cardiac arrhythmias and is also useful in monitoring changes in electrolyte concentrations during the treatment of metabolic diseases that alter electrolyte balance. When evaluat-

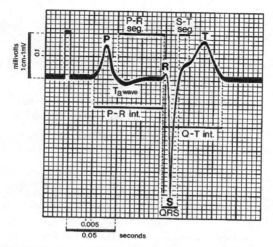

FIG 27.3 Schematic representation of a normal lead II electrocardiographic complex of a racing pigeon. Paper speed 200 mm/s, 1 cm = 1 mV (courtesy of J. T. Lumeij. Reprinted with permission).

ing cardiac enlargement it is best to compare the electrocardiographic findings with those of cardiac imaging techniques.

The electrocardiogram may be of help in evaluating and diagnosing some of the diseases that cause vague signs of weakness, fatigue, lethargy, fever, collapse or seizures. Metabolic, cardiac, neurologic and systemic diseases that produce toxemia can cause one or all of these clinical changes. The electrocardiograph may be used also to monitor heart rate and rhythm in an anesthetized patient. Because the myocardium is very sensitive to hypoxia, the electrocardiogram can serve as a reliable indicator of the oxygenation of the bird. The clinician should realize, however, that cardiac pathology can occur without electrocardiographic changes.

The Electrocardiograph and Recording of the ECG

Regardless of the type of electrocardiograph used, it must be able to run electrocardiograms at a paper speed of at least 100 mm/s. Avian heart rates are so rapid that inspecting and measuring the tracing is less accurate at slower speeds. For routine ECGs, the machine is standardized at 1 cm = 1 mV. When dealing with ECGs with a low voltage, the sensitivity of the machine should be doubled. If the complexes are so large that they exceed the edge of the tracing paper, the sensitivity should be halved. The calibration and the paper speed should always be marked on the electrocardiogram together with the date, time, name and case number of the patient.

It is easiest to perform an ECG on a bird in dorsal recumbency, but right lateral or ventral recumbency is equally effective. Needle electrodes placed subcutaneously are superior to alligator clips for use in avian patients.

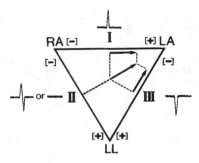

FIG 27.4 If an electrical impulse is traveling in the direction of a lead's negative pole, a negative deflection results and vice versa. If the vector runs perpendicular to a lead, that lead will record either no deflection or an equal number of positive and negative forces. This is called an isoelectric lead.

Lead I in birds is nearly isoelectric. The lead II electrocardiogram in Figure 27.3 is a recording of electrical currents generated during the depolarization and repolarization of the heart. The P-wave signifies that the atria have depolarized, causing contraction and ejection of their complement of blood into the ventricles. The PR-segment indicates the short delay in the atrioventricular node that occurs after the atria contract, which allows complete filling of the ventricles before ventricular contraction occurs. The depression of the initial part of the PR-segment is related to large atrial repolarization forces. In dogs, this is caused by right atrial hypertrophy and is called auricular T-wave or Ta-wave. In racing pigeons, this phenomenon is seen in 83% of healthy individuals and depicts the repolarization of the atria. A "Ta-wave" is also normal in some gallinaceous birds.

In parrots, a slight indication of a Ta-wave may occasionally be noted. The (Q)RS-complex represents ventricular depolarization and contraction with the ejection of blood into the aorta and pulmonary artery. The Q-wave is the first negative deflection, the R-wave is the first positive deflection and the S-wave is the first negative deflection following the R-wave. When there is no R-wave, the negative deflection is called a QS-wave. The largest wave in the QRS-complex is depicted with a capital letter, (ie, Rs or rS). The ST-segment and T-wave depict the repolarization of the ventricles. In clinically asymptomatic racing pigeons and parrots, the ST-segment is often very short or even absent, the S rising directly into the T-wave ("ST-slurring"). When the ST-segment is present, it is often elevated above the baseline (maximum 0.3 mV elevation in the racing pigeon). In mammalian species, these changes are associated with cardiac disease (ie, left ventricular hypertrophy), but the cause of ST-slurring in birds remains undetermined.

The duration (measured in hundredths of seconds) and amplitude (measured in millivolts) of the complexes can be measured. When the machine is standardized at 1 cm = 1 mV each small box on the vertical is 0.1 mV. When the electrocardiograph is recorded at a paper speed of 100 mm/s, each small box on the horizontal is

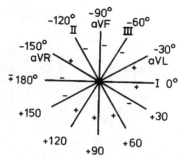

FIG 27.5 Bailey's hexaxial system. The three leads from Einthoven's triangle (I, II, III) and the three unipolar leads (aVR, aVL, aVF) can be redrawn exactly at the same length and polarity by passing each lead through the center point of the triangle. This produces a hexaxial system and angle values can be assigned to both the positive and negative pole of each lead. Now there are six leads, with a positive and negative pole, and each pole has an angle value. This six-lead system is used for determining the mean electrical axis of ventricular depolarization.

0.01 s and when the ECG is recorded at 200 mm/s, each small box represents 0.005 s. The determined values can be compared with reference values (Table 27.1).

ECG Leads

The electrodes are attached to the right wing (RA), the left wing (LA) and the left limb (LL). The right hind limb (RL) of the bird is connected to the ground electrode.

Interpretation of the ECG

Determination of Heart Rate

The marks are spaced so that they are three seconds apart at a 25 mm/s paper speed. To estimate heart rate per minute, the number of complexes that occur in three seconds are counted and multiplied by 20.

Determination of Heart Rhythm

- Is the heart rate normal or abnormal for the species (bradycardia or tachycardia)?
- Is the heart rhythm regular or irregular?
- Is there a P-wave for every QRS-complex, and is there a QRS-complex for every P-wave?
- Are the P-waves related to the QRS-complexes?
- Do all the P-waves and all the QRS-complexes look alike?

Determination of Mean Electrical Axis

The procedure for a rough estimation of the axis is simple and involves three steps:
- Find an isoelectric lead.
- Use the six-axis reference system chart and find which lead is perpendicular to the isoelectric lead (see Figure 27.5).

Table 27.1 Normal Electrocardiograms in Selected Birds

Parameter		Racing Pigeon	African Grey Parrot	Amazon Parrot
Normal heart rate		160-300	340-600	340-600
Normal heart rhythms		Normal sinus rhythm Sinus arrhythmia Second degree AV block	Normal sinus rhythm Sinus arrhythmia Ventricular premature beats Second degree AV block	
Normal heart axis		-83° to -99°	-79° to -103°	-90° to -107°
Normal measurements in lead II	P-wave duration Amplitude	0.015-0.020 s 0.4-0.6 mV	0.012-0.018 s 0.25-0.55 mV	0.008-0.017 s 0.25-0.60 mV
	PR-interval	0.045-0.070 s	0.040-0.055 s	0.042-0.055 s
	QRS complex duration R amplitude (Q)S amplitude	0.013-0.016 s 1.5-2.8 mV	0.010-0.016 s 0.00-0.20 mV 0.9-2.2 mV	0.010-0.015 s 0.00-0.65 mV 0.7-2.3 mV
	ST-segment		Very short or absent Elevation 0.1-0.3 mV No ST depression	
	T-wave	Always discordant to the ventricular complex		
		0.3-0.8 mV	0.18-0.6 mV	0.3-0.8 mV
	QT-interval Unanesthetized Anesthetized	0.060-0.075 s	0.039-0.070 s 0.048-0.080 s	0.038-0.055 s 0.050-0.095 s

• Determine if the perpendicular lead is positive or negative on the tracing and examine the angle value on the six axis reference system. Compare these values with reference values.

When all leads are isoelectric it is not possible to determine the heart axis and the heart is "electrically vertical."

Measuring

All measurements are made on the lead II rhythm strip. Measurements include the amplitude and the duration of the different electrocardiographic complexes (see Figure 27.3). The values found should be compared with the reference values.

P-Wave: With right atrial hypertrophy the P-wave becomes tall and peaked (P pulmonale), and with left atrial hypertrophy the P-wave becomes too wide (P mitrale). There is an increased number of P waves with tachycardia. P pulmonale has been associated with dyspnea induced by aspergillosis or tracheal obstruction. A tall, wide P-wave is suggestive of biatrial enlargement and is common with influenza virus in gallinaceous birds.

PR-Interval: In the normal pigeon ECG, a Ta-wave can be seen in the PR-segment, indicating repolarization of the atria. A small Ta may occur also in some asymptomatic parrots. This finding is considered normal and should not be interpreted as a sign of right atrial hypertrophy as it is in the dog.

QRS-Complex: Two measurements are made on the QRS-complex. The duration is measured from the beginning of the R-wave to the end of the S-wave. The second measurement is the amplitude of the S-wave, measured from the baseline downwards. Low voltage ECGs occur often in birds with pericardial effusion. A QRS-complex that is too wide or too tall indicates left ventricular hypertrophy. Prominent R-waves are suggestive for right ventricular hypertrophy.

ST-Segment: The ST-segment in the avian electrocardiogram is often short or absent. When present, it may be elevated above the baseline, which should not be interpreted as a sign of left ventricular hypertrophy, myocardial hypoxia, myocarditis or hypocalcemia as it is in the dog.

T-Wave: In the normal avian ECG, the T-wave is always in the opposite direction to the main vector of the ventricular depolarization complex, and always positive in lead II. When the T-wave changes its polarity, it suggests that myocardial hypoxia is occurring. The same is true for a T-wave that progressively increases in size (eg, during anesthesia). T-wave changes may also occur in association with electrolyte changes (eg, increased T-wave amplitude with hyperkalemia).

QT-Interval: Prolongation of the QT-interval might be associated with electrolyte disturbances like hypokalemia and hypocalcemia. In African Grey and Amazon parrots, the QT-interval was significantly ($P < 0.05$) prolonged during isoflurane anesthesia (see Table 27.1).

Arrhythmias

Sinus Arrhythmias

The normal rhythm of the heart is established by the SA node. A normal sinus rhythm does not vary in rate from beat to beat. An increase in vagal activity may decrease the heart rate, while a decrease in vagal activity may increase the heart rate. Heart rate may increase during inspiration and decrease during expiration and hence the S-S interval may not be equidistant. The associated rhythm is called sinus arrhythmia.

Sinus arrest is an exaggerated form of sinus arrhythmia and can be diagnosed if the pause is greater than twice the normal S-S interval. A sinoatrial block occurs when an electrical impulse from the sinoatrial node fails to activate the atria. The pauses are exactly twice the S-S interval. A continuous shifting of the pacemaker site in the SA node or the atrium, and hence a continuously changing configuration of the P-wave, is called wandering pacemaker. Sinus arrhythmia, sinus arrest, sinoatrial block and wandering pacemaker have been reported in association with normal respiratory cycles and are considered physiologic in birds.

Pathologic conditions that may induce sinus bradycardia and sinus arrest include hypokalemia, hyperkalemia, thiamine deficiency, and vitamin E deficiency. The conduction abnormalities (SA block, AV block) caused by potassium deficiencies can be corrected by administering atropine, suggesting that potassium increases vagal tone to the SA and AV nodes.

Several toxins have been reported to induce bradycardia, including organophosphorus compounds and polychlorinated biphenyls.

Reflex vagal bradycardia may occur when pressure is exerted on the vagus nerve by neoplasms, and space-occupying lesions impinging on the vagal nerve should be considered when unexplained atropine-responsive bradycardia is seen.

If the sinoatrial node is sufficiently depressed by vagal stimulation, another part of the conducting system may take over the pacemaker function and escape beats may occur. When an electrical impulse originates below the SA node in the atria the configuration of the P-wave will be abnormal, but positive in lead II. When an electrical impulse originates in fibers near the AV node (junctional beat), the P-wave may be absent or negative in lead II, indicating retrograde conduction. With ventricular beats the ectopic focus is localized in the fibers of the ventricle. The QRS complex is usually abnormal (but may be normal) and is unrelated to the P-wave. Atrioventricular nodal escape rhythm has been reported in ducks with sinus bradycardia induced by hyperkalemia.

Atrial Arrhythmias

Atrial tachycardias may be seen as a result of pathologic conditions of the atrium. Sinus tachycardia (two times normal) has been reported in chickens infected with avian influenza virus. When the heart rate is rapid, the P-wave may be superimposed on the T-wave (P on T phenomenon). This phonemenon has been recorded in 16% of normal Amazon parrots and in 6% of African Grey Parrots.

When (paroxysmal) supraventricular tachycardia is associated with valvular insufficiency, digoxin therapy is indicated. It is imperative to differentiate between junctional tachycardia (presence of negative P-waves due to retrograde impulse conduction) and ventricular tachycardia/atrioventricular dissociation (presence of normal P-waves that are usually not followed by a QRS complex; no retrograde impulse conduction to the atrium), because administration of digoxin may potentiate ventricular fibrillation in birds with ventricular arrhythmias.

Atrial fibrillation occurs when electrical impulses are generated in the atrium in a rapid and irregular way, and the atrium is in a state of permanent diastole. Impulses reach the AV node in a high frequency and at irregular intervals, and hence the ventricular rhythm is irregular. The ECG is characterized by the absence of normal P-waves, normal QRS complexes (which may have an increased amplitude and duration because of ventricular hypertrophy) and irregular S-S intervals. Instead of the normal P-waves, baseline undulations (F-waves) may be seen on the ECG.

Digoxin is considered the treatment of choice for atrial fibrillation, but the prognosis should be guarded because of the presence of marked cardiac pathology.

Ventricular Arrhythmias

Supraventricular tachycardias may originate from the sinoatrial node (sinus tachycardia), atrium (atrial tachycardia) or junctional area (junctional tachycardia). Differentiation between sinus tachycardia and atrial tachycardia may be accomplished by measuring the P-P interval. This interval is perfectly equidistant in atrial tachycardia but may be irregular in sinus tachycardia due to vagal effects. Junctional tachycardias can be diagnosed by the presence of inverted P-waves in lead II. The most common cause of sinus tachycardia is nervousness. But it is likely that stress, pain and other known causes of sinus tachycardia in dogs (eg, electrocution) may also precipitate the condition in birds.

Ventricular premature contractions (VPCs) are characterized by QRS complexes that are unrelated to the P-waves. Bigeminy is a rhythm characterized by alternating normal beats and premature contractions.

Ventricular premature contractions in birds have been associated with hypokalemia, thiamine deficiency, vitamin E deficiency, Newcastle disease and avian influenza viruses, myocardial infarction due to lead poisoning and digoxin toxicity.

The rhythm may be regular or irregular in birds with ventricular tachycardia. Positive P-waves can be identified in lead II at a lower frequency. Ventricular capture beats (normal P-QRS complexes in between abnormal PVCs) and ventricular fusion beats (a QRS-complex intermediate between a normal P-QRS complex and a bizarre QRS-complex that is formed by the simultaneous discharge of the ectopic ventricular focus and the normal AV node) are characteristic of ventricular tachycardia.

A special form of ventricular tachycardia is atrioventricular dissociation. In this condition, the atrial and ventricular rhythms are independent of each other, whereby the atrial rate is lower than the junctional or idioventricular rate.

VPCs, ventricular tachycardia and ventricular fibrillation may occur during periods of hypoxia and with the use of halothane. Changes in the configuration of the T-wave should alert the clinician that myocardial hypoxia is present and more severe ECG abnormalities are imminent.

Atrioventricular Node Arrhythmias

Conduction disturbances in the atrioventricular node may lead to various gradations of atrioventricular (AV) heart block. When the impulse through only the AV node is delayed, first degree AV block is present. In second degree AV block some impulses do not reach the ventricles, but the majority of P-waves are followed by a QRS-complex. Third degree AV block or complete heart block is characterized by independent activity of atria and ventricles, whereby the frequency of the atrial depolarizations is higher than the ventricular depolarizations.

First-Degree Heart Block

First-degree heart block has been reported as the result of the administration of various anesthetics such as halothane and xylazine, whereby the PR-interval may increase to three to four times its normal value. The condition is associated with severe bradycardia. Atropine may be used to prevent or reverse the condition.

Second-Degree Heart Block

Second-degree atrioventricular block Mobitz type 1 (Wenckebach phenomenon) has been reported as a physiologic phenomenon in five percent of trained racing pigeons and is seen occasionally in asymptomatic parrots and raptors. In this form of AV block the PR-interval lengthens progressively until a ventricular beat is dropped.

Second-degree AV blocks that can be corrected with atropine have been described in several avian species. This stimulatory effect of atropine on the avian heart suggests that this agent functions, as it does in mammals, to decrease parasympathetic tone to the SA and AV nodes.

Third-Degree Heart Block

Third-degree AV block is characterized by a slow ventricular (escape) rhythm. The ventricular complexes may have a normal configuration or may be idioventricular depending on the site of ventricular impulse formation. The condition should be differentiated from atrioventricular dissociation and ventricular tachycardia whereby there is also no relation between P-waves and QRS-complexes, but wherein the ventricular rate is higher than the atrial rate.

There are no reports on the clinical use of antiarrhythmic agents in avian medicine, and appropriate veterinary or human textbooks should be consulted for further information.

Effects of Anesthesia

General anesthesia is typically associated with a time-related and progressive decrease in heart rate and a corresponding decrease in blood pressure. Methoxyflurane and halothane are both cardiac depressants that sensitize the heart to catecholamines. Halothane, methoxyflurane and ketamine have been reported to cause a decrease in heart rate in some birds and an increase in heart rate in others. Xylazine, acepromazine and hypothermia have all been associated with bradycardia. Atropine can be used to increase the heart rate.

With halothane and methoxyflurane, respiratory and cardiac arrest routinely occur at the same time, and recovery from an anesthetic-induced cardiac arrest is rare. With isoflurane, respiratory arrest typically occurs several minutes before cardiac arrest. Birds with severe arrhythmias induced by an overdose of isoflurane may recover with appropriate intermittent partial pressure ventilation.

The increased PR-interval, first-degree AV block, decreased heart rate and conduction disturbances that occur with halothane anesthesia can be potentiated by the hypothermia that accompanies long-term anesthesia.

Cardiovascular Diseases

Congestive Heart Failure

The pathophysiology of congestive heart failure involves both backward failure and forward failure. Backward failure involves increased atrial and venous pressure due to a failing ventricle, while forward failure involves decreased renal blood flow resulting in sodium and fluid retention.

Pulmonary edema predominates in isolated left ventricular disease. Systemic edema with hepatomegaly and ascites will predominate in isolated right ventricular disease, or when both ventricles are affected.

In birds, the right AV valve (muscular flap) thickens along with the right ventricle in response to an increased workload, and it has been postulated that this predisposes birds to right AV valvular insufficiency and right-sided heart failure.

Clinical Findings

Heart enlargement with a thin left ventricular wall has been reported as a common occurrence in mynah birds. In one study, 12 of 12 mynah birds had an abnormally thin left ventricle and ascites. The predominant clinical sign in affected birds was dyspnea. The heart lesions were associated with liver fibrosis and end-stage iron storage disease.

Treatment

Once congestive heart failure has been diagnosed, the prognosis for long-term survival is guarded, because a specific therapy is not available. A significant prolongation of life, however, can be achieved by providing timely symptomatic treatment. Treatment of congestive heart failure in birds can best be accomplished with the loop diuretic furosemide. The dosage must be adjusted for the individual bird, but 1-2 mg/kg q12-24h is a general starting point. Response to therapy should be rapid and can be best monitored by weighing the patient daily to establish the degree of fluid loss. Dosages should be tapered down to the minimal effective dose, but continuous therapy is required to prevent recurrence of fluid retention.

Side effects of furosemide administration include hypovolemia and hypokalemia. The latter is especially important when diuretics are used together with cardiac glycosides, because these drugs may also lower plasma potassium concentrations. Hypokalemia may increase the frequency of rhythm disturbances induced by cardiac glycosides.

Cardiac glycosides are indicated in congestive heart failure, especially when accompanied by atrial fibrillation. Ventricular tachycardia may be a contraindication because digitalis may induce ventricular fibrillation in these cases. Cardiac glycosides increase the contractility of the heart muscle and delay conduction through the atrioventricular node that can be seen by prolongation of the PR-interval on the electrocardiogram. Arterial pressure, cardiac output and stroke volume are increased, while venous pressure is decreased. A decrease of the heart rate can be seen due to improvement of the circulation and parasympathetic (vagal) stimulation. Signs of toxicity include cardiac arrhythmias and gastrointestinal signs.

Any type of arrhythmia may result from digoxin poisoning. Digoxin therapy should be discontinued immediately if arrhythmias develop, and a lower dose regimen should be established. Diuretic-induced hypokalemia may precipitate digoxin-induced arrhythmias. Only limited information is available with regard to digoxin therapy in birds. A dose of 0.02 mg/kg daily was considered safe and produced satisfactory plasma levels of digoxin in parakeets and sparrows. A dose of 0.05 mg/kg/day was considered safe and produced adequate blood plasma levels in a Quaker Parrot (Monk Parakeet).

Recently, angiotensin converting enzyme (ACE) inhibitors, which reduce the formation of angiotensin II, have gained considerable popularity for the treatment of congestive heart failure in man. There are no reports of the use of these drugs for the treatment of congestive heart failure in birds, but it has been shown that inhibition of endogenous angiotensin II concentrations in quail by captopril can decrease natural water intake.

Vegetative Endocarditis

Endocarditis of the aortic and mitral valves may cause vascular insufficiency, lethargy and dyspnea. Valvular endocarditis is most common in birds with chronic infections (eg, salpingitis, hepatitis and bumblefoot) and has been reported in a large variety of avian species.

Lesions consist of yellow irregular masses on any of the heart valves. The disease is associated with bacteremia, and thromboembolisms may occur throughout the vasculature. Secondary lesions have been described in the liver, CNS, spleen, heart, lungs, kidneys, ischiatic artery and external iliac artery.

Clinical Findings

Valvular endocarditis and vascular insufficiency are frequently associated with lethargy and dyspnea, although the clinical presentation can vary.

Myocardial Diseases

Congenital Heart Disease

Spontaneous cardiovascular malformations like duplicitas cordis, multiplicatis cordis and ectopia cordis have been reported. Intraventricular septal defects are common, while foramen ovale persistence is of little clinical importance. Intraventricular septal defects are usually functionally closed, but in two percent of cases the condition is associated with congestive heart failure. Blood is shunted from left to right, which leads to right ventricular failure and ascites secondary to valvular insufficiency.

Acquired Diseases

In mammals, myocarditis can occur secondary to many common viral, bacterial, mycotic and protozoan infections. Cardiomyopathy has been associated with thyroid diseases, anemia, malnutrition, metabolic disorders, parasitic infections, pancreatitis, toxemias and neoplasia. The pathogenesis of cardiomyopathy and myocarditis in birds is similar to that described in mammals. The liver and myocardium can be sites of excessive iron storage in birds with hemochromatosis.

Fowl plague has been associated with myocardial lesions in a variety of avian species. Myocarditis has been reported as a component of neuropathic gastric dilatation in psittacines. Sarcocysts (muscle cysts containing bradyzoites, the asexual generation of *Sarcocystis* spp.) have been reported in the myocardium of a variety of avian species.

Spontaneous turkey cardiomyopathy (STC, round heart disease, cardiohepatic syndrome) in turkey poults one to four weeks of age is characterized by marked dilatation of the right ventricle with extreme thinning of the ventricular wall.

Myocardial degeneration (round heart disease) of unknown etiology has been described in backyard poultry. The morbidity is very low, but mortality may reach 50%. Lesions consist generally of an enlarged and yellowish heart. A few affected birds may have an excess of gelatinous fluid in the pericardial sac or peritoneal cavity. The disease should not be confused with STC.

Vitamin E and selenium deficiencies are well known as causes for cardiomyopathy in gallinaceous birds. Selenium and vitamin E deficiencies have also been suggested as causes for myocardial and skeletal muscle degeneration in ratites less than six months old that died after a brief period of depression (see Chapter 48). Vitamin E and selenium deficiencies have also been suggested as causes of myocardial degeneration in cockatiels. Affected birds typically have increased activities of SGOT and CPK, decreased heart tone and an increase in pericardial fluid.

Ruptures of the myocardium may occur secondary to degenerative, inflammatory or neoplastic conditions of the myocardium or aneurysms of the myocardial vessels. Myocardial infarctions may result from embolisms originating from valvular endocarditis or heavy metal poisoning.

All conditions that lead to cardiomyopathy or myocarditis may result in increased myocardial irritability and cardiac arrhythmias that can be detected by ECG. Radiographs may reveal cardiomegaly. Electrocardiography has been shown to be effective for diagnosing both spontaneous and furazolidone-induced cardiomyopathy. Characteristic changes include a right axis deviation from negative to positive, ie, from an average of -85 (range -60 to -120) to an average of 70 (range 32-95). The amplitude of the P-wave is increased and the T-wave is negative in leads I, II and III. Similar ECG findings have been reported in psittacine birds with cardiomyopathy.

Treatment of myocardial disease should be aimed at the primary cause. Furthermore, symptomatic treatment is indicated. Digoxin can be used when cardiac output is diminished due to myocardial disease, but is contraindicated when persistent ventricular arrhythmias are present. Digoxin treatment should be discontinued if the severity of an arrhythmia increases.

Epicardial and Pericardial Diseases

Pericardial effusion is a common finding in birds. The accumulated fluid may be a result of cardiac or systemic disease and may be of an inflammatory or noninflammatory nature. Transudates can occur with congestive heart failure and hypoproteinemia. Exudates may be present in a variety of infectious diseases. Fibrinous pericarditis is most common and may lead to adhesions of the epicardium to the pericardium and to constrictive heart failure.

Pericardial effusion may eventually result in heart failure. When a pericardial effusion develops rapidly, the circulatory system will not have time to compensate for the reduced cardiac output, and acute death occurs from cardiac tamponade.

Diagnostic techniques that may be of use in diagnosing pericardial effusion include radiography, electrocardiography, ultrasonography and endoscopy. Ultrasonography is a useful method to demonstrate a pericardial effusion. Electrocardiography may reveal a low voltage ECG.

Fluid for bacteriology, cytology and clinical chemistries can be collected from the pericardial sac, using endoscopy (see Chapter 13). Treatment for pericardial effusion should be both symptomatic and aimed at treating the underlying condition (eg, antibiotics in bacterial pericarditis). Symptomatic treatment can be attempted with furosemide. If sufficient quantities of nonserosanguinous pericardial fluid cannot be removed by conventional means to avoid the occurrence of cardiac tamponade, then it is necessary to create a surgical window in the pericardium.

Atherosclerosis

Atherosclerosis can be defined as a diffuse or local degenerative condition of the internal and medial tunics of the wall of muscular and elastic arteries. The lesions can macroscopically be identified by thickening and yellow discoloration of the arterial wall.

Atherosclerosis has been reported in many avian orders, but Psittaciformes (parrots) and Anseriformes (ducks and geese) appear to be particularly susceptible. Amazon parrots seem to be specifically prone to atherosclerosis, and age appears to be a risk factor.

In birds, atherosclerotic lesions are usually found in the brachiocephalic trunk and abdominal aorta. Lesions in the internal carotid arteries also occur with some frequency. Atherosclerotic lesions in the coronary artery are not as common in birds as in man, but have been reported.

Atherosclerosis and congestive heart failure should be considered in any geriatric patient with lethargy, dyspnea, coughing or abdominal swelling (ascites).

Clinical Changes

Clinical signs associated with atherosclerosis are caused by decreased blood flow through the affected vessels and plaque-induced thrombi that cause vascular accidents.

Clinical signs of atherosclerosis are rarely reported in birds, and the condition is often associated with sudden death; however, subtle and intermittent signs that include dyspnea, weakness and neurologic signs may be present. Regurgitation from an undocumented cause is common. Blood chemistry may reveal elevated plasma cholesterol. Radiologic examination may reveal an increased density and size of the right aortic arch. Nodular densities cranial to the heart may be caused by large arteries with atherosclerotic changes that are seen end on.

Galliformes and Anseriformes may die acutely from dissecting aneurysms that result in aortic rupture secondary to hypertension and atherosclerosis.

Aortic Rupture

Aortic rupture in turkeys is a condition associated with fatal hemorrhage from a ruptured aorta. The precise etiology is unknown, but the disease is associated with hypertension, degenerative changes of the aorta wall (atherosclerosis, qv), copper deficiency and high levels of protein and fat in the diet. Similar lesions may be induced in turkeys by ingestion of the sweet pea (*Lathyrus odoratus*).

NEUROLOGY

R. Avery Bennett

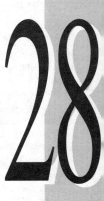

Two of the primary objectives in performing a neurologic examination are to determine if the neuropathy is focal or diffuse, and to localize focal lesions. The examination should be performed in a consistent, logical manner that starts with a complete history (see Chapter 8). Neuropathies are particularly common secondary to trauma, exposure to toxins and malnutrition. Subtle changes in cranial nerve function and abnormal reflexes are difficult to appreciate and interpret in birds. Assessment of segmental reflexes may be difficult in avian patients, making evaluation of muscle tone, strength and atrophy an essential part of the neurologic examination.

Neurologic evaluation of neonates is particularly difficult, and making a "side-by-side" comparison with a "normal" clutchmate is the best way to detect subtle changes. Useful tests include evaluation of the feeding response, menace reflex, use of wings to balance, vocalization, perching ability, pain perception and hopping response.

Mental Status

The patient's mental status and level of consciousness should be evaluated. The bird's ability to perform normal activities and its awareness of its surroundings should be assessed. It is difficult to differentiate between seizures and syncope based on the history; however, either may suggest an intracranial lesion.

Cranial Nerves

An evaluation of the cranial nerves may help localize a focal brain lesion (individual nerves involved) or a generalized encephalopathy (several nerves involved). Olfaction (CN I) is difficult to assess because birds have a poor sense of smell; however, most normal birds will react negatively to noxious odors (eg, alcohol pledget). Birds with CN I dysfunction may exhibit an altered appetite or feeding response.

Failure to avoid obstacles may indicate vision impairment. Bilateral blindness without ocular lesions may indicate neoplasm, abscess or granuloma formation in the brain. The menace reflex can be used to evaluate CN II and VII; however, depending on the circumstances, the absence of a menace response does not always indicate dysfunction of these cranial nerves. The pupillary light response evaluates CN II and III. Because there is complete decussation of the optic nerves at the chiasm, birds do not have a consensual pupillary light response.

Birds have some degree of voluntary control of pupil size because of skeletal muscles in the iris. Excited birds will voluntarily dilate and constrict their pupils. The presence of anisocoria may indicate dysfunction of CN III or a sympathetic neuropathy. Normal eye movements require the coordination of CN III, IV, VI and VIII as well as the cerebellum and brain stem. The presence of nystagmus or strabismus may indicate an abnormality in the vestibular systems. A fundic examination may be performed with the aid of d-tubocurarine. In some birds, intracameral injection of 0.045-0.09 mg d-tubocurarine chloride produces mydriasis within five minutes without systemic effects.

Cranial nerve V is responsible for facial sensation, movement of the mandible and blinking of the eyelids. Diminished beak strength may indicate an abnormality in CN V. Eye blink involves both CN V and VII. A defect in CN VIII will cause deafness or a head tilt toward the affected side. Cranial nerves IX through XII are involved in normal tongue movement, swallowing and beak strength. Dysfunction is manifested by dysphagia. Deviation of the tongue or atrophy of its muscles is observed with damage to CN XII.

Loss of normal physiologic nystagmus may occur with bilateral CN VIII lesions or with severe brain stem lesions. Altered consciousness is usually an accompanying sign with brain stem lesions. Abnormal, spontaneous nystagmus may result from vestibular lesions. Strabismus may indicate vestibular system dysfunction or a lesion in CN III, IV or VI.

Horner's syndrome may occur with intracranial lesions or with a lesion in the cervical sympathetic tract or the brachial plexus.

Locating Lesions

Reflexes are evaluated to help determine if a lesion is central (upper motor neuron) or peripheral (lower motor neuron). Pain perception in the wing requires intact peripheral nerves and the cervical spinal cord. Wing withdrawal is a segmental reflex that is present with intact peripheral nerves, but does not require an intact cervical spinal cord.

The patellar reflex is difficult to assess in birds; however, the withdrawal reflex is also a segmental reflex and should be intact with lesions affecting only the spinal cord.

Conscious proprioception requires an intact peripheral and central nervous system. A lesion in either will result in the bird's knuckling over. The vent response is a segmental reflex, and the sphincter should be responsive to stimulation if a spinal cord lesion is present and the nerve roots are not affected. A crossed extensor reflex generally indicates a lesion in the spinal cord with a loss of normal central inhibitory pathways.

With cervical spinal cord lesions, dysfunction of the wings, legs and cloaca may be observed while head function and cranial nerves appear normal. Weakness in the wings and legs with intact leg and wing withdrawal and vent response would be indicative of a cervical spinal cord lesion. Lesions affecting the thoracolumbar spinal cord will cause leg and cloacal dysfunction without affecting the head, cranial nerves or wings. Cloacal sphincter hypertonia, incontinence and soiling of the vent without signs of head, wing or leg dysfunction are indicative of a lumbosacral spinal cord lesion.

Loss of pain perception indicates a poor prognosis for recovery. It is crucial to differentiate pain perception from withdrawal reflex.

Diagnostic Techniques

The results of the neurologic examination will suggest which diagnostic tests should be performed. A CBC and serum chemistry profile are indicated if an infectious or metabolic neuropathy is considered. Laparoscopy and organ biopsy may be indicated to further define metabolic neuropathies. Serum for viral diseases or chlamydiosis, and blood levels for heavy metals are indicated in some cases. Radiographs are indicated if spinal trauma or heavy metal intoxication is suspected. TSH stimulation test may be helpful if hypothyroidism is suspected. Electromyograms, nerve conduction velocities, spinal evoked potentials and nerve or muscle biopsies are helpful in evaluating neuropathies.

Electrodiagnostics

When available, electrodiagnostic techniques are valuable in avian patients for distinguishing between a neuropathy and a myopathy, localization of neurologic lesions and determining the prognosis for return to normal function.

Neuropathies

Nutritional

Hypovitaminosis E and Selenium Deficiency

Vitamin E is a fat-soluble vitamin and depletion of body stores occurs slowly in adult birds, while young birds may develop clinical signs associated with acute deficiency. In young birds, hypovitaminosis E may cause encephalomalacia, exudative diathesis or muscular dystrophy. Encephalomalacia results in ataxia, head tilt, circling and occasionally convulsions and is particularly common in hatchling budgerigars. Exudative diathesis and muscular dystrophy (white muscle disease) occur also with deficiency of vitamin E or selenium. The myositis associated with hypovitaminosis E may cause clinical changes difficult to distinguish from neurologic signs.

Clinical signs associated with vitamin E and selenium deficiencies include tremors, ataxia, incoordination, abnormal head movements, reluctance to walk and recumbency. Postmortem findings suggestive of encephalomalacia include cerebellar edema or hemorrhage (petechia) with flattening of the convolutions.

Muscular dystrophy is characterized by light-colored streaks in the muscle fibers.

This deficiency has also been incriminated as the etiology of cockatiel paralysis syndrome. This condition appears to occur most frequently in lutino cockatiels infected with *Giardia* sp. or *Hexamita* sp. Vitamin E- and selenium-responsive neuropathies have been reported in a variety of other species including Blue and Gold Macaws, Severe Macaws, Eclectus Parrots and African Grey Parrots.

Clinical signs include slow or incomplete eye blink due to paresis of the lower eyelid, weak jaw muscles, paresis of the tongue, poor digestion with passage of partially digested food, diminished playful activity, hyperactivity, clumsiness and weak grip, low-pitched and weak vocalization, delayed crop-emptying, spraddle leg, death of young in nest, weak hatchlings, increased dead-in-shell, increased egg binding that is not responsive to vitamin A and calcium supplementation and decreased fertility. Cockatiels and other psittacine birds showing these clinical signs have responded to vitamin E and selenium supplementation and antiprotozoal therapy.

Vitamin E deficiency also occurs in piscivorous birds fed an unsupplemented diet of frozen fish (especially smelt). In birds of the family Ardeidae (herons and bitterns), the deficiency manifests initially as fat necrosis accompanied by steatitis. In pelicans, myodystrophy predominates.

Supplementation with injectable and oral vitamin E is the recommended treatment; however, the patient may or may not respond depending on the severity of damage. Muscular dystrophy may resolve with supplementation, but encephalomalacia rarely responds to therapy.

Hypovitaminosis B$_1$ (Thiamine)

Clinical signs of hypothiaminosis include anorexia, ataxia, ascending paralysis and opisthotonos. Opisthotonos ("star-gazing") may result from paralysis of the anterior muscles of the neck resulting in pseudo-hypertonus of the muscles of the dorsal aspect of the neck. Affected birds generally respond within hours of oral or parenteral administration of vitamin B$_1$. A response to treatment provides a presumptive diagnosis. Administration of thiamine is a useful adjunct to therapy in many nonspecific neurologic disorders.

Hypovitaminosis B$_2$ (Riboflavin)

Curled toe paralysis occurs in poultry and is seen in nestling budgerigars with riboflavin deficiency. Other signs include weakness, emaciation in the presence of a good appetite, diarrhea, walking on the hocks with toes curled inward and atrophy of leg muscles. Chicks fed a deficient diet may develop clinical signs as early as 12 days of age. Treatment involves administration of oral or parenteral riboflavin and diet correction; however, many of the changes are irreversible, especially in chronic cases.

Hypovitaminosis B$_6$ (Pyridoxine)

Neurologic signs associated with hypovitaminosis B$_6$ are characteristic, with the bird exhibiting a jerky, nervous walk progressing to running and flapping the wings. The bird then falls with rapid, clonic tonic head and leg movements. These convulsions are severe and may result in death due to exhaustion.

Hypovitaminosis B$_{12}$ (Cyanocobalamine)

Deficiency in a Nanday Conure was reported to cause subacute, multifocal white matter necrosis.

Traumatic

Concussion Lesions

Concussive head trauma is fairly common in free-ranging as well as companion and aviary birds. Injured birds may remain on the bottom of the enclosure and exhibit depression, head tilt, circling or paresis of a wing or leg. Blood may be present in the mouth, ears or anterior or posterior chamber of the eye. Anisocoria and delayed pupillary light response may be present and convulsions may occur if the bird is disturbed.

Fractures of the skull or scleral ossicles may be detected radiographically. In some cases, a bruise might be visualized on the head that is the result of meningeal hemorrhage seen through the cranium. Blood actually leaks into bone and is not subdural. It is very rare for hemorrhage to occur within the brain parenchyma. Unconsciousness with a loss of normal physiologic nystagmus indicates a brainstem lesion with a poor prognosis.

Treatment is supportive and involves maintaining the bird in a dark, quiet, cool area with no disturbances. Dexamethasone appears to be the most important therapeutic agent. The prognosis is guarded-to-poor if the bird is convulsing.

Compressive Lesions

Jugular stasis occurs secondary to thyroid enlargement and results in increased intracranial pressure. Hydrocephalus and intracranial masses cause compressive injury to the brain or spinal cord. With hydrocephalus, the cortex over the lateral ventricles has a "blister-like" appearance at necropsy. Imaging techniques (CT or MRI) and EEG studies may be helpful in diagnosing these conditions.

Spinal Abnormalities

Spinal fractures may be the result of injury or metabolic bone disease and may cause compression of the spinal cord. Tumors may affect the spinal cord by direct invasion or compression. MRI, CT scans and scintigraphy are useful imaging modalities for identifying these lesions, which may not be visible with plain radiographs, especially in the acute phase.

The junction of the fixed synsacrum with the more flexible portion of the thoracolumbar spine is a location susceptible to mechanical stress and vertebral subluxation.

The intervertebral discs of birds differ from those of mammals. They consist of a fibrocartilaginous central region surrounded by a "C"-shaped synovial cavity that extends around the dorsal and lateral margins of the disc. A fibrocartilaginous, wedge-shaped meniscus protrudes into the joint cavity from the dorsal and lateral margins. This zygapophyseal joint has hyaline cartilage with an intervening synovial cavity. With intervertebral disc rupture, this meniscus is driven into the spinal canal along with the fibrocartilaginous disc material.

Dexamethasone and forced rest are the only recommended therapies for birds with spinal lesions. Myelography and spinal surgery have rarely been performed in birds.

Peripheral Nervous System

Trauma

Concussive peripheral nerve trauma occurs as a result of long bone fractures or impact trauma. In many instances, nerve dysfunction is transient; however, as in the case of brachial plexus avulsion, the damage may be permanent.

Brachial plexus avulsion occurs most commonly in traumatized free-ranging birds. Clinically, there is evidence of denervation of the affected wing including lack of pain perception, paralysis with loss of withdrawal reflex and atrophy of the muscles of the affected wing and the ipsilateral pectoral muscles. Signs of Horner's syndrome may be present including ptosis and a dropped "horn" on the affected side of "horned" owls such as Screech and Great Horned Owls. Because of the skeletal muscle in the avian iris, miosis is not a consistent feature of Horner's syndrome. Interruption of the sympathetic pathway from T_1 and occasionally T_2 segments results in these clinical signs.

A long bone fracture may or may not be associated with peripheral nerve injuries. Typically, birds with neurapraxia improve clinically within two to four weeks, while those with axonotmesis and neurotmesis (as with avulsion injury) would not. EMG and spinal-evoked potentials can help determine the degree of injury. If these are not available, it is prudent to treat with supportive care for approximately one month, with weekly evaluation for signs of improved neurologic function.

Abdominal Masses

Compressive peripheral nerve trauma generally occurs secondary to an expanding mass that applies pressure to the nerve. Because the pelvic nerves pass through the renal parenchyma, tumors or infection of the kidneys can damage the nerves. Ovarian tumors, if very large or invasive, have also been reported to damage these nerves. Of 74 budgerigars with abdominal tumors, 64 had paresis of one or both legs. Paresis is usually unilateral in the early stages and is accompanied by abdominal distention.

Egg binding or internal trauma associated with oviposition may result in hemorrhage and swelling around the area of the pelvic plexus, causing a transient paresis or paralysis secondary to neurapraxia.

Circulatory Disturbances

Both peripheral and central neuropathies have been associated with diminished circulation. Atherosclerosis occurs with some degree of frequency in birds. Most commonly, no clinical signs are associated with this condition, and affected birds are simply found dead in their enclosure. In some cases, however, neurologic signs may be observed. Atherosclerosis of the carotid arteries has been described as a cause of ischemia and cerebral hypertension.

Neurologic signs associated with atherosclerosis include a sudden onset of blindness, ataxia, paresis and seizures.

Signs ranging from blindness and ataxia to opisthotonos and seizures have been associated with cerebrovascular accidents and ischemic infarction. MRI, CT scans and EEG may be useful in diagnosing these lesions.

Primary Neoplasms of the Nervous System

Glioblastoma multiforme, choroid plexus tumors, Schwannomas and astrocytomas, pineal body tumors, undifferentiated sarcomas and hemangiomas have been described in the nervous system of companion birds. Clinical signs vary with the location of the neoplasm. Imaging with MRI or CT may be useful in determining the location of the mass; however, all neural tumors are associated with a grave prognosis. Phenobarbital for control of seizures and dexamethasone to decrease cerebrospinal fluid production (thus, intracranial pressure) may provide symptomatic relief.

Pituitary adenoma or pituitary chromophobe adenoma occurs in young (four years old), predominantly male budgerigars with a two to three percent prevalence. These tumors are reported to cause a classic clinical syndrome described as somnolence with occasional convulsions, uncoordinated wing-flapping and clonic leg twitches, followed by unconsciousness. Clinical signs are usually the result of compression of the brain and cranial nerves. Incoordination, tremors and inability to perch have also been reported. Polydipsia and polyuria, cere color change, feather abnormalities and obesity may occur with functional tumors. Exophthalmos, visual deficits, lack of pupillary light response and mydriasis may be present also.

A tentative diagnosis may be confirmed with contrast-enhanced CT scanning of the skull.

Metabolic Neuropathies

Hepatic Encephalopathy

Birds with severe liver disease may demonstrate signs of hepatic encephalopathy. Hepatic lipidosis, mycotoxicosis, hemochromatosis and vaccine-induced hepatopathy have been reported to cause clinical signs of depression, ataxia, diminished conscious proprioception and seizures. With hepatic encephalopathy, these signs usually occur shortly after eating when the blood levels of neurotoxins absorbed from the gastrointestinal tract (and not properly processed by the liver) are high.

Postprandial blood ammonia concentrations may be elevated and can be determined using a conspecific control bird.

Treatment should be directed toward the underlying cause of hepatic failure. Lactulose syrup and a low-protein, high-carbohydrate, high-quality protein diet with a vitamin supplement may provide symptomatic relief while the underlying hepatopathy is corrected. Neomycin sulfate may decrease the formation of ammonia by reducing the quantity of gram-negative bacteria in the colon.

Hypocalcemia

A syndrome characterized by opisthotonos, tonic extension of the limbs and convulsions has been described in young (two- to five-year-old) African Grey Parrots. Initially, an affected bird may seem only uncoordinated and fall from its perch. Eventually, seizure activity is pronounced and may become constant or prolonged. Serum calcium levels are below 6.0 mg/dL with concentrations as low as 2.4 mg/dL reported. Birds demonstrating only intermittent incoordination may still have normal serum calcium levels. This condition has also been observed in Amazon parrots and conures.

At necropsy, the parathyroid glands of affected African Grey Parrots are grossly enlarged, presumably in response to the low serum calcium concentrations.

The etiology and pathogenesis of this condition remains speculative. Affected birds are usually wild-caught and are maintained on a diet deficient in calcium and vitamin D_3 (usually a whole-seed diet). Vitamin A deficiency may also play a role, as hypovitaminosis A has been shown to inhibit osteoclast activity.

Diazepam may be used as an anticonvulsant, but birds generally rapidly respond to the parenteral administration of calcium gluconate. Corticosteroids should not be used in these patients because they increase urinary excretion and decrease intestinal absorption of calcium.

Once the serum calcium concentration has returned to within normal limits, the patient should be placed on a proper diet with calcium and vitamin supplementation. Foods such as dairy products should be encouraged, while those high in fat such as seeds should be eliminated. Serum calcium concentration should be evaluated periodically (every two to four months) to determine if alterations in therapy are indicated. The prognosis for full recovery appears to depend on the severity of damage to the parathyroid glands.

Because it appears that these birds cannot mobilize body stores of calcium, long-term prevention of recurring problems requires that birds receive adequate levels of calcium in proper balance with phosphorus, as well as sufficient levels of vitamins A, D_3 and E.

Hypoglycemia

Hypoglycemia may occur as a result of starvation or malnutrition, hepatopathy, endocrinopathies and septicemia. Blood glucose less than 150 mg/dL (or half the species' normal value) may be an indication of hypoglycemia. Seizure activity usually occurs once the blood glucose level falls below 100 mg/dL. Therapy should consist of 1.0 ml/kg IV of a 50% dextrose solution for acute relief of clinical signs, while the underlying cause of the problem is being determined and corrected. Dextrose solutions (>2.5%) should be administered intravenously with caution because they are hypertonic and may cause tissue damage if perivascular leaking occurs. Dextrose will compromise a patient's acid-base balance and should not be used in dehydrated birds.

Table 28.1   Common Causes of Seizures in Birds

- Nutritional (Calcium, phosphorus and vitamin D_3 imbalances, vitamin E and selenium deficiencies, thiamine deficiency, hypovitaminosis B_6)
- Metabolic (Heat stress, hypocalcemia, hypoglycemia, hepatic encephalopathy)
- Toxic (Heavy metals, insecticides)
- Infectious (Bacterial, fungal or parasitic meningitis or encephalitis)
- Traumatic
- Neoplastic
- Hypocalcemia (African Grey Parrots)
- Hypoglycemic (Raptors)

Seizures and Idiopathic Epilepsy

A typical seizure may consist of a short period of disorientation with ataxia followed by falling to the enclosure floor as a result of the loss of the ability to grip the perch. The bird may remain rigid or have major motor activity for a few seconds or a few minutes.

Idiopathic Epilepsy

Idiopathic epilepsy is used as a diagnosis when other causes of seizures have been ruled out. A syndrome of idiopathic epilepsy has been described in Red-lored Amazon Parrots that has been suggested to have a genetic basis. Seizures of undetermined cause occur with some degree of frequency in Greater Indian Hill Mynahs as well. Mild-to-severe seizure activity may occur in these birds with signs ranging from "periodic trance-like states" and "stiffening up" to grand mal-type seizures.

Diazepam can be used to temporarily interrupt seizure activity. Long-term phenobarbital at a dose of 4.5-6.0 mg/kg PO q12h titrated to effect, appears to be beneficial in reducing the frequency and severity of seizures in these birds. Blood phenobarbital concentration should be determined approximately one month after institution of therapy to evaluate the dosage.

Lafora Body Neuropathy

Lafora body neuropathy has been reported as a cause of fine, continuous myoclonus in one cockatiel and weakness, anorexia and dyspnea in another cockatiel. This disease is characterized by the formation of glycoprotein-containing cytoplasmic inclusion bodies within neurons. This accumulation of glyco-proteins is believed to be the result of a defect in intracellular metabolism.

Xanthomatosis

Xanthomatosis may affect the brain where it appears in association with blood vessels.

Toxic Neuropathies

Heavy Metals

Lead and zinc poisoning are the most common causes of toxicity in birds (see Chapter 37). In addition to common sources of lead contamination, chronic exposure to automobile exhaust has been shown to contribute to the cumulative lead concentrations in body tissues.

Lead adversely affects all body systems by inhibiting enzyme activity and protein formation. Nervous, digestive and hematopoietic systems are most affected. Neurologic changes suggestive of plumbism include lethargy, depression, weakness, ataxia, paresis, paralysis, loss of voice, head tilt, blindness, circling and seizures.

Botulism (Limber Neck)

Botulism in birds is usually the result of ingestion of the exotoxin of *Clostridium botulinum* type C. Botulism is uncommon in companion birds, but occurs with some degree of frequency in waterfowl.

Intoxication occurs following ingestion of contaminated food such as necrotic tissue (plant or animal) or dipterous maggots and other invertebrates. Maggots concentrate the toxin without being affected.

The toxin interferes with the release of acetylcholine at motor endplates causing signs of peripheral neuropathy. All peripheral nerves, including cranial nerves, are affected. The classic clinical sign is a limber neck resulting from paralysis of the cervical musculature. Most birds exhibit hindlimb paresis first, which is characterized by sitting on their sternum with legs extended behind their body. Paralysis of the wings followed by loss of control of the neck and head are observed in the terminal stages. Green diarrhea with pasting of the vent are also common with botulism. Inconsistent clinical findings with botulism are chemosis, swelling of the eyelids and nictitans, ocular discharge and hypersalivation.

Therapy is primarily supportive. Cathartics, laxatives and drenches are used to flush unabsorbed toxins through the gastrointestinal tract. Tube-feeding provides nutritional support for birds that are unable to eat and drink. Antitoxin may be administered intraperitoneally, but it is not commercially available and its benefits are equivocal.

Pesticides

The United States Environmental Protection Agency has registered 36 different organophosphate and 46 carbamate compounds such as carbaryl (Sevin dust), dursban (chloropyrifos), diazanon, malathion, dichlorvos and methyl carbamate. Both of these compound classes are acetylcholinesterase inhibitors that bind to and subsequently inactivate acetylcholinesterase causing an accumulation of acetylcholine at the postsynaptic receptors. Organophosphate bonds are considered irreversible, while carbamate bonds are slowly reversible (spontaneous decay in several days).

Birds are 10-20 times more susceptible to these acetylcholine inhibitors than mammals. Young birds and males are also more susceptible. The development of clinical signs is dependent on the concentration of the pesticide, the route and proximity of exposure, the amount of ventilation, the species of bird and its physical condition.

Acutely, clinical signs are related to excessive stimulation of acetylcholine receptors. Signs include anorexia, crop stasis, ptyalism, diarrhea, weakness, ataxia, wing twitching and muscle tremors, opisthotonos, seizures, bradycardia and prolapse of the nictitans. Bradycardia and dyspnea with crackles and wheezes may occur as the toxicosis progresses. Respiratory failure is usually the cause of death and results from increased mucus secretion, bronchoconstriction and paralysis of respiratory musculature.

The second type of neuropathy is an organophosphate ester-induced neuropathy, which is not associated with an inhibition of acetylcholine. The onset of clinical signs is delayed (7-21 days after exposure) and is the result of a symmetric distal primary axonal degeneration of the central and peripheral nervous systems, with secondary myelin degeneration. Clinical signs include weakness, ataxia, decreased proprioception and paralysis.

Diagnosis of acetylcholinesterase inhibition is usually based on clinical signs and a history of exposure to these compounds. Cholinesterase assay may be performed on blood, plasma, serum or brain tissue. A decrease in acetylcholinesterase of 50% from normal is considered diagnostic. Normal avian plasma cholinesterase levels are reported to be greater than 2000 IU/L. A new cholinesterase test requires only 0.01 ml of serum and results may be available in five minutes.

Intoxication is best treated with atropine, pralidoxime chloride (2 PAM) and supportive care (see Chapter 37).

The exact mechanism of action of organochloride insecticides, such as DDT, is unknown, but clinical signs are usually neuromuscular, resulting from either stimulation or depression of the central nervous system. There is no known antidote for organochloride intoxication. Birds with seizures or other signs of CNS stimulation should be tranquilized or lightly anesthetized with a long-acting agent such as phenobarbital. In cases of CNS depression, stimulants may be beneficial. Cathartics, activated charcoal and general supportive care should be provided as necessary (see Chapter 37).

Therapeutic Agents

Dimetridazole was commonly used to treat trichomoniasis, giardiasis and histomoniasis. Toxicity results in birds with increased water consumption (increased intake of drug). Convulsions, wing flapping and opisthotonos have been reported in budgerigars, goslings, pigeons and ducks.

Other Neurotoxins

Citreoviridin and tremorgens are two types of mycotoxins that primarily affect the neural system. Fusariotoxins and ochratoxins also produce nervous disorders. A syndrome characterized by cervical paresis in free-ranging Sandhill Cranes has been associated with mycotoxicosis.

Domoic acid poisoning was diagnosed as the cause of death in Brown Pelicans and Brandt's Cormorants exhibiting neurologic signs. Twenty-seven of 39 affected birds died within 24 hours. Domoic acid is a neurotoxin produced by marine diatoms. It is an excitatory toxin that binds to both pre- and postsynaptic kainate receptors in the brain, resulting in continuous depolarization of neurons until cell death occurs. It was theorized that this epornitic was caused by the ingestion of contaminated anchovies, which had fed on the diatoms.

Infectious Neuropathies

Fungal

The nervous system may be a secondary site for aspergillosis lesions that may cause ataxia, opisthotonos and paralysis. In infected birds, yellowish, mycotic nodules may be grossly visible within the brain or spinal canal. Fungal granulomas may compress or invade peripheral nerves and cause unilateral or bilateral paresis or paralysis.

Parasitic

Toxoplasma

Toxoplasma gondii infections are reported primarily in Galliformes and Passeriformes with lesions involving the brain and skeletal muscles. Cats are the only host known to excrete infectious oocysts. Considering avian species, it would seem that raptors are most likely to become infected because they prey on the same types of animals as cats. Although toxoplasmosis has been reported in raptors, they appear to be more resistant to infection than other birds.

Clinical signs include anorexia, pallor, diarrhea, blindness, conjunctivitis, head tilt, circling and ataxia. Infection may occur from ingestion of coprophagic arthropods or food and water supplies contaminated with feces from infected cats. A definitive diagnosis is made using a latex agglutination serum test or immunohistochemical staining of affected tissues.

In canaries and finches, toxoplasmosis has been shown to cause loss of myelinated axons in the optic nerve resulting in blindness and conjunctivitis.

Sarcocystis

Sarcocystis infection has been reported in over 60 species of birds, with Old World psittacines apparently more susceptible (see Chapter 36). It is believed that cockroaches and flies may be transport hosts for the parasite. Raptorial species may become infected by ingestion of prey containing the encysted organism.

Schistosomiasis

Granulomatous encephalitis caused by the blood fluke *Dendritobilharzia* sp. has been reported in swans. Neurologic signs included head tilt, circling, weakness and extension of the head and neck.

Baylisascaris sp.

Baylisascaris procyonis is the ascarid of raccoons and is a zoonotic organism that can cause fatal meningoencephalitis in humans. Free-ranging birds are infected by ingesting raccoon feces, while companion birds may become infected by ingestion of food contaminated with parasite eggs. The eggs may remain viable and infective in the environment for years.

Clinical signs are nonspecific and include depression, ataxia and torticollis. The onset may be acute or chronic, possibly related to the number of larvae involved. Treatment with ivermectin has been completely ineffective.

Filaria

Chandlerella quiscali is a filariid nematode of grackles that has been reported to cause cerebrospinal nematodiasis in emus. Gnats are the vectors for natural infection. The gnat is ingested and the larvae migrate into the brain or spinal cord and then into the lateral ventricles of the cerebrum where they mature and produce microfilaria. Affected emu chicks demonstrated torticollis, ataxia, recumbency and death. Circulating microfilaria were not detected (see Chapter 36).

Viral Neuropathies

Paramyxovirus

Clinical signs associated with PMV-1 in companion birds are variable depending on the virulence of the strain and the species of bird affected. In some cases, the only signs may be acute death and high mortality. Other signs are associated with abnormalities of the respiratory, digestive and nervous systems.

Neurologic signs including depression, hyperexcitability, ataxia, incoordination, torticollis, head tremor, opisthotonos, muscle tremors and unilateral or bilateral wing or leg paresis or paralysis occur more commonly in older birds and with chronic infections. Some birds clench their feet while others lose control of the tongue and their ability to grip with the beak.

All reflexes are depressed but neurologic signs are exacerbated by excitement. Seizures and running movements are often observed just prior to death. Neurologic signs generally persist in birds that survive the acute infection.

At necropsy, there may be petechiae on the surface of the cerebrum and cerebellum.

Neuropathic Gastric Dilatation

There is strong evidence that neuropathic gastric dilatation (proventicular dilatation) is caused by a virus. Anorexia, regurgitation, changes in fecal consistency, weight loss, pectoral muscle atrophy and depression are presenting clinical signs. The clinical signs of this disease primarily relate to the gastrointestinal system, with central and peripheral neurologic signs occurring only occasionally. However, the main histologic lesions involve the nervous system.

Avian (Picornavirus) Encephalomyelitis

This picornavirus has been associated with gastrointestinal and neurologic signs in Galliformes, Anseriformes and Columbiformes. Only one serotype is recognized but strains vary in neurotropism. Clinical signs include depression, ataxia, paresis or paralysis, and severe but fine head and neck tremors. Neurologic signs occur only in birds less than 28 days of age.

Polyomavirus (Budgerigar Fledgling Disease)

Although not the primary lesions, tremors of the head, neck and limbs, incoordination and ataxia have been associated with polyomavirus in infected birds.

Reovirus

Reovirus is commonly reported in imported birds and primarily affects African Greys, cockatoos and other Old World Psittaciformes. Clinical signs include uveitis, depression, emaciation, anorexia, incoordination, ataxia, paresis and diarrhea.

Togaviridae

Clinical signs of togaviridae infection include depression, ruffled feathers, decreased appetite, dyspnea, profuse hemorrhagic diarrhea (in emus), ataxia, muscle tremors, weakness, unilateral or bilateral paresis or paralysis, torticollis and death. At necropsy, the cerebral hemispheres may be softened. Vaccines are available and appear to be beneficial in outbreaks.

Marek's Disease

Marek's disease, a lymphoproliferative disease, is caused by a herpesvirus. Peripheral nerve dysfunction occurs secondary to lymphoid infiltrates. Often birds display spraddle leg paralysis with one leg extended forward and the other back. Grossly, the ischiatic nerves appear gray and enlarged with a loss of striations.

Encephalomyelitis in Lorikeets

Encephalomyelitis was described in free-ranging Australian lorikeets. Affected birds demonstrated a progressive bilateral paralysis with clenched feet. A viral or protozoal etiology has been suggested.

Duck Viral Enteritis

Duck viral enteritis is primarily a concern where feral populations of ducks mingle with captive birds. Clinical signs include photophobia, ataxia, seizures, penile prolapse, lethargy, hemorrhagic diarrhea, and serosanguinous nasal discharge. The most notable finding at necropsy is hemorrhagic bands on small intestine.

Duck Viral Hepatitis

Duck viral hepatitis is caused by a picornavirus. Clinical signs include lethargy, seizures, opisthotonos and death. Ducklings suffer the highest mortality, and Muscovy Ducks appear to be resistant to infection with this virus. At necropsy, the liver, spleen and kidneys are enlarged with petechial hemorrhages. It is recommended to vaccinate breeders before the onset of laying.

Bacterial Neuropathies

Listeriosis

Intracranial listeriosis infections cause opisthotonos, ataxia and torticollis. Brain lesions consist of microabscesses.

Chlamydiosis

Occasionally, *Chlamydia psittaci* will cause neurologic signs in birds that survive the acute respiratory or gastrointestinal phase of the disease. Signs include seizures, torticollis, tremors and opisthotonos (see Chapter 34).

Granulomas

Avian tuberculosis can cause neurologic signs if the granulomas occur intracranially or adjacent to peripheral nerves. Osteomyelitis caused by mycobacterium may produce a lameness that could be misinterpreted as a neuropathy. Abscesses, granulomas, encephalitis, myelitis and meningitis may be caused by any bacterial organism. *Salmonella, Streptococcus, Staphylococcus, Pasteurella multocida, Mycoplasma* and *Clostridium* spp. have been isolated. Clinical signs depend on the location and extent of the lesions.

Otitis

Otitis media and interna in companion birds may cause neurologic signs. Otitis interna produces a head tilt and circling toward the affected side.

THERIOGENOLOGY

Kim L. Joyner

Female Reproductive Anatomy and Egg Formation

Ovary

The normal reproductive tract of a mature hen consists of a left ovary and oviduct. The left ovary is located at the cranial end of the kidney and is attached to the abdominal wall by the mesovarian ligament. In young birds the ovary is flattened, in an inverted "L"-shape. It has nearly inappreciable folds and resembles a piece of fat. As birds mature and the gyri become more prominent, small primary oocytes give the ovary a cobblestone appearance. This process occurs by about 25 weeks of age in Blue and Gold Macaws. Ovarian tissue can be more or less melanistic, especially in cockatoos, macaws and some conures. As the breeding season approaches, the follicles undergo a period of rapid growth with the deposition of yolk proteins and lipid produced by the liver. At this point the yellow yolk is clearly visible through the highly vascularized follicular wall.

During the nonbreeding season, the ovarian follicles normally collapse and exhibit atresia. Two kinds of atresia have been described. Bursting atresia occurs when the follicle wall ruptures and yolk is harmlessly released into the peritoneal cavity where it is absorbed. Invasion atresia involves granulosa and theca cells invading the ovum with subsequent *in situ* yolk absorption.

Oviduct

The oviduct consists of five microscopically distinguishable regions: infundibulum, magnum, isthmus, uterus (shell gland) and vagina. Dorsal and ventral ligaments attach the oviduct in the peritoneal cavity. In psittacine birds, the dorsal ligament is clearly visible crossing the cranial division of the kidney.

The cranial infundibulum consists of a thin, nearly transparent finger-like funnel that engulfs the ovum into an ovarian pouch. More distally, the infundibular wall thickens as it becomes tubular. Fertilization occurs in the tubular portion of the infundibulum, where sperm may reside in glandular grooves awaiting the arrival of the ovum. Production of the chalaziferous layer of the albumen and the paired chalazae occurs also in the tubular portion of the infundibulum. Less than an hour later, the ovum exits the infundibulum and enters the highly glandular magnum that is differentiated from the infundibulum by its sudden enlargement in the mucosal folds. It is the largest and most coiled portion of the oviduct and deposits most of the albumen, sodium, magnesium and calcium used in egg development. The egg may remain in the magnum for three hours. Inner and outer shell membranes are added to the developing egg during its one to two hours in the isthmus.

The short uterus has numerous leaf-like lamellae composed of longitudinal folds, consisting of prominent longitudinal muscles and underlying tubular gland cells. This part of the uterus is ovoid in shape and holds the egg during shell deposition. The egg remains in the uterus for 20-26 hours and receives salts, water, the shell and shell pigment. The uterus is highly vascularized during egg laying and must be carefully manipulated during any surgical procedure to prevent excessive hemorrhage (see Chapter 40 for considerations prior to performing uterine surgery).

The S-shaped vagina is the thickest walled portion of the oviduct; it begins at the uterovaginal sphincter muscle and terminates in the cloaca. The vagina does not contribute to the formation of the egg, which passes through the vaginal lumen in seconds during normal oviposition.

Female Hormonal and Physiologic Factors

Developing ovarian follicles consist of concentric layers of yolk, the oocyte, perivitelline lamina, granulosa cells, basal lamina and theca. Ovarian thecal and interstitial cells produce estrogen while the granulosa cells produce progesterone. Increasing concentrations of circulating estrogen stimulate an LH surge that is responsible for the continuation of meiosis two hours before ovulation. At this time, LH causes extrusion of the first polar body, the follicular wall ruptures and ovulation occurs. Extrusion of the second polar body occurs in the infundibulum, and the ovum is formed. The remaining granulosa cells of the ruptured follicle are under the control of LH and prolactin. These cells continue to produce progesterone, which inhibits further ovulation and induces behavioral and physiologic changes associated with incubation and brood care.

In photoperiodic species, day length changes may terminate reproduction; however, in most species a photorefractory state develops that is controlled at the level of the hypothalamus. Long day length as a stimulus is blocked, and serum gonadotropin and gonadal steroid hormones decrease to minimum levels. Photorefractoriness is then terminated by shorter daylight periods.

Hypothalamic control of reproduction is influenced by environmental factors other than light, especially in periodic breeders of equatorial climates. In arid-dwelling species, such as the budgerigar and Zebra Finch, the rostral pituitary is constantly stimulated by the hypothalamus to release gonadotropins except when inhibited by negative external conditions such as drought. During these dry conditions when food would be scarce, the hypothalamic secretions suppress reproductive activity.

In psittacine birds, the laying interval is generally two days. In most Passeriformes, lay intervals are 24 hours, but they can extend up to four to five days in the Andean Condor and up to 44 days in the Brown Kiwi. If progesterone is used to prevent egg laying, it should be administered when a complete clutch has been laid. Premature administration can cause an abnormal ovulatory process that may lead to soft-shelled eggs, mummification, peritonitis and death.

Ovum transport in the oviduct is primarily accomplished by contractions of the oviduct in response to a stretch stimulus. Prostaglandins, which contract the smooth muscle of the oviduct and vagina, may also influence egg transport and expulsion. Arginine vasotocin released by the posterior pituitary stimulates uterus contractility *in vitro*, but it is not clear what role it plays in oviposition. The effect of oxytocin, also produced by the posterior pituitary, in inducing premature oviposition may be mediated *in vivo* by prostaglandins. It is likely that oviposition is a complicated process involving neurohypophyseal hormones, prostaglandins and hormones of the pre- and postovulatory follicles.

Calcium Metabolism

Estrogen increases total plasma calcium by increasing the production of blood calcium-binding proteins. During the laying process in psittacine birds, the calcium levels can become extremely high, reaching levels of 30 mg/dL. Increased intestinal absorption and bone mobilization of calcium are needed to constantly replenish blood calcium in active psittacine hens. For psittacine birds, it is recommended that laying hens be offered at least 0.3% calcium (1:1 or 2:1 ratio with phosphorous) in their diet to prevent bone mobilization, but no more than 1% to ensure that egg shells are not excessively thick.

Calcification of the medullary spaces of the long bones, particularly the femur and tibia, occurs in female birds approximately ten days before egg formation. In budgerigars, the primary sites of medullary calcification are the humerus and femur. If insufficient calcium is consumed, cortical bone will be mobilized. At some point in the mobilization process, calcium deficiency causes a reduction in FSH secretion that stops the laying process. High-fat, low-calcium diets exacerbate a calcium deficiency by decreasing calcium absorption from the intestines. In budgerigars, it is theorized that polyostotic hyperostosis in nonlaying females results from aberrant estrogen metabolism. Affected budgerigar hens have been shown to have normal ovaries and no evidence of hormone-secreting tumors or other endocrine diseases. The liver is responsible for inactivating estrogens, and it has been suggested that impaired liver function may be responsible for this disease.

Other Metabolic Changes

Hematogenic changes associated with egg laying include a slight increase in white blood cell count, packed cell volume, total serum solids and total protein. Alkaline phosphatase levels may also increase due to estrogen stimulation.

Egg Structure and Physiology

Understanding normal egg anatomy allows the clinician to recognize abnormalities and instigate appropriate therapeutic or preventive measures to resolve embryonic death problems and female reproductive disorders.

The germinal disc is a small, circular, opaque white spot on the surface of the yolk that contains cytoplasm and the oocyte. The yolk is classified as either "white" or "yellow" and is layered in strata that are visible when stained with potassium dichromate. The yolk is 50% solids, 99% of which are proteins. Maternal antibodies (IgG) are present in the yolk. It has been demonstrated that vaccinated hens pass anti-PBFD virus antibodies to their chicks and that these antibodies wane to undetectable levels between 30 and 45 days of age.

The albumen is made of the chalaziferous layer, chalazae, and inner, middle and outer layers. At the blunt end of the egg the two shell membranes separate from each other, forming the air cell. The outer layer is adhered to the testa layer of the shell and the inner layer is attached to the dense portion of the albumen. The outermost surface of the egg is covered by a thin, sometimes waxy, cuticle. Microscopic pores in the egg shell allow for passive diffusion of oxygen, carbon dioxide and water during embryo development.

Male Reproductive Anatomy

The paired testes are located within the body cavity ventral to and near the cranial border of the kidney and the abdominal air sac. The testis is attached to the body wall by the mesorchium and is encapsulated by two fibrous coats. In young birds, the testes can appear flattened and pointed when compared to the rounded shape of the mature testicle. Melanistic testes, like melanistic ovaries, can occur in some species of Psittaciformes (Golden Conure, Blue and Gold Macaw, some cockatoos), Passeriformes and Piciformes (Keel-billed Toucans).

Convoluted seminiferous tubules comprised of germ (spermatogonia) and Sertoli cells make up the bulk of the testes and are responsible for spermatogenesis. Leydig cells, also called interstitial cells, produce male androgens and occupy the interstitial spaces between the tubules. The epididymis, considered vestigial in birds, lies along the dorsomedial aspect of the testes and is concealed from view during laparoscopic examination. Spermatozoa exit the epididymis and enter the ductus deferens, which forms a zigzag tubule running parallel with the ureter just medial to the kidneys. The ductus deferens is under hormonal control and is more convoluted during the breeding season. The ductus deferens penetrates the dorsal wall of the urodeum, which functions as a receptacle for sperm. The last two to three millimeters of the ductus deferens project into the urodeum forming a papilla. In passerine birds and budgerigars, the caudal end of the ductus deferens forms the seminal glomus, which enlarges during the breeding season to form a prominent projection in the cloacal wall for the storage of sperm. This prominence allows passerines to be easily sexed during the breeding season.

Although not all avian species have been adequately studied, it is known that ratites, tinamous, Anseriformes, some members of the family Cracidae and one Passeriforme, the Black Buffalo Weaver, have phalli that are intromittent (inserted into the female). Other species have phalli that may become engorged during copulation, but semen transfer occurs by direct cloaca-to-cloaca contact without intromission.

The phallus, if present, is located ventrally in the proctodeum. Dysfunction or disease of the phallus can cause reproductive failure. Psittacine birds do not have a phallus, and copulation is accomplished by an eversion of the cloacal wall, which contains the slightly raised papilla that transfers semen to the everted orifice of the oviduct.

Male Hormonal and Physiologic Factors

FSH initiates the growth of seminiferous tubules and results in increased spermatogenesis. LH promotes development of the testosterone-producing cells of Leydig. Testosterone increases spermatogenesis and growth of accessory reproductive organs, such as the epididymis and cloacal gland. Testosterone also causes manifestation of secondary sexual characteristics such as comb growth, plumage and beak color, structure of feathers, vocalizations and reproductive behavior.

Female Reproductive Disorders

Egg Binding and Dystocia

Egg binding is defined as the failure of an egg to pass through the oviduct at a normal rate. Most companion bird species lay eggs at intervals greater than 24 hours, and individuals within a species may vary by more than one day from the normal oviposition rate. Variability in egg transit times makes it difficult to determine when a problem is occurring.

Dystocia defines a condition in which the developing egg is in the caudal oviduct and is either obstructing the cloaca or has caused oviduct tissue to prolapse through the oviduct-cloacal opening. Egg movement through the oviduct can stop at various locations. The most common anatomic areas for problems to occur are the caudal uterus, vagina and vaginal-cloacal junction.

The pathogenesis of egg binding in a particular case can be multifactorial. The pubic bones are not fused in birds, and pelvic deformities seldom play a role in dystocia. Common causes of dystocias are oviduct muscle dysfunction (calcium metabolic disease, selenium and vitamin E deficiencies), malformed eggs, excessive egg production, previous oviduct damage or infection, nutritional insufficiencies, obesity, lack of exercise, heredity, senility and concurrent stress such as environmental temperature changes or systemic disease. Dystocia can also result from breeding birds out of season, egg production in virginal hens and a persistent cystic right oviduct.

An egg lodged in the pelvic canal may compress the pelvic vessels and kidneys, causing circulatory disorders and shock. An impacted egg may cause metabolic disturbances by interfering with normal defecation and micturition, inducing ileus and renal dysfunction. Pressure necrosis may occur to all three layers of the oviduct wall and lead to rupture.

Clinical Signs

Budgerigars, canaries, finches, cockatiels and lovebirds most frequently have problems with dystocia. This is probably because the presentation of a palpable egg for more than a few hours in small birds is generally more serious than it is in larger birds. Generally, the hen appears depressed, has an abnormally wide stance, is reluctant to fly or perch and may show persistent wagging of the tail and straining movements of the abdomen. Canaries often exhibit drooped wings. Rear limb paresis or paralysis may occur. Egg-related peritonitis, septicemia, leg injuries and abdominal neoplasia show similar clinical signs. Any depression can lead to anorexia, which further compromises the bird's condition.

Hens with dystocia frequently present with depression and secondary complications that require emergency therapy. A complete history including information of past breeding activity and the diet "consumed" will often suggest a pathogenesis. A thorough but rapid physical examination can also establish contributing factors such as obesity, concurrent disease or a malformed egg. Dystocias are most critical in passerines and other small birds, many of which can survive only a few hours without aggressive therapy. Initially the therapeutic plan is to stabilize the patient (see Chapter 15) with an emphasis being placed on correcting the most likely etiology for the dystocia.

In smaller birds the displaced ventriculus may make palpation of an egg difficult. Soft-shelled eggs, shell-less eggs or eggs located cranial to the uterus can also be difficult to palpate. Suspected egg masses must be differentiated from palpable hernias, lipomas or ascites. Radiographs are a useful confirmatory tool but may not delineate a shell-less egg. Radiographically identifying more than one egg in various stages of development is common.

Therapy

The most important consideration in initiating therapy for dystocia is to establish a physiologic normal state. Attempts to remove the egg are secondary to stabilizing a patient in shock. In minimally depressed patients with few complications, the egg will usually pass if the hen is provided with supplemental heat, injectable calcium, selenium, vitamin E, vitamin D_3 and easy access to food and water. Others require subcutaneous or IV fluids, rapidly acting steroids to combat shock, antibiotics to treat sepsis or peritonitis and injectable vitamins and minerals to address further nutritional deficiencies. Prolapsed oviductal or cloacal tissues should be moistened and cleaned with warm, sterile saline washes and water-based antiseptic ointments, such as chlorhexidine. Lubricating tissues surrounding the egg or the cloaca or vagina itself may be of some help to egg expulsion.

The bird should be placed in an incubator at 85-95°F with an inflow of heated, moisturized air. If the egg is not expelled within a few hours, then an injectable prostaglandin (dinoprost tromethamine) can be administered IM or applied topically to the oviductal

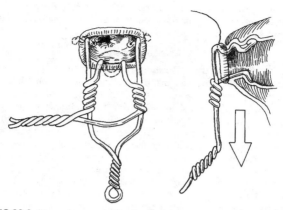

FIG 29.8 A speculum can be used to facilitate evaluation of the cloaca and removal of eggs. 1) opening of the ureter and 2) vaginal opening

tissue. This compound appears to be superior to oxytocin because it has the combined effect of inducing uterine contraction while relaxing the uterovaginal sphincter (see Chapter 18). Prostaglandin or oxytocin should be used only in cases where the uterus is thought to be intact and no adhesions to the oviduct are suspected. A hen receiving these agents must be able to withstand the increased contractions of the oviduct and abdomen that occur following the administration of oxytocin. Clinical signs of oxytocin response include tail pumping, panting, abdominal contractions and elimination of the egg. Increasing and repeated doses of oxytocin can be given if initial injections have no effect. Experimental use of prostaglandins and arginine vasotocin in domestic species has shown that injections of either of these drugs may result in oviposition. Arginine vasotocin likely causes the release of prostaglandins from the uterus. Clinical use of vasotocin in reptiles suggests that this drug may be of some value in birds (0.01-1.0 mg/kg BW). It has been shown that uteri are more sensitive to vasotocin than to oxytocin. Complications of oxytocin or vasotocin use include oviduct rupture.

If medical therapies fail to elicit oviposition, then more aggressive approaches that require manual manipulation of the patient may be necessary. Massaging the abdomen or cervix may help stimulate egg passage or relax the cervix so that the egg can be passed. The egg itself can be digitally manipulated caudally for expulsion. The use of warmed water-soluble solutions or ointments (saline with methyl cellulose) to lubricate the urodeum or vagina is equivocal. Gentle, persistent, caudally directed pressure on the egg may supplement weakened muscular contractions and loosen any recently formed adhesions. Only gentle traction should be used to prevent rupture of the oviduct. As long as the bird remains stable, repeated attempts at digital egg removal should continue. The cervix can be dilated by using a speculum to insert a blunt probe that is advanced in gentle, twirling motions (Figure 29.8). Eggs may be fertile and viable and should be incubated following expulsion. Digital manipulation and contracting therapy should not be used if one suspects ectopic eggs, uterine torsion, uterine rupture, or uterine constrictions due to adhesions (mucosal adhesions to the egg or the opposite uterine wall or serosal adhesions to other abdominal structures).

Ovocentesis

If the bird's condition is deteriorating or if an inappropriate period of time has passed since the dystocia was first noted, then more aggressive therapy such as ovocentesis must be considered. Ovocentesis is performed by aspirating the contents of the egg with a large needle (18 ga). Preferably the egg is manipulated with the use of a speculum so that it is observable and tapped through the cloaca. If this is not possible, the egg is brought in juxtaposition to the abdominal wall so that other organs are not damaged during a transabdominal aspiration procedure. Following aspiration of the egg contents, the egg can be gently collapsed. The risk of tearing the oviduct and producing peritonitis does exist but appears to be minor. The shell fragments and remaining contents of the egg should pass within several days. Fragments that are visible through the cloaca can be gently removed. Some clinicians advocate flushing the uterus post-oviposition with an iodine, chlorhexidine or saline solution to help remove egg fragments and to decrease the incidence of metritis. A Brunswick feeding catheter (3-5 Fr) can be placed through the cervix for this procedure. A course of broad-spectrum antibiotics, chosen based on the results of a Gram's stain collected from the uterus and confirmed as the correct choice by culture and sensitivity, is also recommended.

If the egg is lodged in the caudal oviduct or cloaca and the survivability of the egg is critical, then an episiotomy may be beneficial in delivering the egg. A laparotomy may be necessary to remove egg material or to perform a hysterectomy in cases where the uterus is ruptured or severe adhesions exist. Soft-shelled eggs located cranial to the uterus or ectopic eggs also require surgery.

Many hens with dystocia will attempt to lay another egg. Administration of medroxyprogesterone will stop ovulation, but there are side effects and its use is controversial. Following medroxyprogesterone administration, eggs already present in the proximal oviduct may continue to descend, complicating the bird's recovery, or may stop moving, causing an additional impaction or other complications such as peritonitis and salpingitis. Post-dystocia complications that may require medical or surgical intervention include ruptured oviducts, necrotic oviducts, peritonitis or abdominal hernias. Radiographs are helpful to monitor a hen recovering from dystocia. Abdominal hernias can be difficult to repair, especially if they are chronic in nature. Assisted oviposition may cause a flaccid cervix, allowing reflux of feces and urine into the uterus. Daily flushing and Gram's staining of the uterus to monitor progress following the removal of an egg appear to reduce the occurrence of metritis.

Prolapsed Oviduct and Cloaca

Prolapse of the oviduct may occur secondary to normal physiologic hyperplasia and egg laying or as a sequela to dystocia (particularly in canaries and budgerigars). Usually the uterus protrudes through the cloaca, often together with a partial prolapse

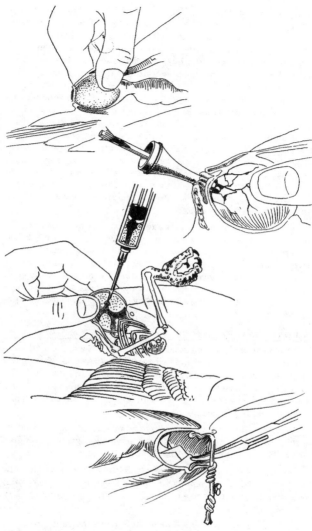

FIG 29.9 a) In many cases of egg impaction, supportive care in conjunction with caudal digital pressure is successful in facilitating the passage of an egg. **b)** If these conservative therapeutic measures are ineffective, then the contents of the egg can be removed (ovocentesis) and the egg can be broken to facilitate oviposition. An otoscope cone or speculum can be used to visualize the egg in the vagina. **c)** If the egg cannot be visualized in the vagina, then ovocentesis can be performed transabdominally. **d)** The egg shell fragments will generally pass in several days. If they do not pass, they can be physically removed from the vagina or cloaca using a speculum and hemostats.

of the vagina and cloaca. Distal portions of the oviduct may also prolapse, and frequently an egg is present. Timely, aggressive therapy is needed to prevent devitalization of uterine tissues and secondary infections. All exposed tissue must be kept as moist as possible and cleaned thoroughly with sterile saline solution. Topical steroid preparations containing antibiotics or dimethyl sulfoxide gel can be used to reduce swelling so that prolapsed tissues can be replaced. If no egg is present, tissue replacement is accomplished by gently guiding the tissues through the cloaca with pressure from a lubricated swab or thermometer. Repeated replacement of tissues may be required, as prolapses often recur. Stay sutures placed in the cloaca or percutaneous retention sutures may prevent further prolapsing while uterine tissues regress in size, abdominal tissues regain structural integrity and the hen has a chance to regain normal muscle tone and strength. The prognosis for birds with uterine prolapses is good as long as they are treated immediately.

If an egg is present in the prolapsed tissue, it must be removed before the tissue is replaced in the abdomen. Digital manipulation or implosion of the egg as discussed under dystocia may be effective. Chronically displaced tissue that contains eggs or egg material may require surgical debridement due to adhesions and shell abnormalities. In severe cases of uterine damage and necrosis, a partial or complete hysterectomy may be necessary, but is best delayed until the bird's condition is stable.

Salpingitis and Metritis

While salpingitis is most common in adult hens, it can also occur in young birds. Salpingitis reportedly occurs less frequently than oophoropathies, obstruction of the oviduct and ectopic ovulation in a variety of avian species. Depression, anorexia, weight loss and abdominal enlargement can occur with salpingitis. A discharge from the cloaca may also occur.

Cockatiel hens that have a history of egg laying followed by mild depression and weight loss may have a low grade salpingitis or focal egg-related peritonitis.

Metritis is a localized problem within the uterine portion of the oviduct. It can be a sequela to dystocia, egg binding or chronic oviduct impaction. Bacterial metritis is often secondary to systemic infections.

Metritis may affect shell formation or uterine contractility or cause infections in embryos (embryonic death) or neonates (weak chicks). Metritis can also cause egg binding, uterine rupture, peritonitis and septicemia. Coliforms, especially *E. coli*, are frequently implicated. Coliform metritis may be complicated by poor diet, and death rates are highest in hens during the ovulatory and egg-laying period.

In more advanced cases, birds may be depressed and have an enlarged abdomen and a palpable turgid uterus. Radiographs often reveal indistinct abdominal detail with a diffuse increase in soft tissue density. Ultrasound has been used in ostriches. An affected ostrich hen may have a history of erratic production, malformed or odoriferous eggs or a sudden drop in production. An odoriferous cloacal discharge may occur, and the WBC may range from 20,000 to 100,000/mm³. Metritis and salpingitis are treated aggressively with parenteral antibiotics, supportive care and therapy for shock (see Chapters 15 and 18). In nonresponsive cases, a laparotomy may be necessary to remove necrotic tissue, inflammatory exudates or egg material. The oviduct may be flushed directly with lactated Ringer's solution (with or without antibiotics) by placing an IV fluid tube or soft catheter into the vagina. Visualizing placement of the tube can be augmented by use of a cloacal speculum.

Oviduct Impaction

Impaction of the oviduct is often a sequela to salpingitis (most frequently), metritis or egg binding. One study found that impactions were nearly always associated with obvious salpingitis in older birds. Impactions may occur from excess secretion of mucin and albumen associated with cystic hyperplasia or inspissated egg material in the magnum. Soft-shelled, malformed or fully formed eggs can impact in the distal oviduct. Cockatiels, canaries and budgerigars are frequently affected, and the condition has been documented in raptors and an African Grey Parrot. Clinical changes are not always obvious and may include a cessation of egg production, progressive loss of condition and alternation between constipation and diarrhea. Chronic deterioration is particularly common if concurrent peritonitis or salpingitis is present. The abdomen may be diffusely or unilaterally (usually left side) enlarged, birds may be reluctant to fly or walk and periodic anorexia may occur. Radiology can be helpful in some cases, but many oviduct impactions can be diagnosed only through endoscopy or exploratory laparotomy or at necropsy. Impacted oviducts may contain obvious egg material, gray or yellow purulent material, calcareous deposits or albumen. Diffuse peritonitis with adhesions can also occur with oviduct impactions. Treatment consists of parenteral antibiotics and in most cases, surgery to clean, repair or remove necrotic portions of the oviduct.

Oophoritis

The normal ovary with mature follicles has yellow, turgid ova. When diseased, the ovum can be wrinkled, black, enlarged, firm or hemorrhagic. In addition, abnormal yolk may appear coagulated or "cooked" and flake off onto the ovary or into the abdominal cavity. Adhesions may exist between follicles and the follicles may be slightly stalked. Bacteremias may cause congestion, distortion and atresia of the follicles. Peritonitis commonly occurs with oophoritis.

Clinical signs of oophoritis include depression, anorexia, chronic wasting and sudden death. Therapy includes supportive care and parenteral antimicrobial agents as dictated by the etiologic agent.

Parasites

Eggs may contain adult ascarids that probably enter the oviduct from the cloaca due to reverse peristalsis. Flukes (*Prosthogonimus ovatus* and related trematodes) inhabit the oviduct of Anseriformes and Galliformes. Heavy infections may cause soft-shelled or shell-less eggs, resulting in salpingitis. Adult flukes less than 1 cm long may be passed in the eggs. Prevention involves the control of aquatic snails and dragonflies that serve as intermediate hosts.

Cloacal Problems

Cloacitis, cloacal strictures, cloacal liths and chronic prolapse of the cloaca can interfere with egg laying and copulation. These conditions may in turn result from traumatic egg laying. The cloaca may become chronically impacted with an egg, resulting in severe cloacitis and abdominal adhesions. Feathers, fat and abdominal lipomas may occlude the vent, inhibiting reproductive ability. Both medical and surgical approaches are helpful in treating cloacal problems (see Chapter 19). It is interesting to note that the cloaca prolapses normally in the Vasa Parrot during the breeding season.

In some cases, cloacal papillomas may interfere with copulation and semen transport. Painful lesions in the cloaca may also discourage individuals from mating; however, healthy chicks can be produced by breeding pairs of psittacine birds where one or both adults have mild to moderate cloacal papillomatosis. The etiology of these lesions is unknown and it is recommended to exclude birds with this condition from a breeding aviary. Affected birds in a collection should be isolated from unaffected birds. Affected parents may or may not produce affected offspring, but regardless, chicks from affected parents should be hand-raised in isolation. Results from various treatment regimes for cloacal papillomatosis vary. A diet low in fat and high in fresh fruit and vegetables with high vitamin A or beta carotene was considered useful in resolving cloacal papillomatosis and cloacal adhesions in one case.

Cystic ova (reported in budgerigars, canaries and pheasants) may be single or multiple and may be noted during laparoscopy in apparently healthy psittacine hens. Ovarian tumors and cystic hyperplasia of the oviduct can occur secondarily. The etiology of this condition and its clinical importance are unknown, but a primary endocrine disturbance is suspected because this lesion is frequently associated with hyperostosis. In affected birds, dyspnea, altered movement and diffuse distention (ascites) of the abdomen are common. Although not always palpable, abnormal ova may be firm, soft, fluctuating or pedunculated. Cysts may rupture, so palpation should proceed carefully. Radiographs may show a diffuse soft tissue density near the cranial lobe of the left kidney. Endoscopically, the ovary may be enlarged with many thin-walled cysts full of straw-colored fluid. Respiratory distress may be eliminated by transabdominally aspirating cystic fluid with a needle and syringe. Cystic ovaries were successfully treated in two budgerigars with oral testosterone. Removal of the ovaries, although technically difficult, may be the only long-term treatment.

[*Editor's Note: This practitioner has had good success internally marsupializing large ovarian cysts in budgerigars. Abdominal ultrasonography is very useful in determining whether abdominal swelling is due to free fluid, cystic structure or solid structures such as tumors or abscesses.*]

Cystic Hyperplasia of the Oviduct

Most reports of cystic hyperplasia of the oviduct are in budgerigars and domestic fowl. The entire oviduct is dilated with a white or brown mucoid fluid, white or creamy masses or occasionally secondary cysts. Cysts also can occur secondary to improper formation of the left oviduct (possible degeneration during embryonic development) or from adhered lips of the infundibulum. The ovary in affected hens may also have cystic changes suggesting an endocrine abnormality. Progressive abdominal distention, ascites and respiratory distress are the most common clinical changes. Palpation and radiographs may reveal the distended oviduct. Abdominal paracentesis may be attempted either for diagnosis or for relief of respiratory distress. Laparotomy will provide a conclusive diagnosis. Hormonal therapy with testosterone may prove effective in resolving the immediate problem, but a hysterectomy may be necessary to prevent future problems.

If a rudimentary right oviduct (or ovary) exists, it may also become cystic. Cysts are of walnut size, contain watery or milky fluid and are situated near the cloaca in domestic fowl. Small cysts may go undetected, but large cysts may place pressure on abdominal organs. Egg binding has occurred secondary to a fully developed right oviduct in a budgerigar. The hen was depressed and thin and had a distended abdomen. Successful bilateral hysterectomies were performed to remove the egg-filled left oviduct and the right oviduct that contained a walnut-sized cyst with gelatinous fluid.

Neoplasia

Budgerigars often have neoplasia in the ovary or oviduct. Ovarian tumors can be very large and represent up to one-third of the body weight. Egg retention, concurrent cysts, ascites and herniation are common sequelae to reproductive tract neoplasias. Changes in secondary sex characteristics (cere color change in the budgerigar) may also occur. Radiographs can be helpful, although an enlarged ovary or oviduct creates an image similar to that seen when uncalcified eggs are present. A confirmatory diagnosis requires exploratory laparotomy and histopathologic examination of biopsy samples. Lymphomatosis is suggested by cauliflower-like growths of the ovary in domestic fowl. A variety of other tumor types has been reported including adenocarcinomas, leiomyomas, leiomyosarcomas, adenomas and granulosa cell tumors. Excisional surgery is the traditional therapy, although prognosis for long-term recovery is poor.

Ectopic Eggs and Non-septic Peritonitis

Egg material may gain access to the abdomen through ectopic ovulation and discontinuous or ruptured oviducts. Ectopic ovulation occurs when the infundibulum fails to engulf an ovum. It may be caused by reverse peristalsis of the oviduct, which occurs during normal egg laying, or by trauma to the oviduct that interferes with normal function.

Restraining or stressing a hen during egg laying has been incriminated as a cause of ectopic ovulation. Peritonitis may or may not develop from ectopic ovulation. If present, it can occur in either a septic or non-septic form. Yolk itself only causes a mild histiocytic response and if free of pathogens will gradually be reabsorbed by the peritoneum.

Depending on the location of rents in the oviduct, completely or partially shelled eggs may be deposited in the abdomen. Ruptured oviducts can result from acute and chronic oviduct impaction, including egg binding, cystic hyperplasia, neoplasia and salpingitis. Large, misshapen eggs may cause uterine disintegration and rupture resulting in ectopic eggs.

Ectopic eggs have been reported in Passeriformes and Psittaciformes. Uncomplicated ectopic ovulation may go unnoticed for a protracted period of time. Abdominal distention, a penguin-like stance and weight loss may be the only clinical changes. Free yolk in the abdomen may be absorbed and systemic antibiotics may be needed until the abdomen clears itself of yolk. The condition may recur if predisposing factors are still present. Excessive accumulations of egg material or fully formed eggs should be removed surgically. Damaged oviduct tissue should be repaired or removed.

Egg-related Septic Peritonitis

Peritonitis is the most frequent cause of death associated with reproductive disorders. It may not be a single disease but part of several syndromes, including ectopic ovulation, ruptured oviducts and salpingitis. It is theorized that it may be the cause instead of the result of a ruptured oviduct. Peritonitis appears to be described most frequently in cockatiels, budgerigars, lovebirds, ducks and macaws.

Presenting clinical signs include sudden death, abdominal swelling, respiratory distress, depression, anorexia and cessation of reproduction. The hemogram may show a severe inflammatory response. Radiology, abdominocentesis and laparotomy are helpful diagnostic aids. Septic peritonitis leading to severe debilitation, sepsis and death can occur if the yolk is contaminated with bacteria. Turbid yellow, green or brown yolky fluid or cheese-like yellowish masses of inspissated yolk material in the abdomen are indications of ectopic ovulation or a ruptured oviduct. Egg-related pancreatitis may cause temporary diabetes mellitus, especially in cockatiels. A temporary stroke-like syndrome has been described in cockatiels with yolk peritonitis, possibly due to yolk emboli. Aspirin may be used as an anticoagulant in cases where yolk emboli are suspected (1 tablet/30 ml water, 0.5 ml/kg PO q8h). The etiologic agent of egg-related peritonitis is often coliforms, especially *E. coli*.

Treatment consists of antibiotics, steroids to reduce inflammation and supportive care (heat, fluids, nutritional supplements). Long-term antibiotic therapy may be necessary and diet correction is advised. Most cases resolve with medical therapy alone, but early diagnosis is essential. If surgery is required to remove egg material or perform abdominal irrigation, the patient should be stabilized first with supportive care and antibiotics.

Chronic Egg Laying

The chronically reproductively active female may exhibit weight loss from constant regurgitation and feather loss or mild dermatitis around the cloaca in association with masturbatory behavior. Removing eggs from the hen effectively induces a form of double clutching and can facilitate the problem. The continuation of egg laying is ultimately hormonally controlled. The most domesticated psittacine birds, cockatiels, lovebirds and budgerigars, are notorious chronic egg layers. Perhaps the high incidence of problems in these species indicates a lack of hormonal balance in controlling egg laying that has occurred due to selective pressures designed to make birds produce continually in a variety of environmental situations.

Hens on a completely nutritious diet can continuously lay eggs for years without deleterious effects. In most cases, however, malnutrition and the progressive stress and physiologic demands of egg laying ultimately will compromise the hen. Calcium deficits lead to abnormal egg production, reduced oviduct inertia and generalized muscular weakness. Egg binding is common in hens that chronically lay eggs. Behavior modification can be attempted to stop the laying cycle (see Chapter 4). The stronger the environmental stimulus to cease egg laying activity, the better. Diminishing exposure to light to only eight to ten hours a day should interrupt the hormonal cycle, and egg laying should cease. Objects stimulating masturbatory behavior or sexually oriented regurgitation should be removed, although many birds will continue reproductive behavior despite this environmental change. Nest boxes and possibly enclosure mates should be removed. Changing the location of the enclosure may also be helpful. Owners may discourage reproductive behavior by decreasing the amount of time spent with a hen until egg laying ceases.

Medical therapy is designed to correct any nutritional imbalances or reproductive tract abnormalities. Mineral and vitamin supplements should be given parenterally and added to the diet. Caloric intake with adequate protein levels should be increased. Despite behavioral and medical therapy, affected hens may continue to lay eggs. The long-term solution in these cases is a salpingohysterectomy (see Chapter 41).

Overproduction

Free-ranging psittacine hens may produce only one, at the most two, clutches per year. Egg production in excess of two clutches a year would thus be considered unnatural. Many captive psittacine birds (particularly Blue and Gold Macaws, cockatoos and Eclectus Parrots) routinely produce four clutches of eggs per year with no apparent side effects; however, continued levels of unnatural clutch production may lead to reproductive tract disease or other disorders precipitated by poor body condition. Overproducing hens may be thin and in poor feather condition, have poor muscular tone and be unable to quickly involute the uterus after egg laying has stopped. To ensure the long-term health of a reproductively active hen, egg production should be limited to two clutches a year in birds exhibiting medical problems secondary to excessive egg production.

Abnormal Eggs

Dietary problems, environmental factors and reproductive tract abnormalities can all result in the production of abnormal eggs. Soft-shelled eggs may be an incidental occurrence or may indicate an underlying nutritional or medical disorder. Nutritional deficiencies of calcium and vitamins A and D_3 have been associated with soft-shelled eggs. Therapy consists of both parenteral and oral nutritional supplements.

Oviduct pathology may also cause abnormal egg production. Suggestive abnormalities include thin-shelled eggs, irregular external calcium deposits, or overly thick-shelled eggs. Uterine infections may cause rough-shelled eggs, which can be corrected by flushing the uterus with appropriate antibiotics.

Metritis, ectopic ovulation and ovarian disease may cause yolkless, small or sterile eggs that appear grossly normal. Inconsistent transient times of the egg passing through the oviduct may cause abnormally sized eggs due to deposition of differing amounts of albumen. A slow passage time of a preceding egg may allow for double ovulation to occur and result in a double-yolked egg.

Male Reproductive Disorders

Toxins

Numerous toxins can affect spermatogenesis in mammals. Reduced spermatogenesis has been reported in Japanese quail exposed to mercury. Copper fungicides in feed have been found to suppress spermatogenesis and induce testicular atrophy.

Cystic testicular degeneration occurs in ducklings given feed with furazolidone.

Anatomical Abnormalities

Testicular atrophy can be caused by orchitis as a result of trauma or genital infection or can be due to progressive infertility. Malnutrition, toxicity or bacteremia may also cause testicular degeneration. Affected birds may demonstrate a lack of libido or be infertile. Therapy is limited to addressing infectious or behavioral problems. If fibrotic or infiltrative changes have occurred, spermatogenesis may be permanently altered.

Orchitis

A variety of bacteria can cause orchitis in birds, including *E. coli*, *Salmonella* spp. and *Pasteurella multocida*. Infections may originate from prolapsed or ulcerated phalli, renal obstruction, cloacitis and septicemia. Clinical signs are similar to those expected for any generalized infection. Antibiotics may be helpful in resolving the active infection but may not prevent or reverse infertility.

Neoplasia

Testicular tumors commonly occur in older budgerigars but can also be found in larger Psittaciformes and other birds.

Sertoli and interstitial cell tumors have been described in birds (see Chapter 25). Lymphoproliferative diseases, such as leukosis, can also affect the testes resulting in infertility. Regardless of the tumor type, testicular neoplasias can involve one or both testes. Unilateral paresis, progressive weight loss and abdominal enlargement are typical clinical signs. Affected birds may have reduced secondary sex characteristics and become more feminine in nature (cere of the male budgerigar turning from a blue to brown color). Metastasis from testicular tumors usually affects the liver. Surgery may be successful if the tumor is easily approached and unilateral and the cock is in good health. Long-term prognosis is guarded due to the possibility of metastasis.

Phallic Prolapse

Birds with a large phallus may develop partial or complete prolapses, which are frequently secondary to trauma, infection or extreme weather fluctuations. Infections may be secondary to mucosal irritation (over-exuberant mating or vent sexing) or fecal contamination.

Exposed tissue should be thoroughly cleaned with a sterile saline solution, carefully debrided and covered with antibiotic cream. Topical DMSO may help reduce swelling, making replacement of the phallus easier and more permanent. Daily therapy and cloacal mattress suture may be necessary to prevent recurring prolapses (see Chapter 41). Systemic antibiotics should be considered due to the possibility of ascending urogenital infections. If large areas of necrosis are present, then surgery is necessary to debride the wound.

Behavioral Abnormalities

Reproductively active males and females (particularly budgerigars and cockatiels) may exhibit masturbatory behavior or excessive regurgitation. These are normal reproductive behaviors that may become pathologic in birds that are isolated. Cockatiel cocks incubate the eggs, and a single male may spend much of the time on the enclosure floor mimicking incubation activities. Removing the bird from its enclosure for long periods of time (with available food and water sources) or changing the enclosure or enclosure location may stop this behavior. In other cases, displaced reproductive behavior may occur in males housed with females. In these cases, the male is often "imprinted" on humans and cannot complete the reproductive cycle with its own species. Exchanging mates may prove helpful, but usually these males should be removed from the breeding program. Human imprinting can also occur in females, and in both genders behavioral abnormalities due to improper imprinting may not be obvious. Indeed, lack of pair-bonding, lack of egg production or infertility may be the only signs associated with the use of hand-raised imprinted birds in a breeding program. The interaction of a chick with its parents and nesting conditions may be critical for successful reproduction in some species (see Chapter 4).

Underproduction

Underproduction is particularly important with endangered species where maximum production is critical to ensure the survival of the species.

If production from a breeding pair does not approach the average, then medical, physical or behavior problems should be addressed. Correction of any medical or physical abnormalities, such as clipping overgrown feathers near the cloaca, dieting overweight birds or treating birds for localized infections can be instituted. The diet should be carefully analyzed and any deficiencies should be corrected. Environmental deterrents to breeding may be determined by using a video camera to observe the pair's daily behavioral patterns. Some changes that may be necessary include repairing birds, improved enclosures, different nest boxes, varied diet, altered climate, different lighting or reducing aviary disturbances induced by humans, other birds or vermin.

Testosterone has been suggested to induce singing in male canaries but can cause serious side effects. Male canaries that do not sing are usually sick or malnourished.

Birds that consistently fail to produce should be removed from the breeding program.

Non-disease Factors Affecting Reproduction

Gender

The most common cause of reproductive failure in companion birds is pairing of two birds of the same gender.

Physical Characteristics

Many species of birds are sexually dimorphic, with visual characteristics that distinguish males from females. Even with monomorphic species, subtle differences may exist that allow determination of gender.

With birds of prey, the female is generally 30% larger than the male, although some size overlap occurs in the intermediate weight ranges. In other groups of birds, the male is generally heavier and has a larger frame than the female. Head size as well as bill breadth, length and depth are often greater in males.

In general, red to brown iris color is more common in female cockatoos; however, this technique is not always reliable, especially in Moluccan, Rose-breasted, Bare-eyed, Goffin's and immature cockatoos. At maturity, wild-type (green) male budgerigars have lavender to dark-blue ceres while females have light-blue to tan or brown ceres. Gender determination based on cere color may not be effective in inbred color mutations. The White-fronted Amazon is clearly sexually dimorphic. Males have numerous red secondary wing coverts while females have few to none.

Vent Sexing

Gender can be determined in most Galliformes, Anseriformes, some game birds, ratites and some species of Cracidae by looking for the phallus on the wall of the cloaca. In Columbiformes and Passeriformes, which have prominent papillae of the ductus deferens, gender can be determined if these structures can be visualized using general anesthesia and a cloacal protractor.

Determining the distance between the pelvic bones (gapped in females, close together in males) has been discussed as a method of gender determination. In larger psittacine birds, this is an unreliable method of gender determination. Some practitioners feel that this is a reliable method for gender determination in mature lovebirds.

Table 29.4   Examples of Sexually Dimorphic Psittacines*

Species	Male	Female
Budgerigar	Cere lavender to dark-blue	Cere pink-brown to light-blue
Cockatiel	Bright yellow face and cheek patch, lacks barring	Tail and flight feathers have barring on underside, monotonous chirp
Cockatoo	Adults have black irides	Adults have reddish-brown irides
Malee, Adelaide Rosella, Red-rumped, Bourke's	Lacks barring when mature	Barring on underside of wings
Red-rumped Parrot	Red rump patch	Green rump patch, paler
Scarlet-chested Parrot	Scarlet breast	Green breast
Regent Parrot, Superb Parrot	Yellow feather patches	Green throughout
Princess Parrot	Coral beak	Brownish beak
Red-bellied Parrot	Red belly	Scattered red feathers on green belly
King Parrot	Red head feathers	Green head feathers
Red-winged Parrot	Blue crown feathers, orange-red iris	Duller green feathers, pale-brown iris
Duchess Lorikeet	Red side rump patch	Yellow side rump patch
Fairy Lorikeet	Blue rump patch	Yellow side rump patch
Josephine's Lory	Red lower back	Green lower back
Whiskered Lory	Red crown	Green crown
Cacatua spp.	Brown to black iris	Red to reddish-brown iris
Eclectus Parrot	Green	Red and purple
Pesquet's Parrot	Red spot behind eye	No red spot
Grey-headed Lovebird	Grey head, neck and breast	Green head, neck and breast
Ring-necked Parakeet	Colored ring around neck	No ring
White-fronted Amazon Parrot	Red alula and primary covert feathers	Slight to no red in primary covert feathers
Mountain Parakeet	Yellow forehead, lores, cheeks and throat	Green forehead, lores, cheeks and throat
Mexican Parrotlet	Blue lower rump and underwing coverts	Yellow-green rump and underwing coverts
Pileated Parrot	Red forehead	Green forehead
African Grey Parrot	Red vent, rump feathers	Grey tips, red feathers

* Not all members within a genus will portray the listed sexual differences. Differences are usually observable only in mature species.

Behavioral Characteristics

Males are generally more aggressive and are responsible for territorial defense. The songs of the male finch, canary and cockatiel differentiate them from females.

Observing copulation in species in which the male completely mounts the female may indicate a successful pair bonding. In New World Psittaciformes, copulation occurs side by side, and homosexual pairs have been observed precisely mimicking this procedure.

Laparoscopic Sexing

Although subject to error when used in young birds with un-differentiated gonads, laparoscopic examination is a definitive method of gender determination when performed by an experienced practitioner (see Chapter 13). Its major advantage over other gender determination techniques is that it allows for direct inspection of abdominal structures, especially reproductive organs, for evidence of disease or dysfunction. Its disadvantage is that it is an invasive procedure that requires anesthesia.

Laboratory Methods

Genetic determination of gender in birds is considered the most reliable of the available noninvasive techniques. One method employs feather pulp as a source of chromosomes.

Determination of gender can also be accomplished by evaluating differences in the DNA composition between males and females. A small volume of red blood cells is necessary for this procedure, and advantages include easy and relatively nontraumatic sample collection and a long sample shelf life without refrigeration.

Environment

Light

The most important factor for reproductive stimulation of free-ranging birds in mid to high latitudes is day length. Lengthening photoperiods elevates LH secretion, which is the primary reproductive hormone.

Climate

High environmental temperature combined with high humidity increases the physiological stress on birds and can decrease reproductive activity. Rainfall triggers courtship behavior in male Zebra Finches.

Season

Effects of environmental conditions on reproduction may be similar in captive birds and free-ranging birds; however, heavily domesticated species like canaries, budgerigars and finches react differently than their free-ranging conspecifics.

Mate Presence

In cockatiels, mate access is essential to ensure nesting behavior. Increases in LH levels necessary for oviposition occurred only in females given full mate and nest box access.

Separating a pair during the nonbreeding season may not affect reproductive success in a subsequent season, and mates will usually reunite, especially if they have previously been reproductively successful.

Mate Selection

In some monogamous birds, such as California Quail and Turtle Doves, forced pairing of mates can result in successful breeding. In other species like cockatiels, forced pairing was found to result in decreased reproductive activity. In some species, force-pairing may result in increased mate aggression.

Aggressive mates can inhibit reproduction by preventing the opposite sex from eating or through direct physical abuse. Aggressive behavior is most noteworthy in cockatoos and is seen occasionally in Eclectus Parrots. Male cockatoos, even in long-term successful pairs, may suddenly attack and sometimes kill their mates. The beak, eyes, skull, feet and cloaca are most commonly traumatized.

Mate Pair-bonding

Pair-bonding refers to the behavioral acceptance that exists between a compatible hen and cock and is evident in all successful pairs. Strong territorial defense coordinated between the male and female, such as lunging at the front of the cage with upraised wings in macaws and tail-fanning with crown and nape feather ruffing in Amazon parrots, are examples of proper pair-bonding.

Evaluating a breeding pair through the aid of video recorders will help identify causes of behavior-induced infertility. Some copulatory efforts may be handicapped by physical, medical or behavioral abnormalities. Birds should be allowed to choose their own mates to increase the likelihood of pair-bonding.

Social Interaction

The presence of other breeding birds is a reproductive stimulus in highly social and colony breeding species. Social birds such as budgerigars should be housed within hearing, if not visual, range of the same species to stimulate successful reproduction.

Social behavior varies during the breeding season in some species. For example, some parrots will feed only in pairs during the breeding season while cockatoos will interact daily with other pairs and feed in larger groups.

In captivity, housing similar species near each other may reinforce the pair bond and strengthen endocrine controls by eliciting territorial defense behavior. In contrast, excessive territorial defense may waste energy and interfere with pair interactions that are critical for reproductive success. Monitoring of a pair's behavior and analysis of enclosure diagrams in multiple-pair and multiple-species aviaries will help define proper housing for each species and individual pair.

Human Interaction

Aviary disturbances and handling birds near the breeding season may disrupt endocrine control of the reproductive cycle or disturb the birds so that mating is not initiated or completed, incubation is interrupted, eggs are damaged or chicks are cared for improperly. Successful territorial defense appears to have a positive effect on reproduction, and males that believe they have defended their nest from humans may be more reproductively active. Although evidence is rather anecdotal, barren pairs have been induced to breed by disturbing, handling or relocating the pairs. Some species of birds are withdrawn and display fear as opposed to aggression when approached by humans, indicating improper territorial defense. These pairs may be more productive once conditioned to human activity or if placed in an isolated, protected area. Annual physical exams can be performed on properly conditioned birds and do not appear to negatively affect reproduction.

Nests

Availability and acquisition of a proper nest site and nesting material may be a strong environmental stimulus for breeding particularly in male cockatiels and finches. In fact, LH surges that stimulate reproduction and spermatogenesis may be induced because of male defense behavior and not because of the presence of a female. The relationship of the perch to the nest box hole (perch ten cm below the hole) played a significant role in reproductive success in budgerigars. This phenomenon may be applicable to considerations of nest box design in other species as well.

Birds are generally classified as being either determinate or indeterminate layers. Determinate layers will lay only a set number of eggs in a clutch regardless of whether any egg is removed or destroyed. Indeterminate layers will continue to lay until they "recognize" the correct number of eggs.

Applying these principles to companion birds, it is logical that if birds are thought to be indeterminate layers, eggs should be removed before incubation starts if production of more eggs is desired. The longer incubation is allowed to proceed the more complete the ovarian regression would be, which would make a hen less likely to lay another clutch. Budgerigars are believed to be determinant layers.

Enclosures

Enclosure design can affect reproduction. Some species of birds appear to breed better in flights as opposed to flight enclosures. The actual dimensions may be important, but longer, wider and higher enclosures may not always be better, as a larger enclosure may represent a territory that a pair feels it cannot adequately defend. Enclosure design in general and nest position, including whether it is within the enclosure, how high it is and whether it is open or obscured by walls, may all influence a pair's feeling of security (see Chapter 2).

Nutrition

Low dietary calcium levels (0.056-0.3%) have been shown to cause a complete cessation of egg laying in gallinaceous birds. Decreased energy intake causes decreased LH levels followed by ovarian atresia. Low-sodium diets also result in cessation of egg laying. Zinc-rich diets decrease feed intake and may directly decrease egg laying by altering metabolism and endocrine functions.

Psittacine birds being fed largely seed diets should be expected to consume low levels of vitamin A, D_3 and E as well as other nutrients (see Chapters 3 and 31). Over-nutrition may precipitate infertility by either mechanically blocking the cloaca or reducing successful ovulation. Abdominal fat and lack of condition may contribute to oviduct inertia and egg-laying problems.

The availability of certain food items and not simply energy consumption may be one of the many stimulants needed to begin or strengthen reproductive activity. Aviculturists can mimic naturally occurring variations in food availability by reducing food intake and variability in the nonbreeding season and then dramatically increasing the quality, quantity and variety of foods before the breeding season. The success of this method is equivocal but suggests the need for further study.

Physical and Medical Characteristics

Adequate exercise is important to reproductive success and decreases the likelihood of reproductive disorders, such as egg-binding. Any physical abnormality or medical condition affecting mobility, balance, the cloacal region or the reproductive tract can cause infertility or decreased reproductive success. Heavy cloacal feathering, such as in Rose-breasted Cockatoos and fancy pigeon breeds, may prevent copulation resulting in infertility. Medications, especially certain antibiotics, can cause infertility or decreased or abnormal egg production. For example, testosterone injections in males can cause infertility, and an entire season of reproduction can be interrupted after the use of injectable doxycycline therapy.

Inbreeding

Males inherit fertility and semen quality characteristics. Some mating behavior is learned and some is inherited. Inbreeding may lead to infertility or decreased production due to genetically controlled physical or behavioral deficits. Lethal and sublethal genes that are more frequently expressed during inbreeding can cause decreased hatching rates.

General

Frequently, the positive environmental factors that stimulate breeding and the negative factors that prevent it cannot be discerned. Successful captive breeding depends on establishing environmentally enriching conditions that stimulate reproductive activity.

Natural Incubation

Natural incubation is a behavior under hormonal control that can be externally affected by many factors. Improper parental incubation can lead to a complete lack of egg development, arrestment of embryo development, late embryo death or abnormal or weak chicks at hatch. Additionally, many species such as macaws tend to be rather nervous in captivity and are notorious for breaking eggs. Minor punctures and hairline cracks can cause the death of a developing embryo. Foster parents or artificial incubation can be used in pairs with incubation problems. Failures in incubation can also originate from embryo-related problems, diet or environmental factors. Studying pertinent egg information and performing thorough diagnostic procedures can help determine the cause of some of these incubation failures.

Information Collection

The attending veterinarian should review existing records concerning the parent's reproductive and medical history and fate of any eggs or chicks. Developing an accurate and consistent record-keeping system and regularly scheduling on-site visits will help identify factors that could explain incubation failures (see Chapter 2).

Reproductive information from each pair including numbers of eggs per clutch, number of clutches per year, time of day eggs are laid, previous fertility and hatchability statistics, causes of egg failure and chick survivability will all help in evaluating a collection. To get a true fertility rate for a pair, one must necropsy all eggs as soon as possible after they are determined to be dead.

Fertility

Documenting if an egg is infertile or was fertile and died in early incubation is the first step in investigating egg problems. Eggs that are fertile but were not incubated or that failed to develop past two to five days of incubation will generally appear infertile when candled. These eggs should be opened to determine if they were fertile. Fresh, infertile eggs have a well organized small blastodisc, which in domestic species can be easily differentiated from the large, sometimes cottony or doughnut-shaped fertile blastoderm. Old, addled or infected eggs in which fertility cannot be determined should not be included in fertility calculations. Additionally, any misshapen, mis-sized or otherwise abnormal eggs that are discarded should not be used in calculating fertility rates. The preferred method would be to include these eggs, as they can be fertile, or to calculate a separate fertility rate for abnormal eggs. Hybrid eggs should also be discounted, as they may have decreased fertility. Fertility rates can be calculated by finding what percentage of the total number of eggs laid were fertile. Undetermined eggs should not be included.

Fertility rates can be useful for discerning problems within a flock or individual pair. Infertility can be a result of behavioral, environmental, nutritional and medical problems. Factors that should be considered include age of the birds, time the pair has been together, time the pair has been in the aviary, enclosure type, enclosure location, production of eggs in the past, past fertility and hatchability, hybrids, inbreeding, date of lay, environmental parameters (temperature, humidity, day length, rainfall) and behavioral characteristics of the pair. Fertility within an aviary should be evaluated on an individual pair and species basis within an aviary. Fertility is normally reduced in older birds, in younger birds and at the beginning and end of a breeding season. Infertility in these cases may be a natural occurrence and not an indication of disease.

Hatchability

Hatchability rates are determined from eggs that were known to be fertile. Including infertile eggs in hatchability statistics will artificially lower hatchability rates and confuse diagnostic efforts. Hatchability rates are calculated by finding the percentage of fertile eggs that successfully hatched.

"Successfully hatched" may or may not include chicks that were weak and died soon after hatching from pre-nursery associated problems. Hatchability rates can be calculated for individual pairs, separate clutches, different species, eggs incubated naturally, eggs incubated artificially and eggs that had various kinds of physical problems or that were manipulated during incubation or hatching. The more precise the hatchability statistic, the more diagnostic the information that is provided.

The number of lethal or chromosomal abnormalities reported in companion bird species is low when compared to domestic species. Evaluating fertility and hatchability statistics from parents and sisters of breeding males may help identify lethal or semi-lethal genes in some family trees. Breeding tests may be required to establish whether such genes are sex-linked or autosomal, dominant or recessive.

Parental Factors

The medical history of each parent should be examined to identify factors that may affect fertility and hatchability. Table 29.6 lists factors associated with embryonic death according to the stage of incubation (first to third trimester). A pair with persistent fertility or hatchability problems should be completely evaluated by performing physical examinations, complete cloacal examinations, cloacal and choanal cultures, Gram's staining and culturing of uterine samples (many uterine problems are anaerobic), complete blood counts, serum chemistries, radiographs, exploratory laparoscopies and evaluation of sperm. Exposure to toxic compounds, either directly or in the food or water, should be considered. Behavioral problems including lack of pair-bonding, inconsistent parental incubation and egg trauma in the nest may also cause hatchability problems.

Diet

Diets should be analyzed for adequate levels of protein, fat, carbohydrates, calorie content, minerals, fiber, calcium and vitamins and for the presence of aflatoxins. Total caloric intake and food selection behavior for each individual bird should be evaluated. Nutritionally deficient hens can produce eggs, but the low level of nutrients may prevent the eggs from hatching. The age of embryonic mortality will usually depend on the degree and type of deficiency or toxicity.

Severe hypovitaminosis A causes a complete cessation of egg production. Partial hypovitaminosis A may cause circulatory collapse and embryo death and has been suggested as a cause of egg binding. Vitamin E deficiencies can cause lethal rings in which the embryo is seen surrounded by a ring of separated tissue. Vitamin D_3 deficiencies can cause small eggs with poorly calcified shells. Ultraviolet light exposure may improve hatchability in these cases while excess D_3 may lead to a complete cessation of egg production. Embryonic hemorrhage is common with deficiencies in vitamins E and K. Vitamin K is also involved with calcium transport, and vitamin K deficiencies can mimic the clinical signs associated with hypocalcemia.

Calcium-deficient eggs exhibit reduced hatchability, poor shell calcification, embryos with rickets and excessive loss of water and

Table 29.6   Causes of Death or Abnormalities in Embryos

FIRST TRIMESTER
- Egg handling
    - Eggs stored too long
    - Eggs stored under incorrect conditions
    - Incorrect egg fumigation or sanitation (dirty hands)
    - Excessive vibrations (jarring)
    - Rapid temperature change
- High temperature in early incubation
- Incubation faults
    - Temperature, humidity, turning
    - Cooling after development has begun
    - Suffocation due to incorrect ventilation
- Inbreeding
- Chromosome abnormalities
- Egg-transmitted infectious diseases
- Parenteral nutritional deficiencies
- Abnormal or aged sperm
- Idiopathic developmental abnormalities
- Drugs, toxins, pesticides
- Cracked eggs
- Small holes in eggs

SECOND TRIMESTER
- Parenteral nutritional deficiencies
    - Riboflavin, vitamin B_{12}, folic acid, biotin, manganese, pyridoxine, pantothenic acid, phosphorus, boron, linoleic acid, vitamin K, vitamin D
- Secondary vitamin deficiencies
    - Antibiotic therapy destroying vitamin-producing flora
    - Diet imbalances, inadequate food intake
- Viral diseases
- Bacterial infections
- Fungal infections
- Egg jarring or shaking in the first trimester
- Incubator faults
    - Incorrect turning, temperature, humidity and ventilation
- Inbreeding resulting in lethal genes

THIRD TRIMESTER
- Malpositions
    - Inadequate or incorrect turning
    - Abnormal egg size or shape
    - Incorrect incubator temperature
- Incubator faults
    - Poor incubator ventilation
    - Egg cooling early in incubation
    - Inadequate or incorrect turning
    - Incorrect temperature
    - Incorrect humidity
- Incorrect hatcher temperature or humidity
- Long storage time pre-incubation
- Infectious disease
- Nutritional deficiencies
    - Vitamin A, D, E, K, pantothenic acid, folic acid
- Lethal genes
- Chromosomal abnormalities
- Idiopathic developmental abnormalities

weight during incubation. The calcium/manganese ratio regulates the rate of hatching, and imbalances of these minerals may cause early or late hatching.

Environmental Factors

Perches should be stable enough for breeding, and nest boxes of suitable size should be easily accessible (see Chapter 2). Nest box size and shape and bedding material should be evaluated. The microclimate of the nesting area, including temperature and humidity, is important for proper incubation and is adversely affected by soiled bedding and improper nest box design. Cultures from bedding material may help identify infectious agents. Ambient temperature, humidity and to a lesser degree rainfall, wind and barometric pressure may affect the success of parental incubation.

Pre-incubation Factors

Non-incubated, fertile eggs will not develop if held at 55-75°F. Cockatiel eggs stored at 55°F and 60% relative humidity did not show decreased hatchability until after three to four days of storage. Eggs can be incubated for two days, removed and placed at 55°F, and placed back in an incubator without a decrease in hatchability. These temperature manipulations are convenient for shipping eggs and for synchronizing hatching times.

Parents may not initiate incubation until more than one egg is laid. Under natural conditions, the failure of a parent to incubate the first egg when temperatures are not within safe preincubation ranges can result in the death of the egg. Exposure of eggs to temperatures that are higher than 55-75°F but below optimal incubation temperatures can cause death of the embryo. Parent behavior, climate and nest box characteristics may be responsible for lack of development or deaths in embryos during the first and last third of development.

Artificial Incubation

Hatchability of artificially incubated eggs is frequently lower than naturally incubated eggs. Eggs that have been naturally incubated for the first five to ten days may have higher hatchability levels than eggs that are artificially incubated for the entire developmental period. The fact that different hatchability rates exist between natural and artificially incubated eggs highlights the need for a wider dissemination of information on successful incubation protocols.

Many aviculturists prefer to use foster parents rather than artificial incubators, particularly during the first week to ten days of incubation. Foster parents must exhibit broodiness and be accepting of the shape, size and color of the foster eggs (see Chapter 6). Bantam and Silkie chickens have been used successfully to foster eggs from many psittacine species. The number of eggs under each foster parent should not exceed the number that the hen can adequately incubate.

Incubation Requirements

Important incubation factors include temperature, humidity, air flow in the incubator and hatcher, egg position during incubation, the angle for egg turning and the number of times per day the egg is turned. Incubator temperature and humidity affect the incubation period, and published incubation periods may vary with different incubation parameters (Table 29.7). Substantial research is necessary to establish the optimal incubator parameters for companion bird species. Most psittacine eggs are incubated at 99.1-99.5°F (37.3-37.5°C) and 80-82°F (26.7-27.8°C) wet bulb, and hatched at 98.5°F (36.9°C) and 88-90°F (31.1-32.2°C) degrees wet bulb. Lower incubator humidities and higher hatcher humidities

Table 29.7   Incubation Periods for Psittacine Species Common in Aviculture

Species	Incubation Period (days)	Pip to Hatch Interval (hours)
African Grey Parrot	26-28	24-72
African parrots (small)	24-26	24-48
Amboina King Parrot	20	24-48
Aratinga conures	24	24-48
Blue-fronted Amazon Parrot	26	24-48
Brotogeris parakeets	22	24-36
Budgerigars	18	12-24
Caiques	25	24-48
Cockatiels	21	24-48
Cockatoos (large)	26-29	24-72
Cockatoos (small)	24-25	24-72
Eclectus Parrot	28	24-72
Goldie's Lorikeet	24	24-48
Grass Parakeet	18	24-48
Green-cheeked Amazon Parrot	24	24-48
Hyacinth Macaw	26-28	24-72
King Parrot	20-21	24-36
Lories	26-27	24-36
Lovebirds	22	24-48
Macaws (medium)	24-28	24-72
Macaws (miniature)	23-27	24-60
Amazona ochrocephala parrots	26-28	24-48
Parrotlets	19	24-36
Pionus parrots	25-26	24-48
Psittacula parakeets	24-26	24-48
Pyrrhura conures	23	24-48
Quaker Parakeet	23	24-48
Red-lored Amazon Parrot	24	24-48
Rose-breasted Cockatoo	22-24	24-72
Palm Cockatoo	28-30	24-72
White-fronted Amazon Parrot	24	24-48

Compiled by Susan Clubb and Keven Flammer

have also been described. Research involving fertile cockatiel eggs determined that 99.5°F (37.5°C) with 56% relative humidity and 98.4°F (36.9°C) with 67% relative humidity were optimal settings for incubation and hatching, respectively.

Temporary shifts in temperature (as long as not excessively hot or cold) probably have no effect on hatchability. Such fluctuations are common when the incubator door is opened and the eggs are candled. It is best to turn off the fan when the incubator door is opened. Daily temperature and humidity charts should be maintained for each incubator. Individual incubators may have hot or cold spots that affect hatchability, and placing numerous thermometers at different locations within an incubator can help to identify these areas. Thermometers and hygrometers should be calibrated frequently to make certain that they are accurate.

A 2°F excess in temperature during the first few critical days of incubation can result in embryonic death. Increasing or decreasing the incubation temperature by 1.4°C caused poor hatchability and increased the incidence of abnormalities in cockatiel chicks. Chicks produced by higher than optimal incubation temperatures were small, weak and dehydrated and frequently had umbilical openings and exposed yolk sacs. Scissor beaks, curled toes and wry necks were also common. Slightly higher temperatures will further increase mortality, and temperatures approaching 104°F (40°C) will kill all embryos.

Marginally lower-than-optimum temperatures may cause a delay in hatching. Temperatures that are constantly a degree or so lower than optimum have been shown to cause an increased number of "late dead" embryos, and if hatching occurs, chicks are weak with large, soft bodies and unabsorbed yolk sacs. Some chicks may be ataxic post-hatching. Hatching may occur several days later than expected. Low humidity results in lower egg weight, larger air cell size and small dehydrated chicks, possibly due to inadequate calcium mobilization for bone development.

Chicks from eggs incubated at high humidities may have excessive amounts of fluid, including residual albumen, that may obstruct the nostrils causing asphyxiation. Eggs should be turned at least five to eight times a day for at least two-thirds of the incubation period. More frequent turning, up to 24 times a day, may improve hatchability in Psittaciformes or with embryos suspected to have a lack of vigor or delayed development. Eggs should be positioned on their sides with the round or air-cell end slightly elevated.

Still-air incubator temperature requirements are usually higher than forced-draft incubators. Placing incubators in a room that maintains a relatively cool (70-80°F; 21-26°C), dry (50-60% relative humidity), environment is ideal. Extreme temperature and humidity fluctuations (5°F or 5% relative humidity) in the incubation room should be avoided. Incubator ventilation, sanitation, abnormal vibrations, improper mechanized egg turning, inaccurate thermometers, inaccurate hygrometers and placement of incubators near walls and windows can all affect incubator function. Incubators with horizontal grill-type turners may be too rough for sensitive embryos. Excessive jarring and shaking, particularly during the early stages of development, can result in embryo death or malformation. Improper egg position and faulty egg turning during development may result in malpositions and incomplete closure of the ventral body wall.

Hatchers should be evaluated in a manner similar to incubators. The success of the sanitation program and the presence of microbial contamination can be estimated with cultures of the incubator surfaces, water trays, egg trays, and incubator room floor, shelves and instruments.

Incubation Preventive Techniques

Prevention of most incubation problems involves correcting the three most common causes for decreased hatchability in artificially incubated eggs: improper temperature, humidity and egg turning. Accurate record-keeping is mandatory for identifying hatching-

Table 29.8   Chick Abnormalities Caused by Incubation Problems

Abnormalities	Possible Causes
Early hatch, thin, excessive vocalizations	Small eggs, species differences, high incubator temperature, low incubator humidity, high incubator or hatcher temperatures (bloody navels)
Late hatch	Large eggs, old parents, eggs stored too long pre-incubation, low incubator temperature, inbreeding
Sticky chicks, albumin present	Low incubation temperature, high incubation humidity, incorrect turning, very large eggs
Dry chicks, stuck to shell	Low humidity during egg storage, incubation or hatching, incorrect turning, cracked eggs, poor shell quality, high incubator temperatures
Small chicks	Small eggs, low humidity during egg storage or incubation, high incubator temperature, high altitude, thin or porous shell, tetracycline used in hen
Weak chicks	Variety of causes including incorrect humidity and parenteral malnutrition
Umbilicus fails to close with varying degrees of unretracted yolk sac	Incorrect incubation temperature, low hatcher temperature, high hatcher humidity, parenteral malnutrition, omphalitis (can be caused by contamination or incorrect incubation temperature), inadequate ventilation
Short, wiry down (species dependent)	Nutritional deficiencies, toxins (eg, mycotoxins), high incubation temperature first two trimesters
Dwarf embryos, stunting in growing chicks	Egg contamination, heredity, parenteral malnutrition, possible hypothyroidism
Short beak, missing beak, face, eye or head abnormalities	High incubator temperature early first trimester, lethal genes, idiopathic developmental abnormalities, parenteral nutritional deficiencies (eg, niacin), low oxygen early first trimester, sulfa drug use in hen, insecticides, herbicides, excess dietary selenium, nicotine, viral
Red hocks	Prolonged pushing on shell during the pipping and hatching, parenteral vitamin deficiencies, thick shells, high incubator humidity, low incubator temperature
Musculoskeletal or neurologic abnormalities	Incorrect incubation temperature (curled or crooked toes, splayed legs), low incubation temperature (bent necks, nervous disorders), high incubation temperature (ataxia, star gazing), low humidity, unsuitable hatching substrate, sulfa drug use in hen, insecticides (scoliosis, lordosis)

related problems. A protocol for carefully evaluating incubator performance and stability should be followed. Pre-conditioning incubators a month prior to breeding season and evaluating daily fluctuations in temperature and humidity in the incubator room and in the incubators may help identify problem areas. The egg-turning mechanism should be checked periodically to confirm that it functions at the correct time interval, maintains the necessary egg angle and does not excessively vibrate the eggs. Excessive vibrations have been associated with reduced hatchability.

Bacterial and fungal agents infrequently cause problems in psittacine eggs, but occasionally a contaminated incubator, hatcher or incubator room can cause high egg losses. Water trays should be removed and disinfected daily and should be filled with distilled water. In the nonbreeding season incubators should be dismantled, and nonsensitive parts should be thoroughly cleaned with a glutaraldehyde solution followed by a long period of air drying. Disinfecting incubators with formalin and potassium permanganate is extremely dangerous and cannot be recommended.

Periodic culturing of newly hatched chicks, eggs and incubator surfaces will indicate if bacterial contamination is occurring. A sterile contact tape can be used to culture nursery surfaces and eggs. An open microbiological agar plate can be placed in an incubator to determine what bacteria are present in the air. Incubators can be tested for the presence of PBFD virus or polyomavirus by taking swabs for DNA probing.

The incubator room should be kept scrupulously clean to prevent particulate matter from contaminating egg shell surfaces. Clothes and shoes worn around other birds should be removed or covered before entering the incubation area. Hands should be thoroughly washed with a disinfectant or gloved before handling eggs. Problems associated with incubation are listed in Table 29.8.

Eggs are relatively resistant to bacterial invasion, but eggs that may have been contaminated with infectious agents should be incubated separately from noncontaminated eggs. Feces and dried particulate matter can be gently sanded off the egg surface, although over-exuberant sanding should be avoided.

Chlorine dioxide foam may be a safe sanitizing agent for contaminated eggs, or eggs can be washed with a warmed iodine solution (104°F) or immersed in warm water baths (110°F) for up to five minutes. Bacterially contaminated eggs can be dipped into a cold water antibiotic solution by warming the eggs to 37°C, and placing them in cold water (4°C) containing 1000 mg/ml of gentamicin solution. Psittacine eggs should not be incubated with eggs from other species.

Monitoring the Embryo

Candling

A candling program allows one to follow developmental progression of an embryo and detect any abnormalities that may occur. Periodic candling will ensure the removal of nondeveloping eggs as soon as they are identified. This increases the likelihood that the cause of an embryo's death can be determined and reduces the possibility of an infected egg contaminating the incubator. Daily candling will improve an individual's ability to recognize developmental stages of the various species.

Candling between the seventh and tenth day of incubation will indicate if an egg is fertile and whether it is developing normally. After the initial candling, eggs can be evaluated every two or three days if desired, and should be examined at least once just before transfer to the hatcher.

Candling naturally incubated eggs should be considered; however, the disadvantages of disturbing the adults and eggs must be weighed against the possible advantages of identifying eggs that need manipulation or intervention for hatching to occur. Candling to determine if the egg is fertile (five to seven days post-laying) followed by evaluation just prior to the expected date of pipping will usually be sufficient for evaluating parent-incubated eggs.

Candling Data: Candling helps identify the degree of egg shell thinning, egg shell cracks, blood rings, meat spots, membrane and blood vessel integrity, heart rate, stage of development, development progression, air cell size and shape, and yolk size, color and shape. Candling later in incubation helps to evaluate malpositions, chick movement, size, shape and location, and internal pip-to-hatch interval. Lack of embryo vitality can be recognized by poor vessel integrity, decreased movement and retarded development. Embryo death in early incubation results in cessation of development, blood rings and loss of membrane and vessel integrity. Late embryo death is somewhat harder to recognize due to the natural opaqueness of the developing embryo, but lack of vessel integrity and movement are indicative of late incubation deaths.

Egg Weights

Eggs should be weighed when they are candled, and weight loss rates can be recalculated throughout the incubation cycle. Air cell dimensions can be evaluated to provide an estimate of weight loss. Eggs from most Psittaciformes should lose an average of 12-13% of their weight from the beginning of incubation to the point of transfer to a hatcher. An additional 3% of weight should be lost during pipping. Desired egg weight loss can be determined using a variety of mathematical formulas. Egg weight loss rates can be used to detect incubation problems and can also be used to manipulate the humidity or egg to ensure proper weight loss.

Egg Necropsy

Every egg that fails to develop or that dies should be necropsied. "Breakout" refers to opening eggs for diagnostic purposes. Candling cannot distinguish very early embryonic deaths from infertile eggs, and the presence of fertility is an important criteria when proceeding with a diagnostic program in avian reproduction. The majority of eggs for necropsy will fall into two distinct age groups: embryonic death at three to five days of incubation, and death perihatching. Early embryonic mortality is common with improper incubation temperature, jarring, inbreeding and chromosomal abnormalities. Deaths at the end of incubation are usually associated with hatching, and the stressful period of switching from allantoic to pulmonary respiration. Factors including improper incubation humidity, temperature and turning are thought to be the leading causes of late embryonic death in psittacines.

Technique: All eggs should be candled before necropsy to determine the best point for entering the egg. This also permits the correlation of candling with necropsy findings. Eggs should be weighed and measured, and external shell characteristics (egg shape, egg size, external calcium deposits, cracks or thinning) should be noted. Pip marks should be evaluated for turning direction, location and size. Chicks normally pip counter-clockwise from the round end of the egg. The egg necropsy should be performed under sterile conditions until cultures have been taken of embryonic fluids and tissues.

The egg is opened over the air cell with sharp-blunt scissors. Shell membranes are examined for abnormalities and then carefully peeled back to expose the internal egg contents. When exposed, the albumen and amnion can be cultured and visible microbial growth may be noted. The chorioallantoic membrane (CAM) normally adheres to the inner shell membranes after the first trimester of development. Adhesions of the embryo to the CAM are abnormal. Eggs that are not necropsied shortly after death may develop adhesions or sticky membranes. Late-term embryos have anatomical differences from adults, but are similar to young chicks.

Internal egg membranes and structures should be evaluated before being altered by manipulation or culture techniques. A ruptured yolk sac can obscure the necropsy field. Color, size and location of the albumen, yolk and allantois are recorded. Presence and characteristics of the circulatory tree are observed. Abnormal odors should be noted.

Enlarging the hole over the round end of the egg is performed by careful removal of egg shell fragments with thumb forceps. If a small chick or no chick is identified, the contents of the egg can be carefully poured into a sterile container. If a well developed chick is present, the position of the air cell with respect to the egg, orientation of the embryo as a whole within the egg, position of the head, beak and neck in relation to the body and position of the beak in relation to the air cell should be evaluated.

Different malpositions have various success rates for hatching in domestic species, and many can hatch unassisted (Table 29.9). Although only six malposition classifications are traditionally discussed, there is an almost endless variety of malpositions that can occur, some of which are very subtle and require close inspection.

Psittaciformes appear to have different malpositions than domestic species. Frequently the head appears on an even plane with the right wing, and the entire body may be rotated such that the spine is on a horizontal plane with the short axis of the egg. The significance of this malposition is not known. Common causes of malpositions include turning problems, incorrect position in the incubator, oxygen deprivation, excess CO_2, lack of embryo vigor and delayed development.

If a chick can be seen in the egg, it should be weighed, measured and staged according to standards. Remaining albumen, chorioallantoic membrane blood vessels and ruptured yolk or allantoic contents may adhere to the shell once the chick is removed. If size permits, the chick should have a full necropsy performed, being careful to keep the yolk sac membrane intact. Special attention should be given to the hatching muscle for size, edema and hemorrhage. Other gross evaluations, including skin color and hemorrhage, musculoskeletal deviations, internal hemorrhages and contents of the mouth, nares, crop and esophagus, should be made. The liver may be hemorrhagic from exuberant kicking, especially if a chick was malpositioned.

The hatching muscle (Muscularis complexus) is a primary storage site for lymph in the embryo and is normally enlarged perihatching. Lungs are evaluated for evidence of air intake or for the presence of fluid, although this differentiation usually requires histopathology. Tissues should be fixed in formalin for histopathologic evaluation. Eggs can be frozen for future analysis of toxic substances.

Table 29.9   Classic Malpositions of Chick Embryos

Malposition 1:	Head between the thighs. Failure of the chick to lift and turn its head to the right in the middle of the last trimester. Completely lethal. Incidence increased by high incubation temperature.
Malposition 2:	Head in the small end of the egg. Chick is upside down in the egg. Hatchability reduced by 50% in domestic species. Incidence increased by incubator egg position and low temperature.
Malposition 3:	Head is under the left wing. Chick rotates its head to the left as opposed to the right. Usually lethal. Incidence increased by incubator egg position, temperature and parenteral nutrition.
Malposition 4:	Beak is away from the air cell. Upward turned aspect of the maxilla and egg tooth is not near the air cell; however, the rest of the embryo is normally positioned. Slightly reduced hatchability. Incidence increased by incubator egg position.
Malposition 5:	Feet over head. Usually lethal.
Malposition 6:	Head is over the right wing. Normally the head is under the right wing in domestic species. Psittacines may normally hold the head in the same plane as the wing. Reduced hatchability slightly in domestic species. Incidence may be increased by parenteral malnutrition.

Microbiology of Eggs

External egg structures discourage but do not stop microorganisms from entering the egg. Bacteria located in an egg could suggest environmental contamination that occurred after embryonic death. If the necropsy is performed immediately following embryonic death, finding bacteria in the embryo can indicate bacteremia or an infected ovary or oviduct in the hen. Bacterial contamination of an egg usually originates from the atmosphere, the nesting area or the surface of the cloaca.

Egg structures are affected by bacteria in different ways. The source of persistent egg infections may be identified by culturing the hen's cloaca, nest box contents, the exterior egg shell, albumen, yolk and embryonic tissues. Gram-positive bacteria occur mostly on the surface of the egg, and the insides of contaminated eggs contain mostly gram-negative bacteria. Chicks that are infected in the egg usually die with macroscopic yolk lesions (coagulated yolk and yolk sac hemorrhages). In other cases, embryos may die before the production of macroscopic changes in the yolk and a histological examination is necessary to establish the presence of an infection.

Egg Therapeutics

Treatment of bacterially infected eggs is possible although preventing infections is more effective. Medical intervention should be attempted only in those cases where the embryo is at risk of dying. Perpetuation of weak genetic lines in companion birds may be exacerbated by assisting in the hatching of troubled eggs.

Pre-incubation

Defects in egg shells can be repaired by using sparing amounts of Elmer's glue, surgical glue or paraffin. Thick or excessively large applications of these substances can retard air exchange or create difficulty for the chick during hatching. It has been suggested that large defects can be covered with egg shell remnants from other eggs, although the prognosis for these eggs should be considered poor. Tremulous air cells resulting from trauma or weak shell membranes may indicate blastoderm shock and ruptured shell membranes. Eggs with tremulous air cells usually have reduced hatchability but should not be discarded because embryos may develop and hatch normally. These eggs should be hand-turned as should all eggs with suspected shell or membrane defects.

Incubation

Manipulation of eggs before the point of hatching should be limited. The most frequently used techniques are designed to change the weight loss of an egg. Eggs can be moved to higher or lower humidity incubators based on weight loss. Eggs can also be gently sanded or have small holes placed in them over the air cell to increase weight loss. Paraffin can be used to partially cover the egg to reduce weight loss although no more than 60% of the area above the air cell or total air cell surface should be coated. Sealing a large portion of the air cell may decrease oxygen intake and cause the embryo to invert within the egg. Eggs that have had their shell altered should be hand turned to keep the sealant intact and to reduce chances of damaging the shell. Irregular or weak vascular patterns may be corrected by increasing the turning frequency.

Injecting sterile lactated Ringer's solution into severely dehydrated eggs has proven successful in some cases. Injection of sterile water into the small end of the egg (albumen) during the first half of incubation led to addled eggs in one study but was of benefit if given later in incubation. Replacement volumes to be given are calculated from egg weight deficits. Injecting antibiotics (piperacillin 200 mg/ml, 0.02 ml for macaw eggs, 0.01 ml for cockatoo eggs) into bacterially contaminated eggs has been attempted with some success. If done properly, injecting gentamicin into the albumen was not found to lower hatchability.

Small dental drills or needle puncture holes can be used to make a pathway for delivering injections into either the small end of the egg or over the air cell. Holes should be resealed with paraffin or glue. Pre-incubatory egg injections with 2.4 mg of tylosin and 0.6 mg of gentamicin was successful in eliminating *Mycoplasma meleagridis* from turkey poults.

Late Incubation

As the chick develops, the head comes to lie under the right wing, with the tip of its beak directed towards the air cell. When the air cell drops and enlarges, the hatching process has begun and a chick begins the transition from chorioallantoic circulatory respiration to pulmonic respiration. As the circulation to the allantois no longer has the capacity to meet the embryo's needs for gas exchange, the chick begins to move its head to the air-filled end of the egg. This stage of hatching can be observed only by candling. The CO_2 level in the embryo rises causing the neck muscles to twitch, and the embryo will penetrate the membrane into the air cell. At this point, the embryo begins to breathe air, and the patent right-to-left cardiovascular shunts close. The muscle twitching also occurs in the abdominal musculature initiating retraction of the yolk sac into the coelomic cavity. As the chick becomes more active and depletes the oxygen in the air cell, its carbon dioxide level increases to 10%, producing even stronger muscle contractions of the neck until the beak creates a puncture in the shell. At this point the chick is breathing room air and vocalizations can be heard.

Once eggs have started to pip and are transferred to the hatcher, they should be left undisturbed. As it hatches, the chick alternates between jerking head movements, which continue to chip the shell, and prolonged muscle contractions of the neck and back, which straighten the neck and force the body to rotate slightly counterclockwise.

Premature intervention in the hatching process can cause embryonic death. Proper intervention at the correct time can definitely result in a hatched chick that would have otherwise died. The amount of assistance required is difficult to determine but it is generally best not to rush the hatching process, but to gently assist each stage as necessary. Pip-to-hatch intervals are 36-48 hours in most species and hatching times of less than 24 hours and greater than 80 hours usually indicate a problem. Chicks that pip one-fourth to one-half of the egg and then stop for an extended period of time, or that reverse direction and return to the pip site, usually require assistance.

Chicks can be safely removed from their eggs if the yolk sac and blood vessels have retracted. In general, chicks that have made one quarter of a turn during pipping can usually be safely removed from the egg. Chicks can bleed to death or rupture their yolk sacs if removed prematurely, although in some cases minor bleeding and a partially unabsorbed yolk sac must be accepted to remove a chick before death occurs. Candling or dampening the inner shell membrane with sterile water will help elucidate the position of unretracted blood vessels. Once chicks pip internally, it is important that they have an unoccluded path for air intake. Malpositioned chicks or chicks with delayed albumen ingestion may need egg shell fragments removed and fluid cleared from their nares.

If drawdown fails to occur, little can be done to assist the chick. The transition from allantoic respiration to breathing air is delicate and timely. Forcing the process will result in the death of the chick. If internal pip has occurred but external pip does not, a small hole can be safely created in the air cell to provide a source of fresh air. If there are no signs of external pip after 36 hours from drawdown, a breathing hole should be created. The breathing hole need only be a few millimeters in diameter and can be created using a bur with or without magnification depending on the size of the egg.

To perform an ovotomy, the egg is candled and the air cell identified and marked with a soft pencil. The shell over the air cell is cleaned with dilute chlorhexidine or povidone iodine. It is important to keep the ovotomy site totally over the air cell where there are relatively few blood vessels in the outer shell membrane. If the shell is opened over any other area of the egg, severe, life-threatening hemorrhage may occur. Vessels that are regressing take on a ghostlike appearance and are often only partially filled with blood.

If, after providing a breathing hole, external pip still does not occur, the shell should be removed over the air cell. This procedure is usually performed 48 hours after drawdown or early on the scheduled hatch date if it is accurately known. Using a bur, the shell is removed without disrupting the outer shell membrane, which lies directly below and attached to the shell. A circular area of shell 0.5-1.5 cm in diameter should be removed, depending on the size of the egg. Once the shell has been removed, the outer shell membrane should be moistened with saline on a cotton-tipped applicator. Once moistened, the membrane becomes translucent, making it easy to identify any vessels that might need to be coagulated using bipolar radiosurgical forceps. After the vessels are coagulated, the membrane can be opened with the bipolar forceps revealing the chick within the air cell.

If the chick has entered the air cell, there will be a small nick in the inner membrane through which the beak has penetrated allowing respiration. The inner membrane is generally moister and more translucent than the outer shell membrane, except in the area where the beak has penetrated. In this region, the vessels retract and the membrane will usually appear dry and white. The inner shell membrane is delicate and highly vascular. The membrane should be carefully manipulated to prevent tearing. The entire exposed inner shell membrane will rapidly desiccate and should be kept moist by adding drops of warm, sterile saline or lactated Ringer's solution. Small quantities of fluids should be used to keep the chick from drowning. If the membrane is opaque, it is not properly hydrated.

For a successful hatch to occur, there must be an increase in CO_2 within the air cell to stimulate the chick to struggle, which ensures retraction of the yolk sac and the break out from the egg. The hole created in the shell can be partially sealed to allow this increase in CO_2 to occur. A stretchable, wax type test tube sealant can be used to effectively seal the hole created in the shell. The edges should be smoothed out and the egg returned to the incubator. An alternative solution is to place the egg in a small plastic bag with moistened sterile gauze. The bag can be partially sealed to allow an increase in CO_2 to develop, and the moistened gauze will ensure adequate humidity.

Chicks that are slightly malpositioned may create an external pip below the air cell. Strong chicks will continue to move their head toward the air cell creating additional external pips along the way. Appearance of more than one external pip may be an indication that the chick is malpositioned and may need assistance. If the pip is properly located, the egg should be returned to the incubator with the pip up. If the pip is on the opposite end of the egg from the air cell, it is likely that the chick is inverted and will need major assistance. If the pip is close to, but not within the air cell, intervention is indicated (see Chapter 41).

Embryo Extraction

Embryos that enter the air cell prematurely may defecate inside the shell causing a compromise in the normal metabolic management of waste.

When sufficient time has passed that the risk of fecal contamination is high or if the chick appears to be weakening based on decreased vocalizations and movements, the hole in the shell and shell membranes should be enlarged to allow gentle extraction of the chick's head and neck. The chick should be grasped by the beak and gently pulled out of the shell to allow visual inspection of the yolk sac. If the inner shell membranes have not adequately retracted, the yolk sac will still be visible, (incompletely absorbed). If no feces are found, the chick is gently replaced and the egg is sealed to allow hatching to proceed. The chick should be re-evaluated every one to three hours for the presence of feces. If the chick appears weak, oral administration of 5% dextrose solution may be beneficial. This can be alternated with lactated Ringer's solution to provide additional electrolytes. Because embryos are very susceptible to drowning, it is best if the solution can be placed into the esophagus or ingluvies using a 1 mm diameter silicone catheter or metal feeding tube. Excessive quantities of fluid should be avoided to prevent the accumulation of fluids in the allantois, which may increase the potential for membrane ruptures or delayed yolk sac absorption.

Once feces are observed within the shell, the chick should be removed. The chick is gently extracted with care taken to control hemorrhage from any unretracted vessels. The major attachment of the chick to the shell is in the area of the umbilicus where the vessels of the inner shell membrane attach to the yolk sac and umbilicus. The chick is extracted to a point where these vessels are visible and a vascular clip can be easily applied. The vessels are transected using radiosurgery and the chick is completely removed from the shell.

Aggressive hatching assistance is indicated for inverted chicks to prevent their dying of hypoxia or drowning. The earliest indication that a chick is inverted is an external pip at the small end of the egg. In approximately one of three inverted chicks, the air cell will have drawn down far enough to supply the chick with air. This is beneficial as the key to saving inverted embryos is providing air and enough time to allow retraction of the yolk sac. A breathing hole should be created over the air cell, which will change the pressures within the egg and allow the embryo to slide down into the large end of the egg and the air cell to migrate to the small end of the shell. The original pip site should be enlarged, with care taken not to damage the vessels within the membranes. If bleeding occurs it should stop in ten seconds. Sustained bleeding of chorioallantoic membranes can be stopped by applying pressure with sterile swabs or with the careful and specific application of a chemical coagulant such as silver nitrate. Experimentally, excessive bleeding can be controlled by placing injectable vitamin K sparingly on the bleeding CAM. A small amount of air (depending upon the size of the egg) may be injected into the egg through the original pip site to infiltrate under the membrane and expand it in any areas not trapped by the shell.

The egg should then be returned to the incubator with the pip site elevated at a 45° angle. Air should be injected through the pip site every two hours for the first day. On the second day, the pip site should be enlarged. The membranes should be left dry allowing the shell to separate from the membranes more easily. During the second and third days, the membrane should be gently and very gradually torn around the pip site allowing vessels to retract between manipulations. Eventually, as the shell is removed from the small end of the egg, the yolk sac should be visualized to determine if it has retracted. Once the end of the shell and its associated membranes are removed and the yolk has retracted, the chick will usually emerge without further assistance.

Unabsorbed yolk sacs are best left unattended and allowed to fully retract. This may require leaving a chick in the egg for several hours longer than normal so that the shell protects this fragile sac. Small umbilical protuberances can generally be ignored although the chick should be handled carefully until the umbilicus is sealed. Frequent application of disinfectants such as iodine solutions will prevent infections of the umbilicus and yolk sac. Larger protuberances can be carefully placed into the abdomen with the aid of a swab dipped in a water-based sterile ointment. The umbilicus is then sutured or surgically sealed with glue.

Surgical ligation and removal of the yolk sac may be needed in cases with a persistent or very large external yolk sac (see Chapter 48). Chicks that require amputation of the yolk sac can survive but have higher mortality levels. The chick is anesthetized with isoflurane to prevent traumatic injuries to the yolk sac and a hemostatic clip is applied to the umbilicus between the chick and the yolk sac. Two sutures (8-0 to 10-0) are placed to aid in closure of the umbilical opening with care taken to place them shallow enough to avoid penetrating umbilical vessels. The hemostatic clip is outside the body and an occlusive dressing is applied to protect the umbilicus. Occasionally, herniation of intestinal contents can occur through the umbilical opening while the chick is still within the egg. The prognosis is poor in these cases, although surgical resolution of the hernia should be attempted. Exteriorized tissues should be adequately cleaned with sterile saline and kept moist with the application of ointments if necessary. Umbilical openings can be surgically enlarged if necessary to replace herniated intestines (see Chapter 41).

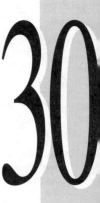

NEONATOLOGY

Keven Flammer
Susan L. Clubb

Care of pediatric patients is becoming an important segment of avian medicine as legislation and economic factors continue to restrict the importation of wild-caught psittacine birds. Because most birds entering the pet trade come from domestic sources, it is to the advantage of avian practitioners to become knowledgeable in avicultural and pediatric medicine.

Altricial species such as psittacine birds, song birds and pigeons are helpless at hatch. Most altricial birds are born naked with their eyes closed and depend totally on their parents for food and warmth. Neonates lack a fully competent immune system and are more susceptible to disease than older birds. Because they are helpless, the conditions under which they are maintained, the diet they are fed and the amount of parental care they receive all have a profound influence on their health.

Options for Raising Birds

Chicks can be raised by their parents, by avian foster parents or by humans (hand-raised). Each of these options has particular advantages and disadvantages.

Parent-raising

Allowing the parents to raise their own offspring has some advantages if the parents provide adequate care. It saves the considerable labor associated with hand-feeding, and parent-raised chicks usually develop faster. Parent-raised birds may also acquire species-specific behavioral traits that may be lacking in hand-raised chicks. It is known that hand-raising does not prevent normal breeding behavior, and many aviculturists believe that hand-raised chicks are better adapted to captivity and will breed sooner than chicks raised by other means.

Captive parents do not always provide optimal care and may traumatize, fail to feed, improperly feed or abandon chicks, especially if there are disturbances in the aviary. Chicks that are parent-raised beyond the pin-feather stage are also more difficult to tame and are less suitable as pets. Many aviculturists elect to hand-raise the larger, more expensive psittacine birds. Parent-raising is most often used with small, highly productive species such as cockatiels, love-birds and budgerigars where the cost of hand-raising is difficult to recover upon sale of the bird.

Fostering

Fostering refers to moving eggs or babies from one nest to another. Fostering is necessary when chicks are from neglectful or abusive parents or when there are large differences in the sizes of the chicks or between the times the eggs hatch. Fostering may also be used to increase production by removing eggs from a productive pair, which will stimulate them to lay more eggs. Fostering may spread disease, and the medical histories of both sets of parents should be established before considering cross-fostering.

Hand-raising

Aviculturists may hand-raise birds for the following reasons:
• To produce a tame bird that will socialize with people.
• To increase production by encouraging a pair of birds to lay additional clutches.
• To raise offspring hatched from artificially incubated eggs.
• To save sick or abandoned offspring.
• To reduce the burden of parental care on a compromised parent.
• To prevent or reduce the transmission of diseases from the parents to the neonate.

The disadvantages of hand-raising include the intensive labor required to feed birds and the threat of disease outbreaks that can occur when multiple nestlings from different pairs are concentrated in a nursery. Hand-raised birds seldom gain weight as quickly in the initial week of growth as parent-raised chicks; however, they usually compensate later and wean at a normal weight.

Problems Associated with Parent-raised Birds

Nestling birds are most likely to have medical problems during the first week of life, at fledging and at weaning. Monitoring the condition of parent-raised offspring in the nest box can be difficult. Nest boxes should be constructed with a small door that can be used for viewing the chicks and examining the eggs. A fiberoptic light and mirror may be helpful.

Chicks receiving adequate parental care will have food in their crops and yellowish-pink skin. Chicks that have empty crops, act listless and are cool to the touch are receiving inadequate care and should receive immediate attention. These chicks may be hypothermic, hypoglycemic, dehydrated or have bacterial or yeast infections. The solution to many of the problems associated with parent-raised neonates is to remove them for hand-raising.

Parental Problems

Parenting is a learned process and captive birds do not always make ideal parents, especially with the first few clutches. Parents may eat, traumatize or abandon the eggs or the chicks. Some parents never learn to provide adequate care; others may learn to provide improved care with subsequent clutches. Disturbances in the aviary will increase parental problems. Most psittacine birds lay eggs every two to three days and start incubation when the first egg is laid. Highly productive species such as cockatiels may lay an additional clutch before fledging chicks from the previous lay. These adults may remove the feathers from the chicks in an attempt to encourage them to leave the nest.

Nestling Problems

Any factor that decreases the vigor of the chicks (disease, cold, competition) can decrease their chances of being properly fed. Often the older and more vigorous chicks will compete most efficiently for food and parental attention, causing younger chicks to be neglected and undernourished.

Environmental Problems

Nestlings in a hot, cold or damp nest box may be stressed, fail to beg for food or be abandoned. Improper nest material may be ingested or inhaled or may support the growth of bacteria and fungi. Rats, snakes and other predators may consume nestlings or disturb the parents and prevent regular feedings. Disturbances of the nest box may cause parents to neglect or traumatize chicks.

Injuries

Nestlings may be injured by their parents, other nestlings or improper nest box construction (eg, exposed nails, slippery nest material). Poor nutrition can cause metabolic bone disease and make the chicks more susceptible to fractures. Many of the larger psittacines are territorial and may traumatize the nestlings when defending the nest. To prevent these injuries, the nest box can be equipped with a sliding door over the entrance hole to exclude the parents from the nest box while chicks are being examined. Chicks may also traumatize each other, most frequently injuring the beak, face and wing tips.

Infectious Diseases

Microbial infections (gram-negative bacteria, chlamydia, viruses and yeast) and internal parasites (eg, giardia and trichomoniasis) are frequent causes of mortality in nestling birds.

Ill nestlings should be pulled for hand-feeding and appropriate treatment. These birds should be raised separately from other neonates and should not be fed by the same person who cares for the other birds in the nursery. If this is not possible, some microbial infections can be treated by offering medicated food to the parents who will then feed it to the nestlings. Fortunately, adult birds are often less selective of their diet while feeding offspring and may accept foods that they would ordinarily refuse. Parents preferentially feed nestlings soft, moist food, which should be offered fresh two to three times daily. Only highly susceptible microbial infections can be treated by offering medicated food to the parents, because it is difficult to achieve adequate antibiotic concentrations in the chick by using this technique (see Chapter 17). It is also possible that a parent could feed toxic amounts of the antimicrobial agent to the chicks. Viral infections such as polyomavirus and psittacine beak and feather disease virus (PBFD) can also affect parent-raised chicks.

External Parasites

Red mites (*Dermanyuss gallinae*), Northern fowl mites (*Ornitysluss sylvarium*), fire ants, Africanized bees and mosquitoes can infest the nest box and cause discomfort, anemia and even death of chicks. Adding a small amount of 5% carbaryl powder to the nest material will aid in control, but care should be taken in areas where insect vectors (eg, cockroaches) might carry *Sarcocystis* sp. If cockroaches enter the nest box and die from the insecticide, they may be eaten by either the parents or nestlings and subsequently transmit *Sarcocystis* sp. Insecticides should be used only if indicated by the infestation of a parasite. They should not be used prophylactically.

Hand-raising Birds

Husbandry and Preventive Medicine

When faced with a neonatal health problem, it is essential for the clinician to carefully evaluate the environmental conditions, hygiene practices and feeding methods in the nursery. Possibly one of the most overlooked factors in raising healthy psittacine chicks is providing them with ample rest periods in which they are not disturbed between feedings.

Nursery Design

The nursery should be separated from any contact with adult birds, and the aviculturist should take steps to prevent disease transmission from the adult flock. It is best to have separate caretakers for the adults and the babies. If this is impossible, the aviculturist should shower and change clothes between caring for adults and young. It is advantageous to have several potential nursery rooms in case there is a disease outbreak. If possible, valuable or endangered species should be raised in a room separate from common species that have a high incidence of infectious diseases (eg, budgerigars, cockatiels, lovebirds and conures). The nursery room(s) should have adequate temperature control and be self-contained.

Table 30.1 Guidelines for Nursery Management

1. Every nursery should have a separate room where sick birds can be isolated. This room should not share air flow with the primary nursery. Nestlings showing signs of disease should be immediately moved from the primary nursery and isolated.

2. If a baby leaves the nursery for any reason and is exposed to other birds, it should not be returned to the primary nursery.

3. A nestling should never be added from another facility.

4. The same people should not care for both the adults and the neonates, unless special precautions are taken to avoid disease transmission.

5. Visitors, especially people who own birds, should be restricted from entering the nursery. People can act as mechanical vectors of infectious agents.

6. Ideally, every bird that is sold should be tested for microbial diseases, PBFD virus and polyomavirus before shipment.

7. Thorough cleaning of nursery facilities and equipment is better than partial cleaning followed by the use of disinfectants. Disinfectants are toxic, and exposure to the nestlings should be minimized (both direct contact and fumes).

8. Proper feeding practices can minimize problems.
   a. Use a proven diet and constantly evaluate growth by assessing development and comparing weight gains with a growth chart.
   b. Store dry nestling diet in a cool, dry, rodent-free area. Opened food containers should be stored in the freezer.
   c. Feeding formula should be carefully measured and mixed, and the temperature checked before feeding.
   d. Mix food fresh for each feeding. Do not store mixed food in the refrigerator and feed it at a later time.
   e. Use an individual syringe for each nestling.
   f. Never feed a bird and place the syringe back in the feeding formula.

Age at Time of Removal from the Nest

For most species, nestlings less than two to three weeks of age are easiest to adapt to the hand-feeding process. Older birds may be fearful of people and more difficult to feed, while younger chicks more readily accept hand-feeding but must be fed more frequently.

Housing

Chicks should be housed in brooders in order to provide the precise temperature and humidity control required for optimal development of young neonates. Inside the brooder the chick should be kept in a small plastic container lined on the bottom with soft, absorbable paper toweling to aid in support and provide security. Slick surfaces can cause leg deformities. Chicks can also be housed in containers with a raised floor made of plastic-coated wire. The mesh must be small enough to prevent the leg (especially the tibiotarsal joint) from extending through the wire.

Partially feathered chicks can be housed in open plastic pans or aquariums if the nursery is properly heated. Fully feathered chicks are capable of flight and should be kept in secure enclosures.

Temperature and Humidity

The relative humidity for tropical species should be above 50%. Temperature should be adjusted for the behavior of the particular bird. Birds that are too hot will pant and hold their wings away from their bodies; those that are too cold will huddle, shiver and may have slow crop-emptying times. Chicks housed at temperatures outside the optimal range will grow more slowly. Some suggested temperatures for psittacine chicks are provided in Table 30.2.

Table 30.2	Suggested Ambient Temperature Ranges for Psittacine Chicks
Recent hatchlings	92-94°F
Unfeathered chicks	90-92°F
Chicks with some pin feathers	85-90°F
Fully feathered chicks	75-80°F
Weaned chicks	68-75°F
The actual temperature should be adjusted to the needs of the individual chick.	

Substrate

The substrate on the floor of the "nest" should absorb moisture from the droppings, provide firm footing and not cause major digestive problems if ingested. Cloth diapers or unfrayed cotton woven towels and coated wire screens can be used with few problems. Problem substrates include tissue paper (provides poor traction), soft, crumpled or shredded paper, wood shavings or chips (cause impactions if ingested), sawdust (causes respiratory problems if inhaled), and coarse pelleted bedding (causes GI irritation or blockage if ingested).

Housing Multiple Chicks

Nestlings seem to grow best if they are housed with their clutch mates; however, chicks should be separated if there are substantial differences in body size, or if a bird becomes ill. Housing birds from different clutches together is discouraged because of the threat of disease transmission.

Chick Identification

Chicks should be assigned individual identification numbers upon entering the nursery and identified by closed banding or transponder implants when they are large enough. At a minimum, the aviculturist should record the following information in a log book: egg number if artificially hatched, identification of siblings and parents and location of the parents' enclosure.

Diets

A diet containing approximately 25-30% solids (70-75% water) should be fed to nestlings older than one or two days. It may be beneficial to feed a more dilute diet for the first day after hatching because the chick will be using the contents of its yolk sac for nutrition. Inexperienced hand-feeders should actually weigh the solid and liquid portions of the diet to ensure a proper dilution is fed. Evaluating a cooked diet according to visual consistency is inaccurate. Cooked starches may cause the formula to appear thick even though the percentage of solids is very low. The food should be warmed to 101-104°F and the temperature measured with an accurate thermometer. The instructions provided with commercial diets should be carefully followed. A hot plate or coffee maker should be used for heating formula. The use of a microwave oven for heating food frequently results in severe crop burns.

Feeding Methods

Most aviculturists now use syringes for feeding, although bent spoons or crop tubes are occasionally used. Catheter-tipped syringes are especially popular. Hungry nestling birds display a feeding response that consists of rapid, thrusting head movements and bobbing up and down. These movements can be stimulated by touching the commissures of the beak or pressing lightly under the mandible. While the bird is displaying this behavior, the glottis is closed and large amounts of food can be delivered quickly with less fear of passing food into the trachea. If a neonate resists feeding or a feeding response is not displayed, the chance of tracheal aspiration is greater. If a young bird that is not eating on its own refuses to eat for two to three feedings in a row, it may be having a medical problem that should be evaluated. As some birds get older, they display less of a feeding response and are more difficult to feed. This may be an indication that weaning is beginning to occur. If an older bird resists feeding, that feeding should be skipped. The chick may be hungrier and more willing to eat at the next scheduled feeding. A long, soft tube can be used to feed re-calcitrant birds. Short tubes should not be used, as they may become detached from the syringe and swallowed.

Feeding Amounts and Frequency

Birds one to five days old should be fed six to ten times daily; chicks with eyes closed, four to six times daily; chicks with eyes opened, three to four times daily; and birds with feathers emerging, two to three times daily. Chicks less than one week old may benefit from around-the-clock feeding, but it is not necessary to feed older chicks through the night. The last feeding can be given between 10:00 p.m. and 12:00 a.m. and the first between 6:00 and 7:00 a.m. The crop should be filled to capacity and allowed to nearly empty before the next meal. The crop should be allowed to completely empty at least once each day (usually in the morning following the final night feeding). It is important to feed young birds the maximum amounts of food early to stimulate good growth and increase crop capacity. However, excessively large meals in very small birds can predispose them to regurgitation and subsequent aspiration.

Weaning

Some birds wean themselves at the appropriate body weight by refusing to be hand-fed, but many others must be encouraged to wean (particularly cockatoos and large macaws). Several weeks prior to the expected age of weaning, the bird should be offered a variety of foods such as corn, cooked vegetables, various fruits, soaked monkey chow, formulated diet, spray millet, hulled seeds and peanut butter and jelly sandwiches. Seeds with hulls and large chunks of food should be avoided because at this stage the bird may consume them whole. Most birds will pick up and play with food long before they actually consume the material. It is best to accustom a weaning baby to a wide variety of formulated diets and fresh fruits and vegetables. If birds are weaned onto a specific diet, it is important that a new owner continue feeding the same diet until the bird is accustomed to its new surroundings and the diet can be safely changed.

When the bird is at the right weight and development or consuming some solid food, the midday feeding should be gradually eliminated, followed by the morning and then the evening meals. If the bird was fed properly to begin with, weight loss in the range of 10-15% of the peak body weight may be expected during the weaning process. If the bird was underweight to begin with, any weight loss may be abnormal. Subclinical illness (especially gram-negative bacterial infections of the alimentary tract) may become apparent during weaning. Clinical signs could include excessive weight loss, slowed crop-emptying times, depression, diarrhea, regurgitation or simply a failure to wean. If problems are noted, weaning should be postponed and the underlying problem diagnosed and treated.

Some birds will resist hand-feeding before they are capable of maintaining adequate body weight on their own. This is especially common in malnourished birds that are stunted in growth but of weaning age. It may be necessary to tube-feed these birds, because forcing them to hand-feed increases the risk of aspiration and causes severe stress.

Hygiene

Careful control of environmental sources of pathogenic bacteria and yeast are essential for maintaining healthy chicks. The most important sources of microbial contamination include the food, water supply, feeding and food preparation utensils, other birds in the nursery and the hand-feeder. If microbial infections are repeatedly encountered in a nursery, these areas should be cultured in order to identify and eliminate the source of contamination.

The diet should be mixed fresh before each feeding. As a guide, the standards for cleanliness in a nursery should be higher than the feeders would maintain for themselves. Opened containers of dry baby formula should be stored in sealed containers in the freezer. Powdered baby formula that has been mixed with water should never be stored and fed to babies in subsequent feedings. Hands should be washed between birds or groups of birds to avoid transmitting diseases. A separate syringe should be used for each bird and the syringes should be filled in advance. Under no circumstances should a syringe used to feed a bird be dipped back into the food for a refill; this will result in the spread of infectious agents throughout the nursery. Quaternary ammonium products containing a detergent are recommended for disinfection since they will cause less drying of the syringe plunger than Clorox. The syringe plunger should be periodically removed and scrubbed to avoid a build-up of food and pathogens. Feeding implements must be thoroughly rinsed to reduce exposure of chicks to residual disinfectants.

New Additions

New additions to the nursery should be placed in separate brooders, fed last and monitored carefully until it is apparent that they are healthy. It is prudent to culture the cloaca of new birds at the time they enter the nursery to diagnose and eliminate potential microbial infections that might spread to other chicks. A cloacal swab can also be submitted to make certain that the neonates are not shedding polyomavirus. Detecting an infectious agent in a newly introduced chick also indicates that the parents and egg incubator should be evaluated. In this manner, chicks can be used to monitor the health of the adult collection.

Evaluating Nestling Birds

History

Avicultural clients should be asked to prepare a written summary prior to taking a nestling psittacine chick to the veterinarian. The history should include the following:
1. The past breeding and health history of the parents and condition of the chick's siblings.
2. Problems during incubation or hatching if the chick was artificially incubated. (Chicks that have problems hatching frequently grow poorly during the first few weeks of life and may be stunted).

3. Brooder temperature, substrate, hygiene practices (including exposure to any disinfectants) and condition of other birds in the nursery.
4. The type of diet, percent solids content, how the diet is prepared, amount and frequency of feedings and implement used to feed the chick.
5. The identification number and method used to identify the chick.

Body Weight Charts

One of the most valuable tools for evaluating nestling birds is a chart recording daily body weight. Birds should be weighed prior to the morning feeding when the crop and GI tract should be relatively empty. At most stages of development, juvenile birds should gain a certain amount of weight daily. Failure to gain this amount of weight is cause for concern. See Table 30.5 for suggested normal growth rates for selected psittacine species.

Developmental Characteristics

Recording developmental characteristics, such as the date the eyes open, the first appearance of head, wing and tail feathers and any other physical changes will help in assessing the growth of a chick. Delayed developmental characteristics usually indicate delayed overall growth and stunting.

Physical Examination

A thorough physical examination is as important in nestlings as it is in adults. During the examination, chilling and stress should be avoided by warming hands, warming the room and keeping handling times to a minimum. Birds with food in the crop should be handled carefully to avoid regurgitation and aspiration. The heart and lungs should be auscultated to detect cardiac murmurs and moist respiratory sounds. The eyes and ears should be carefully examined to evaluate normal development and opening. It is normal to have a clear discharge from the eyes when they open. In macaws, the eyes usually open between 14 and 28 days following hatching; in cockatoos, between 10 and 21 days; and in Amazon parrots, from 14-21 days. The ears are open at hatching in Old World Psittaciformes, and open from 10-35 days of age in neotropical species.

Posture

Until weaning, neonates sit on their hock joints, rather than up on their feet, using their protuberant abdomen to create a tripod stance. Young birds may be uncoordinated and splay their legs when trying to walk. This should be considered normal unless a limb is held consistently in an abnormal position.

Body Conformation

Nestlings have relatively little muscle mass and a large, protuberant abdomen. The pectoral muscles are almost nonexistent. As the bird ages, the muscle mass will increase, but even at weaning they will be thinner than in an adult. Body mass in young

Table 30.5 Sample Weight Gains (g) of Selected Hand-raised Psittacine Birds and Normal Adults

Species	Age (days) 0	3	7	12-14	14	21	28	35	42	49	Adult
Cockatiel	4-6	5-6	12-14		45-65	72-108	80-120	80-90	80-95	90-110	90-110
Golden Conure	7-11	10-12	12-23		20-25	30-100	45-150	90-240	125-270	180-310	262
Green-cheeked Amazon Parrot	10-14	15-22	30-50		90-135	200-250	225-310	280-350	290-350	***	360
Lilac-crowned Amazon Parrot	11-13	15-20	25-35		75-140	160-240	250-300	300-350	310-350	***	360
Blue-fronted Amazon Parrot	14-17	20-25	35-60		100-170	240-280	280-370	350-420	380-440	380-430	432
Yellow-headed Amazon Parrot	12-21	16-30	25-50		75-200	140-300	230-450	270-580	310-560	380-565	568
Yellow-crowned Amazon Parrot	12-15	15-33	25-55		70-170	175-260	250-360	350-440	400-480	***	500
Yellow-naped Amazon Parrot	11-18	16-35	28-75		60-100	170-360	275-500	420-600	500-650	500-650	596
Eclectus Parrot	12-20	16-35	23-60		60-150	110-240	190-350	260-440	300-450	320-480	432
African Grey Parrot	11-17	15-211	25-40		70-120	135-250	240-335	300-440	380-470	435-500	554
Red-vented Cockatoo	11	16-20	25-30		70-100	145-200	230-280	250-300	275-350	230-350	298
Citron-crested Cockatoo	12-15	15-23	26-84		78-144	148-265	208-366	292-430	319-445	320-464	357
Bare-eyed Cockatoo	8-14	11-35	18-70		48-170	99-308	167-363	238-415	283-410	289-415	375
Goffin's Cockatoo	8-11	10-15	20-45		70-100	125-240	175-275	220-325	250-350	250-350	255
Lesser Sulphur-crested Cockatoo	8-15	12-22	25-60		65-120	140-250	225-320	280-340	315-380	320-410	450
Rose-breasted Cockatoo	7-12	10-17	15-40		35-100	70-200	115-300	175-370	220-400	240-423	403
Medium Sulphur-crested Cockatoo	12-15	18-25	35-70		65-140	160-250	240-350	340-450	400-525	450-550	465

Table 30.5 Sample Weight Gains (g) of Selected Hand-raised Psittacine Birds and Normal Adults

Species	Age (days) 0	3	7	14	21	28	35	42	49	Adult
Major Mitchell's Cockatoo	9-13	13-22	25-55	55-130	140-220	210-300	270-375	290-450	340-500	423
Umbrella Cockatoo	12-20	15-20	25-55	75-150	170-300	280-400	350-530	450-600	500-725	577
Triton Cockatoo	11-19	15-30	30-70	90-170	200-325	290-475	400-650	450-750	490-800	643
Moluccan Cockatoo	16-22	21-30	35-55	90-170	190-300	330-450	470-650	600-750	680-825	853
Greater Sulphur-crested Cockatoo	16-20	18-35	35-80	100-200	220-330	370-525	450-625	500-725	550-880	843
Yellow-collared Macaw	9-15	12-20	25-35	60-90	110-160	190-240	230-280	250-290	270-300	250
Red-fronted Macaw	12-16	18-25	25-45	70-130	140-250	230-360	330-470	405-530	465-580	490
Caninde Macaw	14-22	19-25	30-45	70-120	165-250	275-420	420-600	520-725	600-800	752
Military Macaw	17-26	24-45	35-170	85-300	220-425	360-650	500-800	600-950	680-1050	925
Scarlet Macaw	17-26	25-45	40-65	90-175	200-400	380-625	540-800	720-1050	830-1150	1001
Blue and Gold Macaw	16-27	25-40	40-100	90-250	200-450	350-650	525-900	670-1100	800-1200	1039
Green-winged Macaw	17-28	30-55	45-80	100-250	225-450	400-650	610-900	830-1030	990-1190	1194
Buffon's Macaw	20-26	25-35	40-70	100-170	250-500	450-750	650-900	850-1100	1050-1350	1290
Hyacinth Macaw	20-27	25-35	45-75	110-180	250-400	450-600	600-750	800-1000	900-1200	1355

Weight ranges are provided as suggestions only, as growth of an individual chick is dependent on hatch weight, body structure, sex, diet and feeding and husbandry.

nestlings is best assessed by noting the thickness of the muscle and subcutaneous fat covering the elbows, toes and hips.

Skin

Normal nestlings have yellowish-pink skin with a supple, warm feel. Dehydrated nestlings will have dry, hyperemic skin that feels sticky to the touch. Nestlings with white, cool skin are either hypothermic or moribund and need immediate attention. Some flaking of the skin is normal; excessive amounts of flaking indicate dehydration or exposure to high temperature, low humidity or malnutrition.

Feather Growth

The first feathers appear on the head, wings, and tail, followed by feather emergence on the rest of the body. Gross discrepancies in the pattern of feather development may indicate stunted growth. Feather dysplasia (eg, pinched-off feathers, constrictive bands, blood in the rachis) or epilation may indicate polyomavirus, PBFD virus, adenovirus or bacterial folliculitis. Neonates being treated with antibiotics may also have abnormally developed feathers.

Crop

The crop should empty at least once daily; overstretched, damaged and atonic crops will not empty properly. The crop should be palpated for foreign objects and trapped, doughy food, and examined externally for redness or scabs that might indicate a burn or puncture.

Droppings

Nestlings often have polyuric droppings. This usually results from the liquid diet they are fed.

Diagnostic Procedures

Clinical Pathology

The clinical pathology of nestling psittacine birds is poorly documented; however, recent publications have established reference intervals for some species. In general, nestling birds normally have lower packed cell volumes (20's-30's), lower total protein (1-3 g/dL), and higher white blood cell counts (20,000-40,000) when compared to adults of the same species (see Appendix). Young chicks also have lower plasma concentrations of albumin and uric acid and higher concentrations of alkaline phosphatase and creatine phosphokinase. It is very important to note these age-related differences in hematology so that misinterpretation of laboratory values does not result in the unnecessary treatment of a normal chick.

Microbiology

Young birds are highly prone to microbial infections and cloacal cultures, and fecal Gram's stains should be routinely evaluated during development. Normal aerobic cloacal flora is gram-positive and consists of *Lactobacillus, Corynebacteria, Staphylococcus,* non-hemolytic *Streptococcus* and *Bacillus* spp. Common pathogens include gram-negative bacteria and yeast. Many commercial diets contain nonpathogenic brewer's yeast that can be seen on Gram's stains of the crop or feces. Yeast that is contained in the diet should not be budding (an indication that the yeast is alive). Choanal cultures can be used to evaluate the microflora of the upper respiratory tract.

Radiography

The anatomic differences of nestling birds must be considered when interpreting radiographs. The proventriculus and ventriculus are normally much larger than in an adult and may fill most of the abdominal cavity, especially if food is present. Intestinal loops may also be filled with food. Filling of the digestive tract with food reduces the volume of the air sacs. Growth plates in the bones may be open and the general muscle mass will be reduced.

Endoscopy

The techniques and indications for endoscopy are similar to those for adults. An endoscope can be used to identify foreign bodies, inhaled food or aspergillosis in the trachea. Flexible or rigid endoscopes are useful for visualizing the crop when foreign bodies or burns are suspected. The proventriculus and ventriculus are best visualized with flexible scopes passed per os. Great care must be used when scoping the coelomic cavity of nestling birds because the relatively large digestive tract reduces the free space in which the scope can be safely introduced to the air sac. The bird should be fasted for several hours (depending on age) before attempting this procedure. Indications for laparoscopy include surgical sexing, documentation of aspiration or pneumonia and identification of abdominal or thoracic masses not confined to the digestive tract. Nestling birds can be endoscopically sexed as young as six weeks of age.

Common Problems of Neonates

Neonatal Problems

Failure to Absorb the Yolk Sac

The yolk sac is a diverticulum of the intestine and is internalized into the abdomen just prior to hatch. Following hatch, the yolk is normally absorbed and provides nourishment and maternal antibodies during the first days of life. Once the yolk is absorbed, only a small remnant of scar tissue should remain. A common cause of death in artificially hatched chicks during the first week of life is retention of the yolk sac, which may be associated with primary or secondary infections of the navel (omphalo-vitellitis).

Yolk sac infections can occur secondary to infections of the navel if it is poorly internalized prior to hatching. Alternatively, bacteria can multiply in the hatching egg following fecal contamination of the shell. Affected animals have enormous yolk sacs that are 20-40% of the total body weight. The navel may be thickened, prominent and necrotic. Failure of yolk absorption is reported primarily in ratite and waterfowl chicks, but also occurs in companion birds. The normal interval for complete absorption of the yolk varies in different species. The yolk sac is no longer visible at six days in macaws, is absent in the ostrich in eight or more days and is palpable in emus for approximately seven days. Birds with unabsorbed yolk will have enlarged, doughy abdomens, and the large yolk sac may be visible through the abdominal wall or via radiography. Dyspnea, exercise intolerance, depression, anorexia and inability to stand have also been reported.

Stunted Growth

Possible causes of stunting include:

- Improper feeding: unbalanced nutrition, not feeding enough volume, not feeding frequently enough and feeding a diet with low total solids.
- Poor environmental conditions in early development: low or high temperature, low humidity.
- Diseases: any disease may cause a chick to expend energy fighting the disease, rather than using energy for growth. Clinical and subclinical microbial diseases caused by gram-negative bacteria and yeast are commonly implicated. These organisms may be secondary problems indicating primary viral infections, environmental inadequacies, immunosuppression or malnutrition. Stunted birds may also be infected with polyomavirus or PBFD virus.
- Hyacinth Macaw, Palm Cockatoo and Queen of Bavaria Conure neonates appear to have a higher incidence of stunting than other species, possibly because they have dietary requirements that are not met with commonly used diets. Currently, these species do best when fed high-fiber, high-fat formulated diets throughout development, with the addition of nuts at weaning.

Malnourished birds can often be salvaged by correcting the underlying problems and gradually increasing their plane of nutrition. If the stunting is mild and the cause is corrected early, many birds will wean normally. Moderate stunting may result in a smaller bird with a globose head and slender beak. If the stunting is severe, the bird may survive for a long time without growing but will eventually die. Euthanasia should be considered for nestlings that are confirmed positive for PBFD virus.

Congenital Abnormalities

Reports in the literature would suggest that budgerigars, cockatiels and African Grey Parrots have a greater incidence of congenital deformities than do other psittacine species.

Documented cases of congenital abnormalities in psittacine chicks include bilateral anophthalmia in a budgerigar, varying degrees of cryptophthalmus and ankyloblepharon in four cockatiels, congenital extra-hepatic biliary cysts in an African Grey Parrot and familial cataracts in Scarlet Macaws. Skeletal deformities are considered to be the most common congenital abnormalities in psittacine birds, but specific cases rarely have been reported in the literature. Other reported, but poorly documented, deformities include hydrocephalus, and abnormalities of the pelvis, hock, feet, sternum and jaw, stifle and hips, tarsus, long bones of the legs and the beak.

Choanal atresia was diagnosed in an African Grey Parrot and an Umbrella Cockatoo with histories of chronic (four months and four years, respectively) ocular nasal discharge since hatch.

Infectious Diseases

Microbial Infections

The interpretation of culture results in nestling birds is controversial. Strains of *E. coli, Klebsiella* and *Enterobacter* spp. vary widely in pathogenicity; many cause disease, but some strains can be isolated from completely normal chicks. Some veterinarians believe that gram-negative bacteria and yeast should be treated only if a nestling is showing clinical signs of disease with or without an elevated white blood cell count. Other veterinarians believe all gram-negative bacteria and yeast are potential pathogens and should always be eliminated by antimicrobial therapy. The authors' personal opinions lie in the middle. If only a few organisms are cultured in a healthy nestling, treatment should be delayed unless clinical signs are evident.

Treatment of microbial infections in nestling birds should be approached in the same manner as in adults (see Chapter 17), with a few special considerations. Medication is more easily delivered via the oral route because nestling birds are fed and handled frequently. If possible, antibiotics should be administered when the alimentary tract is relatively empty. Food in the alimentary tract reduces the absorption of most antibiotics, and calcium in the diet will significantly reduce the absorption of tetracyclines. However, some oral antibiotics cause local GI irritation (eg, trimethoprim/sulfonamide combinations and doxycycline), and birds will regurgitate unless the drug is administered with a small amount of food. A bird should not be fasted for antimicrobial administration if this will reduce the number of feedings and slow growth. If injectable drugs must be used, the subcutaneous route is preferred, because young nestling birds have little muscle mass and it is difficult (but not impossible) to deliver intramuscular injections. Injections should be carefully given into the pectoral muscle of young chicks, as the sternum is soft and easily penetrated with a needle. To prevent secondary yeast infections, neonates should be screened with fecal Gram's stains, or nystatin should be administered prophylactically.

Viral Infections

Polyomavirus is the most common viral infection described in psittacine nurseries. The onset of clinical signs is usually acute and includes crop stasis, listlessness, regurgitation and vomiting. Hemorrhages may be observed on the skin, and injection sites and broken or plucked feathers will bleed excessively. Most birds are nonresponsive to therapy and die within 24-48 hours. Survivors fail to gain normal weight, are prone to secondary microbial infections and often fail to wean. Feather abnormalities can occur that are grossly similar to those seen with PBFD virus infections. A more common and subtle clinical presentation has been identified. Slow growth, abnormal flora (gram-negative and yeast), beak malalignment, leg deformities and hepatomegaly may be the only clinical signs present.

Polyomavirus can be controlled in an aviary by testing adult birds and raising neonates from carriers separately from neonates from non-carriers. Neonates can be tested as they are pulled from the nest to determine if they are shedding polyomavirus. Shedders should be raised separately from non-shedders.

[*Editor's Note: Recently, a polyomavirus vaccine has become available and shows great promise for controlling this disease.*]

Psittacine beak and feather disease also occurs in neonates. Cockatoos and African Grey Parrots are most commonly affected. Clinical signs are most often seen in older, fully feathered chicks just prior to or at the time of weaning. The onset is subacute and clinical signs include weight loss, listlessness and feather abnormalities. Many neonates showing clinical signs will have reduced red and white blood cell counts. The course of disease is often chronic. PBFD virus can be eliminated from a collection by testing adult birds and removing those that are subclinically infected.

Any neonate that is transferred from a facility should be tested negative before shipment. This will protect the aviculturist from allegations that they sold a subclinically infected bird.

Other viral infections are rarely reported in nestling birds. Herpesvirus infection (Pacheco's disease) occasionally causes nursery outbreaks. Poxvirus occurs primarily in lovebirds and imported South American psittacines such as Amazon and Pionus parrots. Poxvirus outbreaks may occur in tropical regions (eg, southern Florida) with high bird and mosquito populations.

Diseases of suspected viral etiology are occasionally observed in pediatric patients. Neuropathic gastric dilatation has been described in birds of all ages. Care should be taken when interpreting juvenile bird radiographs since the proventriculus is normally larger than in adults.

Avian viral serositis is a neonatal problem characterized by the accumulation of serous fluid in the abdominal cavity. Large amounts of fluid may accumulate and cause severe abdominal distention. Liver, bursal and lymphoid necrosis may also occur. This problem has been suspected to be caused by a togavirus that is related to eastern equine encephalomyelitis virus.

Table 30.7   Procedures During a Nursery Disease Outbreak

1. **Plan ahead:** Aviculturists should have a plan before an outbreak occurs. At least three separate nursery rooms will be required in a disease outbreak. Friends and families can sometimes be enlisted to take birds into their homes and feed them, but it is best if they are trained before they are actually needed.

2. **Isolate clinically ill birds:** At the first signs of illness, a chick should be isolated in a separate room, preferably one with air flow that is separate from the main nursery. Some aviculturists will question why isolation is necessary because the sick bird has already exposed the rest of the nursery to the disease. Sick birds should be immediately isolated because they shed higher quantities of infectious agents than asymptomatic carriers. Isolation of clinically ill birds can greatly reduce the load of infectious material in the nursery.

3. **Do not bring new birds into the nursery:** New hatchlings should go to a separate nursery room to avoid exposure. Ideally, a separate caretaker would be available for these birds.

4. **Maximize good hygiene practices:** If good hygiene practices are not in effect, they should be implemented immediately. Great care should be taken to reduce disease exposure when feeding chicks. If the same feeders must feed ill and healthy chicks, they should shower between groups and wear separate protective clothing in each room.

5. **Determine the cause:** Polyomavirus is the most common cause of nursery outbreaks; PBFD virus, chlamydial, yeast and some bacterial infections can also spread rapidly through a nursery. In some cases, it is best to sacrifice and necropsy an ill nestling to rapidly determine the etiology of the disease problem. This may provide information that can save the other birds. Many microbial infections are secondary to diseases that are difficult to diagnose (such as polyomavirus, PBFD virus and chlamydia).

6. **Treat the birds:** If microbial infections are identified, treatment should be initiated with appropriate drugs. If viral infections are identified, consider euthanasia or isolate sick birds and provide supportive care.

7. **Eliminate the cause:** Find and treat or eliminate asymptomatic disease shedders. Investigate hygiene and feeding practices if microbial infections are confirmed.

8. **Consider all-in all-out procedures:** Consider the primary nursery to be an isolation area. Do not add new birds until all nestlings that were exposed to the disease are moved to another area. This practice is essential with diseases with a long incubation or latency period (eg, polyomavirus and PBFD virus).

9. **Decontaminate the environment:** During the outbreak, clean the facility, brooders and air control system frequently to decrease environmental contamination. At the end of the outbreak, thoroughly clean and disinfect the room before using it as a nursery. If polyomavirus or PBFD virus was encountered, pay particular attention to cleaning the air control system (see Chapter 32).

10. **Do not sell chicks until proven healthy:** As noted above, many diseases (especially polyomavirus and PBFD virus) have a long incubation period. Some birds that are infected early in development will not show clinical signs until weaning. Ideally, neonates should not be sold until they are tested for these two viral diseases.

Parasitic Infections

With a few exceptions, internal parasites are an infrequent cause of disease in nestling psittacines in the United States, but are commonly found in countries where parrots are raised in flights with dirt floors. Trichomonas and giardia are frequent causes of death in young budgerigars, cockatiels, finches and Columbiformes. Coccidia are commonly recovered from lories, lorikeets, passerines, Columbiformes, and finches; their importance appears to depend on the chick's immune status. *Atoxoplasma serini* is a common cause of mortality in juvenile canaries. The safety of many parasiticidal drugs has not been investigated in nestling birds, and care should be exercised when selecting a treatment regimen. For example, furacin has a low therapeutic index in lory neonates (see Chapter 37).

Disorders of the Alimentary Tract

Pharyngeal and Esophageal Trauma

Damage to the pharyngeal or esophageal wall can occur during metal tube- or syringe-feeding when a nestling lunges against the feeding instrument. When a puncture occurs, food may be deposited into the subcutaneous tissues and will often migrate caudal to the puncture site. Liquid food can drain all the way to the base of the crop and be confused with crop contents. If the puncture is in the pharyngeal cavity, food will usually collect in the space ventral to the mandibles. The bird should be stabilized, and the food pockets surgically opened, curetted and thoroughly flushed (see Chapter 41). Antimicrobial therapy designed for both gram-positive and gram-negative organisms should continue for at least 14 days.

Air in the Crop

Bubbles or filling of the crop with air is usually caused by aerophagia. It occurs most often in stunted birds that beg constantly for food, but has also been observed in young birds of many species (especially cockatiels). Slowly delivering food will contribute to aerophagia because the chick attempts to gulp the feeding formula faster than the food is provided. Some inexperienced hand-feeders will confuse this condition with crop stasis, subcutaneous emphysema and filling of the cervicocephalic air sac. Air is easily distinguished from food or fluid by transilluminating the crop. Visualization of blood vessels in the crop wall can help differentiate between air located in the crop and air located in the subcutaneous space.

Feeding a nutritious formula at a steady rate will correct the problem in some birds. If aerophagia is persistent, the ingested air can be carefully removed ("burped out") and the bird immediately fed before it can gulp more air. In some cases it may be necessary to tube-feed these neonates.

Crop Stasis

The crop stasis problem is usually related to generalized gut stasis (often caused by a yeast or gram-negative bacterial infection) rather than a primary crop disorder, but there are numerous possible etiologies.

Causes of crop stasis include:
- Primary crop disorders: foreign bodies, crop infections; crop atony caused by overstretching; crop burns; crop impactions caused by fibrous food, large food chunks (eg, raw carrots) or bedding; and dehydration of food in the crop leading to formation of a concretion or doughy mass.
- Delayed transit time or obstruction of the distal gut: intestinal ileus due to generalized infection, neuropathic gastric dilatation, polyomavirus, GI foreign bodies or hypothermia.
- Cold food.

The crop should be examined and gently palpated to determine if it is atonic or burned, or if foreign material or an impaction is present. A CBC, serum chemistries, cloacal culture and radiographs are indicated if the bird has clinical signs of disease. Whole body radiographs can be used to evaluate the distal alimentary tract and barium contrast studies can be used to determine gastrointestinal transit time. The crop can be swabbed or flushed for culture and cytology.

A bird with crop-emptying problems should be fed carefully. The crop should not be overstretched, as this will cause atony and compound the problem. Mild cases of crop stasis caused by a dehydrated food mass or overfeeding can often be solved by administering a small amount of warm water and gently massaging the crop. If the food does not pass in three to five hours, the crop should be emptied and flushed with warm saline. To flush the crop, a lubricated soft feeding tube with an open end is gently passed into the crop, and a small amount of saline is flushed in and out to draw crop material into the syringe. It may be necessary to palpate the tube and direct it toward the food mass and away from the crop wall. When moving or withdrawing the tube, negative pressure on the syringe should be released to make sure the tube does not attach to the crop wall and cause damage.

Crop stasis caused by generalized ileus is a serious problem that requires immediate attention. Complete stasis may be one of the early signs associated with fatal diseases such as polyomavirus, PBFD virus, septicemia or sarcocystis infection. With these progressive diseases, treatment may not be successful. If the stasis is caused by a microbial infection (yeast, bacteria or chlamydia), intensive medical management may be effective (Table 30.8).

Table 30.8   Treatment for Crop Stasis

1. Empty and flush the crop with LRS using a feeding tube. Repeat every six to twelve hours if the crop does not empty. Digestive enzymes are often beneficial.

2. Give intravenous, intraosseous or subcutaneous fluids. Most birds with crop stasis are dehydrated and require parenteral fluid administration. A Gram's stain of a crop swab can be used to determine the microbial agents that are present.

3. If a generalized microbial infection is suspected, start treatment with a broad-spectrum antibiotic and antifungal drug. Cephalosporins and penicillins are the safest drugs to use; aminoglycosides and sulfas should be avoided due to potential dehydration and renal toxicity. Injectable antibiotics should be used if there is severe stasis because oral antibiotics would not be properly absorbed. Oral antifungals (nystatin) should be used because the parenteral antifungal drugs (eg, amphotericin B) may be toxic. If chlamydiosis is diagnosed, a single SC injection of oxytetracycline or doxycycline IV can be used to initiate therapy, followed by oral doxycycline (see Chapter 17).

4. If the bird has generalized ileus, a motility stimulant such as metoclopramide or D-panthenol can be administered. Response to these stimulants is highly variable.
   [Editor's Note: This practitioner has had good success using cisapride dosed at 0.5-1.5 mg/kg PO q8h.]

5. Once the crop starts to partially empty and the bird is stabilized, limited feeding should resume. The bird should be fed a liquid, complex carbohydrate, medium-fiber-content diet until the crop is emptying normally (see Chapter 15). Gerber's oatmeal with applesauce and bananas baby cereal mixed 50:50 by volume with water works well. The bird should be fed less volume, more frequently. As the crop starts to empty normally, the diet that is normally fed should be gradually substituted (provided it is nutritionally adequate). It is important to restore normal feeding as

quickly as possible because dilute baby food diets do not provide sufficient nutrition for growth. Subcutaneous fluid administration and antibiotics should continue until the bird is clinically normal.

6. If the crop is overstretched or atonic it is beneficial to apply a "bra" to elevate the crop and facilitate emptying. The bra can be constructed from elastic bandage material or baby tube socks and should be applied while the crop is full to make sure it is not too tight. The neonate should be confined to a small container for a few days if it objects to the bra and falls over backwards. Most chicks will eventually accept the bra.

7. Parenteral nutrition would be beneficial in cases of crop stasis; however, at the time of this publication this is still a highly experimental procedure and specific recommendations are speculative at best (see Chapter 15).

Crop Burns and Fistulas

Severe burns can result from a single, overly heated meal (eg, greater than 120°F), or by repeated exposure to food that is slightly hot (115°F). Birds will readily accept hot food, and the feeder may not recognize a problem for days to weeks after the burn occurs. If one bird in a nursery has a crop burn, all of the other neonates should be carefully examined to determine if they have also sustained injuries.

Mild burns result in tissue swelling, erythema and blister formation, and can be treated with antibiotics and topical application of soothing vitamin A and E ointments. The bird should be fed reduced volumes more frequently during the healing process.

Severe crop burns cause greater tissue damage. In the early stages the crop will adhere to the overlying skin; the skin will be hyperemic and the site may be covered with a scab. Eventually the crop may fistulate, and food and water will leak from the crop soiling the bird's chest. Bird owners are frequently puzzled by this odd phenomenon. Crop fistulas are treated by removing the scab, surgically excising the necrotic portion of the skin and crop and then separating and individually closing the crop and skin (see Chapter 41). The timing of surgery is important. Birds with this condition are often debilitated and should receive supportive care and enteral alimentation to build their strength prior to anesthesia and surgery. Ideally, the tissues surrounding the fistula should be given as much time as possible to heal before surgery, and the scab should be left in place as long as possible to encourage wound contraction that will reduce the size of the fistula. If surgery is attempted before the tissues surrounding the burn have healed, it is difficult to accurately assess the extent of devitalized tissue that must be debrided. Surgical adhesives can be used to close the crop and allow feeding or a pharyngotomy tube can be passed (see Chapter 41). It has been estimated that it takes seven to ten days following a burn to determine the extent of tissue injury.

Large crop defects (greater than one-third the size of the crop) can be difficult to repair. Closure frequently results in a reduced crop capacity. Following repair, the bird should be fed small amounts of food frequently to prevent reflux and aspiration. The amount of food offered can be gradually increased to stretch the crop. If the esophagus was involved, a pharyngotomy tube may be necessary to allow feeding yet protect the wound during healing. An alternative to a pharyngotomy tube is to place a mushroom-tipped jejunal catheter in the crop and tunnel it subcutaneously up the side of the neck. If it is impossible to close the skin over the defect, the wound should be covered with a permeable dressing and allowed to heal as an open wound.

Regurgitation

Hand-fed birds (especially macaws and African Grey Parrots) commonly regurgitate at weaning, and it is important to differentiate this relatively normal phenomena from a pathologic condition. Causes of regurgitation include overfeeding, crop stasis, alimentary tract infections (especially candidiasis), alimentary tract foreign bodies, blockage of the alimentary tract and use of some drugs such as trimethoprim-sulfa compounds and doxycycline. Treatment consists of correcting the underlying cause.

Foreign Body Ingestion or Impaction

Nestling birds are curious and may ingest foreign objects. Preventing neonates from consuming foreign bodies is far easier than treating them. The feeder should be very selective about the objects the birds are allowed to contact.

If a consumed foreign object is located in the crop, the bird should be treated immediately to prevent the object from entering the proventriculus. It is much easier to retrieve objects from the crop than the proventriculus, and birds have a remarkable capacity for passing even relatively huge objects such as feeding catheters into the proventriculus. Some objects can be "milked" up the esophagus and retrieved from the caudal oral cavity with forceps. Forceps can also be introduced into the crop to retrieve foreign bodies, with or without the aid of endoscopy. Objects can also be retrieved via an ingluviotomy incision (see Chapter 41).

Objects in the proventriculus or ventriculus can be tolerated for long periods but should be retrieved if they have the potential to erode the stomach wall or can be digested, resulting in toxicity. Foreign bodies may be removed using an endoscope, or forceps can be passed into the proventriculus via an ingluviotomy incision with the aid of air insufflation (via a rubber catheter) (see Chapters 13, 15). The endoscope must be carefully passed to prevent rupture of the thoracic esophagus or proventricular wall. The proventriculus and ventriculus can also be opened surgically as described for adult birds (see Chapter 41).

Proventricular or ventricular impactions caused by grit or bedding material are serious and require urgent attention. Mild accumulation of material in the ventriculus (that does not impede passage of ingesta) can be treated by hydrating the patient and administering laxatives (dioctyl sodium sulfosuccinate or psyllium or digestive enzymes). Psyllium should be limited to no more than one percent of the dry weight of the tubed formula to prevent it from causing an impaction. If this does not work, mineral oil should be administered into the crop, followed 30 minutes later by a large volume of barium sulfate (10-15 ml/kg) that may help force the mineral oil through the GI tract by gravitational pressure. The patient should be kept well hydrated with SC fluids due to the hygroscopic nature of barium sulfate. Serial radiographs can be used to evaluate the success of the therapy. If this treatment fails, proventriculotomy (see Chapter 41) or gastric lavage (see Chapters 13,15) can be attempted but both are associated with a guarded prognosis.

Intestinal Intussusception

This condition is occasionally reported in macaws and is associated with diarrhea and possibly intestinal hypermotility. In severe cases the ileum may telescope into the colon and protrude through the cloaca. Mild cases are diagnosed radiographically and may respond to antimicrobial and supportive therapy. Severe cases with a visible cloacal prolapse are usually fatal. Successful jejunostomy and jejunocloacal anastamosis have been reported.

Disorders of the Respiratory Tract

Upper Respiratory Infections

Nestling birds can pass food through the choanal slit, resulting in clogged nostrils and upper respiratory problems. These can be treated by removing the food plug with a feathered wooden applicator (see Chapter 8) or dull needle, and gently flushing the nares with saline until clear. Microbial infections of the upper respiratory tract are treated in the same manner as in adult birds (see Chapter 22). [*Editor's Note: Smooth ear curettes of various sizes (00-2) make an excellent tool for cleaning debris from the choanal slit and nares.*]

Aspiration Pneumonia

Aspiration occurs most often in birds that are reluctant to feed or if the aviculturist introduces food when there is no feeding response. If large amounts of food are inhaled, the bird will die from asphyxiation. Rapid placement of an air sac cannula and aggressive antimicrobial (eg, trimethoprim-sulfa, ketoconazole) and steroid therapy may save the patient, but the prognosis is poor. Some birds respond to such aggressive treatment and die months later due to a chronic fungal infection. If small amounts of food are aspirated, the event may not be noted at the time but the bird may later develop a foreign body pneumonia. An affected bird will show poor weight gain, a persistently elevated white blood cell count and may or may not show respiratory signs. Often, the pneumonia may be noted only by radiology or at necropsy.

Miscellaneous Disorders

Hepatic Lipidosis

In most cases, hand-fed birds gain weight slower than parent-fed birds, and the hand-feeder should be instructed to maintain the maximum weight gain possible. Umbrella Cockatoos, Moluccan Cockatoos and Blue and Gold Macaws may be an exception to this recommendation. In these species, and possibly others, it is possible to overfeed (especially in the later development stages) and cause massive weight gains and hepatic lipidosis. It has been suggested that multiple deficiencies of fiber, vitamins and minerals and nutritional excesses combine to cause this problem. Affected birds are usually dyspneic, especially when food in the digestive tract places additional pressure on the respiratory system following feeding. The abdomen is usually protuberant and the pale, enlarged liver may be visible through the skin. In these cases, the amount of food fed should be *gradually* reduced and small meals should be fed more often to avoid respiratory distress. Hyperthermia will aggravate the respiratory distress and should be avoided. If identified early, the birds may wean normally, but in severe cases the liver will be massively enlarged and the bird will die. This condition can be prevented by feeding a proven diet and comparing the bird's weight gain to established growth charts. If the bird is normal in body size but substantially heavier than the upper limit on the chart, the possibility of hepatic lipidosis should be considered.

Hepatomas

Hepatic hepatoma has been described primarily in macaws, and may occur when blunt trauma ruptures the liver and causes hemorrhage. The trauma may occur when the bird is lifted with pressure over the liver or it may simply be idiopathic. Affected birds are pale with extremely low hematocrits and may be saved by repeated blood transfusions within the first few days following the traumatic event.

Gout

Deposition of uric acid crystals in the tissues is called visceral gout and is usually due to end-stage renal disease. Clinical signs include crop stasis and vomiting followed by death. Excess vitamin D_3 results in dystrophic calcification of numerous organs including the kidney, which then may result in gout (see Chapters 3, 21). Macaws seem to be particularly sensitive to excessive dietary consumption of vitamin D_3 and calcium.

Wine-colored Urine

Reddish urine and urates have been described in juvenile African Grey Parrots and some Amazon and Pionus parrots. It can be distinguished from hematuria by a fecal occult blood test. It occurs sporadically with several hand-feeding formulas, and the pigment may be more pronounced on some bedding materials, especially certain brands of paper towels. This condition has not been associated with pathology or other clinical signs.

Musculoskeletal Disorders

Leg Deformities

Orthopedic problems in nestling birds are poorly understood and the causes are believed to be multifactorial. Nutritional deficiencies (especially of vitamin D_3 and calcium), trauma and housing the birds on slippery surfaces are the most common causes. Genetic and incubation abnormalities probably also occur. Polyomavirus may be a common underlying cause. In general, leg deformities are challenging to repair and the earlier the diagnosis and the younger the bird, the better the prognosis (see Chapter 42).

Spraddle or Splay Leg: Mild deformities can be treated by packing the bird in a deep cup with tissue or towel padding to take pressure off the legs. More severe deformities and those in older birds require a fixation device in addition to packing in a cup. The chick can be taped over a foam rubber pad or sanitary napkin, or placed in a piece of foam with slits cut for the legs. As an alternative, the legs can be hobbled together with elastic tape at the tarsometatarsus and if needed across the tibiotarsus. The hobble should be changed every two to four days to allow growth.

Valgus Deformity (Bowing of the tibiotarsus with lateral rotation of the femur or tibiotarsus): This is usually caused by premature closure of one side of the growth plate of the proximal or distal tibiotarsus. Surgically closing the opposite side of the growth plate or periosteal stripping to even out the growth, followed by a dome osteotomy and realignment of the tibiotarsus may be necessary. The osteotomy is best performed after the bones have ossified. Macaws and cockatoos should be approximately 65-70 days old before attempting an osteotomy procedure.

Toe Malposition

Malposition of digits in neonatal birds is believed to be secondary to malnutrition. Reducing the dietary protein content and slowing the growth of some chicks may aid in correcting the problem. Affected chicks should receive parenteral and dietary vitamins and mineral supplements including vitamins A, D_3, E, B complex, C, K_1, calcium, iodine, selenium, iron, copper and cobalt. Other proposed etiologies include virus infection and improper incubation.

Improving the substrate is also beneficial. The chick should be placed in a smaller, padded environment such as a teacup lined with a towel. This will help diminish the tendency for the legs to splay and the toes to curl. In many cases, taping the affected toes in a normal position is necessary. Generally, the affected digits should be maintained in the supported position for approximately as long as they were malpositioned (usually a maximum of several days). If the condition is recognized early, corrective measures may be required for only a few hours. This must be monitored closely as deformities can be caused by leaving bandages or splints on too long.

A corrective shoe may be made from a piece of firm material such as thin cardboard or radiographic film. The shoe should be made to properly fit the foot of the affected individual with a notch in the shoe into which each toenail will be placed. Once the shoe is made, the foot is placed in the shoe and each digit is taped into a normal position using very thin strips of masking tape. A hydroactive dressing may be used to make a corrective shoe. The material is cut to fit the foot as described above. The plantar aspect of each toe is placed on the sticky surface of the hydroactive dressing in a normal position. A second piece of hydroactive dressing is applied dorsally to sandwich the toes in place and to maintain reduction. This material is especially appropriate as it is soft, unlikely to cause pressure problems and easy to remove.

Constricted Toe Syndrome

This condition is most commonly reported in Eclectus Parrots, macaws and African Grey Parrots. The lesion consists of an annular ring of constriction that eventually causes swelling and necrosis of the distal segment of the toe. The etiology is unknown but may be related to low brooder humidity or fracture of the digits. If the degree of constriction and swelling of the distal segment is mild, warm water soaks and frequent massage may restore circulation and correct the condition. If a fibrous annular ring is present, it should be carefully incised and accumulated serum and tissue debris gently debrided (see Chapter 41). The toe should be soaked in warm, dilute, povidone-iodine solution and bandaged. A DMSO dressing may reduce inflammation and antibiotic ointments help soften and prevent reformation of the annular ring. If the distal segment is severely swollen or necrotic it should be surgically removed, preferably at a joint proximal to the constricting lesion. Toe constrictions can often be prevented by keeping susceptible species on non-desiccating surfaces and in brooders where the humidity is maintained above 50%. Commercial forced air brooders with rapid air changes tend to desiccate the chicks and should be avoided.

Stifle Subluxation

Stifle luxation or subluxation in both juvenile and adult birds has been reported. Rigid fixation of the stifle by applying a KE apparatus to the distal femur and proximal tibiotarsus may fuse the joint and permit limited, but less painful ambulation. The knee should be fixed in a slightly flexed position. Tolerance of the device is variable and it should be left in place for 30-40 days in large birds and 21 days in smaller species. Flunixin can be used for one to three days after placement and removal of the fixation device to reduce pain and inflammation.

Beak Problems

Lateral Beak Deviation (Scissors Beak)

Lateral deviation of the upper beak is most often diagnosed in macaws. If noted early (ie, a few days after hatch), the lower beak should be trimmed in a ramp-like fashion to encourage the upper beak to slide over to the side opposite the curvature. Differences in the height of the occlusal surfaces of the mandibular beak should be corrected, and digital pressure should be applied to the beak two to four times daily to gently push the beak back in position. If the beak is calcified or if conservative therapy fails, a ramp built from dental acrylic over a stainless steel mesh can be attached to the lower beak to apply pressure to correct the upper beak (see Chapter 42). The acrylic device should be left in place for one to twelve weeks, depending on the bird's age and the severity of the defect. Correction of severe beak deformities in older birds is seldom complete, but substantial improvement can be made.

Mandibular Prognathism

Mandibular prognathism (underbite), in which the upper beak tucks within the lower, is seen primarily in cockatoos. If the beak is still soft, physical therapy may correct the condition. A finger or loop of gauze can be used at each feeding to apply traction and extend the maxillary beak rostrally. The cartilaginous extensions should be clipped if they are contracted. If the beak is calcified, physical therapy combined with trimming of the lower beak to allow the upper to extend into a notch may help. If this fails, a dental acrylic prosthesis can be applied to the rostral end of the maxillary beak to stretch the maxilla and force it over the mandibular beak (see Chapter 42).

Compression Deformities of the Mandible of Macaw Beaks

If noted before the beak calcifies, it can be corrected by trimming beak tissue from the lateral walls and manually reshaping the lower beak. Once the beak calcifies, it is difficult to repair.

Traumatic Subluxation of the Premaxilla-frontal Joint

Juvenile birds will occasionally subluxate the upper beak when playing or flying. The upper beak will usually be displaced dorsally, and fractures of the premaxilla or frontal bone may be apparent. It is extremely painful, and the bird should be anesthetized while the beak is placed back in a normal position (see Chapter 42). Most birds have been reported to heal well, although some may need to be hand fed for a few days. Antibiotics and anti-inflammatory drugs should be used where indicated.

Integumentary Problems

Feather Stress Bars

Stress bars are horizontal defects in the feathers that occur when there is endogenous release of corticosteroids or when corticosteroids are administered during feather growth (see Chapter 24). Large numbers of stress bars may indicate malnutrition, stunting or a disease problem.

Feather Dysplasia

Malformed feathers, feathers that fail to grow, and feathers that are easily epilated are most often caused by polyomavirus or PBFD virus. Hyperthermia, drug reactions and bacterial folliculitis are less common causes.

Occluded Ear Openings

Occlusions of the external openings of the ears are most often seen in macaws, (especially Military Macaws). Macaws are born with a thin membrane covering the ear canal that should start to open between 12 and 35 days of age. If the canal fails to open, it should be explored with blunt forceps and an opening surgically created if necessary. If a small hole is found, it can often be enlarged by stretching it with the tips of a pair of hemostats. Occasionally the canal will become infected and fill with inspissated pus. This material should be removed by curettage and flushing, cultured for bacteria and fungus, and the ear treated with appropriate topical and systemic antibiotics. *Pseudomonas* sp. is a common contaminant and ointments containing an aminoglycoside antibiotic should be used until culture results are available.

Eyelid Malformation

Malformation of the eyelids resulting in a narrow aperture is occasionally seen in cockatiels. Several surgical techniques and means of chemical debridement have been attempted with little success. In all reported cases, the aperture closed following treatment. Affected birds can often adapt to this handicap (see Chapter 26).

■ MALNUTRITION

Patricia Macwhirter

The diet of every avian patient should be carefully evaluated, even if the bird appears clinically to be well nourished. Marginal nutritional inadequacies frequently occur (see Chapter 8), and correcting the diet will improve a bird's general health and its ability to resist infectious diseases. Gastrointestinal malabsorption, hepatitis or renal disease can increase nutrient requirements so that diets that are sufficient in healthy birds may be insufficient for unhealthy birds.

Birds with signs of malnutrition have often developed strong preferences for unbalanced diets. Most seed diets, for example, contain excessive levels of fat and may be deficient in vitamins A, D_3, E, B_{12} and K_1, plus riboflavin, pantothenic acid, niacin, biotin, choline, iodine, iron, copper, manganese, selenium, sodium, calcium, zinc and some amino acids (eg, lysine and methionine).

Birds can be encouraged to accept new foods by offering them first thing in the morning when the appetite is strongest. Favorite items can be withheld until later in the day. New foods may also be mixed with the bird's normal familiar diet. Some birds may be encouraged to eat an unfamiliar food if they can observe its consumption by other birds.

While a diet change is occurring, it is important that the bird be carefully monitored for weight loss. Radical, unsupervised changes in the diet can lead to starvation. Ketosis was seen in some cockatoos that refused to eat during the transition to formulated diets. Ketonuria can be demonstrated by a reagent strip examination of the urine.

Clinical Conditions Associated with Malnutrition

Obesity

Obesity is the most common and the most severe malnutrition-related problem recognized in avian practice. In some cases, obesity will be secondary to the overconsumption of food in a bird attempting to consume missing nutrients. However, in most cases, obesity in companion birds is a result of feeding excess quantities of improper foods (eg, cookies, crackers, sweets) or high-oil seeds (sunflower, safflower, hemp, rape, niger), a lack of exercise and increased food intake due to boredom.

Fresh fruit and vegetables have lower calorie densities than dried foods or seeds and should make up a sizable portion of a low-energy diet. Decreasing caloric intake can also be achieved by restricting feeding times (eg, ten minutes in the morning and evening) rather than offering food ad lib. Ideally, companion birds should be fed pelleted or extruded foods supplemented with small quantities of fresh fruit and vegetables. Some formulated diets may be helpful in controlling obesity and fatty liver problems.

Some species, such as Rose-breasted Cockatoos, Sulphur-crested Cockatoos, Amazon parrots and budgerigars, are particularly prone to becoming obese and may develop secondary lipomas, fatty liver degeneration and heart disease. Hypothyroidism, which can be associated with low dietary iodine, has been correlated with obesity and lipoma formation, particularly in budgerigars. In birds that are confirmed to have hypothyroidism, thyroxine supplementation is recommended (see Chapter 23).

Low Body Weight/Poor Growth

Low body weight or poor growth can be the result of inadequate food intake, which in turn can be caused by an insufficient quantity of food, inappropriate diet, unfamiliar food items, infrequent feeding, weaning onto solid foods too early, or loss of appetite, maldigestion or malassimilation of food caused by medical problems.

Low body weight or poor weight gain independent of organopathy can generally be corrected by placing the bird on a high-energy diet (high in fat and carbohydrates). Digestive enzymes and fiber hemicellulose may increase the digestibility and absorbability of the diet.

Diets for Birds with Malabsorption and Diarrheal Syndromes

Parasites, bacterial infections, mycotoxins and pancreatic disease may interfere with the absorption of nutrients from the digestive tract. In addition to correcting the primary problem, these birds need foods that are easily digested and absorbed to facilitate healing of the gastrointestinal tract. Lactose and excessive amounts of green vegetables should be avoided. Diets should be moderately low in fiber and provide easily digested carbohydrate (eg, canary seeds, millet, panicum, corn or hulled oats) and a moderate amount of highly digestible protein. Vitamin and mineral supplementation, particularly of vitamins A and E, may be needed. The addition of digestive enzymes to the diet may be useful (see Chapter 18). In some cases, feeding a small quantity of grit may improve digestion and aid absorption, but should be supplied only in low quantities to prevent gastrointestinal impaction.

Polyphagia

Occasionally birds will overeat fibrous food or grit, causing crop or ventricular impactions. These problems are more likely to occur if young birds are suddenly introduced to new food items (unhulled seeds, particularly). ingestion and impaction (see Chapter 48).

Feigned polyphagia, in which a bird hulls seeds and appears to be eating but the crop remains empty, may occur in some birds that are very weak or that are offered inappropriate food items. Vitamin E and selenium deficiencies have been suggested as possible causes of this problem. Clients should not rely on the husking of seeds to indicate food intake. Monitoring body weight and fecal output is more effective.

Polydipsia/Polyuria

Nutritional causes of polydipsia and polyuria include hypovitaminosis A, calcium deficiency, excess protein, hypervitaminosis D_3, excessive dietary salt, dry seed diet, formulated diets or a high percentage of dietary fiber.

Digestive Disorders

White plaques in the mouth or swelling in the salivary ducts may be associated with hypovitaminosis A.

Oral paralysis in cockatiels may be related to vitamin E and selenium deficiencies and a malabsorption syndrome secondary to giardiasis.

Cold food, a cold environment or infrequent feeding of large amounts of food may increase the risk of crop impaction in juvenile or debilitated birds. Degeneration of ventricular musculature has been associated with vitamin E and selenium deficiencies and calcinosis due to hypervitaminosis D. Crop liths may develop in birds on marginal diets. The etiology is undetermined.

Diarrhea may occur in birds fed low-fiber or high-fat foods, particularly highly processed human foods (eg, cakes, desserts, crackers). Bacteria or parasitic enteritis may occur in birds that eat foods contaminated with excrement.

Nutritional cases of malabsorption or maldigestion (passing undigested food) include vitamin E and selenium deficiencies (sometimes associated with giardia infection), excess oil in the diet or dehydration. A lack of grit has been frequently discussed as a cause of maldigestion; however, companion birds on formulated diets do not appear to require grit.

Birds should not be offered grit on an ad libitum basis. If offered free choice, some birds may overconsume grit, leading to crop, proventricular or ventricular impactions. Birds showing compulsive grit consumption should be evaluated for hepatopathy, pancreatitis, renal dysfunction and general malnutrition.

Respiratory Disorders

Dyspnea (extended neck) and wheezing may be associated with goiter, particularly in budgerigars. Hypovitaminosis A leads to squamous metaplasia of epithelial surfaces causing obstruction of respiratory passages or sinusitis. Dyspnea may be caused by calcium or vitamin D_3 deficiency if severe enough to demineralize bone, causing thoracic or spinal deformities.

Plumage Abnormalities

Dark, horizontal lines (stress marks) on feathers have been associated with nutritional deficiencies (particularly methionine) and indicate that a release of corticosteroid hormone occurred while the feather was developing. Molting abnormalities, retained feather sheaths and dry flaking beaks have also been associated with overall nutritional deficiencies.

Feather picking may be initiated by dry, flaky, pruritic skin, which in turn can be caused by nutritional deficiencies, particularly deficiencies of vitamin A, sulfur-containing amino acids, arginine, niacin, pantothenic acid, biotin, folic acid and salt. Excessive dietary fat has been incriminated as a possible cause of self mutilation.

Deficiencies of minerals such as calcium, zinc, selenium, manganese and magnesium may be associated with brittle, frayed feathers and dermatitis. Arginine deficiency may cause wing feathers to curl upward in chicks.

Birds lacking a dietary source of carotenoids may develop muted feather or skin colors, while dietary supplementation of carotenoids in birds with suitable genetic backgrounds will result in increased depth of color.

Porphyrins are aromatic compounds synthesized by birds that may produce colors such as red, green or brown. Porphyrins are less sensitive to dietary influences than carotenoids, but both are present in edible blue-green algae, and enhanced feather coloration would be expected in birds fed a diet containing this material.

Melanin occurs in granules in the skin and feathers and produces black, brown and red-brown colors. This pigment is derived from tyrosine in an enzymatic reaction requiring copper. Consequently, deficiencies of tyrosine (or other related amino acids) or copper could interfere with melanin production and cause dark-colored feathers to become lighter.

A change in feather color from green to yellow is usually caused by a loss of structural blue color, which may be associated with essential amino acid deficiencies. While this color change is commonly seen in nutritionally deficient Psittaciformes, the exact nature of the deficiency has not been clarified, and it is possible that more than one amino acid could be involved.

Feather color may change from blue to black, green to black or grey to black in birds that are sick or malnourished. These color changes are associated with altered keratin structure in the spongy layer that prevents normal light scattering.

Skin Changes

Plantar corns and pododermatitis have been associated with biotin and vitamin A deficiencies, particularly in obese birds. Edema of subcutaneous tissues has been seen with vitamin E and selenium deficiencies. Exfoliative dermatitis on the face and legs has been associated with biotin, pantothenic acid, riboflavin or zinc deficiency.

Skeletal and Muscular Disorders

Demineralized, bent bones and pathologic fractures may occur in birds with hypovitaminosis D and calcium, phosphorus or magnesium deficiencies or imbalances.

Slipped tendon of the hock (perosis) may occur with manganese, biotin, pantothenic acid or folic acid deficiencies. Obese birds that are not allowed sufficient exercise and birds fed high-mineral diets may be prone to this condition. In some cases, surgical correction is possible (see Chapter 46).

Enlargement of the hock, without tendon slipping, may occur with zinc deficiency.

Neurologic Signs

Seizures or localized paralysis have been associated with salt toxicity and low levels of thiamine, calcium and vitamin E. Leg paralysis has been associated with calcium, chloride or riboflavin deficiency.

Cervical paralysis has been associated with a folic acid deficiency. Jerky leg movements have been associated with pyridoxine deficiency.

Sudden collapse or fainting has been associated with hypoglycemia in raptors or in other species when a bird has not eaten and is acutely stressed. Syncope is characteristic of advanced hypocalcemia in African Grey Parrots.

Frequently, companion birds that are switched from an unbalanced all-seed diet to a balanced formulated diet will undergo a corresponding change in behavior characterized by decreased biting, screaming and chewing, and increased activity and playfulness.

Reproductive Disorders

Calcium, vitamin E and selenium deficiencies may be associated with egg binding.

General Ill Health or Sudden Death

Fatty liver infiltration may occur due to high fat diets, fatty acid or B vitamin deficiencies and high-energy diets in exercise-deprived birds.

Gout may be a precipitating cause or an end result of systemic diseases. Ascites may be associated with excessive dietary levels of iron in birds susceptible to iron storage disease (hemochromatosis). Atherosclerosis may be associated with diets high in fat and cholesterol.

Aortic rupture has been associated with copper deficiency in poultry and is suspected to occur in ratites.

Immune Response

Adequate levels of both B complex (particularly pantothenic acid and riboflavin) and vitamin E have been shown to improve the body's response to pathogens. In poultry, vitamin C and zinc are involved in T-cell response, and vitamin C stimulates macrophages and helps to counter the immunosuppressant effects of stress. Low vitamin A levels may result in a suboptimal immune response and have been associated with the occurrence of aspergillosis in psittacines.

Deficiencies of Specific Nutrients

Excess Dietary Protein

Starter rations for turkey poults or pheasants may contain nearly 30% protein, but young ratites, waterfowl and psittacine birds require much lower levels. Using a high-protein diet in these latter species may result in clinical problems such as airplane wing in ducks, deformed legs in ratites, poor growth rates in psittacine birds and increased susceptibility to disease in all species.

Inappropriate calcium levels in the diet may compound problems caused by excessive dietary protein. A group of macaw neonates being fed a human, high-protein baby cereal with added vitamins and calcium showed suboptimal growth rates.

Nutritional data collected in juvenile cockatiels indicated that a protein level of 20% was optimal for this species. Levels over 25% produced transient behavioral changes such as biting, nervousness, rejection of food and regurgitation.

Diets for Birds with Renal Disease or Gout

Birds with renal disease or gout should be provided diets that decrease the workload of the kidneys and slow the loss of renal function. These diets should be lower in protein and meet energy needs with non-protein calories. Calcium, phosphorus, magnesium, sodium and vitamin D_3 levels should be reduced to avoid renal mineralization. Vitamin A should be present in adequate amounts to ensure proper function of the mucous membranes lining the ureters. B vitamins should be increased to compensate for losses associated with polyuria.

Protein and Amino Acid Deficiencies

Insectivorous birds require higher protein levels than granivores and generally require live food such as crickets or mealworms. If these insects are reared exclusively on bran, their total body protein may be low, and consequently the level and quality of protein that they provide to birds will also be low. Feeding crickets that have been raised on dried dog food or encouraging insectivores to consume artificial diets with appropriate levels of high quality protein prevents the problem.

Lysine deficiencies have been associated with impaired feather pigmentation in poultry, but not in cockatiels.

Methionine deficiency has been associated with stress lines on feathers and fatty liver change. Cystine and methionine act as sources of glutathione, which has a sparing effect on vitamin E.

Fats and Essential Fatty Acids

Fats provide a concentrated source of energy. Linoleic and arachidonic acids are essential fatty acids needed for the formation of membranes and cell organelles. In mammals, lipogenesis occurs mainly in adipose tissue while in birds, it nearly all occurs in the liver.

Lipogenic liver function in birds predisposes them to the occurrence of conditions involving excessive accumulation of liver fats.

Fatty liver syndromes of undetermined etiologies are common in companion birds. In addition to fatty liver, excessive levels of fat in the diet are known to cause obesity, diarrhea and oily feather texture, and to interfere with the absorption of other nutrients such as calcium. Poor growth and reduced resistance to disease also occur with essential fatty acid deficiencies.

Ventricular erosion may occur in birds fed highly polyunsaturated fatty acids (such as those present in cod liver oil), if the fatty acids are not protected by an adequate dietary level of vitamin E. Because of these problems, fish liver oils are not recommended as dietary components in companion birds. Soybean oil is a good source of fatty acids that is less likely to spoil.

Atherosclerosis may be induced by diets high in saturated fats and cholesterol.

Carbohydrates

Exercise-deprived birds on high-energy diets may develop fatty liver infiltration even though carbohydrates, rather than fats, form the major component of energy consumed.

Small companion birds (eg, finches) may collapse from hypoglycemia if they are deprived of food for even short periods. Food restriction prior to anesthesia should not exceed several hours. Raptors that are fed small quantities of food as part of their training program may experience hypoglycemic collapse and may require emergency therapy with oral or parenteral glucose.

Vitamins

Most birds require the same vitamins as mammals with the exception that vitamin D_3 (not vitamin D_2, as in mammals) is the active form of this compound. Exogenous vitamin C is required in fruit-eating birds such as bulbuls, but seed-eating species are generally able to synthesize vitamin C.

Birds with vitamin deficiencies may have life-threatening clinical signs (eg, seizuring associated with thiamine deficiency) or simply appear ruffled and in poor condition. Vitamins A, C, E and B complex are all involved with immune responses, and deficiencies in these compounds may increase the severity of infectious diseases.

Fat-soluble Vitamins

Vitamin A: Vitamin A is formed in the liver from beta carotene. It is involved in mucopolysaccharide biosynthesis and is needed for the formation of normal mucous membranes and epithelial surfaces, for growth, for vision, for the development of the vascular system in embryos, for the production of adrenal hormones and for the formation of red and orange pigments in feathers. Numerous clinical problems may be associated with hypovitaminosis.

Small white pustules may be seen in the mouth, esophagus, crop or nasal passages. If squamous metaplasia causes blockage of salivary ducts, small swellings (often symmetrical) may be noted dorsally around the choana, around the larynx and laterally under the tongue or mandibles. White caseous material may accumulate in the bird's sinuses, particularly if hypovitaminosis A is associated with a concurrent sinus infection. Squamous metaplasia may also lead to thickening and sloughing of part of the lining of the syrinx with subsequent partial or complete tracheal obstruction. Xerophthalmia occurs if squamous metaplasia affects the eyes. There may be lacrimation, and caseous material may accumulate under the eyes. In chicks, acute hypovitaminosis A has been associated with weakness, incoordination and ataxia. These symptoms must be differentiated from "crazy chick disease" caused by hypovitaminosis E.

In mild cases of hypovitaminosis A, particularly in budgerigars, the only clinical signs may be polyuria and polydipsia, but squamous metaplasia may be seen histologically along the gastrointestinal and urinary tracts. Kidney damage and gout may occur if squamous metaplasia causes partial or complete occlusion of the ureters.

Reduced egg production is common in hens with hypovitaminosis A. In cocks, hypovitaminosis A may cause decreased sperm motility, reduced sperm counts and a high level of abnormal sperm.

Hypovitaminosis A may cause hyperkeratosis of the plantar skin of the metatarsal and digital pads.

Hypovitaminosis A should be initially treated with parenteral supplementation, which establishes rapid blood levels and does not rely on intestinal absorption. In limited clinical trials, some birds may respond just as quickly to supplementation of the diet with spirulina. Oral administration in the food and modification of the diet to include natural sources of beta carotene is recommended. Zinc levels in the diet should be sufficient to allow for normal vitamin A function. Liver disease may decrease the bird's ability to store vitamin A.

Vitamin D: Vitamin D helps to stimulate gastrointestinal absorption of calcium, has a hormonal effect on regulation of calcium and phosphorus excretion in the renal tubules and may be involved in controlling alkaline phosphatase in the blood. An increase in alkaline phosphatase may be an early indication of hypovitaminosis D_3.

Vitamin D precursors in the uropygial gland may be spread on the feathers, activated by UV light and then consumed during preening activities. This process requires natural sunlight or appropriate artificial ultraviolet light. Hypovitaminosis D_3 can easily occur in birds raised indoors. It is advisable to supplement indoor birds that do not have access to natural sunlight with exogenous vitamin D_3.

Signs of vitamin D_3 deficiency parallel those of calcium deficiency. Adult hens may show thin-shelled or soft-shelled eggs, decreased egg production and poor hatchability. Seizuring or leg weakness may occur due to pathologic bone fractures or if an already low blood calcium level is further exacerbated by metabolic demands of egg laying.

Hypovitaminosis D_3 in neonates is characterized by demineralized and easily broken bones. Leg bones will frequently be bent into grossly distorted positions. The sternum may be bent laterally or indented. The spinal column may undergo lordosis or fracture easily, causing pressure on nerves and subsequent paralysis.

Clinical evidence suggests that young macaws may be particularly susceptible to hypervitaminosis D. Nephrocalcinosis, suspected to be associated with hypervitaminosis D, has been reported in a dove, a toucan, a cardinal and a variety of Psittaciformes. Neonatal birds are best fed proven formulas (see Chapter 30).

Vitamin E: Vitamin E is an antioxidant that acts to prevent fat rancidity and fatty acid degeneration in foodstuffs, as well as acting in concert with selenium and sulfur-containing amino acids to prevent peroxidative damage to cell membranes.

If accompanied by deficiencies in sulfur-containing amino acids or selenium, hypovitaminosis E may result in skeletal muscle dystrophy as well as muscular dystrophy of the heart or ventriculus. Electrocardiographic changes may accompany heart muscle dystrophy. Undigested seed in the droppings may occur with ventricular muscular dystrophy. Degeneration of the pipping muscle may occur in neonates, resulting in decreased hatchability. Exertional rhabdomyolysis or spraddle legs may be associated with vitamin E and selenium deficiencies (see Chapter 48).

Hypovitaminosis E may cause encephalomalacia in poultry and other species.

Deficiencies in vitamin E and selenium may cause exudative diathesis, which results in edema of ventral subcutaneous tissue in poultry. Prolonged hypovitaminosis E may cause testicular degeneration in males, and in hens it may result in infertility or early embryonic deaths.

Birds suspected of hypovitaminosis E should receive parenteral supplementation. Mild conditions may respond dramatically to this treatment. In cases where there is irreversible nerve or muscle damage, response is poor (see Chapter 18).

Vitamin K: Vitamin K is required for the synthesis of prothrombin. Deficiency of vitamin K results in prolonged prothrombin time and delayed blood clotting. Affected birds may exsanguinate from minor traumatic injuries. Bacterial flora in the intestine are the natural source of vitamin K. Clinical problems associated with bleeding or petechia from pulled feathers may respond to injectable vitamin K, but naturally occurring hypovitaminosis K has not been proven in companion birds. Sulfaquinoxaline has been reported to induce hypovitaminosis K in poultry, and it is possible that long-term antibiotics used in aviary birds could do likewise.

Water-soluble Vitamins

Thiamine (Vitamin B₁): Thiamine deficiency may lead to loss of appetite, opisthotonos, seizures and death. Deficiency of thiamine is uncommon in birds on a seed diet because seeds and grains generally contain sufficient thiamine. Thiamine deficiency-induced seizures and neurologic signs may occur in carnivorous birds fed solely on meat or day-old chickens, and in fish-eating birds fed fish containing thiaminase.

Response to treatment in thiamine deficiency cases can be dramatic. Affected birds will respond within minutes to injectable thiamine. Response to oral thiamine may also be rapid.

Riboflavin (Vitamin B₂): In young chicks, riboflavin deficiency causes weakness and diarrhea, but the bird's appetite remains normal. Affected birds have toes curled inward both when walking and resting. The skin is rough and dry.

Older birds are more resistant to riboflavin deficiency than juveniles. Heterophil counts may increase and lymphocyte counts decrease. Primary wing feathers may be excessively long.

Niacin (Nicotinic Acid): Clinical signs of niacin deficiency are fairly nonspecific and include poor feathering, nervousness, diarrhea and stomatitis. Niacin deficiency has not been described in Psittaciformes.

Pyridoxine (Vitamin B₆): Chicks with pyridoxine deficiency may show depressed appetites, poor growth, perosis, jerky movements and spasmodic convulsions. As with riboflavin deficiency, heterophil counts may increase while lymphocyte counts decrease.

Pyridoxine deficiency was suspected in juvenile rheas that developed "goose-stepping" gaits.

Pantothenic Acid: Symptoms of pantothenic acid deficiency in chicks are similar to those of biotin deficiency and include dermatitis on the face and feet, perosis, poor growth, poor feathering and ataxia. Severe edema and subcutaneous hemorrhages are signs of pantothenic acid deficiency in developing chicken embryos. Similar signs have also been seen in developing ostrich embryos. High incubator humidity may contribute to this problem. Cockatiels reared on pantothenic acid-deficient diets failed to grow contour feathers on their chests and backs, and many died at three weeks of age. Affected birds had the appearance of feather-picked chicks.

Biotin: Natural sources of the vitamin are the same as those for pantothenic acid, and signs of biotin deficiency may parallel those of pantothenic acid: dermatitis on the face and feet, perosis, poor growth, poor feathering and ataxia. Biotin deficiency may also be associated with swelling and ulceration of the foot pads, and biotin-deficient embryos may show syndactylia and chondrodysplastic changes in the skeleton. Although egg yolk is a rich source of biotin, uncooked egg white contains a biotin antagonist called avidin, and biotin supplementation of a diet containing raw egg white may not correct the deficiency unless the biotin-binding capacity of the egg white has been exceeded. Mycotoxins may also interfere with biotin uptake.

Folic Acid: In poultry, folic acid deficiency has been associated with embryonic mortality, deformation of the upper mandible, poor growth, macrocytic anemia, bending of the tibiotarsi and perosis. Folic acid is synthesized by bacteria in the digestive tract, so antibiotic therapy, particularly with sulfonamides, could induce a deficiency.

Choline: A deficiency of choline caused poor growth and perosis in juvenile turkeys and chickens. In older birds, fatty liver infiltration may occur. Cockatiels reared on choline-deficient diets showed unpigmented wing and tail feathers but no signs of perosis.

Vitamin C: Bulbuls and fruit-eating birds may require exogenous vitamin C (ascorbic acid) but in chickens, and probably most species of seed-eating birds, vitamin C is synthesized in the liver. Signs of vitamin C deficiency have not been documented in companion birds.

Minerals

Calcium and Phosphorus

Calcium in the diet is used for bone formation, egg shell production, blood clotting, nerve impulse transmission, glandular secretion and muscle contraction. Phosphorus is important in many body functions including bone formation, the maintenance of acid-base balance, fat and carbohydrate metabolism and calcium transport in egg formation.

If calcium utilization exceeds absorption from the intestine over a prolonged period of time, parathyroid hormone excretion will increase and the parathyroid glands will enlarge. This condition, called secondary nutritional hyperparathyroidism (SNH), allows normal blood calcium levels to be maintained. High levels of phosphorus or low levels of vitamin D in the diet may exacerbate SNH. Symptoms of the syndrome may include weakness, polydipsia, anorexia and regurgitation. In breeding hens, SNH may result in decreased egg production, production of soft-shelled eggs, egg binding and fragile bones (see Chapter 23).

Hypocalcemic seizures associated with severe parathyroid enlargement and degeneration occur as a syndrome in African Grey Parrots. Affected birds are generally between the ages of two to five years. Abnormal clinical pathology findings include leukocytosis and hypocalcemia. Calcium levels may be below 6.0 mg/dL and sometimes as low as 2.4 mg/dL. At necropsy, there is no apparent calcium mobilization from bones as would be expected when blood calcium levels decease in normal birds. Affected birds have difficulty in mobilizing calcium from body stores, and should be supplemented constantly with dietary calcium.

Diets for Birds with Hypocalcemia: Calcium syrup may be used in the drinking water, sprinkled on seeds or soft foods or administered directly. Foods containing high levels of calcium such as bones, cheese or yogurt may be provided. Calcium powder may be sprinkled on soft food. High-fat seeds (eg, sunflower, safflower) may interfere with calcium uptake from the intestine. Levels of vitamin D_3 in the diet should be evaluated and supplemented if needed.

High-calcium diets are generally required only until normal body reserves are restored. The addition of psyllium to the diet may increase the absorption of calcium. Long-term consumption of high levels of calcium may interfere with manganese or zinc absorption and may result in renal calcium deposition, reduced numbers of glomeruli per kidney and subsequent renal failure.

Hypocalcemic seizures are rare in species other than African Grey Parrots. Occasionally, companion birds on an all-seed diet will be presented with seizuring caused by hypocalcemia. These birds usually respond dramatically (within minutes) to intramuscular calcium and multivitamin therapy.

Muscle meat is low in calcium and high in phosphorus with a ratio of 1:20. Carnivorous birds fed an all-meat diet, day-old chicks or pinky mice may show signs of calcium deficiency and SNH. Feeding whole adult mice, older chicks, quail or rats to carnivorous birds should provide better calcium balance. It is important to provide variety in the type of food fed.

Long bone deformities in juvenile birds, particularly ratites, may be associated with high protein, low calcium diets; however, reducing dietary protein and supplementing calcium may not always correct the problem. In these situations, the overall suitability of the diet, including the calcium to phosphorus ratio, the level of magnesium and electrolytes and the energy level in the diet should be evaluated. The birds should be encouraged to exercise more and the rate of weight gain should be reduced (see Chapter 48).

Excess phosphorus consumption can exacerbate SNH. Decreases in egg production, poor egg shell quality and rickets could occur with phosphorus deficiency, but this is unlikely because the mineral is very widely distributed in common food items.

Magnesium

Magnesium is necessary for bone formation, for carbohydrate metabolism and for activation of many enzymes. Its metabolism is closely associated with that of calcium and phosphorus. Deficiencies in young chicks may result in poor growth, lethargy, convulsions and death. Excessive amounts may cause diarrhea, irritability, decreased egg production and thin-shelled eggs.

Iron

Iron deficiency may result in hypochromic, microcytic anemia. Normal levels of non-heme iron in the plasma are necessary for feather pigmentation.

Diets for Birds with Anemia: Birds with anemia should receive a diet that is high in energy and protein, and be supplemented with B complex vitamins (including B_{12}, pyridoxine, niacin and folic acid), iron, cobalt and copper.

Diets for Birds with Hepatopathies: Iron storage disorders have been reported in a variety of non-psittacine species, particularly Indian Hill Mynahs, birds of paradise, hornbills and toucans. In some cases, the disease has been correlated with diets high in iron, and problems with the condition decreased when dietary iron levels were lowered to less than 40 ppm (see Chapters 20, 47).

Liver disease may decrease the absorption and storage of fat-soluble vitamins A and D and inhibit the synthesis of vitamin C necessitating supplementation. Other objectives in designing diets for birds with liver disease include reducing the work load on the liver (fat conversion, gluconeogenesis, deamination and nitrogen conversion), preventing sodium retention and hypokalemia, restoring liver glycogen and minimizing the possibility of hepatic encephalopathy. The diet should contain a readily available energy source such as dextrose or other easily digested carbohydrate. Canary seeds, millet, panicum, corn or hulled oats are relatively high in carbohydrate and low in protein and fat. These should be used in preference to sunflower seed, rape or niger, all of which are much higher in fat and protein and lower in carbohydrate. Birds with hepatopathy should be offered a variety of fresh fruit and vegetables that are generally high in easily digestible carbohydrates. These fruits and vegetables should be organically grown to prevent exposing the compromised liver to pesticides. The diet should contain a low level of protein of high biologic value such as chopped hard-cooked egg, cottage cheese or cooked chicken. For carnivorous birds, purine-containing foods (offal) should be avoided. The bird should receive a sufficient volume of food to meet caloric needs (see Chapter 20).

Copper

Copper is necessary for heme synthesis and is an important component of several enzymes.

Selenium

In addition to having a vitamin E-sparing effect in the prevention of ventricular myopathy, white muscle disease and exudative diathesis, selenium is also linked with exocrine pancreatic function and the production of thyroid hormones.

Manganese

Manganese is required for normal bone and egg shell formation and for growth, reproduction and the prevention of perosis.

Zinc

Zinc is needed for the formation of insulin and many enzymes in the body. In poultry, zinc deficiency may cause short, thickened long bones, enlargement of the hock, dermatitis and impaired T-cell function.

Iodine

Iodine is needed for the formation of thyroxine and related compounds in the thyroid gland. Iodine deficiency may result in goiter (enlargement of the thyroid glands).

Clinical signs of goiter are the result of pressure on organs adjacent to the gland. A loud, wheezing respiration with neck extended may occur if there is pressure against the trachea. Crop dilation and vomiting may occur if the goiter obstructs the outlet to the crop. Iodine-deficient budgerigars are particularly prone to goiter. Goiter has occasionally been reported in other species of birds (see Chapter 23).

Birds with goiter must be handled with care. Excessive stress may cause regurgitation and subsequent aspiration of vomitus. Conservative therapy should include the administration of a drop of iodine orally each day. Injectable iodine and dexamethasone may be necessary in more advanced cases. Once stabilized, the bird should be changed to a formulated diet.

Excess dietary iodine has also been reported to induce goiter (eg, birds consuming iodine-based cleaning agents). High levels of iodine may also antagonize chloride, depress growth rates and induce CNS signs.

Budgerigars with thyroid tumors may have clinical signs identical to those seen with goiter. While goiter will generally respond quickly to iodine supplementation, thyroid tumors will not. It has been suggested that iodine-deficient diets may be associated with signs of hypothyroidism (eg, lethargy, obesity or dermatitis); however, these signs are rarely seen in companion birds with goiter (see Chapter 23).

Potassium

Potassium is widely distributed in food of both plant and animal origin. Symptoms associated with deficiency are unlikely to occur, but in chickens these may include decreased egg production, egg shell thinning, muscle and cardiac weakness, tetanic convulsion and death.

Sodium and Chloride

In psittacine birds, it has been suggested that salt deficiency may play a role in some cases of self-mutilation. Sodium deficiency alone may cause a decrease in cardiac output, hemoconcentration, reduced utilization of protein and carbohydrates, soft bones, corneal keratinization, gonadal inactivity and adrenal hypertrophy.

Demineralized bone formation was seen in a variety of juvenile Australian parrots fed a homemade mineral block containing apparently adequate calcium and phosphorus levels, but an excess level of salt. The problem stopped when the mineral block was removed.

Excessive amounts of salt may be acutely toxic. Affected birds show intense polydipsia, muscle weakness and convulsions.

Water

Budgerigars and Zebra Finches (species that evolved in desert regions) have been reported to survive several months without drinking, apparently relying on water derived from metabolic sources. On the other hand, healthy companion birds may consume significant amounts of water daily and become distressed if water is withheld.

Some birds that have not evolved for desert living (eg, canaries), may die if they do not drink water for 48 hours. The addition of any compound to the drinking water can cause these birds to stop consuming water, resulting in a rapid dehydration and death.

VIRUSES

Helga Gerlach

In general, viral infections remain untreatable. Nonspecific supportive care, antimicrobials to prevent secondary bacterial and fungal infections and good nutritional support, including the supplementation of vitamin C, remain the only available therapeutic regimens for most viral infections. Newly emerging concepts in the use of antisense RNA will undoubtedly result in more specific therapies for many infectious diseases (see Chapter 6). Interferon has been suggested for treatment of viral infections. Paramunity inducers have proven effective with some viral diseases. Acyclovir has proven to be effective with some strains of avian herpesvirus and may have positive effects in treating poxvirus infections. Substantial viral disease outbreaks may be prevented by having a working knowledge of the transmission routes and pathogenesis of a particular virus, by using specific diagnostic tests to detect clinical or subclinical infections, by practicing sound hygiene and by maintaining closed aviaries.

Diagnostic Principles

There are several procedures that can be used to confirm the presence of a viral infection: 1) Isolation of the pathogen from the test material; 2) Demonstration of viral particles or inclusion bodies by histopathology; 3) demonstration of viral antigen (Ag) in infected tissues using viral-specific antibodies (Ab); 4) Demonstration of viral nucleic acid in infected tissues using viral-specific nucleic acid probes; 5) Indirect demonstration of a viral infection by detection of humoral antibodies. A viral disease can sometimes be demonstrated by a rise in antibody titers in paired serum samples.

Viral-specific nucleic acid probes are more sensitive than other techniques and allow the detection of small concentrations of virus as well as the ability to detect the presence of viral nucleic acid before substantial histologic changes may have occurred.

Virus Identification

Direct identification of a virus by electron microscopy is possible only with a relatively high concentration of the virus (generally >10^6 particles/ml). As a rapid but insensitive survey, fresh tissue samples fixed on grids (stained with osmium or another appropriate stain) can be examined by electron microscopy for the presence of viruses. Viral-specific nucleic acid probes allow the detection of very small concentrations of a virus in infected tissues or contaminated samples (crop washing, feces, respiratory excretions). Analytic methods such as electrophoresis without blot systems (Ab-dependent with blots), chromatography and nucleic acid probes are the most sensitive methods of demonstrating virus. They function independent of Ag-Ab reactions. The recent advances in genetic engineering will certainly have profound effects on virus detection in the future. DNA probes are currently available for detecting polyomavirus and psittacine beak and feather disease virus. Other similar diagnostic tests will ultimately be developed. All other methods of virus identification are based on changes induced by the virus, such as histologically discernible inclusion bodies. Viral-specific antibody preparations can be used to confirm the presence of a virus.

Indirect Virus Identification

Indirect virus identification techniques require the demonstration of specific antibodies in a patient's serum. To differentiate between Ab's that have been induced by prior exposure to an agent and those caused by a current infection, it is necessary to test two serum samples collected at two- to three-week intervals. A rise or fall in Ab concentrations or a switch from IgM to IgG are indicative of an active infection.

Table 32.2   Characteristic Histologic Lesions and Diagnostic Techniques of Selected Avian Viruses

Virus	Characteristic Lesions	Diagnostic Methods
Adenovirus	Basophilic intranuclear inclusions	Histopathology, serology (AGID)
EEE	Non-suppurative encephalitis, "descending" encephalitis	Histopathology, serology (HI)
Herpesvirus	Basophilic to eosinophilic intranuclear inclusion bodies (Cowdry type A)	Histopathology, virus isolation (Ab titers inconsistent)
Papillomavirus	Hyperkeratotic epidermis, intranuclear inclusions	Histopathology
Polyomavirus	Enlarged cells containing clear basophilic or amphophilic inclusions	Histopathology suggestive, virus isolation, viral-specific DNA probes (detecting shedders and confirming infections), *in situ* hybridization of tissues
PBFD virus	Basophilic intranuclear inclusions in epithelial cells, basophilic intracytoplasmic inclusions in macrophages	Histopathology, viral-specific DNA probes (detecting symptomatic or asymptomatic infections in blood), *in situ* hybridization of tissues
Paramyxovirus		Electron microscopy (EM), serology (HI), viral isolation
Poxvirus	Epithelial ballooning degeneration, intracytoplasmic inclusions (Bollinger bodies) pathognomonic, intranuclear inclusion bodies	Histopathology, viral culture, virus detection in feces by culture or EM
Reovirus	Necrotizing hepatitis, rarely intranuclear inclusion bodies	Virus isolation

Serologic cross-reactions caused by closely related antigens or epitopes with an identical structure can cause false-positive results when using indirect virus identification techniques.

Avipoxvirus

Members of the Poxviridae family (Avipoxvirus genus) cause a variety of diseases in birds. These large DNA viruses (250-300 nm) induce intracytoplasmic, lipophilic inclusion bodies called Bollinger bodies (pathognomonic). These inclusion bodies may be identified in affected epithelial cells of the integument, respiratory tract and oral cavity.

The genus *Avipox* seems to be restricted to birds. Most of the members of the genus seem to be species-specific, but some taxons appear to be able to pass the species, genus or even family barrier. Although certain poxvirus strains will experimentally infect variety of host species, cross-immunity may not always be inducible.

Various *Avipox* spp. demonstrate serologic cross-reactions (VN and ID). Hemagglutinins are not produced. Species differentiation is based on host spectrum, plaque morphology of primary isolates, thermostability, optimal propagation temperature, serology, cross-immunity and ultrastructural characteristics.

Poxvirus lesions have been documented on the feet, beak and periorbitally in numerous Passeriformes.

Transmission

Transmission occurs through latently infected birds and biting arthropods in the habitat. In many areas, mosquitoes serve as the primary vectors, and infections are most common during late summer and autumn when mosquitoes are prevalent.

Direct transmission of the virus between birds is linked to traumatic injuries induced by territorial behavior, which allows the virus access to the host through damaged epithelium.

Pathogenesis

Most members of the Poxviridae stimulate the synthesis of DNA in the host's epithelial cells resulting in hyperplasia of the affected epithelium. Avipoxvirus cannot penetrate intact epithelium. Traumatic lesions that may be induced by biting insects (mosquitoes, mites and ticks) can cause sufficient damage to the epithelial barrier to allow viral entrance to the host. Infections may be restricted to the portal of entry, or viremia and subsequent distribution to target organs may occur.

Avian poxvirus infections, particularly in a flock situation, can remain latent for years. Nonspecific stress factors are associated with viral reactivation.

Clinical Disease and Pathology

The course of the disease is generally subacute, and it takes three to four weeks for an individual to recover. Flock outbreaks require two to three months to run their course. Clinically recognized symptoms include:

Cutaneous Form ("Dry Pox"): The cutaneous form is the most common form of disease in many raptors and Passeriformes but not in Psittaciformes. Changes are characterized by papular lesions mainly on unfeathered skin around the eyes, beak, nares and distal to·the tarsometatarsus. The interdigital webs are most frequently affected in waterfowl and the Shearwater. As lesions progress, papules change color from yellowish to dark brown and develop into vesicles that open spontaneously, dry and form crusts. Spontaneous desquamation may require weeks and occurs without scarring in uncomplicated cases. Pigmented skin will frequently be discolored following an infection. Secondary bacterial or fungal colonization of lesions can substantially alter the appearance and progression of the disease.

In some cases, vesicles may not form and papules become hyperplastic, remaining in the periorbital region, nares, sinus infraorbitalis or on the tongue. Blue-fronted Amazons and Indian Hill Mynahs frequently develop ocular lesions.

Diphtheroid Form ("Wet Pox"): Poxviral lesions that occur on the mucosa of the tongue, pharynx and larynx (rarely in the bronchi, esophagus and crop) cause fibrinous lesions that are grey to brown and caseous. Disturbing the exudates covering these lesions will induce severe bleeding. Multiple foci that coalesce may prevent a bird from swallowing food or result in dyspnea (or asphyxiation) if the larynx is involved. Oral lesions are frequently seen in Psittaciformes, Phasianiformes, Bobwhite Quail, some Columbiformes and Starlings.

Cutaneous and diphtheroid lesions may occur in the same bird or either or both types of lesions may be noted in a flock outbreak. The septicemic form can also occur in conjunction with either cutaneous or diphtheritic forms of this disease.

Septicemic Form: An acute onset of ruffled plumage, somnolence, cyanosis and anorexia characterize septicemic poxvirus infections. Most birds (mortality rates of 70-99%) die within three days of developing clinical signs. Cutaneous lesions are rare and antemortem documentation of infections is difficult. Septicemic infections are most common in canaries and canary and finch crosses. Canarypox frequently causes a desquamative pneumonia with occlusion of the air capillaries resulting in dyspnea.

Tumors: Some Avipoxvirus strains have oncogenic properties. Passeriformes and Columbiformes that survive infections are prone to tumor formation. These rapidly growing, wart-like efflorescent tumors of the skin are generally void of normal epithelium and hemorrhage readily when disturbed. Bollinger bodies are usually present in the neoplastic tissue but viable virus may not be demonstrated. Surgical removal of the skin tumors is an effective therapy.

Specific Poxviral Symptoms

Psittacine poxvirus infections have been documented in numerous South American parrots and parakeets. *Amazona* spp. and *Ara* spp. are most severely affected. Ocular lesions begin as dry areas on the eyelid that become crusty with exudate, sealing the lids closed. Secondary infections frequently cause keratitis, followed by ulceration, perforation of the globe, panophthalmia and finally ophthalmophthisis.

Cutaneous lesions in raptorial birds from most regions are relatively mild and self-limiting. In contrast, cutaneous lesions in Persian Gulf falcons are characterized by inflammatory necrotic processes that inhibited feeding. In some of these birds, CNS signs including somnolence, anorexia, opisthotonus, tonic-clonic cramps of the tail muscles and paresis and paralysis of the feet occurred.

Poxvirus infections in lovebirds usually cause cutaneous lesions although diphtheroid lesions ("wet pox") have also been described. Morbidity and mortality in lovebirds may reach 75% of the at-risk population.

Poxvirus infections in 10- to 60-day-old ostrich chicks are characterized by small vesicles containing yellowish fluid on the eyelids and face. Lesions become dry and form a scale within six to ten days of forming. Diphtheroid lesions may also occur on the larynx, oral mucosa and the base of the tongue.

Diagnosis

A definitive diagnosis of poxvirus can be made through the histologic demonstration of Bollinger bodies in biopsy samples of suspect lesions. Culture is usually necessary to document the septicemic or coryzal forms of the disease.

Control

Birds that recover from pox should be protected from further disease for at least eight months, but many reports indicate shorter durations of immunity. Vaccination is the best method for controlling poxviral infections. Taxon-specific vaccines are available for only a few of the avian poxviruses. Vaccines are commercially available for psittacine poxvirus, and should be considered to prevent infections in high-risk populations (imported birds, pet shop birds exposed to imported birds, areas with high densities of mosquitoes). The manufacturer's guidelines for vaccination should be carefully followed. Canaries (and crosses) should be immunized with an appropriate vaccine. Only healthy flocks of these birds should be vaccinated. The use of a vaccine in an actively infected flock of canaries and other birds may result in recombination between the field and vaccine virus strains, inducing a severe disease in the entire flock.

Fowlpox vaccine has been found to provide protection for ostriches. Vaccination at 10-14 days old is recommended in areas with high densities of mosquitoes.

Herpesviridae

Herpesviridae are 120 and 220 nm diameter, double-stranded DNA viruses. Herpesvirus is not always restricted to a specific host or tissue. Crossing over a host- or tissue-specific barrier can alter the pathogenicity of the virus considerably. Herpesviruses primarily infect lymphatic tissue (either B- or T-cells), epithelial cells (skin, mucosa, hepatocytes) and nerve cells. As a group, herpesviruses generally induce latent and persistent infections (for weeks, months, years or lifetime) in an adapted host with irregular periods of recrudescence and shedding. Latently infected birds can remain asymptomatic for years.

Because humoral antibodies decrease with time, indirect diagnosis of herpesvirus infections by detection of antibodies may give false-negative results. Herpesviruses generally produce Cowdry type A intranuclear inclusion bodies in target cells.

The Herpesviridae family is divided into three sub-families:

- α-Herpesvirinae (hemorrhagic lesions)
- β-Herpesvirinae (necrotic lesions)
- τ-Herpesvirinae (lytic/neoplastic lesions)

Transmission

Transmission routes for avian herpesviruses in companion birds have not been thoroughly investigated. Vertical transmission has been confirmed only with budgerigar herpesvirus and duck plague herpesvirus. Budgerigars infected experimentally with Pacheco's disease virus shed virus with the feces for 48 hours post-infection.

Experimentally infected birds that remained asymptomatic shed virus in the feces for approximately three weeks. Rapid spread through the aviary is common with virulent strains. The acute onset of clinical signs in several members of the flock may occur three to five days after the initial case is recognized.

Pathogenesis

Infectious Laryngotracheitis (ILT)

The herpesvirus responsible for ILT is distributed worldwide and appears to be serologically uniform. Strain virulence varies widely from apathogenic to highly virulent. Unlike other herpesviridae, natural transmission is exclusively aerogenic. The virus has an affinity for respiratory epithelium, and viremia does not develop.

Clinical Disease, Pathology and Diagnosis

Virulent strains of ILT cause severe dyspnea, gasping and coughing-like sounds. Expectoration of bloody mucus is common, and infected birds shake their heads to expulse the mucus. Affected birds become progressively weak and cyanotic and die from asphyxiation. A similar clinical picture has been described in canaries.

Depending on the chronicity of the infection, postmortem findings may include hemorrhagic or fibrinous inflammation of a thickened mucosa of the larynx, trachea and in some cases, the bronchi. Caseous plugs or fibrinonectrotic pseudomembranes may also be noted.

Immunodiffusion, VN, IF and ELISA can be used to identify isolates. In infected birds, precipitating antibodies can be demonstrated as early as eight to ten days post-infection. The occurrence of intranuclear inclusion bodies in the respiratory epithelial cell is indicative, but confirmation of the disease requires virus isolation.

Control

Cell-adapted vaccines that have a considerable residual pathogenicity and may induce vaccinal reaction are available for chickens.

Amazon Tracheitis (AT)

The AT virus shares a serologic relationship with ILT and is considered a mutant of this virus. A herpesvirus pathologically similar to the ILT virus has been described in Bourke's Parrots.

Clinical Disease, Pathology and Diagnosis

Varying species of Amazon parrots develop similar clinical disease following natural infection. Peracute, acute, subacute and chronic (up to nine months duration) infections have been described. Fibronecrotic ocular, nasal or oral discharges accompanied by open-beaked breathing, rales, rattles and coughing are common. As a rule, the disease in Bourke's Parrots takes a less florid course.

Pharyngeal or laryngeal swabs submitted for culture are suitable for confirming a diagnosis.

Duck Plague (DP — syn. Duck Virus Enteritis)

Duck plague virus seems to be distributed worldwide with the exception of Australia, and has been documented in free-ranging and captive Anatidae (ducks, geese and swans). The disease is characterized by damage to the endothelial lining of vessels resulting in tissue hemorrhage, gastrointestinal bleeding and free blood in body cavities. Intermittent virus shedding in clinically healthy birds has been noted for up to five years.

Clinical Disease, Pathology and Diagnosis

Peracute death may occur without clinical signs. A more acute course is characterized by polydipsia, photophobia, nasal discharge, serous to hemorrhagic lacrimation, anorexia, cyanosis and greenish, watery (occasionally hemorrhagic) diarrhea. Mature birds generally have a more prolonged course of disease. Many birds swim in circles and are unable to fly. Paralysis of the phallus, convulsions or tremor of the neck and head muscles are occasionally noted. Affected free-ranging waterfowl may sit on the water with neck and head in extreme extension.

Postmortem lesions differ according to species susceptibility, degree of virus exposure and virulence of the infecting strain. Suggestive lesions include petechia and ecchymosis on the epicardium, serous membranes and the large blood vessels of the body; annular hemorrhagic bands on the mucosa of the intestinal tract; necrosis in the cloacal wall and long parallel diphtheroid eruptions or confluent necrosis in the lower third of the esophagus. Nonspecific lesions include necrotic foci in the liver and hemorrhage of developing egg follicles.

A definitive diagnosis requires virus isolation. VN is recommended for virus identification and to demonstrate antibodies in the host.

Pacheco's Disease Virus (PDV)

Pacheco's disease virus (PDV) has been described all over the world and is associated with a systemic, in many instances acute, disease that affects the liver, spleen and kidneys.

Susceptibility to PDV seems to be restricted to the Psittaciformes. Patagonian and Nanday Conures are frequently discussed as asymptomatic carriers that intermittently shed virus; however, any bird that recovers from a PDV infection should be considered a carrier.

There are indications that inclusion body hepatitis in Psittaciformes (described and diagnosed as Pacheco's disease) is caused by several herpesviruses that are serologically distinct from the "original" virus.

Clinical Disease

PDV generally induces an acute, nonspecific disease characterized by somnolence, lethargy, anorexia, ruffled plumage and intermittent diarrhea, polyuria and polydipsia. Biliverdin staining of liquified feces and urates is indicative of the severe liver necrosis caused by the virus. Sinusitis, hemorrhagic diarrhea, conjunctivitis and convulsions or tremors in the neck, wings and legs have occasionally been described. Stress factors are thought to induce recrudescence in asymptomatic carriers resulting in virus excretion and an epornitic in exposed birds. In other cases, only a single bird may suddenly die while the rest of the flock remains unaffected. Old World Psittaciformes appear to be more resistant to PDV than do New World Psittaciformes.

Pathology and Diagnosis

With peracute or acute disease, birds are in generally good condition at the time of death. A massively swollen, tawny, light-red or greenish-colored liver with subserosal hemorrhages or necrotic foci is common. The spleen and kidneys are also distinctly swollen, and the intestinal mucosa may be hyperemic. Virus identification is possible by VN, ELISA and IF. Precipitation with the ID is useful as a screening test. The use of monoclonal antibodies allows differentiation between the various PDV serotypes. Antibodies to PDV are difficult to demonstrate and provide no clinically relevant information.

Treatment

Acyclovir has been shown to be effective for treating at least some strains of PDV. The recommended treatment regimen is to administer the water-soluble powder at a dose of 80 mg/kg q8h by gavage tube. Severe muscle necrosis will occur if the intravenous product is injected IM. If gavage administration is not practical, the powdered acyclovir can be added to the food at a dose as high as 240 mg/kg. Treatment is most effective if started before clinical signs develop. Acyclovir may cause considerable nephrotoxicity, and this drug should be administered carefully in patients with nephropathies.

Control

An inactivated PDV vaccine is commercially available in the USA. There have been frequent reports of granulomas and paralysis following the use of this vaccine, particularly in cockatoos, African Grey Parrots and Blue and Gold Macaws. The vaccine is intended for use in high risk patients (import stations, pet shops that handle birds). The instructions for use provided by the manufacturer should be carefully followed.

Budgerigar Herpesvirus

A vertically transmitted herpesvirus has been isolated from the feathers of budgerigars. The virus is occasionally recoverable from parenchymatous organs, blood or feces. Decreased egg hatchability is the principal problem associated with this virus, which is serologically related to the pigeon herpesvirus, but not to Pacheco's disease virus or related strains. Most isolates of this virus have been from so-called "feather dusters." Virus isolated in cell culture can be identified using antibodies in the VN or ID tests.

Inclusion Body Hepatitis in Pigeons (Infectious Esophagitis)

This herpesvirus has a worldwide distribution, and various strains show morphologic, pathogenic and serologic differences (plaque formation in CEF). Small plaque variants are less pathogenic or apathogenic. The large and small plaque-forming viruses may be two different strains. Falcons and owls might also be susceptible and could be infected through contact with diseased pigeons.

Transmission can occur through contact with contaminated feed or water, through direct contact between mates and through parenteral feeding of offspring.

Clinical Disease, Pathology and Diagnosis

In the flock, morbidity is typically 50%, with a 10-15% mortality rate. Serous rhinitis and conjunctivitis are usually the first clinical signs of disease. Small diphtheroid foci on the pharynx and larynx (which develop into so-called sialoliths) are indicative of an active infection. Mild diarrhea, anorexia, vomiting and polydipsia may also occur. Affected squabs may die within one to two weeks or slowly recover. Tremors, ataxia and an inability to fly may occur in some birds. Recurring trichomoniasis is common in flocks with endemic herpesvirus.

Contagious Paralysis of Pigeons (PHEV - Pigeon Herpes Encephalomyelitis Virus)

The distribution of the virus is undetermined.

Clinical Disease, Pathology and Diagnosis

Affected birds develop progressive, chronic central nervous signs that start with incoordination and end with an inability to fly and paralysis.

Inclusion Body Hepatitis of the Falcon (FHV - Falcon Herpesvirus)

Falcon herpesvirus seems to be distributed in the northern hemisphere of the Old and New Worlds. There is a close antigenic relationship between FHV and the pigeon and owl herpesviruses. Field cases of falcon herpesvirus have been described in the Peregrine Falcon, Common Kestrel, Merlin, Red-necked Falcon, Prairie Falcon and American Kestrel. Experimentally, the African Collared Dove, immature budgerigar, Striated Heron, Lone-eared Owl, Screech Owl, Great Horned Owl and Muscovy Duck have been shown to be susceptible.

The falcon herpesvirus has an affinity for reticuloendothelial cells and hepatocytes. There is no confirmed information on the natural transmission of this virus. It has been suggested that the consumption of infected prey may be involved in transmission.

Clinical Disease, Pathology and Diagnosis

Generally, an acute disease develops with mild to severe depression, weakness and anorexia. Mortality may approach 100%. At necropsy, light-to-tan colored necrotic foci are seen in the liver, spleen, bone marrow and lymph follicles of the intestine.

Hepatosplenitis Infectiosa Strigum (OHV - Owl Herpesvirus)

Owl herpesvirus has a limited host spectrum and occurs in free-ranging and captive owls. The virus is distributed across Europe, Asia and the United States. Natural infections are mainly seen in owls with yellow- or orange-colored irises including: Eagle Owl, Great Horned Owl, Striped Owl, Long-eared Owl, Snowy Owl, Little Owl, Tengmalm's Owl and Forest Eagle Owl.

In contrast to other avian Herpesviridae, OHV affects both epithelial and mesenchymal cells. Virus is excreted from the oral cavity and in urine. Consumption of infected prey should be considered a potential method of transmission. Compared with other avian Herpesviridae, the incubation period for OHV is prolonged (seven to ten days) rather than the more typical three to five days.

Clinical Disease and Pathology

Clinical signs including depression, anorexia and weakness may last for two to five days. Infrequently, yellowish nodules the size of millet seeds may develop on the pharyngeal mucosa. These lesions may be secondarily infected with *Trichomonas* spp. In captivity, mortality rates may approach 100%. The demonstration of antibodies in free-ranging owls indicates that birds can survive infections. Leukopenia has been described during active infections.

The necropsy reveals numerous necrotic foci in the liver, spleen and bone marrow. Other suggestive lesions include diphtheroid (frequent) and hemorrhagic (rare) enteritis, diphtheroid stomatitis, esophagitis, proventriculitis and laryngitis (less frequent) as well as single necrotic foci in the lungs and kidneys. Moniliform necrotic nodules may be found along the jugular vein, probably emanating from the remains of thymic tissue.

Table 32.5 Survey of Avian Herpesviridae

Disease	Susceptible Species
Subfamily - α	
Infectious laryngotracheitis	Chickens, pheasants, peafowl, canaries
Amazon tracheitis	Genus *Amazona*, Bourke's parrot
Duck plague (syn. Duck virus enteritis)	Ducks, geese, swans
Subfamily - β	
Pacheco's disease virus, "Pacheco's disease-like" virus	All Psittaciformes considered susceptible to varying degrees. At least three different serotypes. Host spectrum of two recent isolates is unknown.
Budgerigar herpesvirus	Budgerigar, pigeon, Double Yellow-headed Amazon
Pigeon inclusion body hepatitis (Esophagitis)	Pigeons, falcons, owls, budgerigar
Pigeon herpes encephalomyelitis	Pigeons
Falcon herpesvirus inclusion body hepatitis	Peregrine Falcon, Prairie Falcon, Common Kestrel, American Kestrel, Merlin, Red-necked Falcon Experimentally susceptible birds (see text)
Owl herpesvirus (Hepato-splenitis infectiosa strigum)	Eagle Owl, Great Horned Owl, Forest Eagle Owl, Snowy Owl, Striped Owl, Long-eared Owl, Little Owl, Tengmalm's Owl. Experimentally susceptible birds
Bald Eagle herpesvirus	Bald Eagle
Lake Victoria cormorant virus	Little Pied Cormorant
Crane inclusion body hepatitis	Demoiselle Crane, Crowned Crane, Whooping Crane, Sandhill Crane
Stork inclusion body hepatitis	Black Stork, White Stork
Colinus herpesvirus	Bobwhite Quail
Subfamily - not classified	
Marek's disease virus	Gallinaceous birds
Turkey herpesvirus	Gallinaceous birds
Canary herpesvirus	Canary
Gouldian Finch herpesvirus	Gouldian Finch
"Local" herpesvirus causing papilloma-like lesions on feet	Cockatoo, Macaw
Herpesvirus associated with papilloma	Conures

Diagnosis

The necrotic foci in the liver, spleen, intestine and along the jugular vein should be differentiated from those caused by mycobacteriosis. Although the morphology is strikingly similar, the foci caused by herpesvirus are soft and are not demarcated from the surrounding tissue. In comparison, mycobacteria-induced tubercles are caseous, crumbly and normally well demarcated. Trichomoniasis-induced diphtheroid pharyngitis appears similar to that caused by herpesvirus. Additionally, *Trichomonas* spp. and fungi can be secondary invaders of pharyngeal lesions induced by herpesvirus.

The bone marrow of the femur is the best tissue to submit for virus isolation. Differentiation of OHV, FHV and PHV requires electrophoresis to delineate strain-specific proteins.

Gouldian Finch Herpesvirus

An uncharacterized virus suggestive of herpesvirus has been identified by electron microscopy in clinically affected Crimson Finches, Red-faced Waxbills and Zebra Finches. In a mixed species aviary, Gouldian Finches died from lesions caused by a herpesvirus, while other Passeriformes in the collection remained unaffected. Mortality in Gouldian Finch flocks may reach 70% of the birds at risk.

Clinical Disease and Pathology

Listless birds with ruffled plumage develop increasingly severe dyspnea with minimal discharge from the nostrils. Swollen and edematous eyelids and conjunctivae may be sealed with crusts in the lid cleft. Despite severe dyspnea, affected birds may continue to try to eat, although sometimes unsuccessfully. Death is common five to ten days following the first clinical signs.

Necropsy findings included severe emaciation even though some affected birds continued to eat. Swollen eyelids and conjunctivae, serous discharge in the conjunctival sacs and fibrinoid thickening of the air sacs were the only characteristic findings. Apart from congestion, parenchymal organs appeared normal.

Other Herpesviruses

A herpesvirus has been described in lovebirds with malformed feathers, but the involvement of this virus in causing the lesions has not been determined.

Papilloma-like lesions thought to be caused by a herpesvirus have been described on the feet of cockatoos.

Histopathology is consistent with squamous papillomas. Electron microscopy has been used to demonstrate virus particles suggestive of herpesvirus. A herpes-like virus was observed by electron microscopy in association with a cloacal papilloma in an Orange-fronted Conure.

Papovaviridae

The Papovaviridae family of viruses consists of two genera, *Papillomavirus* and *Polyomavirus*, both of which are double-stranded DNA viruses.

As a group, the papovaviruses tend to cause persistent infections that become active following stressful events.

Papillomavirus

Papillomavirus has been associated with the formation of benign epithelial tumors (papillomata) on the skin and epithelial mucosa of many mammalian species.

Clinical Features

The first demonstration of a papovavirus in a non-mammalian species involved the recovery and characterization of a papillomavirus from proliferative skin masses found on the legs of finches in the family Fringillidae. The virus appears to be rare in other avian species.

A papillomavirus was demonstrated in a Timneh African Grey Parrot with proliferative skin lesions on the head and palpebrae.

Papillomatous lesions have been diagnosed histologically from proliferative growths originating from skin overlying the phalanges, uropygial gland, mandible, neck, wing, eyelids and beak commissure from various Psittaciformes including Amazon parrots, African Grey Parrots, Quaker Parakeets, cockatiels and budgerigars. While a viral etiology has been assumed for these epidermal proliferations, virus has not been demonstrated in association with any of these lesions.

Histologic lesions suggestive of papillomas have been described at numerous locations along the avian gastrointestinal tract. These papillomatous lesions most frequently occur at the transition between mucosa and cutaneous epithelium in the cloaca.

Grossly, papillomatous lesions may appear as large, distinct masses or may occur as numerous small, raised lesions covering the mucosa. These friable growths may be pink or white and have a tendency to bleed easily when bruised. Acetic acid (5%) will turn papillomatous tissue white, helping to identify suspect lesions. Many internal papillomatous lesions are not recognized until necropsy. Suspicious lesions in the oral or cloacal cavity can be viewed directly.

Attempts to demonstrate papillomavirus in suspect lesions by electron microscopy, low stringency southern blotting techniques or immunocytochemical procedures have all failed. Attempts to induce lesions in Amazon parrots, macaws and cockatoos using homogenized lesions have also been unsuccessful; however, the disease has features that suggest an infectious agent. Chronic irritation of the cloacal mucosa with epithelial cell hypertrophy or hyperplasia could result in a histologic lesion that morphologically resembles those induced by papillomavirus and has been suggested as an alternate cause of these lesions. Herpes-like virus particles were described in a cloacal papilloma in a conure. Malnutrition, particularly with respect to vitamin A, has been suggested to potentiate lesions.

Histologic examination is necessary to confirm a diagnosis in any suspect lesions. Amazon parrots with papillomatous lesions have been described as having a high incidence of malignant pancreatic or bile duct carcinomas.

Therapy

Suggested therapeutic measures for cloacal papillomas have been based on the physical removal of the masses through cryotherapy, radiocautery or surgical excision. These procedures have been performed alone or in combination with the use of autogenous vaccines. None of the proposed therapies is consistently effective, and papillomatous tissue often recurs. The use of autogenous vaccines has been described but is generally not effective. Spontaneous regression of papillomatous tissue has been described.

Staged cauterization with silver nitrate sticks may prove to be the easiest, safest and best way to remove papillomatous lesions from the cloaca. Lesions should be exteriorized by inserting a moistened cotton swab followed by carefully rubbing a small area of the lesion with a silver nitrate stick. The silver nitrate should be immediately inactivated with copious fluids to prevent the liquified material from burning unaffected mucosal tissues. The procedure is repeated at two-week intervals until the lesions have been removed.

Epizootiologic evidence has been used to suggest that intestinal papillomas are caused by an infectious agent even though no etiology has been confirmed. Mutual preening and sexual contact have been suggested as methods of transmission. Until further information on the etiology of this disease is available, it is prudent to isolate birds with lesions from the remainder of a collection.

Polyomavirus

Budgerigar fledgling disease (BFD) is caused by the first avian polyomavirus to be characterized. Polyomaviruses recovered from several species of Psittaciformes have been shown to be similar by comparing restriction maps of viral DNA and by using viral-specific DNA probes.

Transmission

Some asymptomatic adults produce persistently infected young, while others have neonates that intermittently may develop clinical signs and die.

Experimental data and observations with the natural disease suggest that polyomavirus transmission may occur by both horizontal and vertical routes. Parents may transmit virus to offspring through the regurgitation of exfoliated crop epithelial cells. Virus can replicate in the epidermal cells of the feather follicles resulting in the presence of virus in "feather dust," which may enter a susceptible host through the respiratory or gastrointestinal tract. The recovery of viral DNA from the cloaca suggests that the virus could be shed from gastrointestinal, renal or reproductive tissues.

Aviary personnel, technicians, veterinarians, pet owners and any aviary equipment should be considered important vectors for this environmentally stable virus.

Findings in support of vertical transmission include the identification of intranuclear inclusion bodies in one-day-old budgerigars and the occurrence of infections when eggs from parents that consistently produce diseased neonates are cross-fostered to parents producing normal young.

Theoretically, a persistently infected hen could pass maternally derived antibodies, virus or both to its young. The clinical status of the chick could then depend on the level of maternally derived antibodies and the stage of immunocompetency when viral exposure occurs. Chicks that have protective levels of maternal antibodies as well as infections derived from the parents may serve to infect susceptible neonates in the nursery. Persistent infections with intermittent shedding and vertical transmission are also suspected to occur in finches and result in early embryonic death.

The incubation period is not known. Affected budgerigar fledglings show peak mortality rates between the 15th and 19th day of life. In larger parrots, death may occur from 20-140 days of age, with most deaths occurring between 20-56 days of age.

Pathogenesis

The age of a bird at the time of viral exposure may be a major factor in the pathogenesis of polyomavirus infections. Budgerigars that die shortly after hatch have more severe and widespread lesions than do birds in which the morbid state is more prolonged. It is theorized that persistently infected birds may be those that are infected before they are immunocompetent.

Field studies have shown that birds that die from avian polyomavirus frequently have antibodies to the virus. Massive hepatocellular necrosis (with intranuclear inclusion in hepatocytes) is the most frequent histologic lesion in larger psittacine birds that die from avian polyomavirus.

The BFD virus can replicate in a variety of target cells of many avian species including chicken embryo cells. Following the primary viremia, inclusion bodies can develop in most internal organs as well as the skin and developing feathers. The highest virus concentration is usually found in the brain. The virus has been associated with immunosuppression through its ability to destroy or inhibit the normal development of lymphoid tissue.

Polyomaviruses in mammals are natural tumor inducers. There has thus far been no association between polyomavirus infections in birds and an increased incidence of tumors.

Clinical Features

An avian polyomavirus appears to be distributed worldwide, but there are some apparent strain differences. Avian polyomavirus appears to infect a wide variety of Psittaciformes, Estrilidae and Ploceidae including macaws, Amazon parrots, conures, White-bellied Caiques, parrotlets, African Grey Parrots, lovebirds, Ring-necked Parakeets, Eclectus Parrots, Scarlet-chested Parrots, Bourke's Parrots, cockatoos and finches.

Budgerigars: Neonates from infected flocks may develop normally for 10-15 days and then suddenly die with no premonitory signs. Other infected hatchlings may develop clinical signs, which include abdominal distention, subcutaneous hemorrhage, tremors of the head and neck, ataxia and reduced formation of down and contour feathers.

Infected budgerigars may die rapidly once clinical signs develop, and reports on mortality rates vary from 30-100% of affected hatchlings. Survivors may exhibit symmetrical feather abnormalities characterized by dystrophic primary and tail feathers, lack of down feathers on the back and abdomen and lack of filoplumes on the head and neck. Birds often die acutely with the crop and gastrointestinal tract full of food. Surviving fledglings frequently have dystrophic feathers (French moult). Affected birds are unable to fly and are often called runners or hoppers. Similar feather lesions can be caused by the psittacine beak and feather disease (PBFD) virus. In general, feather lesions in budgerigars caused by polyomavirus resolve after several months, while those induced by PBFD virus will continue to progress.

In North America and Europe, lesions attributable to French moult are thought to be caused either by the polyomavirus or by the PBFD virus. Investigations in Australian budgerigars have demonstrated that clinical signs associated with French moult are associated with the PBFD virus and not with avian polyomavirus.

Other Psittaciformes: In larger psittacine birds, polyomavirus infections may cause peracute death with no premonitory signs or acute death after development of clinical changes including depression, anorexia, weight loss, delayed crop emptying, regurgitation, diarrhea, dehydration, subcutaneous hemorrhages, dyspnea and polyuria. Intramuscular injection sites or damaged feathers may bleed profusely. Neurologic signs characterized by ataxia, tremors and paralysis have been described in some Psittaciformes. Clinical signs are common at the time of weaning, and infected fledglings typically die 12-48 hours after developing clinical signs. Infections may occur in both parent-raised and hand-raised neonates. In one outbreak, mortality rates in exposed neonates ranged from 31-41% of the at-risk population. Infected birds that recover are thought to become asymptomatic virus carriers.

Table 32.8   Gross Lesions Associated with Polyomavirus Infections

Heart	
Budgerigars	Hydropericardium, cardiomegaly, myocardial hemorrhage
Other Psittaciformes	Myocardial hemorrhage, epicardial hemorrhage, pale myocardium
Liver	
Budgerigars	Hepatomegaly, yellow-white foci
Lovebirds	Pallor, congestion, mottled hemorrhage
Other Psittaciformes	Hepatomegaly, red and yellow mottling, friable
Finches	Swollen, pallor, mottled, hemorrhage
Spleen	
Lovebirds	Small, pallor
Other Psittaciformes	Splenomegaly, friable
Finches	Splenomegaly, congestion
Gastrointestinal Tract	
Budgerigars	Intestinal hemorrhage
Other Psittaciformes	Intestinal hemorrhage
Finches	Serosal or subserosal intestinal hemorrhage
Kidney	
Budgerigars	Swelling, pallor or congestion, white foci, petechiation
Other Psittaciformes	Pallor, swollen
Finches	Perirenal hemorrhage
Skin	
Budgerigars	Subcutaneous hemorrhage, feather dystrophy
Other Psittaciformes	Feather dystrophy, petechial hemorrhage, ecchymotic hemorrhage
Other	
Budgerigars	Ascites, lung congestion
Lovebirds	Increased serosal fluids
Other Psittaciformes	Pale skeletal muscle, ascites, serosal and subcutaneous hemorrhage, pallor

Table 32.9   Histologic Lesions Associated with Polyomavirus Infections

Heart	
Budgerigars	Coagulative necrosis, mycardial degeneration, inclusion bodies
Lovebirds	Enlarged endothelial cells
Other Psittaciformes	Myocarditis, epicardial hemorrhage, inclusion bodies (myocardium)
Finches	Myocarditis, inclusion bodies

Liver	
Budgerigars	Coagulative necrosis, vacuolar degeneration, inclusion bodies
Lovebirds	Hepatic necrosis, hemorrhage, inclusion bodies
Other Psittaciformes	Hepatic necrosis, inclusion bodies
Finches	Kupffer's cell hyperplasia, hepatocellular necrosis, periportal heterophils and lymphocytes, vacuolar degeneration, inclusion bodies (hepatocytes, Kupffer's cells)

Spleen	
Budgerigars	Lymphatic atrophy, inclusion bodies, (reticuloendothelial [RE] cells)
Lovebirds	Lymphoid depletion, necrosis, inclusion bodies
Other Psittaciformes	Karyomegaly of RE cells, multifocal necrosis, inclusion bodies
Finches	Macrophage hyperplasia, necrosis, lymph depletion, inclusion bodies

Gastrointestinal Tract	
Budgerigars	Inclusion bodies (crop, intestines)
Other Psittaciformes	Serosal hemorrhage, epithelial desquamation of crop and esophagus, inclusion bodies (esophagus, proventriculus, intestines)
Finches	Necrosis and plasma cell infiltrates of lamina propria, enlarged vacuolated epithelial cells, inclusion bodies, mainly enterocytes

Kidney	
Budgerigars	Focal nephrosis, vacuolar degeneration, inclusion bodies (renal tubular epithelium)
Lovebirds	Enlarged endothelial cells, enlarged epithelial cells, karyomegaly of renal tubules
Other Psittaciformes	Membranous glomerulopathy, thickened glomerular capillaries, inclusion bodies, (glomerulus interstitium, collecting tubules)
Finches	Inclusion bodies (endothelium, tubular epithelium)

Skin	
Budgerigars	Ballooning degeneration (follicular epithelium, lateral and axial plate cells, epidermis) follicular and epidermal hyperplasia, inclusion bodies (epidermis, follicular epithelium, uropygial gland)
Other Psittaciformes	Ballooning degeneration and karyomegaly in epithelium of growing feathers, inclusion bodies (follicular epithelium)

Other	
Budgerigars	Bone marrow necrosis, lymphatic atrophy, cerebellar lesions (particularly in the Purkinje cells), inclusion bodies (pancreas, adrenals, lung, gonads, brain)
Other Psittaciformes	Generalized hemorrhage, bursal medullary necrosis, bone marrow necrosis, inclusion bodies (bone marrow, pancreas, adrenals, skeletal muscle, lungs)
Finches	Bone marrow necrosis, inclusion bodies

A chronic form of polyomavirus has also been described and is typified by weight loss, intermittent anorexia, polyuria, recurrent bacterial or fungal infections and poor feather formation. Birds that recover appear normal, although some birds have been found to die months later from renal failure. The feather abnormalities that are relatively common with polyomavirus infections in budgerigars have been less frequently described in other psittacine birds.

In the Eclectus Parrot, transient gastrointestinal stasis, melena and abdominal pain have been described in older chicks. Occult hematuria has been suggested as an indication of a polyomavirus infection in this species. Cloacal swabs from suspect patients can be screened for the presence of polyomavirus nucleic acid using viral-specific DNA probes. Affected birds may have increased activities of LDH, AST and alkaline phosphatase.

Finches: Lesions suggestive of a polyomavirus infection have been described as a cause of acute mortality in two- to three-day-old fledgling, young adult and mature finches. Affected birds had nonspecific signs of illness 24-48 hrs before death. Many of the fledglings that survived had poor feather development, long tubular misshapen lower mandibles, and fledged several days later than normal young.

Diagnosis

A confirmed diagnosis requires immunohistochemical staining of suspected lesions using viral-specific antibodies or the detection of viral nucleic acid using polyomavirus-specific DNA probes. The VN can be used to identify virus isolated in cell culture.

Immunodiffusion and virus neutralization techniques have been used to demonstrate polyomavirus antibodies in exposed birds. Subclinical carriers that intermittently shed polyomavirus have been thought to maintain high antibody titers in serial serologic assays. Based on these suppositions, the demonstration of sustained high antibody titers has been used to screen for polyomavirus carriers; however, polyomavirus-specific DNA probes have been used to demonstrate that there is no correlation between the shedding of polyomavirus in excrement and the titers of neutralizing antibodies.

Viral-specific DNA probes have been used to demonstrate polyomavirus nucleic acid in various tissues including liver, spleen, kidney, cloacal secretions, intestinal secretions, serum and blood. Viral nucleic acid occasionally can be detected in the blood or serum of some infected birds; however, the best antemortem sample for detecting polyomavirus shedders in larger psittacine birds is a cloacal swab. Testing birds twice per year (before and after the breeding season) is recommended to detect intermittent viral shedders.

DNA probes can also be used to detect viral nucleic acid in fresh tissues from birds that are suspected to have died from polyomaviral infections.

Therapy

In chicks that are hemorrhaging, injection of 0.2-2.5 mg/kg bodyweight of vitamin K IM may be helpful and can increase survival rates favorably, although prognosis in birds with heavy hemorrhaging is poor.

Control

Manual removal of any organic debris followed by the use of appropriate disinfectants is required to prevent or contain outbreaks. Sodium hypochlorite (5%) is thought to be effective against the BFD virus at a concentration of 50 ml/L of diluent. A polyomavirus DNA probe test can be used to screen walls, caging, air circulating ducts and equipment in the home or hospital to determine if this virus is contaminating a bird's environment.

With the highly infectious nature of avian polyomavirus, particularly to young Psittaciformes, closed breeding operations that do not allow visitors should be encouraged. A cloacal swab of any bird that is being added to a collection should be analyzed during the quarantine period to determine whether a bird is shedding polyomavirus. All birds being sold from an aviary should be tested to determine if they are shedding polyomavirus before shipment. Birds also should be tested for viral shedding during the post-purchase examination.

A bird that is shedding polyomavirus could be maintained as a pet if it does not expose other birds, particularly neonates, to the virus. Breeding birds shedding polyomavirus should be separated from the remainder of the collection, and offspring from these birds should be raised separately from birds that are not shedding the virus. Offspring from shedders should also be raised separately from birds that are not shedding the virus.

A killed avian polyomavirus vaccine was found to induce virus-neutralizing antibodies in Blue and Gold Macaw chicks that were sufficient to protect them from subsequent challenge. This suggests that a vaccine could be effective in preventing infections. [Editor's Note: Recently, a commercially-produced polyomavirus vaccine has become available.]

Depopulation of budgerigar aviaries experiencing outbreaks followed by restocking with seronegative birds has been suggested as a method of controlling enzootic infections in this species. It has been suggested that polyomavirus-free budgerigar nestlings can be produced by interrupting the breeding cycle, removing all but the older breeding birds and disinfecting the aviary. Depopulation is not a practical nor recommended procedure for controlling polyomavirus in larger Psittaciformes.

Circoviridae

Psittacine Beak and Feather Disease Virus

A chronic disease characterized by symmetric feather dystrophy and loss, development of beak deformities and eventual death was first described in various species of Australian cockatoos in the early 1970s.

The disease has been diagnosed in numerous Psittaciforme species in addition to cockatoos.

The virion size and nucleic acid characteristics described for the PBFD virus are similar to those found for the chicken anemia agent (CAA) and for the apparently nonpathogenic porcine circovirus (PCV).

A virus that morphologically resembles PBFD virus has been described in pigeons. When compared to PBFD virus, the pigeon circovirus is antigenically unique and has some differences in nucleic acid sequence.

Epizootiology

Histologic or clinically suggestive lesions of PBFD have now been described in 42 species of Psittaciformes. Psittacine beak and feather disease has been documented only in Psittaciformes.

Transmission

Psittacine beak and feather disease virus was recovered in the feces and crop washings from various species of psittacine birds diagnosed with PBFD. While the concentration of PBFD virus demonstrated in the crops of positive birds was low, the possibility of an adult transmitting the virus to neonates during feeding activities that involve the regurgitation of food and exfoliated crop epithelium deserves consideration. High concentrations of the virus also can be demonstrated in feather dust collected from a room where birds with active cases of PBFD are housed.

Artificially incubated chicks from a PBFD-infected hen consistently develop PBFD suggesting that vertical transmission of the virus occurs.

Pathogenesis and Immunity

PBFD is a progressive disease with temporary remission in the occurrence of new lesions in the periods of nonmolting. The lesions of the beak may progress during the intermolt period. It has been suggested that the virus depends on the multiplication of the host cells for its replication.

The clinically apparent form of PBFD virus is considered fatal. Most infected birds survive less than six months to one year after the onset of clinical signs, though some birds have been known to live over ten years in a featherless state. Death usually occurs either from changes induced by secondary bacterial, chlamydial, fungal or other viral agents, or from terminal changes that necessitate euthanasia.

The predilection for birds to die from secondary or opportunistic pathogens has been interpreted to indicate an immunosuppression that is thought to be induced by damage to the thymus and bursa.

PBFD-positive birds with inclusion bodies located only within the nucleus of infected epithelial cells have been found to spontaneously recover. On the other hand, larger psittacine birds with intracytoplasmic inclusion bodies located in macrophages usually succumb to the disease. Because the macrophage is critical for the initial processing and presentation of viral antigen to the immune system, it can be postulated that the determining factor in whether an infected bird develops a chronic fatal PBFD virus infection, or develops a protective immune response is based on how the body processes the virus before it begins to persist in the cytoplasm of macrophages.

Some birds exposed to the PBFD virus remain clinically normal and develop HI and precipitating antibody titers. The factors that determine whether a bird mounts an immune response or is fatally infected could depend on the age at the time of exposure, the presence and levels of maternal antibodies, the route of viral exposure and the titer of the infecting virus.

Incubation Period

The minimum incubation period is 21-25 days. The maximum incubation period may be months to years.

Clinical Disease

Clinical (and pathological) signs may vary greatly. Generally, PBFD is a disease of young birds (up to three years), but older individuals (up to 20 years of age) may also develop clinical lesions.

Based on markedly different clinical presentations, peracute, acute and chronic forms of PBFD have been described. The type of clinical disease appears to be influenced by the age of the bird when clinical signs first appear.

Peracute disease is suspected in neonatal psittacines that show signs of septicemia accompanied by pneumonia, enteritis, rapid weight loss and death. The peracute syndrome appears to be particularly common in young cockatoos and African Grey Parrots. Peracute cases of PBFD may be missed if a complete necropsy and thorough histologic exam are not performed on young of susceptible species that die suddenly.

The acute form of PBFD, commonly called French moult in Australia, is most frequently reported in young or fledgling birds during their first feather formation after replacement of the neonatal down, and chicks as young as 28-32 days of age have been described with classic lesions.

Acute infections are characterized by several days of depression followed by sudden changes in developing feathers, including necrosis, fractures, bending, bleeding or premature shedding of diseased feathers. In some acute cases of PBFD, birds with minimal feather changes may be depressed, develop crop stasis and have diarrhea, followed by death in one to two weeks. Gross feather lesions in the acute form of the disease can be quite subtle with only a few feathers showing dystrophic changes. This clinical picture is particularly common in young Sulphur-crested Cockatoos and lovebirds. In African Grey Parrots a nonregenerative anemia is reported (PCV=14-25%) with typical inclusion bodies in the bone marrow; however, it has not been determined if these changes are caused by the PBFD virus or if they are a result of secondary pathogens.

Chicks that develop clinical lesions while the majority of feathers are still in a developmental stage exhibit the most severe feather pathology. These birds may appear totally normal one day and exhibit 80-100% feather dystrophy within a week.

Chronic PBFD is characterized by the progressive appearance of abnormally developed feathers during each successive molt. Gross changes include retention of feather sheaths, hemorrhage within the pulp cavity, fractures of the proximal rachis and failure of developing feathers to exsheathe. Short, clubbed feathers, deformed, curled feathers, stress lines within vanes and circumferential constrictions may also be present. Replacement feathers become increasingly abnormal, and if birds live long enough they will eventually develop baldness as the feather follicles become inactive.

In older birds, the first sign of PBFD is the replacement of normal powder down and contour feathers with dystrophic, necrotic, nonviable feathers that stop growing shortly after emerging from the follicle. The disease then progresses to involve the contour feathers in most tracts, followed by dystrophic changes in the primary, secondary, tail and crest feathers.

Clinical changes in the beak and oral mucosa of PBFD-positive birds are characterized by progressive elongation, transverse or longitudinal fractures, palatine necrosis and oral ulceration. If the powder down feathers in cockatoos are dystrophic, the beak may appear to be semigloss or gloss black, instead of its normal grey color.

Classically, beak deformities develop in birds following a protracted course of PBFD where substantial feather changes have occurred; however, some individuals develop severe beak lesions with relatively minor feather pathology, and cracking of the hard corneum at the distal portion of the beak may be the initial complaint requiring veterinary attention.

Pathology

At necropsy, internal lesions are variable and differ with age and the type of secondary infection. In young birds, the cloacal bursa may be small with poorly developed folds and the thymus may reveal small lobes with pale necrotic tissue. In mature birds the spleen is frequently small and depleted of lymphocytes, and occasionally necrosis of the reticular cells can be observed. Extracutaneous inclusions demonstrated to be PBFD virus were found mainly in macrophages in the beak, palate, esophagus, crop, nail, tongue, parathyroid gland, bone marrow, Kupffer's star cells of the liver, spleen and thyroid gland. In the intestinal tract inclusion bodies were mainly found in epithelial cells.

Inclusion Bodies

Basophilic intranuclear and intracytoplasmic inclusion bodies have been consistently demonstrated by hematoxylin and eosin staining.

Immunohistochemical staining with viral-specific antibodies was used to confirm that intracytoplasmic basophilic inclusion bodies and some intranuclear inclusion bodies observed in hematoxylin and eosin-stained tissue sections contain PBFD viral antigen.

Diagnosis

PBFD should be suspected in any psittacine bird with progressive feather loss involving malformed feathers. Because several viruses may result in similarly appearing intranuclear inclusion bodies, a confirmatory diagnosis of PBFD requires the use of viral-specific antibodies to demonstrate PBFD virus antigen or the use of DNA probes to detect PBFD virus nucleic acid. Viral-specific DNA probes are most sensitive for detecting PBFD virus and can be used on biopsy samples to confirm an infection or on blood samples from a live bird to detect viremia.

The hemagglutination-inhibition (HI) test was found to provide a rapid, specific technique to assess the immunologic response of psittacine birds to the PBFD virus. Precipitating antibodies can be demonstrated using an agar-gel immunodiffusion test. A suitable culture system for the PBFD virus has yet to be discovered.

The recommended sample to submit for DNA probe detection of active or subclinical (birds that are showing no feather abnormalities) infections is whole anticoagulated blood (0.2-1.0 ml of blood in heparin). In addition, in birds that have feather abnormalities, biopsy samples of diseased feathers should be placed in 10% formalin and held for further diagnostic testing should any be needed.

Therapy

Numerous therapeutic trials have been attempted for PBFD virus-infected birds. Recoveries have been reported principally in birds with only intranuclear inclusion bodies. While feather lesions can be tolerated as long as the animal is kept in a controlled environment, beak lesions (also nail lesions) can be painful, particularly when secondarily infected. Euthanasia is suggested under these conditions. Secondary infections should be treated accordingly, and special examinations for cryptosporidiosis might be indicated.

Control

The chicken anemia agent (CAA), which is similar in ultrastructure and DNA composition to the PBFD virus, has been found to be environmentally stable, and infectivity remains unchanged when the virus is heated to 60°C for one hour and following treatment with detergents, enzymes and many commercial disinfectants. While the environmental stability of the PBFD virus is unknown, it would be prudent to consider its stability to be similar to that described for CAA. Psittacine neonates, which seem to be most susceptible to the PBFD virus, should definitely not be exposed to areas that may have been contaminated by feces or feather dust from a PBFD-positive bird.

In an effort to reduce the number of cases of PBFD, all birds of a susceptible species should be tested to determine if they are latently infected with the PBFD virus. This is particularly true with respect to breeding birds, birds being sent to pet shops and birds being evaluated during post-purchase examinations.

The DNA probe can also be used to screen walls, caging, air circulating ducts and equipment in the home or hospital to determine if PBFD virus is contaminating these surfaces.

A negative DNA probe test for PBFD virus indicates that viral nucleic acid was not detected in the submitted sample. A positive DNA probe test for PBFD virus indicates that viral nucleic acid has been detected in the submitted sample. A positive test in a bird that has feather abnormalities suggests that the bird has an active PBFD viral infection. A positive blood test in a bird that does not have feather abnormalities may indicate that the bird is latently infected or that it recently has been exposed to the PBFD virus and is viremic. A bird that tests positive and has no feather abnormalities must be retested in 90 days. If the bird is still positive, then it should be considered to be latently infected. A negative test 90 days later would indicate that the viral nucleic acid was no longer detected in the blood and that the bird has probably eliminated the virus.

A companion bird that is diagnosed as a PBFD virus carrier can live a long life when provided a stressor-free environment and supportive medical care. These birds should be restricted from contact with other susceptible birds, particularly neonates. PBFD virus-infected birds should not be maintained in breeding facilities or where they may expose susceptible neonates or adults. Infected birds should be removed from the breeding collection and nursery immediately.

It is likely that a widespread and continued testing and vaccination program can be used to control this disease in companion birds.

Adenovirus

Aviadenovirus are divided into three groups according to common group antigens as detected by virus neutralization, growth in cell culture and nucleic acid characteristics.

Group I: Fowl adenovirus (FAV) consists of 12 serotypes (numbered 1-12) that have been isolated from chickens, turkeys (3 serotypes), pigeons, budgerigars, Mallard Ducks, guineafowl, pheasants, geese (3 serotypes) and Muscovy Ducks.

Group II: Turkey hemorrhagic enteritis virus, marble spleen disease virus and chicken splenomegaly virus. The common group antigen is distinct from that of group I.

Group III: contains only the virus associated with infectious salpingitis (Galliformes) and a similar virus isolated from ducks. This virus subtype shares some common antigenic sites with group I adenoviruses. This group of aviadenoviruses has hemagglutination activity.

Adenovirus particles are 70-90 nm, nonenveloped and contain double-stranded DNA. Adenovirus replicates in the nucleus producing basophilic intranuclear inclusions.

Aviadenovirus are distributed around the world, and many avian species of all age groups are known to be susceptible.

Transmission

Transmission is known to occur through the oral route, and inhalation is suspected. The virus is excreted mainly in the feces. Egg transmission plays a role in the maintenance of infections in a flock. A breeder hen may pass either virus or antibodies to the egg. The primary change in infected eggs is reduced hatchability.

Pathogenesis

Aviadenovirus is generally considered to be an opportunistic pathogen. Reoviridae have been implicated as factors in nondomesticated avian species. Some highly virulent strains of aviadenovirus are capable of producing disease alone (hydropericardium syndrome). Aviadenovirus can trigger secondary infections by inducing mild histopathologic lesions without clinical signs.

Clinical Disease and Pathology - Group I

Group I strains have been associated with respiratory signs, anemia, inclusion body hepatitis, intestinal disease, pancreatitis and nephropathies. In other cases, adenoviruses have been isolated or detected by inclusion bodies or electron microscopy from birds with CNS signs.

Gross lesions are nonspecific including tracheitis, swelling of the liver or kidneys and catarrhal enteritis. Liver lesions vary with the virulence of the strain, but may include vacuolated degeneration of the hepatocytic cytoplasm with lymphocytic infiltration in Glisson's triangles. In more severe cases, hepatocytes show intranuclear eosinophilic inclusions, which increase in size and become basophilic before developing a halo around the inclusion.

Species-specific Considerations

Guineafowl: The main lesion is necrotic pancreatitis, but some respiratory signs (air sacculitis) also occur. Intracerebral infections induce clonic-tonic type CNS signs.

Japanese Quail: An adenovirus was isolated from chicks with CNS signs.

Quail Bronchitis (QB): Mortality can reach 90% in young birds up to six weeks of age.

QB is highly infectious and spreads to young quail mainly through direct contact. Vertical transmission should be expected, although this route has not yet been confirmed.

Clinical signs include sudden death or signs of respiratory disease, such as tracheal rales, coughing, ballooning skin over the infraorbital sinus, sneezing, increased lacrimation and conjunctivitis.

Pigeons: Pigeons have been described with clinical signs of anorexia, a "crouching position" for one to two days, ruffled plumage, slimy green droppings, polydipsia, polyuria, watery overload of the crop, vomiting and respiratory distress.

Goshawk: FAV 1 was isolated from a free-ranging Goshawk that experienced clonic-tonic type CNS signs and died shortly after being recovered from the wild.

Psittaciformes: Pancreatitis and nephropathies have been the two main lesions described in lovebirds.

Adenovirus-like intranuclear inclusions have also been described in the otherwise normal renal tubular epithelium of clinically normal lovebirds. In other birds, numerous inclusions were associated with tubular necrosis and subacute interstitial nephritis.

Adenovirus-like particles have been connected with acute onsets of mild diarrhea and lethargy in Eclectus Parrots. Hepatitis with subcapsular hemorrhage and enteritis (in some birds hemorrhagic) were the main lesions. Irregular, discrete interstitial pneumonia and rapid death were also described.

Basophilic intranuclear inclusions were observed mainly in enterocytes of *Pionus* spp. and *Neophema* spp. with persistent torticollis and other CNS signs. Clinical changes were similar to those described with paramyxovirus infections.

Adenovirus was isolated from two budgerigars with individual histories of enteritis and sudden death.

An epizootic of adenovirus-induced hepatitis has been described in a group of Psittaciformes in a collection of zoo birds. Affected birds included Green-cheeked Amazon, Patagonian Conure, Eastern Rosella, Hyacinth Macaw and a Lesser Sulphur-crested Cockatoo. Hepatitis and enteritis suspected to be caused by adenovirus has been described in Moluccan and Rose-breasted Cockatoos.

Waterfowl: An epornitic of adenovirus was described in captive Muscovy ducklings in France. Affected animals were lame and emaciated. Birds began to die suddenly at about 35 days of age, and mortality rates averaged 1-1.5% of the flock daily for about ten days. Tracheitis (diphtheroid) accompanied in some cases by bronchitis and pneumonia was described in 10% of two- to three-week-old Muscovy ducklings in another outbreak.

Diagnosis

Virus isolation is best achieved from the feces, pharynx, kidneys and liver. Adenovirus-specific DNA probes have been developed for demonstrating viral nucleic acid in infected tissues and clinical samples.

Group-specific antibodies can be demonstrated by ID and ELISA. With the number of adenovirus serotypes, a monovalent vaccine would be of questionable value. Vertical transmission and the continuous cycle of viremia followed by antibody production in infected birds makes it exceedingly difficult to produce uninfected offspring.

Group II

The adenovirus that cause hemorrhagic enteritis in turkeys, marble spleen disease (MSD) in pheasants, and chicken adenovirus group II splenomegaly are considered serologically identical.

In the Common Pheasant, MSD virus replicates mainly in reticular cells of the spleen. Young birds are most frequently infected between ten to twelve weeks of age. Acute death may occur without clinical signs or preceded by a brief period of anorexia and dyspnea caused by severe pulmonary edema. Grossly, the spleen may be enlarged two to three times its normal size and is frequently mottled with multiple, grayish, confluent foci. The lung may be congested, edematous and in rare cases, hemorrhagic.

Suspected adenovirus infections in White and Pearl Guineafowl are characterized by acute pulmonary edema, splenomegaly and ascites.

Diagnosis

The clinical and pathologic signs are suggestive of the disease. The principal rule-outs are various intoxications and reticuloendotheliosis. The agent forms intranuclear inclusion bodies, particularly in splenic cells, and the presence of viral particles consistent with adenovirus can be demonstrated by electron microscopy. Adenovirus-specific DNA probes designed to document infections in Psittaciformes can also be used in pheasants and chickens.

Group III

The natural host of adenovirus group III appears to include various ducks from Europe and Asia that are asymptomatically infected. Virus recovery is necessary for a definitive diagnosis. Cloacal swabs or material from the female genital tract are good diagnostic samples. HI using virus-specific antibodies can be used to confirm the presence of the virus in a cell culture.

Unclassified

Viral particles suggestive of adenovirus have been demonstrated electron microscopically from captive American Kestrels with hemorrhagic enteritis. The antigen does not react with aviadenovirus group II antibodies. Clinical signs include melena, regenerative anemia and high mortality. Gross lesions include hyperplasia of the white pulp in the spleen and petechiation in the mucosa of the esophagus, colon and coprodeum. In addition, disseminated intravascular thrombi and necrosis of the myocardium may be evident.

A disease that clinically mimics MSD has been described in Blue Grouse. The disease has not been experimentally reproduced and it is uncertain if an adenovirus is involved. Clinical signs are lethargy, ruffled plumage, foamy, watery diarrhea and death.

Parvoviridae

The family Parvoviridae consists of nonenveloped, single-stranded DNA viruses of hexagonal morphology with an estimated 32 capsomeres and a size of 19-25 nm. Avian parvoviruses induce intranuclear inclusion bodies of the Cowdry A type, and form syncytia in cell cultures.

Goose Parvovirus Infection (Derzsy's Disease)

Transmission and Pathogenesis

This virus is highly infectious, and transmission is possible horizontally via oral and nasal routes and transovarially by freshly infected, non-immune breeder geese. Non-immune goslings or Muscovy ducklings between 1-21 days of age are most susceptible to infection. Following entry into the host, virus is distributed to the target organs including the liver, spleen, heart, adrenal gland, thyroid gland and thymus.

Clinical Disease and Pathology

Anorexia and polydipsia followed by cessation of water intake are the earliest clinical signs. Goslings appear chilled and occasionally develop conjunctivitis, diarrhea and diphtheroid membranes on the tongue. Somnolence, weakness and giddiness occur prior to death (up to 100% mortality). In older birds that survive, down feathers may fall out, particularly on the neck, wings and back. The skin may be hyperemic and the uropygial gland swollen.

Gross lesions include hepatomegaly with subcapsular petechial hemorrhage and bile congestion together with a small, limp spleen and a highly enlarged thyroid gland.

Diagnosis

Liver, pancreas and thyroid glands are suitable material for virus isolation. Virus identification can be carried out with VN, ELISA or IF. Antibodies appear five to ten days following infection and persist for approximately one year.

Parvovirus infection of the gosling is a hepatic disease (with intranuclear inclusion bodies), small spleen and changes in the thyroid gland.

Control

Because maternal antibodies successfully prevent the disease in goslings, vaccination of the breeder geese at least six weeks before the beginning of egg production is recommended. Breeding geese without antibody titers should be vaccinated twice. A booster vaccination might be necessary for the second half of the breeding season to prevent hepatitis in goslings hatched late in the breeding season.

Myocarditis and Encephalopathy in Canaries

Myocarditis and encephalitis were described in association with a virus that morphologically resembled parvovirus in three adult canaries from different origins. It is unusual, however, that a parvovirus would cause disease in an adult bird.

Hepadnaviridae

The Hepadnaviridae virion is 40-60 nm in diameter with an icosahedric, enveloped, symmetric nucleocapsid consisting of one highly immunogenic protein. The virus contains partially double-stranded circular DNA.

Related avian taxons (formerly duck hepatitis B group now in the newly formed genus Avihepadnavirus) have been described in the Pekin Duck and domestic goose. Avihepadnavirus is less oncogenic than mammalian strains. It has been suggested that avian strains require co-carcinogenic factors to induce neoplasms. Infection with Avihepadnavirus is a triggering factor for clinical and pathologic changes of the new duck syndrome (see Chapter 33).

Generally, infections are subclinical in ducks and geese. Transmission takes place vertically and leads to chronic viremia without the development of humoral antibodies.

Reoviridae

The family Reoviridae consists of three genera: Orthoreovirus, Orbivirus and Rotavirus.

Avian Orthoreovirus

The genome is a double-stranded RNA segregated into at least three size classes. The virus replicates in the cytoplasm of the host cells. Hemagglutination activity is not present in avian strains. Because frequent cross-reactions are reported, it seems that avian orthoreovirus strains exist as antigenic subtypes rather than as distinct serotypes.

Avian orthoreoviruses occur worldwide; the current host range includes chickens, pheasants, quail, turkeys, ducks, geese, pigeons, birds of prey, Psittaciformes and other companion and aviary birds.

Transmission

Ingestion of viral particles is probably an important route of infection, but respiratory transmission is also possible. Vertical transmission is epornitically fundamental in chickens and turkeys.

Pathogenicity

The pathogenesis of orthoreovirus infections has not been clearly defined. Many strains may induce latent infections, which may impair the immune system and result in immunosuppression.

Development of humoral antibodies may provide protection from the disease; however, fecal shedding occurs in persistently infected birds even though antibody titers are present.

Clinical Disease and Pathology

Psittaciformes: The clinical signs reported in Psittaciformes vary among infected hosts. An infected cockatoo (species not given) and Grey-cheeked Parakeet developed nonspecific clinical signs including emaciation, incoordination, labored breathing and diarrhea. Enteritis, liver congestion, necrosis and in some cases, a swollen spleen are common pathologic changes in African Grey Parrots (mortality up to 100%). Chronic respiratory infections have been described in Amazon parrots.

African Grey Parrots may develop uveitis, although this is rare in uncomplicated reovirus infections.

Ophthalmic lesions are characterized by a fixed, dilated pupil and reticular hemorrhages followed by uveitis, hypopyon and fibrous exudates in the anterior and posterior chambers.

It has been suggested that Old World Psittaciformes are highly susceptible to orthoreovirus, while New World Psittaciformes may be infected but are more resistant to disease. Clinical pathology associated with infections include anemia, leucopenia (with 90-100% lymphocytes), hypoalbuminemia, hyperglobulinemia and increased levels of AST and LDH late in the disease process. In many cases, orthoreovirus is not the only infectious agent involved in a disease process, complicating the interpretation of lesions; however, African Grey Parrots have been infected with isolated virus, fulfilling Koch's postulates.

Pigeons: In infected pigeons, the most frequent clinical signs are diarrhea and dyspnea. A catarrhal enteritis is a common necropsy finding. A serologic survey in Belgium and West Germany revealed carriers of antibodies among homing pigeons as 8% and 16%, respectively.

Muscovy Ducks and Mullards: Mullards are a cross between Muscovy Ducks and Mallards. While Mallards are resistant to the disease, Mullards are highly susceptible. At necropsy, pericarditis and air sacculitis of the anterior air sacs are the main findings, frequently accompanied by hyperplasia of the spleen and perihepatitis.

Geese: A reovirus has been found to cause infectious myocarditis in geese. Five- to twenty-one-day-old goslings may develop clinical signs following infection. Older birds appear to be resistant.

Finches (Estrildidae and Ploceidae): Clinical signs in finches are associated with enteritis and swelling of the liver, which can be severe enough to be noted through the abdominal skin. At necropsy, disseminated yellowish, greasy or soft foci, which histopathologically represent focal coagulative necrosis, can be observed.

Diagnosis

Cloacal swabs and samples from the rectum and affected parenchymatous organs are best for viral isolation. Demonstration of viral antigen in affected tissues is possible by IF.

Control

Commercially available vaccines for poultry are ineffective in Psittaciformes because of antigenic variance among strains. An inactivated vaccine produced from a reovirus recovered from parrots was found to reduce losses associated with an outbreak.

The use of chlorhexidine in the drinking water (20 ml per gallon of water) was thought to reduce the transmission of reovirus infection in a flock of African Grey Parrots. Long-term use (up to 30 days) may be necessary, and there were no observable side effects from this length of chlorhexidine exposure.

Orbivirus

Orbivirus is a genus of the Reoviridae that depends on insects such as culicoides, phlebotomus and ticks for transmission. An orbivirus has been isolated from a cockatiel and a budgerigar. The cockatiel died suddenly and at necropsy displayed degeneration of the myocardium, a swollen liver and spleen and cloudy air sacs. In the case of the budgerigar, dyspnea, photophobia and ruffled plumage was observed prior to death. Postmortem examination revealed atrophy of the pectoral muscles, catarrhal enteritis and a slightly swollen liver. Experimentally infected budgerigars developed severe greenish diarrhea for four to eight days with no pathologic lesions noted on postmortem examination. Infected birds seroconverted, and reisolation of the virus was possible from the feces.

Rotavirus

Rotaviruses are distributed worldwide and have been documented in chickens, turkeys, Helmeted Guineafowl, pheasants, ducks, pigeons and lovebirds. Avian strains are resistant to ether, chloroform, sodium deoxycholate, pH 3 and 56°C for 30 minutes. The persistence of infectivity in the environment is not known.

Transmission and Pathogenesis

Rotavirus is excreted in the feces in high numbers, and can be transmitted by both direct and indirect contact. Ingestion may be the most important portal of entry. Infections in three-day-old poults suggest egg transmission, which has not been proven.

Rotavirus is a cause of enteritis and diarrhea in a variety of mammalian and avian species. The virus replicates mainly within the enterocytes of the small intestines. Because viral replication causes lysis of the host cell, the intestinal absorption in infected birds is dependent on the number of infected enterocytes. A decrease in the absorption of D-xylosis has been suggested as an indicator of enterocyte damage. Birds that overcome infections develop intestinal immunity via IgA and humoral antibodies (IgG), which are also transferred via egg yolk to the chick. Humoral antibodies do not protect against infection, even in the newly hatched chick. Cell-mediated immunity is necessary for full protection. Incubation periods are short (one to three days) in chickens and turkeys.

Clinical Signs and Pathology

Infected ducks do not develop clinical or pathologic signs of disease. A short-term (five- to eight-day), self-limiting, transmissible enteritis has been described in the Helmeted Guineafowl. Pheasants and partridges, especially those infected as chicks, may develop diarrhea and stunting and have increased levels of mortality (up to 30%). In infected pigeons, a watery diarrhea may occur. Rotavirus antibodies have been demonstrated in approximately 10% of the pigeons examined. A rotavirus isolated from a lovebird caused the death of a chicken embryo following yolk sac inoculation. The lovebird showed no clinical signs.

Diagnosis

Because many avian strains have not been grown in cell culture, electron microscopy is still a common method of identification. The demonstration of viral RNA by means of electrophoresis is also possible. Serologic diversity among strains, difficulties in propagating the virus and the widespread occurrence of the virus make the detection of antibodies to the virus difficult to interpret.

Birnaviridae

The virus of the infectious bursal disease is a member of this family. Disease is seen only in chickens. The virus destroys mainly the cloacal bursa of growing chicks causing a passing or (rarely) permanent immunosuppression (refer to textbooks on poultry disease).

Coronaviridae

The family Coronaviridae contains only the genus Coronavirus. Recognized taxons are the infectious bronchitis virus (IBV), turkey coronavirus and at least nine mammalian species. A coronalike-virus isolated from Japanese Quail has not yet been characterized. Isolates from guineafowl and pheasants are serologically different from chicken strains. Coronavirus has been reported as a cause of disease in Psittaciformes. Coronavirus contains a single-stranded RNA.

IBV is distributed worldwide and is not antigenically uniform. Chickens are the main host and may develop respiratory signs, interstitial nephritis, visceral gout or egg shell problems with decreased albumen quality.

Coronal enteritis is distributed primarily in turkey-raising countries, and the turkey is the only recognized host.

Pheasants: IBV has been isolated from pheasants in Great Britain with some regularity.

In adult birds, reduced egg production, poor egg quality, slight to moderate respiratory signs and low mortality associated with egg peritonitis, urolithiasis, visceral gout and swollen kidneys are typical. Mortality is highest in eight- to ten-week-old birds (up to 40%) with renal lesions being conspicuous.

Guineafowl: IBV has been recovered from guineafowl with enteritis and hepatopancreatitis. Anorexia and high mortality in young birds were common in affected flocks. Emaciation, pancreatitis, enteritis, dehydration and nephritis are common findings at necropsy.

Psittaciformes: Two coronavirus strains have been isolated from parrots (one unspecified species and a Cape Parrot). The two parrot strains appeared to be in the same taxon (which was not related to IBV and several mammalian coronaviruses).

Preliminary studies indicated that the virus is pathogenic for both chickens and budgerigars. Principal lesions were associated with necrotic hepatosplenitis.

Pigeons: IBV has been isolated from racing pigeons.

Clinically affected pigeons showed ruffled plumage, dyspnea and excess mucus at the commissures of the beak. Eleven birds died during the first 24 hours following clinical signs. At necropsy, the birds were in average condition and had recently eaten, but the linings of the crop and esophagus were ulcerated. Mucoid pharyngitis and tracheitis were seen, and the lower intestines contained fluid.

Ostrich chicks: A coronavirus was identified by electron microscopy in a group of two-week-old ostrich chicks with enteritis.

Japanese Quail: A coronalike-virus was isolated from Japanese Quail with respiratory signs.

Togaviridae and Flaviviridae (Arbovirus A and B)

These viruses are spheroid, enveloped, single-stranded RNA. Most of the Togaviridae and Flaviviridae isolated from birds are arthropod-borne viral taxons, which implies that they can be transmitted by arthropod vectors and that the virus in question can replicate in the arthropod host. In birds, ornithophilic arthropods are the main vectors.

Eastern and Western Equine Encephalomyelitis (EEE, WEE)

EEE (genus Alphavirus of the Togaviridae) is mainly transmitted by *Culiseta melanura*, but may also be transmitted by other mosquitoes (*Aedes* spp. and *Culex* spp.). For WEE (genus Alphavirus of the Togaviridae) the main vector appears to be *Culex tarsalis*. Viral isolates or antibodies against both EEE and WEE viruses have been recovered from more than 60 avian species.

Pathogenesis

The virus can be ingested by mosquitoes with the blood of infected hosts from 24 hours post-infection throughout the viremic period (average two to five days) and transmitted to new hosts 7-20 days later. The hemagglutinating virus is probably distributed by erythrocytes through the whole body including the brain. Encephalomyelitis mainly develops in young birds. Infections principally occur through insect bites, but horizontal spread following feather picking and other forms of cannibalism have been shown to occur in pheasants.

Clinical Disease, Pathology and Diagnosis

Outbreaks of EEE are seen mainly in pheasants, but also have been documented in ducks, Chukars, turkeys, Whooping Cranes, emus, finches and pigeons. These birds may die peracutely or acutely with mortality of up to 80%, depending on the age. An age-linked resistance has been demonstrated in pheasants beginning at 28 days. Clinical changes in a group of infected Lady Gouldian Finches included severe paresis and dyspnea. Lesions caused by WEE are rare, but are essentially the same as those due to EEE: depression, incoordination, paresis and paralysis, torticollis, tremor, polydipsia and somnolence. Clinical chemistry tests reveal anemia with normal numbers of leukocytes. AST, LDH and uric acid values are distinctly elevated.

At necropsy, EEE and WEE lesions are similar (swollen liver, mucoid duodenitis, dehydration) in most species. Pheasants typically develop a neurotropic disease, while lesions in chickens are mainly myocardiotropic. Histopathology reveals a nonpurulent encephalitis with edema, meningitis, perivascular infiltrates, diffuse gliosis (also in the spinal cord) and necrosis in the cerebral cortex.

In Lady Gouldian Finches, necropsy findings included consolidation in the lungs and a pale liver and kidney.

Diagnosis

Homogenates of blood, liver, spleen and brain are best for virus isolation. The virus can be identified in cell culture by HI, ELISA, radioimmune assay or molecular hybridization.

Control

Control of insects, mites and ticks is important in preventing infections. Sentinel birds (some pheasant chicks) may be used to indicate the presence of infected mosquitoes.

Several recommendations have been made to vaccinate ratites in endemic areas with an inactivated equine EEE vaccine. Neither the efficacy nor safety of this vaccine when used in ostriches has been established. Written permission should be obtained from the insurance carrier of an ostrich before vaccination is carried out. The recommended vaccination protocol includes vaccination at three months of age followed by a booster one month later and every six months thereafter.

Zoonotic Potential

Human disease is rare and occurs following bites from infected mosquitoes. EEE and WEE both cause an acute infection of the CNS ranging from mild meningoencephalitis to lethal encephalitis or encephalomyelitis. In endemic areas, extensive vaccination of horses has reduced the levels of infection in humans.

Venezuela Equine Encephalomyelitis (VEE)

The causative agent of VEE is a member of the genus Alphavirus (Togaviridae). Birds play a minor role; the main reservoir is rodents. Vectors are *Culex* spp. with preference for rodents. However, in swamp areas some egrets and herons are known to be carriers. The main avian reservoir is the Striated Heron.

Human cases are characterized by a general benign course with acute but short fever, headache, myalgia, arthralgia, lymphadenopathy and frequently exanthema, but rarely CNS signs or hemorrhage.

Avian Viral Serositis (AVS)

A toga-like virus is suspected to cause a disseminated serositis in some Psittaciformes.

The host spectrum currently includes several juvenile macaw species, macaw hybrids and a Rose-ringed Parakeet. All naturally affected birds came from nurseries or were parent-raised on farms where neuropathic gastric dilatation was endemic, and many of the contact birds were known to have died from this disease.

Clinical Signs and Pathology

Affected birds die acutely or lose weight and have distended abdomens containing ascitic fluid. Some birds develop respiratory distress.

At necropsy, the presence of serosal fluid in the abdomen with or without fibrinous clots was the prominent finding. In some cases, the liver was swollen and the lungs edematous.

The importance of this virus for parrots and any role this virus may play in neuropathic gastric dilatation (proventicular dilatation) require further investigation.

Rubivirus, German Measles

Rubivirus (formerly rubellavirus) is classified as a member of the Togaviridae. It is not known to cause disease in any avian species. However, antibodies indicating a carrier state with possible shedding of the virus have been found in urban pigeons. Because rubivirus is a human pathogen, the occurrence of antibodies in free-flying urban pigeons suggests that these birds may be a reservoir for human infections.

Israel Turkey Meningoencephalitis (ITM)

ITM virus belongs to the Flaviviridae. *Aedes aegypti* and *Culex molestus* are the main vectors. The disease was initially described in northern Israel (in season with its vectors), but has now been documented in southern Israel and South Africa. The main host is the domesticated turkey, which under field conditions becomes sick after ten weeks of age.

Clinical changes include progressive paresis and paralysis and spastic, uncoordinated movements. Mortality averages 10-30%, but can reach 80% in some flocks.

Louping III Virus Infection

The Louping Ill virus belongs to the Flaviviridae and is serologically related to the Siberian tick encephalitis virus (Russian spring-summer encephalitis) and the Central European tick-borne encephalitis virus. *Ixodes ricinus* ticks are the main vector. The established avian host spectrum includes the Willow Grouse and the subspecies Red Grouse, Rock Ptarmigan, capercaillie, Black Grouse and the Common Pheasant. The first three birds discussed are very susceptible and usually develop CNS signs.

St. Louis Encephalitis (SLE), Japanese B-Encephalitis (JBE), Murray Valley Encephalitis (MVE)

The agents belong to the family Flaviviridae. They occur on three different continents and are serologically related. There are more than 30 species of susceptible birds that do not become sick. Avian reservoirs include Brown-headed Cowbird, House Sparrow, some egret and heron species, and in Australia, ibises and cormorants. The human disease is similar to EEE.

Rhabdoviridae

Birds are not considered natural reservoirs for the rabies virus, but they can nonetheless develop active infections while remaining asymptomatic.

In one survey, rabies virus titers were detected in six orders of birds representing 22 species. Twenty-three percent of the raptors had titers and eight percent of the non-predatory scavengers including starlings, crows and ravens had rabies antibody titers. These findings suggest that viral exposure occurs through contact with infected prey species.

The self-limiting nature of the virus in avian species is believed to be due to a rapid production of antibodies.

Clinical Disease and Pathology

The clinical course in species naturally and experimentally infected can take 2-42 days. A short excitable period with jumping, crying, trying to flee, aggressiveness toward humans and epileptiform convulsions is followed 24 hours later by ataxia, weakness of the limbs, falling on the flanks and, finally, flaccid paresis (including head and neck). Two weeks later somnolence, apathy, compulsive movements and death can occur. Spontaneous recovery has also been reported.

There has been no documented case of human rabies from an avian exposure.

Paramyxoviridae

Members of this family have nonsegmented single-stranded RNA of negative polarity and an enveloped, helical, capsid symmetry.

Avian Paramyxovirus

Newcastle disease virus (NDV) is the type strain for avian paramyxoviruses. Numerous, serologically different strains of this virus have been isolated worldwide. Hemagglutination inhibition (HI) tests, neuraminidase inhibition tests, serum neutralization tests and comparison of structural polypeptides have resulted in the identification of nine serotypes (PMV-1 to PMV-9).

PMV-1

PMV-1 consists of NDV and related strains that are serologically, molecular biologically and pathogenically unique. They are found in Columbiformes and some Psittaciformes.

Newcastle Disease

NDV is serologically uniform and isolates are divided based on their virulence and epizootiologic importance (velogenic, mesogenic or lentogenic). Virulence is host-specific and varies considerably with experimental infections in other species.

Some mammals are susceptible to NDV, and humans may develop a severe conjunctivitis.

Transmission

Virus enters the host mainly through the respiratory and gastrointestinal tracts. Vertical transmission can occur, but is rare with velogenic strains because viremic hens usually stop laying.

The most common carriers (reservoirs) include free-ranging waterfowl, Pittidae, Psittaciformes, some Passeriformes and Strigiformes.

Clinical Disease and Pathology

Lentogenic, mesogenic and velogenic strains of NDV produce varying clinical disease in chickens. The clinical expression varies widely in other birds, even between two species of the same genus. Several clinical presentations are characteristic.

- Peracute death; several hours of depression caused by viremia.
- Acute gastrointestinal disease (VVND); voluminous greenish diarrhea accompanied by anorexia, lethargy and cyanosis.
- Acute respiratory disease; upper respiratory exudates, rales and dyspnea.
- Acute gastrointestinal and respiratory disease.

Chronic central nervous system (CNS) disease characterized by opisthotonos, torticollis, tremors and clonic-tonic paralysis of the limbs.

Affected birds typically have petechia on serosal surfaces and fatty tissues and on the mucosa of the larynx, trachea and proventriculus. Egg follicle hemorrhage may also be noted in protracted cases. Hemorrhagic necrotizing enteritis, mainly within the jejunum, is common with virulent strains. Lymphatic tissue in association with the hemorrhagic lesions forms "boutons," which are pathognomonic in Phasianiformes. Birds with CNS signs may have no gross lesions, or hyperemia of the brain may occur.

Diagnosis

For the rule-out list, infectious and noninfectious causes of gastrointestinal or respiratory tract disease should be considered. One differentiating factor is that ND is not associated with sinusitis. CNS lesions are typical for ND in a variety of bird species. As a rule, the incubation time is prolonged in these cases, and histopathologic lesions may be difficult to document. Comparable clinical signs may be seen with chlamydiosis (meningitis), salmonellosis (encephalitis purulenta) encephalomalacia, lead toxicity and calcium deficiencies. Histopathologic differentiation is only possible following thorough examination of a variety of affected tissues.

Antemortem diagnosis of NDV can be performed by culturing virus from feces or respiratory discharge (swabs) from affected birds. The number of samples required for a diagnosis depends on the size of the flock, the clinical signs (CNS) and the quarantine situation.

Treatment

Hyperimmune serum (2 ml/kg body weight IM) can be used to protect exposed birds but is of no benefit once clinical signs are present. CNS signs occur in the presence of humoral antibodies. Use of B vitamins and anticonvulsants for treating NDV-induced nonpurulent encephalitis is discouraging; in controlled studies, there was no difference in treated or untreated groups. Following improvement (which may take a year), any disturbance or stressful event may cause a bird to have severe convulsions or tremors.

Control

NDV occurs worldwide and many free-ranging birds can function as carriers. Effective vaccination regimes would be helpful in controlling infections in aviaries, breeding farms and zoo collections; however, ND is a notifiable disease in many countries and governmental regulations may control vaccination protocols. Most birds in orders other than Phasianiformes must be vaccinated parenterally for an effective antibody response to occur. Inactivated vaccines produced for chickens are useful, provided that there are no governmental regulations that restrict vaccination. Oil-adjuvanted vaccines have been shown to cause abscesses surrounding the injection site in some birds and must be used with caution. Abscesses secondary to subcutaneous infections are easier to treat than those that occur following IM injections.

Live vaccines produced for chickens (and used for other Galliformes) should not be used in other avian orders. The potential infectivity of the vaccine strain of virus in a nonadapted host has not been determined. Vaccines administered to Psittaciformes in the drinking water have been shown to be ineffective.

As a general consideration in an active outbreak, emergency vaccination with Hitchner B_1 and truly apathogenic LaSota strains is possible via ocular or nasal drops (five chicken doses per bird). These strains function as competitive inhibitors, and the local protection induced cannot be determined by an increase in humoral antibodies.

PMV-1 Pigeon

A PMV-1 strain that is closely related to NDV but serologically, biochemically and pathogenically unique was first recognized in domesticated pigeons in the late 1970s, probably having arisen in the Middle East. The virus reached Europe by 1981 and spread all over the world, affecting particularly racing and show pigeons.

Clinical Disease and Pathology

Affected Columbiformes have nondescript clinical signs including polydipsia, polyuria, anorexia, diarrhea and vomiting. These frequently unrecognized acute signs are followed by clonic-tonic paralysis of the wings (more rarely the hind limbs), head tremors and torticollis. In contrast to ND, flaccid paresis and paralysis may occur, probably from a peripheral neuropathy. Other less frequent signs are unilateral blepharedema, egg deformation, embryo mortality and dystrophic molt. Dyspnea, which is common with ND, does not occur.

Diagnosis

Procedures designed for isolating NDV are effective for PMV-1 pigeon. The HI test can be used to differentiate between NDV and PMV-1 pigeon. Final differentiation is possible only by the use of monoclonal antibodies.

Treatment

Vaccination with live vaccines may exacerbate latent chlamydia or pigeon herpesvirus infections.

Inactivated vaccines are preferable for pigeons. In an active outbreak, vaccination with an inactivated vaccine will decrease the length of the disease and mitigate the clinical signs. Once CNS signs develop, vaccination is of no value; however, spontaneous recoveries do occur.

Control

For vaccination, homologous, inactivated oil emulsion vaccines are commercially available. Annual boosters are necessary. All birds in a loft, and competitive traveling groups of homing pigeons, should be vaccinated. Squabs from hens vaccinated three months before laying may not have protective antibodies. Squabs can be vaccinated with homologous vaccine by four weeks of age. Inactivated NDV vaccines provide only six months of protection.

Vaccines are best applied subcutaneously in the neck. Intramuscular injections in homing pigeons can cause severe irritation of the pectoral muscles. To prevent fatal hemorrhage from the plexus subcutaneous collaris (see Chapter 44), injections must be given in the caudal third of the neck, near the middle of the dorsal aspect.

Twirling Syndrome

This disease of uncertain etiology has been described in the African Silverbill, Zebra Finch, Gouldian Finch and related species. Clinically, the sudden onset of torticollis and circling is conspicuous, but depression and weight loss are also evident. Clinical signs typically occur within one week of shipment from their place of origin. Some birds will be affected while others from the same shipment remain unaffected. Mortality may reach 20%. Some birds recover completely while others retain a permanent head tilt. Individual companion birds are also known suffer from this disease. WBC may range between 2,000 and 14,000. Antibiotic therapy does not change the course of the disease. Pathology and histopathology have failed to implicate a specific etiologic agent, but a virus is suspected. PMV should always considered in Passeriformes with neurologic signs.

Orthomyxovirus

The family Orthomyxoviridae consists of avian influenzavirus (AIV) and all other influenzavirus taxons. Orthomyxoviridae are segmented RNA viruses with helical symmetry. Influenzavirus can be classified into two groups designated A and C. The specificity is provided by the nucleoprotein and matrix antigens.

Many avian species, particularly large congregations of migrating birds, may serve as main reservoirs for virus recombination.

Influenza C is usually restricted to humans, but there are exceptions. During a human outbreak of influenza (formerly called B) in Hungary, 4.1% of zoo and free-ranging birds examined had antibodies against the same virus type.

Avian Influenza A (AIV)

Infections with influenza A virus can cause subclinical to mild respiratory diseases, loss of egg production or generalized acute lethal disease. Acute lethal infection in domesticated chickens is called fowl plague and is a reportable disease in many countries.

Influenza A virus is divided into subtypes according to the antigenicity of its hemagglutinin and neuraminidase. Thirteen hemagglutinins and nine neuraminidases have been distinguished to date (H1 to H13 and N1 to N9).

AIV is distributed worldwide and has a large host spectrum that includes domesticated ducks and geese, free-ranging ducks and geese, chickens, turkeys, guineafowl, chukars, quail, pheasants, sandpipers and sanderlings, turnstones, terns, swans, gulls, herons, guillemots, puffins and shearwaters. Latent infected carriers also occur. AIV has been isolated from captive birds including Indian Hill Mynahs, various Psittaciformes (Sulphur-crested Cockatoo, African Grey Parrot, budgerigar), Passeriformes, Accipitriformes and Musophagiformes (Lady Ross's Turaco, Purple-crested Turaco, White-crested Turaco, Black-billed Turaco, Guinea Turaco).

Diagnosis

The differential diagnosis list should include respiratory and gastrointestinal pathogens as well as PMV, *Chlamydia* sp. and *Mycoplasma* spp.

A definite diagnosis depends on the isolation and identification of the strain in question. Fowl plague-like conditions caused by highly virulent strains may be suspected due to the acute to peracute course and the hemorrhages at necropsy. Swabs from the cloaca and the upper respiratory tract are suitable for direct virus demonstration from live birds. Parenchymatous organs (lungs, liver, spleen, brain) provide the best postmortem sample for virus isolation. Samples are to be placed in sterile transport medium containing high levels of antibiotics to inhibit bacterial growth and shipped at no more than 4°C.

Retroviridae

Avian retrovirus is separated into two genera. Avian type C retrovirus group (avian leukosis-related viruses) includes avian sarcoma and leukemia virus (SLV). The type species is avian leukosis virus. A type C retrovirus that is unrelated to SLV is the causative agent of the lymphoproliferative disease (LPD) in turkeys. The avian reticuloendotheliosis virus is now a species within the genus mammalian type C viruses in the subgenus reticuloendotheliosis viruses.

The genome consists of a negative-sensed, single-stranded RNA. Retrovirus is further characterized by a reverse transcriptase (revertase) that is necessary for the formation of a DNA provirus during viral replication, which takes place in the cytoplasm.

Avian Sarcoma/Leukosis Virus (SLV)

The host spectrum is dependent on autosomally transmitted susceptibility or resistance of avian cells to receptors of avian retroviral subgroups (susceptibility = dominant, resistance = recessive). Genetic resistance can be selected for or manipulated.

Subgroups may produce varying types of tumors, and many neoplasms occur in connection with defective viral strains that require a helper virus for replication. Despite high rates of infection (more than 50% in some flocks), few birds (1-3%) actually die from a neoplastic disease. The types of neoplasias induced by the avian SL group include fibrosarcoma/mesenchymoma, chondroma, osteochondrosarcoma, osteopetrosis, mesothelioma, endothelioma, hemangioma, undifferentiated stem-cell leukosis, lymphoid leukosis, myeloblastosis/monocyte leukosis, myelocytosis, myelocytomatosis, erythroblastosis (medullary or leukemic), nephroblastoma, renal adenoma/adenocarcinoma, ovarian cystadenoma/adenocarcinoma, thecoma, granulosa cell tumor, seminoma, hepatoma, pancreatic adenoma and carcino/fibrosarcoma of the intestinal mesentery.

Transmission

Vertical transmission by gonadal cells (virus in the albumen of the egg) or virus genome (also incomplete) in the haploid egg and semen cells is important. Horizontal infection takes place through contaminated feces and saliva, and antibodies are produced that are not protective. Lifelong infections are common.

Clinical Disease and Pathology

A clinical diagnosis depends on identifying visible or palpable tumors. The patient's general condition and ability to fly are frequently undisturbed for a relatively long time. Abdominal enlargement and dyspnea caused by the space-occupying tumors can occur in advanced cases. A massively distended liver may be palpable. Hematology, especially differential smears, are frequently nondiagnostic because avian leukosis rarely results in a leukemic blood picture (ie, tumorous blood cells or their precursors in the peripheral blood). An increase in leukocytes (heterophilia, lymphocytosis and monocytosis) is common. In many instances, the lymphocytes are mature, but in Amazon parrots and chickens, bow-formed pseudopodia may be visible. The AST may be increased if the liver is affected.

SLV causes a variety of non-neoplastic conditions, of which immunosuppressive disorders and suppression of thyroid function are the most important. The latter is considered one cause of stunting in growing chickens. At necropsy, multiple tumors of the liver and spleen, more rarely the kidneys, subcutis, periorbital cavity, heart, lungs, ovary, intestine and cloacal wall are seen. A retained cloacal bursa is suggestive. Affected organs are diffusely swollen with or without a grayish mottled surface and a soft consistency.

Diagnosis

Neoplasms induced by other agents are solitary, while SLV generally causes multiple tumors. In chickens, Marek's disease virus usually affects younger birds and involves nervous tissue, which is rare with SLV-induced tumors (see Chapter 25).

Plasma, serum and neoplastic tissues are best for demonstrating the presence of virus. The virus can also be isolated from oral washings, feces, feather pulp and from the albumen of freshly laid eggs. Samples should be shipped immediately in cooled containers because the virus is heat labile. Antemortem diagnosis can be determined using biopsy, endoscopy or differential blood smears.

Treatment and Control

Treatment is generally ineffective in advanced cases. Experimental application of an androgen analogue "mibolerone" in chicks between the 1st and 49th days of life has been shown to prevent leukosis. The drug is anabolic and had no deleterious effect on egg production. This drug has not been investigated in companion birds. Selection of genetic resistance in the presence of the virus is a useful tool and should be applied wherever possible.

Erythremic Myelosis in Conures (Hemorrhagic Conure Syndrome)

This condition has been recognized as an endemic disease in Blue-crowned Conures, Peach-fronted Conures, Orange-fronted Conures and Patagonian Conures. Periodic recurrence of eventually fatal bleeding is characteristic of the disease. During these bleeding episodes, proliferations of erythroblasts are present in the hepatic sinus and in the pancreas. Normal bone marrow is replaced by immature red blood cells suggesting erythroleukosis. A viral etiology (retrovirus) has been suggested, but has not been proven. Calcium deficiencies are believed to trigger the disease.

Clinical Disease, Pathology and Diagnosis

Epistaxis, dyspnea, severe weakness, intermittent polyuria and diarrhea and occasionally ataxia are common. Clinical pathologic changes include packed cell volume of approximately 26%, leukocytosis represented by heterophilia (84%), severe polychromasia and anisocytosis, decrease of the total protein, hypoglycemia and hypocalcemia, elevated creatinine and large numbers of immature erythrocytes in the peripheral blood.

At necropsy, multiple pulmonary hemorrhage, development of pseudocysts in the pectoral muscles and pericarditis are common.

Avian Reticuloendotheliosis Virus (REV)

REV differs from SLV and is related to certain mammalian REV. As with SLV, several subspecies or subgroups that are closely related, but differ in antigenicity and pathogenicity exist. These include reticuloendotheliosis virus (Twiehaus), duck infectious anemia virus, spleen necrosis virus, chicken syncytial virus (CSV), nonclassified isolates from Muscovy Duck, visceral lymphomatosis of the Common Shelduck and racing pigeon (serologic evidence in 0.1% of examined sera).

Some of the viruses in this group have oncogenic properties and induce tumors principally of lymphoreticular or reticuloendothelial cells. Occasionally, these viruses are associated with other neoplasms such as histiocytic sarcoma, fibrosarcoma or myxosarcoma. Non-neoplastic lesions due to degenerative-inflammatory processes are common. As with SLV, defective strains that require helper viruses to replicate do occur.

The natural hosts are probably turkeys and waterfowl; however, chickens, ducks, geese and Japanese Quail are also susceptible to natural infection. Experimental infection is possible in pheasants and guineafowl.

Transmission and Pathogenesis

Horizontal transmission occurs among young birds when viremic animals shed the virus via feces or in body fluids. Mosquitoes, particularly *Culex annulirostis*, are reported to be capable of transmitting the virus after feeding on a viremic bird. Vertical transmission is possible, but only at a low rate with eggs (albumen) and semen. The virus replicates primarily in the reticular and endothelial cells along the capillary walls.

In contrast to SL, most REV-induced neoplasms occur in young birds, although some chronic cases have been reported. Infection with REV induces a transient or permanent disturbance of the immune system.

Diagnosis (All REV)

The lack of characteristic lesions, variability of lesions and similarity of lesions caused by different etiologies make diagnosis difficult. Direct and indirect methods of viral demonstration are necessary. Heparinized blood, plasma, leukocytes or homogenates from tumorous tissues are suitable for virus isolation.

Picornaviridae

Picornaviridae are the second smallest RNA virus known. They are nonenveloped, have a cubic morphology with 32 capsomeres and single-stranded RNA. Five genera (Enterovirus, Hepatovirus, Rhinovirus, Aphthovirus and Cardiovirus) can be distinguished.

Avian Encephalomyelitis (AE)

The classification of AE is still uncertain. The four virus-specific proteins are larger than those usually associated with Picornaviridae. The AE virus is distributed worldwide. The main host is the chicken, but natural infections have been documented in pheasants, Japanese Quail, waterfowl and turkeys. Antibodies following natural infection (without clinical disease) were found in partridges, probably Rock Partridge and Red-legged Partridge, as well as pheasants and turkeys. Egg transmission plays the main role in epornitics. Horizontal transmission distributes the virus within the flock inducing latent carriers. Flocks infected during the breeding season will produce two to four infected clutches.

Clinical Disease and Pathology

Survivors can develop ocular lesions including enlargement of the eyeball, marked opacity of the lens, seemingly fixed pupils and total blindness. Blindness may also occur in Black Grouse and capercaillie raised with AE-vaccinated chickens. In domesticated turkeys, 1% of the poults may show CNS signs including tremors, ataxia and incoordination. About 30% of the sick turkeys may die.

Differential Diagnosis and Diagnosis

Encephalomalacia (vitamin E and selenium deficiencies) is the main rule-out. Diagnostic therapy might be indicated. Intoxications, particularly those with a heavy metal (lead) must be considered. In pheasants, infections with Togaviridae are possible in the appropriate season.

Control

Several types of vaccine are available.

Duck Virus Hepatitis (DH)

Three types of DH infection are distinguished.

Type I has a worldwide distribution and causes high mortality (up to 100%) in domesticated *Anas platyrhynchos* ducklings, mainly during the first week of life. A distinct age resistance (three to six weeks) is seen in which younger birds are protected by maternal antibodies.

Type II has been isolated only in East Anglia, United Kingdom. In contrast to Types I and III, it is an astrovirus (antigenically different from astrovirus isolated from chickens and turkeys) that has been associated with 10-50% mortality in ducklings, depending on their age. All the recorded outbreaks have initially involved ducks kept in open enclosures, so that all free-ranging birds and gulls are suspected to be vectors.

Type III has been isolated only in the United States. The virus is not related to Type I. Diseases are generally less severe than those caused by type I with mortality rates rarely exceeding 30%. *Anas platyrhynchos* ducklings appear to be the only susceptible species.

Control

Viral-specific convalescent serum can be used in newly hatched ducklings. A vaccine is available for Type I that can be used in breeder stock to ensure high titers of maternal antibodies. A live avirulent vaccine can also be used in ducklings in the face of an outbreak. Recovered ducklings are considered immune.

Viral Enteritis in Cockatoos

Free-ranging Sulphur-crested Cockatoo and galah (Rose-breasted Cockatoo) chicks (seven to nine weeks old) developed profuse diarrhea and wasting and died shortly after being captured. The incidence of this disease (1,000-2,000 birds) is considered to be 10-20% annually in which galahs represented the higher percentage of affected birds. Clinical signs included yellow-green and mucoid feces beginning two to seven days after capture. Affected birds were anorexic, depressed, lost weight and became dehydrated following the onset of diarrhea. All affected birds eventually died or were euthanatized after one to four weeks of clinical disease. The birds failed to respond to treatment with various antibiotics and electrolytes.

Particles with the morphologic features of an enterovirus were detected in 18 out of 31 birds by electron microscopy. Because no virus could be isolated in embryonated chicken eggs, as is frequently the case with entero-like virus, the etiologic importance of the particles could not be determined.

Diseases with Infectious Characteristics but Uncertain Etiology

There are many clinical conditions that suggest a viral infection, and new ones are certain to be recognized with the advent of better diagnostic methods.

Neuropathic Gastric Dilatation (NGD)

This disease has been observed since 1977. It is suggested that the problem has been imported with macaws from Bolivia. The various *Ara* spp. are considered most susceptible but the disease has been described in many other Psittaciformes. A disease with clinical and histologic lesions similar to those described with Psittaciformes has also been confirmed in free-ranging Canada Geese.

Several possible viral agents have been described by electron microscopy, but none has been confirmed as the etiologic agent. [*Editor's Note: In 1996 it was reported that a virus fulfilling KOCH's postulate for NGD was found by researchers. At press time the viral family had not been identified.*]

Pathogenesis

Generally, this is a disease of young birds (nestlings to juveniles), but adults may also develop clinical signs. The destruction of the intramural ganglia of the proventriculus, ventriculus and to a lesser extent the descending loop of the duodenum explains the loss of peristalsis followed by obstruction of the proventriculus, atrophy of the ventricular wall and insufficiently digested food. The obstruction of the proventriculus can cause vomiting. The involvement of autonomic ganglia of the heart, brain, particularly the cerebellum and medulla oblongata, and the spinal cord may cause acute death with 100% mortality in affected birds. It has been suggested that the neurologic lesions may be caused by an autoimmune reaction.

Clinical Disease and Pathology

NGD is a chronic disease that may be associated with an acute onset of clinical signs. Clinical signs vary with the host and the severity of the condition, but generally include depression, progressive weight loss, vomiting or the passing of undigested food in the droppings. Some birds have an excellent appetite yet continue to lose weight. Anorexia may occur shortly before death. Polydipsia and polyuria may occur as well as neurologic signs such as leg weakness, incoordination and lameness. Diarrhea may occur late in the disease process and is usually the result of secondary bacterial or fungal enteritis.

The hemogram reveals a two- to three-fold increase in leukocytes (heterophils, monocytes and basophilic granulocytes). The negative caloric balance results in hypoglycemia and anemia. An elevation in creatine phosphokinase (CPK) levels has been suggested as a diagnostic tool; however, CPK concentrations are not believed to increase from damage to smooth muscles, and atrophy of striated muscle usually does not cause increased CPK activities.

Necropsy findings include emaciation, cachexia and a distended, frequently impacted proventriculus, ventriculus or crop. Erosions and ulcerations with or without hemorrhage can be observed on the proventricular mucosa, occasionally even causing ruptures. The muscular layer of the hypotrophic ventriculus appears whitish in color.

Diagnosis

In the experience of the author, about 10% of dead birds with signs indicative of NGD are not suffering from that disease (see Chapter 19).

Any cause of intestinal blockage can cause similar-appearing clinical changes and gross necropsy findings. Antemortem diagnosis requires histopathologic examination of biopsies of the ventriculus, which is difficult to sample. The absence of histologic lesions with suggestive clinical signs can indicate that the proventricular dilatation is of another etiology, or that the biopsy sample was collected from unaffected tissue.

Treatment and Control

Apart from hygienic considerations, symptomatic treatment can be attempted consisting of removal of stagnant ingesta, feeding soft or liquid feed and control of secondary infections. Supportive care has been efficacious in keeping birds alive for more than one year. In breeding flocks, affected birds should be removed as soon as possible. Birds that are in contact with patients that have confirmed infections should be placed in quarantine for at least six months together with cockatiel fledglings or breeding pairs as sentinels. New additions to the aviary should be quarantined for at least six months; however, this quarantine period may be insufficient to detect latently infected birds.

Nephroenteritis of the Domestic Goose

This disease has been described in Hungary and was differentiated from goose hepatitis and goose myocarditis. Although the agent has not been isolated to date, it is possible to reproduce the disease with filtrated material from the kidneys and intestine of sick goslings.

Clinical Disease and Pathology

Affected goslings seem to develop normally. The watery feces observed at the onset of the disease is frequently overlooked. Lethargy occurs only a few hours prior to death. Eight to ten hours before death, the feces become malodorous, fibrinous or bloody. In natural outbreaks, the peak of the mortality (up to 100%, but dependant on age) is reached at between 18-21 days of age.

Table 32.17 Reference Data on Common Avian Viruses

Virus	Incubation	Environmental Stability	Disinfectants	Control
Adenovirus	Natural infection 24-48 hours, slow spread in flock	Stability varies with isolate, resistant to many disinfectants, resistant to chloroform, 60-70°C, pH 3, pH 9	Formalin, aldehydes, iodophors (requires 1 hour of contact)	No vaccine, vertical transmission, continuous infectivity cycle
EEE & WEE virus	1-7 days	Stable when refrigerated	0.2% formalin, 3% phenol	Horse vaccine for pheasants
Enterovirus	1-7 days transovarial, 11 days with horizontal transmission	Extremely stable, resistant to chloroform, pH 3, 56-62°C for hours	1% formaldehyde, 2% caustic soda, 2% calcium hypochlorite (3 hours), 5% phenol, undiluted Clorox	AE vaccine, several types
Herpesvirus - PDV	Natural outbreak, 3-7 days, experimental, 48 hours	Unstable, cell associated or mucus coated virus more stable, 56°C for 1-5 minutes	Most disinfectants probably effective	Killed vaccine
Herpesvirus - AT	Experimental, 3-4 days			ILT vaccine protects chickens from AT, efficacy of ILT vaccine in Amazon parrots is unknown
Budgerigar herpesvirus	Unknown	Unknown		Interrupt breeding to increase Ab titers
Herpesvirus - DVE	3-4 days			Live attenuated vaccine, protect ponds from free-ranging waterfowl
Herpesvirus - ILT	6-15 days			Chicken vaccine, but not for pheasants

Table 32.17   Reference Data on Common Avian Viruses

Virus	Incubation	Environmental Stability	Disinfectants	Control
Herpesvirus - PHV	Experimental, 7 days Natural outbreaks, 5-10 days	56°C for 30 minutes		Experimental vaccines decrease clinical signs
Herpesvirus - FHV/OHV	Experimental, 3-10 days depending on virus and host			No vaccine, avoid mixing infected and non-infected birds, artificial incubation and hand-rearing
Influenza	Few hours to 3 days, varies with virulence, route of exposure and avian species	Unstable	Most disinfectants	Ultraviolet radiation, temperature increases
MSD pheasants Adenovirus Group II	6 days with oral infection			Oral vaccination of chicks (4-6 wks), chicks with THE or avirulent MSD
Newcastle disease virus	Experimental, 3-7 days, 25 days in some	Daylight, up to 4 weeks room temperature, 56°C sensitive	Lysol, cresol, phenol, 2% formalin, oxygen, cleaving compound, resistant to most disinfectants	
Orbivirus	Experimental, 4-8 days	Extremely stable	pH 3, resistant to lipolytics	
Papillomavirus	Unknown, probably prolonged	Stable, ether, temperature extremes	See text	
Polyomavirus	Unknown, suspected to be days to weeks	Stable, 56°C for 2 hours	Chlorine dioxide, phenolic disinfectants, Clorox	Experimental vaccine protects macaws from BFD virus

Table 32.17 Reference Data on Common Avian Viruses

Virus	Incubation	Environmental Stability	Disinfectants	Control
Parvovirus	5-15 days, varies with age and antibody titer	Stable, resistant to organic solvents, pH 3, 56°C for 3 hours, Na hypochlorite, H_2O_2 (1%)	Resistant to many disinfectants	Vaccinate breeder geese six weeks before egg laying (IM vaccine)
PBFD virus	Experimental (min 2-4 weeks), maximum unknown, may be months to years	Probably very stable, CAV stable to 60°C for 1 hour	Unknown	Experimental killed vaccine effective
Poxvirus	Varies (virus strain and host species) generally 1-2 weeks, canaries 4 days (10-12 days for hybrids)	Stable in soil for one year	Steam, 1% KOH, 2% NaOH, 5% phenol	Homologous or heterologous vaccines (see text)
Reovirus	Psittacine infected IM shed virus 2 days PI, geese 3-6 days, experimental, 3-9 days post-infection	Stable, pH 3, H_2O_2, 60°C for 8-10 hours	70% ethanol, 0.59% iodine, aldehydes/alcohols (2 hours)	Experimental inactivated vaccine may be effective
Retrovirus	Unknown	Unstable, stable pH 5 to pH 9, moderate ultraviolet radiation stability	Lipid solvents (detergents), thermostable, freeze-thawing destroys	

BACTERIA

Helga Gerlach

Bacterial infections may be primary or secondary. This differentiation is important for the evaluation of a disease process. After becoming established, many secondary invaders are able to maintain a disease process independent of other infectious agents or predisposing conditions. The companion bird clinician must determine the importance of bacterial isolation for a specific bird species and a specific disease process. Some specific points may guide the clinician in interpreting bacterial culture results (Table 33.1).

Gram-negative Bacteria of Clinical Significance

As a group, intestinal bacteria can be part of the normal flora or pathogenic organisms that are not routinely found in the GI tract; in some cases, normal flora can become secondary pathogens. When a bacterium leaves the mucosal surface and penetrates the intestinal wall, it then can induce systemic disease, including septicemia and death. The Enterobacteriaceae are considered the most important avian intestinal pathogens, but other groups, such as *Aeromonas, Pseudomonas, Alcaligenes, Bordetella* spp. and related organisms, as well as *Vibrio* and *Campylobacter,* may also colonize the gastrointestinal tract.

Enterobacteriaceae

Enterobacteriaceae are able to propagate in the environment if they are in the proper conditions. Enterobacteriaceae are ubiquitous and considered to be part of the autochthonous intestinal flora in many mammals, including humans and some species of birds (Table 33.2).

Isolation of Enterobacteriaceae from the respiratory or reproductive tracts is abnormal. This group of bacteria can colonize most avian tissues, where it is frequently considered as a secondary pathogen. In some cases, Enterobacteriaceae can function as primary pathogens. Substantial differences exist in the virulence of the various Enterobacteriaceae. The genera *Enterobacter, Hafnia, Serratia* and *Proteus* are of a low pathogenicity. *Serratia marcescens* is increasingly found in large parrots with chron-

Table 33.1 Guides to Interpretation of Bacterial Culture Results

- Isolation of an organism in an almost pure culture (approximately 80% of the colonies present) may indicate that the bacteria is a component in the disease process.

- Isolating large numbers of bacteria in almost pure culture from the heart tissue is suggestive of bacteremia, and the isolated agent should be considered part of the disease process.

- Isolating a bacteria that is part of the autochthonous flora may indicate that it is functioning as an opportunistic (secondary) pathogen.

- If the isolated organism has pathogenicity markers, it is probably involved in the disease process. It is not possible to determine if the bacteria is a primary or secondary pathogen.

- Isolating bacteria from parenchyma with pathologic or histopathologic lesions suggests that the agent contributed to the disease process.

- Isolating a bacterium without identifying other microorganisms (virus, chlamydia, other bacteria, fungi, protozoa) suggests that the agent is a primary pathogen. Finding virus or chlamydia suggests that the bacterium may be a secondary pathogen. Isolation of bacteria from a bird with fungi and protozoa suggests that the bacterium is a primary pathogen.

- Obtaining mixed cultures or identifying individuals within a given flock with different bacterial isolates suggests secondary infections are occurring.

- Isolating small to moderate numbers of bacteria from the liver or kidney can be "normal," because birds have hepatic and renal portal circulations and lack lymph nodes that filter blood before it drains into the liver and kidney. Because lymph follicles are distributed throughout these organs, defense responses actually occur within the parenchyma and not externally, as in mammals. These organs should not be expected to be sterile, but should be expected to contain autochthonous flora. The number of organisms isolated at necropsy depends on the time of death and the method of handling the body (eg, storage, preservation).

Table 33.2 Birds in which Enterobacteriaceae is not Normal

• Psittaciformes (parrots, parakeets)	• Gruiformes (cranes)
• Fringillidae (finches)	• Otididae (bustards)
• Ploceidae (weaver finches)	• Sphenisciformes (penguins)
• Astrildae (waxbills)	• Ciconiiformes (storks, ibises)
• Accipitriformes (hawks, vultures)	• Tetraoninae (grouse)
• Falconiformes (falcons)	• Musophagiformes (turacos)
• Strigiformes (owls)	• Trochiliformes (hummingbirds)

ic debilitating diseases. Predisposing factors seem to include previous antibiotic treatment and immunosuppression.

Escherichia (E.)

E. coli is the most commonly encountered member of this genus; in many avian species it is considered to be a more important pathogen than salmonella. This genus contains a number of species that may be motile or nonmotile, encapsulated or nonencapsulated. In experimental transmission studies, all lysine decarboxylase-negative *E. coli* strains have been found to be virulent in birds.

Clinical Disease and Pathology

Colisepticemia is characterized by an acute onset of lethargy, anorexia, ruffled plumage, diarrhea and polyuria. *E. coli* septicemia usually involves the kidneys, although clinical signs of renal involvement may or may not be present. CNS involvement is rare. Ocular lesions occasionally occur and include exudation of fibrin into the anterior eye chamber or uveitis. Serofibrinous arthritis can occur as a sequela in some infected birds. Fibrinous polyserositis, the severity of which depends on the chronicity of the infection, may be noted at necropsy. Catarrhal enteritis is common but nonspecific. The most consistent histologic lesion is serofibrinous inflammation with plasma cell infiltration in the liver and kidneys.

Localized enteritis caused by *E. coli* is a result of enterotoxin production, which induces an increased secretion of fluids. The resulting diarrhea causes a substantial loss of electrolytes and proteins and induces dehydration and cachexia. Some strains of *E. coli* are capable of colonizing and destroying the intestinal epithelium. These strains typically induce a pseudomembranous or ulcerative enteritis. Clinically infected birds die peracutely or develop nonspecific signs associated with enteritis. Infections with these strains are usually diagnosed on postmortem examination.

Coligranulomatosis (Hjaerre's disease) is particularly common in Phasianiformes including chickens, turkeys, peafowl, partridges and capercaillie. Coligranulomas are thought to occur when other agents damage the intestinal mucosa and allow a secondary infection with specific *E. coli* serovars.

Affected birds develop diarrhea, polyuria and chronic weight loss. Granulomatous dermatitis is occasionally noted. Grayish foci of varying sizes in the liver, intestinal subserosa and spleen or kidney are typical findings at necropsy. Acid-fast staining should be used to rule out mycobacteriosis.

E. coli can cause a primary rhinitis but is generally a sequela to infections elsewhere in the body. Air sac lesions can be severe and may extend to the peritoneum, causing a fibrinous polyserositis. Except in geese, *E. coli* pneumonia is rare.

Hens can develop *E. coli* infections characterized by fibrinous salpingitis or oophoritis originating from organisms that ascend from the cloaca or by imprint metastases from infected air sacs. Infections are usually chronic in nature, with untreated birds eventually dying from salpingoperitonitis. Genital tract infections in males are less common, but when they do occur they usually result in orchitis and permanent sterility.

Diagnosis

Specific diagnosis requires culturing the organism from infected tissues.

Treatment

The ability of a selected drug to penetrate target tissues or granulomas must be considered. Parenteral antibiotics are necessary for treating most *E. coli* infections. In addition to antibiotics, therapeutic considerations should also include administration of avian lactobacilli in an effort to lower the intestinal tract pH and help establish a proper autochthonous flora. Lactulose may also be helpful in lowering the intestinal pH. Providing a nutritional diet is important in improving gastrointestinal physiology in malnourished birds.

Salmonella (S.)

Most strains are motile and grow on common media. Most vertebrates can be infected with some *Salmonella* spp. However, the host susceptibility and development of carrier states vary widely among species. Free-ranging birds can be subclinical carriers and serve as a reservoir for the aviary. In addition to free-ranging birds, rats, flies and other vermin may also serve as vectors of salmonella. Avian species without ceca or with involuted ceca appear to be more susceptible to salmonella infections than birds with fully functioning ceca. Bacteroides and *Spherophorus* spp. are considered autochthonous cecal flora, and these gram-negative anaerobes may function as natural antagonists for *Salmonella* spp.

Transmission

Salmonella enters the host principally through the oral route. Contaminated dust from feces or feathers may be involved in aerogenic spread in some cases. Egg transmission can occur with fully walled and L-form salmonella.

Pathogenesis

One of the characteristics of the group Enterobacteriaceae is that they all produce endotoxins. Salmonella is no exception, and some cases of food poisoning are linked to this bacterium. Indirect death through endotoxin contamination of food is rare in birds; most avian salmonella problems are associated with direct infections. Virulent strains are those that can penetrate an intact intestinal mucosa, and nonvirulent strains are those that require a mucosal lesion to enter a host. Nonvirulent strains often colonize the gut, resulting in asymptomatic infections and intermittent shedding. Once virulent or nonvirulent strains have passed the mucosal barriers, they induce a septicemia that results in an immune response or colonization in tissues and eventual death of the bird.

Clinical Disease and Pathology

Acute diseases are characterized by nonspecific signs including lethargy, anorexia, polydipsia (sometimes followed by polyuria) and diarrhea. In subacute to chronic cases, CNS signs, arthritis (particularly in pigeons), dyspnea and indications of liver, spleen, kidney or heart damage are common. With high-dose infections, conjunctivitis, iridocyclitis and panophthalmia may occur.

Postmortem lesions include dehydration, degeneration or necrosis of skeletal musculature, gastroenteritis (occasionally with ulcers and granulomas), enlargement of the liver and spleen (with or without disseminated small whitish foci), bile congestion and nephropathy. Chronic infections usually cause pericarditis or epicarditis fibrinosa, granuloma formation in the liver, spleen and kidney, and degeneration or inflammation of the ovary or testis. Fibrin filling the cecal lumen is a common finding.

Treatment

Whether or not to treat salmonella infections in companion birds is controversial. The author believes that clinically affected birds and companion birds that are identified as carriers should be treated because of public health hazards. Therapy should include appropriate antibiotics (based on sensitivity) and lactobacillus products. In general, the frequently encountered salmonella strains are sensitive to commonly available antibiotics, but some strains from free-ranging birds (particularly from seagulls) demonstrate varying degrees of antimicrobial resistance. CNS signs and chronic infections tend to be refractory to therapy. Flock management of salmonella should concentrate on preventing egg transmission by identifying and removing subclinically infected breeders. Treating birds that have egg-derived infections is extremely difficult.

Treatment of L-forms can be attempted with clindamycin (100 mg/kg body weight) or a combination of erythromycin and ampicillin (both components at the full dose).

Control

Proper hygiene is the best tool for preventing salmonella outbreaks. The effective control of flies, rodents and other vermin is essential. Regular cleaning and disinfection of the aviary and nursery, along with proper storage of food, are all important in preventing salmonellosis.

Citrobacter (C.)

The three species of *Citrobacter* (*C. freundii*, *C. amalonaticus* and *C. diversus*) are less commonly encountered than other members of the Enterobacteriaceae.

Citrobacter spp. cause serious secondary infections in weaver finches and waxbills. A rapid bacteremia followed by acute death occurs when the organism penetrates the intestinal mucosa. Ostriches, particularly chicks and young birds, also appear to be very susceptible to *Citrobacter* spp. Infected birds of any species may die without any clinical signs, or they can exhibit a brief period of depression and diarrhea prior to death. Postmortem changes indicate septicemia (petechiation of the heart, musculature and parenchyma). Surviving birds frequently become carriers. Therapeutic decisions should be based on appropriate culture and sensitivity. Neomycin delivered by gavage is often effective in clearing intestinal infections. In flock outbreaks, the same drug administered in the drinking water may be helpful in controlling infections.

There have been no reported cases of citrobacter infections in humans derived from exposure to infected birds.

Klebsiella (K.)

K. pneumoniae and *K. oxytoca* are frequently recovered from birds in which they can function as primary pathogens, particularly in weaver finches, or they can be involved as opportunists in immunosuppressed or stressed patients. These organisms are nonmotile Enterobacteriaceae, and most members of the genus are encapsulated.

Klebsiella spp. bacteremia usually results in the colonization of the kidney, causing renal failure. In chronic infections, the lungs may also be involved.

Encephalomyelitis is occasionally noted in terminal cases. While systemic klebsiella infections are most common, local infections involving the sinuses, skin, oral cavity and crop may also oc-

cur, particularly in Psittaciformes. The diagnosis is made by isolation and identification of the organism.

Yersinia (Y.)

The genus *Yersinia* currently consists of eleven species. Unlike
other Enterobacteriaceae, which are strictly rod-shaped, *Yersinia*
spp. form ovoid-to-coccoid rods that replicate in the environment
at extremely low temperatures (+4°C) if provided the proper
sources of organic nitrogen.

Y. pseudotuberculosis appears to be the most important avian
pathogen. *Y. pseudotuberculosis* infects a wide range of hosts, including many bird species and various mammals, particularly rodents and including humans. Toucans, toucanets, aracaris, bar-
bets and turacos appear to be extremely susceptible.

Clinical Disease and Pathology

Y. pseudotuberculosis may be associated with peracute, acute or
chronic clinical disease. Peracute death without clinical signs is
common in infected Piciformes and Musophagidae. Clinical signs
associated with acute disease include lethargy, dehydration, diarrhea and dyspnea. Emaciation, wasting and flaccid paresis or
paralysis are common with subacute or chronic cases. Birds with
a wasting syndrome appear similar to animals infected with tuberculosis. Infected ducks frequently develop tarsal joint swelling.
Canaries may be severely dyspneic prior to death.

Gross changes associated with peracute infections include
swelling of the liver and spleen and bloody-to-fibrinous exudate
into the body cavity. Submiliary-to-miliary, sharply demarcated
grayish foci within the liver, lungs, spleen and kidneys are common with the acute course. Chronic infections are characterized
by granuloma formation in organs and the skeletal musculature.
Ulcers in the proventriculus, ventriculus and duodenum may occur in infected canaries.

Diagnosis

Definitive diagnosis requires isolating the organism from affected tissues. Placing contaminated samples in a cool environment for two weeks may help in recovering *Y.* spp.

Treatment

Birds with the peracute to acute forms of yersiniosis usually die
before therapy can be instigated. Parenteral drug administration
is required if therapy has any chance of being successful. Treating
chronic cases is difficult because granulomas prevent antibiotics
from reaching the yersinia organisms nestled in the center of
necrotic debris. Flock outbreaks can be prevented by treating clinically unaffected animals and applying strict sanitary measures.

Pseudomonas (Ps.) and Aeromonas (Ae.)

These two gram-negative rods are taxonomically unrelated but
nevertheless have characteristics that make it best from a clinical
perspective to discuss them together. Both bacteria are frequently found in aquatic environments and can propagate in cool water
(20°C or lower). Both bacteria will grow on common media and in-

duce β-hemolysis on blood plates. These hemolysins are potent toxins and are capable of damaging many cells in addition to erythrocytes. *Ps. aeruginosa* produces a blue-green diffusible pigment and has a sweetish odor.

Clinical Disease and Pathology

Virulent strains of these bacteria can cause a septicemia that induces diarrhea, dehydration and dyspnea followed by acute death. Infected skin lesions are edematous or necrotizing. Localized infections may occur in the upper respiratory tract, causing rhinitis, sinusitis and laryngitis. Hemorrhages and coalescent necrosis in the liver, spleen and kidney are the most common postmortem findings. Catarrhal to hemorrhagic enteritis with edema and fibrinous inflammation of the serosal membranes may also be noted.

Diagnosis and Control

Aviary outbreaks of pseudomonas are most common when organic material contaminates the water supply, allowing a proliferation of the organisms in the drinking water. Routine cleaning of food and water containers, along with any external water pipes, is an important control measure.

Alcaligenes (Ac.) and Bordetella (Bo.)

The genera *Alcaligenes* and *Bordetella* are taxonomically related. Both genera are widely spread in the environment. *Alcaligenes* is found mainly in aquatic environments. *Ac. faecalis, Bo. avium* and *Bo. bronchiseptica* infect a wide variety of birds in many orders. Psittaciformes and turkeys as well as many finches seem to be particularly susceptible to these bacteria.

At necropsy, tracheitis, bronchopneumonia and air sacculitis are common findings with subacute to chronic courses of bordetella, whereas alcaligenes infections are characterized by coalescent liver necrosis in addition to respiratory disease.

Campylobacter (C.)

C. jejuni may appear in different forms including a short comma, S-shaped, long spiral or coccoid form. The latter is usually an indication of degeneration. Colony formation takes 72-96 hours at 37-42°C in a microaerobic environment.

Clinical Disease and Pathology

Clinical signs are generally associated with subacute to chronic hepatitis and include lethargy, anorexia, diarrhea (frequently with yellowish stained feces) and emaciation. High mortality has been noted in finches, especially among fledglings. Heterophilia and thrombocytophilia are the most consistent changes in the CBC.

At necropsy the liver is enlarged, pale or greenish in color and is congested, with or without hemorrhage.

Treatment and Control

There are discrepancies between the antibiograms and clinical recovery. Erythromycin or tetracyclines, dehydro- or streptomycin (never in Psittaciformes) or furane derivatives (not in waterfowl) can be tried. Diseases frequently recur despite therapy.

Vibrio (V.)

The genus *Vibrio* comprises numerous species that are not easy to differentiate. *V. cholerae* is of utmost importance as a zoonotic organism.

Spirochaetaceae

Borrelia (Bor.) anserina (syn. *Spirochaeta gallinarum*) is a gram-negative, helical motile organism that stains with Giemsa.

Transmission

The main vectors for transmission are ticks, in which the organism can be passed transovarially and survive for over a year.

Clinical Disease and Pathology

Acute cases are characterized by a high fever (bacteria generally cause a low body temperature), anorexia, depression (droopy, cyanotic heads), yellowish diarrhea, lethargy, ataxia and paralysis. Morbidity is high, and mortality may range from 10-100% depending upon the susceptibility of the host. Spontaneous recovery may occur around the sixth day postinfection. Chronic disease is characterized by anemia, paralysis and dyspnea.

At necropsy, a mottled, severely enlarged liver is characteristic except in pheasants. In these birds the spleen may be small or normal in size. The liver shows hemorrhages and necrotic foci. Mucoid hemorrhagic enteritis, serofibrinous pericarditis and swollen kidneys may also be seen.

Diagnosis

Blood smears stained with Giemsa or examined by darkfield microscopy are useful for diagnosis. Culturing *Bor.* sp. is very difficult.

Pasteurella (P.)

The family of Pasteurellaceae currently includes the genera *Pasteurella, Actinobacillus* and *Haemophilus*. All three genera can be pathogens in birds.

Pasteurella spp. characteristically exhibit bipolar staining in tissue smears or from first culture passages when fixed in methanol and stained with methylene blue. There are presently eleven species within this genus, but others will undoubtedly be added. *P. multocida,* which causes fowl cholera, and *P. gallinarum* are two of the most commonly encountered species.

Transmission

Pasteurella infections in birds principally occur in the respiratory tract. Transmission can occur through direct contact with contaminated aerosols or through mechanical vectors such as blood-sucking mites. Infected rodents and free-ranging birds are considered important reservoirs. Cats should always be considered to be carriers of *P. multocida,* and any bird that has been mouthed by a cat should be treated with antibiotics immediately.

Clinical Disease and Pathology

Acute forms are characterized by cyanosis, dyspnea and diarrhea followed by death. Excess mucus may be present around the nostrils or beak. Birds that survive acute disease often develop respiratory rales, sinusitis, conjunctivitis or swelling of the sinus infraorbitalis. Arthritis and CNS signs have been reported in some chronic cases. Granulomatous dermatitis has been noted in raptors, owls and pigeons.

Postmortem findings with acute disease may be absent or limited to petechiae or ecchymoses of the parenchymal organs. Prolonged cases are characterized by exudative serositis (mainly white, in contrast to yellow with *E. coli*) and the formation of necrotic foci in infected organs. Catarrhal to fibrinous rhinitis, necrotic pneumonia, sinusitis, blepharoconjunctivitis and tracheitis are common with chronic courses. Following bacteremia, *Pasteurella* may colonize numerous tissues, resulting in arthritis, osteomyelitis, otitis media and granulomatous dermatitis. Granulomas may also be noted in the liver and spleen.

Treatment

Septicemic birds rarely survive, even when treated intensively. Parenteral administration of broad-spectrum, long-acting sulfonamides can be tried. The combined use of antibiotics and hyperimmune serum has proven to be beneficial. Treating birds with chronic forms is very difficult because of the irreversible damage that occurs to parenchymal organs.

Actinobacillus (At.)

Actinobacilli are polymorphic rods that may exhibit bipolar staining similar to Pasteurellae.

Clinical Disease and Pathology

Many infected birds die acutely. Birds with a more chronic course typically develop joint lesions. Species-specific strains that infect geese morphologically resemble *P. influenzae*. This organism has been referenced as a cause of chronic disease in the gosling, characterized by emaciation, failure to thrive, poor feed conversion and arthritis.

Diagnosis and Treatment

Isolation and identification of the causative agent is necessary for diagnosis. Tetracyclines and chloramphenicol are indicated for initial therapy. Sensitivities for many strains are difficult to interpret because of oversized inhibition zones. In young geese, antibiotics must be given during the first week of life or lesions become too extensive to be reversed.

Haemophilus (H.)

Chickens are considered to be the only definitive host of *H. paragallinarum*, which is the agent of coryza contagiosa gallinarum.

Clinical Disease and Pathology

Haemophilus infections generally cause a rhinitis that results in a serous-to-mucoid or even fibrinous exudate. Conjunctivitis and sinusitis may also occur. The most common postmortem finding is catarrhal-to-fibrinous rhinitis. Bronchopneumonia and air sacculitis are frequently described but are usually the result of concomitant infections (virus, other bacteria, *Candida* spp.).

Gram-positive Bacteria of Clinical Significance

Staphylococcus (S.)

Staphylococcus infections can induce sporadic or enzootic disease in many avian species.

Members of the genus *Staphylococcus* (apart from *S. aureus*) are commonly recovered from many avian species and are considered part of the autochthonous flora. When present in diseased tissue, they are generally considered to be secondary invaders.

S. aureus

Avian strains of virulent *S. aureus* are relatively species-specific and rarely induce disease in mammals. Isolation of the organism can frequently be accomplished from the skin and the mucosa of the respiratory or digestive tract of clinically normal birds.

Clinical Disease and Pathology

Staphylococcus can induce a wide range of clinical and pathologic lesions, including high embryonic mortality, yolk sac or umbilical inflammation, septicemia, arthritis-synovitis, osteomyelitis, vesicular dermatitis, gangrenous dermatitis and bumblefoot.

Staphylococcus septicemia may be characterized by nonspecific clinical signs including lethargy, anorexia, a kyphotic posture, ruffled plumage and sudden death. The acute occurrence of necrosis to the distal digits or adnexa of the head and neck is suggestive of a thrombi-inducing infection, which can be sequela to staphylococcus septicemia. During the initial phases of the ischemic process, the involved digits may be swollen, congested and painful, and many affected birds exhibit lameness. The acute onset of tremors, opisthotonos and torticollis can often be linked to staphylococcus-induced necrosis in the CNS. Gross lesions associated with staphylococcus septicemia include petechiae and ecchymoses of internal organs. Chronic infections may result in endocarditis valvularis.

Arthritis-synovitis, characterized by the formation of serofibrinous or fibrinous inflammation of the synovial membranes of tendon sheaths and articular bursae, is frequently noted with staphylococcal infections in gallinaceous species. Any joint may be involved but there appears to be a predilection for colonization of the tarsal and metatarsal joints. Following antibiotic therapy, staphylococcus may be present in its unstable L-form, which is difficult to treat.

In immature birds with active growth plates, *Staphylococcus* frequently localizes in the epiphyseal area with secondary invasion of the bone marrow, resulting in osteomyelitis. Endogenous osteomyelitis is considered to be impossible after consolidation of the growth plate. Infection of the growth plates often leads to chronic skeletal abnormalities. Infections are frequently localized to the proximal epiphyses of the femur, tibiotarsus, tarsometatarsus and fifth to seventh thoracic vertebrae. Vertebral injury may lead to clinical changes described as "kinky back."

Staphylococcus-induced vesicular dermatitis is characterized by the formation of vesicles containing yellowish exudate that form brownish to blackish crusts following rupture. Concomitant infection with poxvirus (or other immunosuppressive agents) may be involved in the disease process.

Staphylococcus-induced gangrenous dermatitis is initially recognized by the occurrence of subcutaneous edema and hemorrhage followed by inflammation the skin. Affected skin is typically blackish and smudgy and feather loss is common. *Clostridium perfringens* or another *Clostridium* sp. is a common secondary invader. Both *Staphylococcus* and *Clostridium* require a triggering factor (often damaged epithelium) to enter the tissue. Gangrenous dermatitis is rare in most bird species.

Advanced bumblefoot is a necrotizing abscess on the plantar surface of the foot. Depending on the location and chronicity of the abscess, infection may or may not extend to neighboring joints, tendon sheaths and bones. The condition is frequently described in raptors but may occur in other avian species. The precise pathogenesis of bumblefoot is undetermined (see Chapter 16). Although staphylococci are frequently isolated from these lesions, they are by no means the only bacteria that can be recovered from diseased tissue.

Streptococcus (Sc.) and Enterococcus (Ec.)

Streptococci and enterococci consist of numerous species that readily grow on most commonly used media. These organisms are ubiquitous (mainly in dust and air), and some strains can survive for long periods in the environment.

Sc. and *Ec.* are considered part of the autochthonous flora of the skin and the mucosal surfaces of the digestive, respiratory and reproductive tracts. *Sc.* and *Ec.* transition from normal flora to disease-inducing agents depends on the functional state of host defense systems.

Clinical Disease

The clinical diseases caused by pyogenic streptococci and other streptococci and enterococci are relatively similar. Clinical presentation can be peracute to chronic, with birds surviving six to eight weeks in the chronic form. Omphalitis in recent hatchlings is typical with egg transmission or infections obtained from the hatchery.

Septicemia may lead to a peracute apoplectiform death or severe depression followed by death in two to three days. Other signs such as diarrhea, dyspnea, paresis, conjunctivitis and sinusitis (Japanese Quail) may develop.

Chronic disease is typified by inflammation of joints, tendon sheaths and adnexa of the head. Fibrinous joint lesions, with or without abscess formation, can occur several months after the initial infection. Birds that survive systemic infections may develop cardiac valve insufficiency secondary to endocarditis. This condition is difficult to diagnose and often presents as chronic dyspnea.

Group C *Streptococcus* has been associated with pneumonia secondary to bacteremia in a variety of avian species.

Ec. group D is frequently implicated as a cause of pneumonia in various bird species, particularly Passeriformes, and primarily infects young birds. In canaries, *Ec. faecalis* can cause a tracheitis and chronic respiratory disease that manifests clinically as changes in the voice (more "sparrow-like") or complete voice loss.

Treatment

Aggressive treatment with parenterally administered antibiotics is the recommended therapy. Pyogenic streptococci are generally sensitive to penicillins, erythromycin, tylosin, spectinomycin, clindamycin and pleuromutilin. Enterococci have varying antimicrobial sensitivities. Chronic joint and tendon sheath infections are difficult to resolve and may require a combination of surgery, joint lavage and prolonged antibiotic therapy. Streptococci in synovial membranes are frequently in their L- or protoplastic form. Treatment in these cases consists of ampicillin and erythromycin or enrofloxacin.

Mycobacterium (M.)

All bird species that have been experimentally exposed have been found to be susceptible to *M. avium*. Shedding from an infected host occurs primarily in the feces and urine, causing contamination of the soil or water supplies within the aviary.

Transmission

Avian mycobacteriosis primarily involves the alimentary tract. Transmission occurs mainly through contaminated feces, although aerogenic routes of transmission are possible. Arthropods can serve as mechanical vectors of *M. intracellulare* and *M. avium subsp. avium*.

Clinical Disease

In some bird species the clinical course is atypical, and acid-fast rods have been detected more or less accidentally. This is particularly the case with small Passeriformes, especially the Hooded Siskin. Clinical signs associated with mycobacteriosis are highly variable. Adult birds usually develop a chronic wasting disease associated with a good appetite, recurrent diarrhea, polyuria, anemia and dull plumage. Immature individuals frequently develop subclinical conditions. Intermittent switching lameness may occur as a result of painful lesions in the bone marrow. Arthritis, mainly of the carpometacarpal and the elbow joints or tubercle formation of the muscles of the thigh or shank can be seen occasionally. These clinical changes are particularly common in Falconiformes and Accipitriformes. Skin over the affected joint is often thickened and ulcerated. Tubercle formation in the skin is rare, but when it is present, pinpoint to pigeon egg-sized nodules filled with yellow fibrinous material may be noted. Granulomas may be seen within the conjunctival sac, at the angle of the beak, around the external auditory canal and in the oropharynx. Mycobacteriosis should be suspected when tumor-like lesions recur after surgery.

Pathology

The presence of miliary to greater-than-pea-sized nodules in the wall of the intestinal tract and in the liver, spleen and bone marrow are characteristic of *M. avium* infections. Granuloma formation can occur in any organ but is generally localized to the intestinal tract and reticuloendothelial organs.

Diagnosis

The demonstration of acid-fast rods in tissues or on cytologic preparations is suggestive of mycobacteriosis. False-negative staining can occur by not obtaining an adequate sample. The demonstration of acid-fast rods in the feces has been suggested as a useful diagnostic tool in subclinical birds. Mucus present in the feces can interfere with test results, and samples should be processed with one of the sputum solvents used in human medicine before staining. The most consistent results can be obtained by centrifuging the feces and then spreading the surface of the pellet on a slide for staining. This test is relatively insensitive and requires the presence of approximately 10^4 bacteria/g of feces to be positive. Culture is required to make a distinct diagnosis.

Treatment and Control

Birds that are definitively diagnosed (biopsy of affected tissue with histopathology and culture) with *M. avium* or *M. intracellulare* infection should be euthanatized. Contact birds should be removed from the contaminated area, quarantined for two years and tested every 6-12 weeks to determine if they are reacting. Birds that remain negative (also not shedding the agent with the feces) and are in good physical condition following the quarantine procedure can be considered free of the disease.

The transmission of *M. avium* to humans is possible. However, transmission is probably dependent on inherent resistance, the immune status of the person in question, the frequency of exposure and the number of bacteria per exposure. [*Editor's Note: If treatment is elected the owner should be made fully aware of the zoonotic potential. Requiring a signed release form is probably appropriate.*]

Erysipelothrix (E.)

Erysipelothrix rhusiopathiae can induce an acute-to-subacute septicemic disease. Infections are most commonly discussed in ducks and geese but can occasionally occur in other avian species including Psittaciformes.

Pathogenesis

E. rhusiopathiae infections are most common in waterfowl and fish-eating birds during cold weather when food is scarce and energy requirements are high.

Clinical Disease and Pathology

E. rhusiopathiae usually causes peracute death. If clinical signs occur, they may include lethargy, weakness, anorexia and hyperemia or bruising of the featherless, nonpigmented skin. Greenish discolored droppings, dyspnea and nasal discharge have been reported in some cases. In the Marabou Stork, infections have been characterized by inflammation and necrosis of the cutaneous adnexa of the neck.

Petechiae in the subcutis, musculature and intestinal mucosa are common gross lesions in diseased birds. The liver and spleen are friable and discolored (red to black).

Diagnosis

Diagnosis is confirmed by isolating *E. rhusiopathiae*. The best samples for isolation (if the tissues are fresh) are liver or spleen. In severely autolytic cases, bone marrow samples may be the most diagnostic.

Listeria (L.)

Listeria spp. may infect a number of avian species, including Psittaciformes. Canaries appear to be more susceptible to infections than other birds.

Clinical Disease and Pathology

Clinical disease is usually associated with sporadic deaths in a collection. Epornitics can develop in canaries and related birds that are maintained in dense populations. Chronic infections can induce lesions in the heart, liver and, rarely, the brain. If clinical signs are noted, they are generally associated with CNS signs and include blindness, torticollis, tremor, stupor and paresis or paralysis. Subacute-to-chronic cases usually cause a severe monocytosis (10-12 times normal).

The presence of serofibrinous pericarditis and myocardial necrosis is considered suggestive of *Listeria*.

Diagnosis

A confirmed diagnosis requires the isolation of *L. monocytogenes* from affected tissues. Appropriate transport media are necessary for proper shipment of samples.

Clostridium (Cl.)

The genus *Clostridium* includes a group of ubiquitous bacteria that are considered to be autochthonous flora in raptors and in birds with well developed ceca, including Phasianiformes (gallinaceous birds) and Anseriformes.

Pathogenesis

Clostridium spp. produce more potent toxins than any other bacterial genus.

Necrotic or Ulcerative Enteritis

Clostridia-induced enteritis can occur in many avian species. Flock outbreaks are most commonly associated with Phasianiformes, especially those within the subfamilies Tetraoninae (grouse) and Odontophorinae (New World quail) or captive and free-ranging lorikeets. Ulcerative gastritis, not enteritis, is the most common form of clostridial infection reported in the ostrich.

Necrotic enteritis usually occurs in young birds after the second post-hatching week. Adult birds are more resistant. In the acute form of the disease, clinical changes include diarrhea (with or without blood) and polydipsia, followed by death within a few hours. Birds with chronic lesions exhibit retarded growth and weight loss before dying.

Pathologic changes include diffuse or focal hyperemia of the mucosa, which develops into necrotic areas or ulcers. These lesions are most common in the upper jejunum. Lesions start as pinpoint foci and progress to include a necrotic center with a wall and a reddish halo. Ulcers may coalesce and perforate the intestinal wall. Swelling and necrosis of a grayish liver, spleen and kidney are common.

Gangrenous Dermatitis

Gangrenous dermatitis can be caused by *Cl. perfringens* type A, *Cl. septicum,* or *Cl. novyi.* These organisms can directly colonize damaged skin. Microscopic epithelial lesions caused by abrasions, avipoxvirus or staphylococci can become secondarily infected with *Clostridium* spp. The patient's immune status may also play a role in the overall pathogenesis.

The sudden occurrence of regional feather loss with a blue-red or almost black skin discoloration is a characteristic lesion. Affected skin may also be edematous and painful as a result of gas accumulation in the tissue. Sick animals typically develop toxemia and die within 24 hours. With screamers (genus *Chauna*), their corneous-lined bony wing spurs can cause prick-like skin injuries predisposing them to clostridial diseases.

The occurrence of emphysema, edema and hemorrhages (with or without necrosis) in the subcutis, skeletal musculature and myocardium are characteristic necropsy findings.

Botulism (syn. Limberneck)

Cl. botulinum neurotoxins are typically ingested in contaminated foods. Rarely, clinical disease may result from primary colonization of the alimentary tract. *Cl. botulinum* has been found to produce six thermolabile exotoxins (designated A to F). High concentrations of clostridium toxins are common in decaying meat and vegetation. Fly larvae (maggots) that feed on decaying material are resistant to the toxins but can serve as a source of intoxication for those species that eat maggots. With a few logical exceptions, most birds are probably susceptible to *Cl. botulinum* toxins. Vultures seem to be resistant to the toxins. Some raptors (that eat carrion) have a reduced susceptibility.

Flaccid paralysis of the skeletal musculature (including the tongue) is the characteristic clinical change. Bulbar paralysis, feather loss and diarrhea may be noted in some birds. Birds with substantial clinical signs usually die, although a few can spontaneously recover.

Confirming a diagnosis requires using mouse animal models to demonstrate the presence of toxins in serum, filtered liver or kidney from an affected animal.

Tetanus

A few cases of *Cl. tetani* intoxication in birds have been reported in older literature. There have been no cases of tetanus reported in birds using more confirmatory diagnostic tests. Generally, birds are considered to be highly resistant to *Cl. tetani*; cases reported in older literature may have been incorrectly diagnosed.

Other Gram-positive Rods

Bacillus spp., *Corynebacterium* spp., *Streptomyces* spp. and *Lactobacillus* spp. are commonly recovered from avian-derived samples. Because these organisms are frequently isolated from clinically normal birds, they are considered to be components of the autochthonous flora. Megabacterium is considered to be a pathogenic organism, although little information is currently available on its involvement in avian disease. *Bacillus* spp. isolated from birds are difficult to differentiate, and most have not been described taxonomically. *Bacillus anthracis* has not been associated with clinical disease in birds, presumably because their high body temperature inhibits the production of the pathogenic toxins. Vultures, and to a lesser extent raptors, are known to be mechanical vectors.

None of the *Corynebacterium (Co.)* spp. that have been isolated from birds has been found to be pathogenic.

Streptomyces spp. can occasionally be isolated from the avian respiratory system.

Lactobacillus spp. can be identified on the mucosa of the intestinal, respiratory and reproductive tracts of many avian species. In birds that do not possess Enterobacteriaceae as a normal component of the gut flora, lactobacillus seems to play an important role in inhibiting colonization of Enterobacteriaceae.

Isolation of megabacteria is difficult, and biochemical descriptions that would allow appropriate taxonomic classification have not been performed. This organism has a unique morphology and is a large (1 x 90 mm) gram-positive rod.

Some researchers believe that megabacterium is the causative agent of progressive weight loss ("going light syndrome") in budgerigars. The name "going light syndrome" should provisionally be replaced by megabacteriosis, because weight loss is a clinical sign of a variety of chronic diseases. Experimental infections with pure cultures of megabacterium induce disease only in English standard budgerigars and not in the normal breed. These findings suggest that birds vary in susceptibility to the organism, and other factors are involved in the pathogenesis. The host spectrum includes canaries and related finches, cockatiels, lovebirds, chickens and young (3-week-old) ostriches.

Clinically infected birds develop chronic emaciation over a 12- to 18-month period that may or may not involve intermittent periods of recovery. Severely affected birds may pass digested blood in the feces. Contrast radiography typically indicates a sandglass-like retraction between the proventriculus and ventriculus. This finding is considered highly suggestive of megabacteriosis. Megabacterium is shed in the feces and can be detected by gram-stained samples from severely sick birds.

At necropsy, a proventriculitis or proventricular ulcer with or without hemorrhages can be observed. Lesions are most common in the pars intermedia gastris. The organisms lie densely together in the necrotic tissue foci. There is usually little inflammatory cellular reaction associated with the organism, which can be seen readily at low magnification from proventricular scrapings. Impression smears from the liver and spleen may be useful in detecting the bacteria, which can be encapsulated in the tissues. There is no treatment because of resistance to all antibiotics commonly used.

Table 33.8   Differential Diagnosis of Bacterial Infections

Arthritis or Synovitis
  Staphylococcus
  Actinobacillus sp.
  E. coli
  E. rhusopathiae (ducks and goose)
  Mycobacterium avium
  Mycoplasma spp.
  Pasteurella multocida
  Salmonella spp.

CNS Signs
  Listeriosis
  Chlamydiosis
  E. coli
  Klebsiella pneumoniae
  Listeria monocytogenes
  Salmonella spp.

Dermatitis
  Pseudomonas/Aeromonas spp.
  Clostridium spp.
  Staphylococcus spp.

Enteritis
  E. coli
  Aeromonas sp.
  Most enteric organisms
  Pseudomonas spp.
  Salmonella spp.
  E. rhusiopathiae
  Chlamydiosis
  Listeria sp.
  Pasteurella spp.

Hepatitis
  Most bacteria that cause
    septicemia
  Campylobacter
  Pasteurella spp.
  Chlamydiosis
  Salmonella spp.

Pseudomonas enteritis
  Clostridium spp.

Respiratory Disease
  Alicalgenes
  Enterobacteriaceae
  Pasteurella spp.
  Cytophaga (duck septicemia)
  Pasteurella spp.
  Haemophilus
  Chlamydiosis (eg, psittacines,
    Columbiformes)
  Salmonella spp.

Septicemia
  E. coli
  Many bacteria
  Listeria spp.
  E. rhusiopathiae
  Pasteurella spp.
  Salmonella spp.
  Yersinia pseudotuberculosis
  Pseudomonas/Aeromonas
  Most Enterobacteriacae
  Staphylococcus (mimics numerous
    other infectious agents)
  Streptococcus/Enterococcus
  Borrelliosis (high tick areas)

CHLAMYDIA

Helga Gerlach

The genus *Chlamydia* currently consists of two antigenically related species, *C. trachomatis* and *C. pneumoniae,* which are restricted to humans, and *C. psittaci,* which has a wide host spectrum among birds (most Psittaciformes and at least 130 non-Psittaciformes), mammals (horse, cattle, sheep, roebuck, domesticated cat, guinea pig, dog) and humans. *C. psittaci* can be highly contagious and induces a disease called psittacosis in parrots and ornithosis (by legal definition) in all other animals and man. Because the same agent is involved, the use of the term chlamydiosis to describe infections caused by this organism should be encouraged. Chlamydiosis is a reportable disease in many countries.

C. psittaci is an obligate intracellular bacterial parasite that contains DNA and RNA and has a rudimentary cellular wall that does not contain muraic acid or peptidoglycan. This organism is capable of autonomic synthesis of species-specific enzymes, but depends on the host cell for energy (by means of adenosine triphosphate and nicotinamide adenosine diphosphate) and probably some amino acids, particularly tryptophan. These requirements prevent chlamydia from growing on cell-free media.

Pathogenicity

The pathogenicity of chlamydia cannot be fully explained by the direct damage to the host cells. The most important virulence factor is a toxin, which occurs with various degrees of intensity in the different strains and is closely bound to the outer membrane of the elementary bodies.

The outcome of an infection is dependent on the ratio of elementary bodies to macrophages. Lethal lytic reactions occur in phagocytes infected with high numbers of virulent chlamydial particles. Low doses of a virulent strain are rapidly inactivated by mononuclear and polymorphonuclear phagocytes. If the macrophage is damaged, the chances of the chlamydial organism to survive are reduced. Low doses of a nonvirulent strain do not stimulate an appropriate lytic reaction, resulting in macrophages that are converted into long-lived epithelioid cells that remain chronically infected (see Chapter 5).

It is a high probability that infected macrophages transfer their "inclusions" during mitosis in the bone marrow onto the progeny cells. Lifelong carriers may be the result.

Stability of Chlamydia

The infectious elementary bodies, which can be stained as described by Giemsa, Gimenez, Stamp, Macchiavello's or Castaneda, can survive outside the host (protected by proteinaceous material) and inside host cells for several weeks.

Transmission

Elementary bodies present in feather dust and dried feces are primarily dispersed through air circulation. Ingestion of elementary bodies results in infection of the intestinal epithelial cells. Vertical transmission through the egg has been documented in domesticated ducks, Black-headed Gulls and budgerigars, and has been suggested in turkeys. Chlamydia can usually be detected in the feces ten days prior to the onset of clinical signs.

Cockatiels are frequent carriers of chlamydia and can shed the agent in the feces for more than one year following an active infection. Infected ducks have been shown to shed chlamydia in the feces for 100 days, and harbor the organism on the nasal mucosa for 170 days.

Clinical Disease and Pathology

Clinical Signs

Young birds exposed to high doses of a virulent strain develop acute systemic infections frequently resulting in death. Clinical signs can include rough plumage, low body temperature, tremor, lethargy, conjunctivitis, dyspnea, rales, coryza (pigeons) and sinusitis (budgerigars). Emaciation, dehydration, yellowish-to-greenish droppings (suggesting liver involvement), or grayish, watery droppings may also be noted. Death ensues within 8-14 days. Spontaneous recovery is rare. Survivors may have poorly formed feathers.

Subacute or protracted diseases are typical for all avian species with a reduced susceptibility or for those infected with a moderately virulent strain. Progressive emaciation, greenish diarrhea, occasional conjunctivitis and high levels of urates in the droppings are common. Clinical signs may be subtle and overlooked. Psittaciformes occasionally develop CNS signs, including paroxysmal or continuous clonic-tonic convulsions, tremors and opisthotonos. Untreated birds die within a few weeks.

A distinct, sometimes recurrent, keratoconjunctivitis with no other, or only subtle, signs has been described for small Australian parakeets (especially in the genus *Neophema*), pigeons, ducks, and European finches. Diseases in *Neophema* spp. are frequently refractory to therapy. Conjunctivitis and nasal discharge are characteristic of chlamydiosis in domestic pigeons. Mortality rates of the ophthalmic form are about 10%, but can reach 100% if untreated. Conjunctivitis may be the predominant clinical sign in infected domestic ducks and geese. Mortality, particularly in duck-lings, can range between 10-80%.

Chlamydiosis in ratites can cause clinical and pathologic lesions of a rather nonspecific type. High mortality has been reported in ostrich chicks infected with *C. psittaci*. The chronic course is clinically inconspicuous, although anemia is common and LDH and AST levels may be increased five to ten times. Birds with persistent infections may not be recognized until they infect other animals or their caretakers. The documentation of infections in nestlings from an apparently healthy breeding pair is also suggestive of latently infected adults.

Gross Lesions

Gross lesions can vary as widely as the clinical disease. Acute lesions are characterized by hepatomegaly, fibrinous peritonitis, air sacculitis, perihepatitis, pericarditis, bronchopneumonia, enteritis and nephrosis. Splenomegaly is frequently discussed as a common finding in chlamydiosis. However, fibrinous air sacculitis is more indicative of chlamydiosis in Psittaciformes and pigeons.

Splenomegaly may not occur with chlamydiosis at all. In sexually active males, chlamydial-induced orchitis or epididymitis results in permanent infertility. Oophoritis is rare.

Subacute to chronic lesions are characterized by anemia caused by a panmyelopathy in the bone marrow and tissue deficiencies of heterophils and macrophages. The pathogenesis of the panmyelopathy is undetermined. Chronic cases are characterized by proliferation of connective tissue (up to cirrhosis) in the liver and kidney. Pancreatic necrosis has been described particularly in budgerigars and pigeons.

Differential Diagnosis

The clinical and pathologic presentation of chlamydiosis is so variable that it can normally be ruled out only with laboratory investigations. The more common rule-outs include infections with herpesvirus, paramyxovirus, influenza A virus and Enterobacteriaceae, particularly salmonellosis. The CNS signs should be differentiated from Newcastle disease and salmonellosis, and the conjunctivitis in ducklings and goslings from influenza A infections and mycoplasmosis.

Diagnosis of Chlamydiosis

Diagnostic Methods

Cytology

Conjunctival smears of birds with conjunctivitis can be stained for intracellular inclusions called Levinthal-Cole-Lillie (LCL) bodies. As a rule, smears contain heterophils, some lymphocytes, some plasma cells and occasionally macrophage-like cells containing intracytoplasmic LCL bodies. Since LCL bodies are difficult to detect, a positive test is confirmatory while a negative smear does not rule out chlamydiosis. Immunofluorescent methods using commercially available conjugates are more sensitive.

Every veterinary hospital should be able to perform cytologic evaluation of imprint slides including postmortem samples of the liver, spleen and air sacs (see Chapter 10).

Table 34.1 Clinical Pathology Findings Associated with Chlamydiosis

Parameter	Change
WBC	Elevated (2-3 times normal)
Hct	Decreased (20-30%)
Heterophils	Normal
Lymphocytes	Decreased to normal
Monocytes	Normal
Eosinophils	Normal
Basophils	Normal
CPK	Elevated (>2 time normal)
LDH	Elevated (>2 times normal)
AST	Elevated (>3 times normal)
Total protein	Slight increase
Uric acid	Normal
Bile acids	Elevated (>2 times normal)

Culture

Culture of chlamydia is routinely performed in McCoy cell line, Buffalo Green Monkey cells or chicken embryo fibroblasts. Cell culture is sensitive and able to detect small numbers of chlamydia within two to three passages. For isolation, parenchymal organs (liver, spleen, lungs, kidneys,) and feces should be shipped in transport medium.

Antigen Detection Systems

Highly sensitive and specific ELISA test systems are available for detecting chlamydial antigen or anti-chlamydial antibodies. An antigen test kit developed for human *C. trachomatis* has been used successfully for *Chlamydia psittaci*, which has the same group-specific antigens. Comparisons between this test kit and cell culture indicated that false-negative results occurred with ELISA when insufficient numbers of chlamydial particles were present in the sample. False-negative cell culture results occurred when chlamydial organisms were no longer viable.

In evaluating 7,000 cloacal swabs for the diagnosis of chlamydiosis, it was determined that the antigen ELISA is sensitive, quick to perform.

Extremely high concentrations of avian *Staphylococcus aureus* (more than 10 or more than 1.5 x 10^9/ml suspension) can cause false-positive ELISA results. *Actinobacillus salpingitidis*, which is rarely found in feces, and *Acinetobacter calcoaceticum* can also cause false-positive results. *Staphylococcus hyicus*, a non-avian staphylococcus, has also been implicated in false-positive reactions.

Antibody Tests

Detection of anti-chlamydial antibodies using complement fixation (CF) was proven to be unsuitable because birds produce mainly non-CF antibodies following a chlamydial infection. The C1 of guinea pig complement, which is a critical component of the

CF test, is incompatible with the serum of many avian species. A test that functions independent of the species in question was necessary for serologic diagnosis of chlamydiosis in the class Aves. An inhibitory ELISA (= BELISA) that recognizes four times more infected birds than CF has been developed.

The relationship between CF and BELISA indicates that high anti-chlamydial antibody titers detected by CF and BELISA are indicative of a positive reaction; low titers are diagnostic only with BELISA. Ten months following an experimental chlamydial infection, CF antibodies decrease considerably, while BELISA shows a continuous increase. This finding suggests that the composition of the antibodies detected varies and that only those antibodies detected by BELISA are stimulated by the permanent intracellular presence of chlamydia.

The high sensitivity of BELISA has shown that *C. psittaci* antibodies are more widely distributed than previously thought. Sustained detection of antibodies by BELISA suggests that chlamydia may cause a lifelong persistent infection, which is difficult to eliminate with treatment.

Treatment of Chlamydiosis

Therapeutic Agents

Many countries have instigated governmental regulations for treatment and control of chlamydiosis to prevent zoonotic infections. The following therapeutic considerations address only the scientific aspects of treating chlamydiosis, and the reader should be aware of local laws governing therapy. Several antibiotics have *in vitro* activity against chlamydia, but only the tetracyclines and enrofloxacin have been used successfully *in vivo*, the latter only in limited trials.

The tetracyclines alter the replication of chlamydia by inhibiting the synthesis of enzymes, the growth and fission of the reticulate bodies and possibly the reorganization of the elementary bodies. The host defense mechanisms must be intact to remove damaged chlamydial elements before they can recover and begin replicating. Providing the immune system with the time necessary to remove these damaged reticulate and elementary bodies is one reason for long-term anti-chlamydia therapy.

Tetracyclines are effective only against actively metabolizing microorganisms, ie, during growth or fission. This drug is not effective in treating latently or persistently infected birds in which the chlamydia is located inertly in macrophages. Strains of chlamydia that are resistant to tetracyclines are still rather rare (one strain from ducks > 75 μg tetracycline), but strains with reduced sensitivity continue to be recognized. It has been shown that there is no direct correlation between the blood level of tetracyclines and therapeutic efficacy. Thus, the suggested blood level of >1 μg/ml cannot be assumed to equate with successful treatment.

Some chlamydial strains can develop resistance to tetracycline if exposed to subtherapeutic levels for prolonged periods of time.

In acutely sick birds chlamydial organisms undergoing rapid metabolism, and treatment with tetracyclines leads to immediate cessation of shedding and a clinical recovery in accordance with the severity of the parenchymatous lesions. In these birds, elimination of *Chlamydia psittaci* is possible; however, under practical conditions, not likely.

Chlortetracycline

Chlortetracycline (CTC) for oral application can be administered in soft mixed feed (cooked grain with or without egg [yolk, albumen]), in commercial parrot pellets or on dehulled seeds covered with CTC. The latter is recommended (500 ppm) for budgerigars and small finches. Food containing 5,000 ppm of CTC is normally provided, although there are many avian species, particularly among the Psittaciformes, that reach effective blood levels with CTC concentrations of 2,000-2,500 ppm. Birds will generally consume more food when it contains a lower concentration of CTC. Birds that have been shown to do well with food containing lower concentrations of CTC are listed in Table 34.3.

Chlortetracycline is renally excreted and should be used cautiously in patients with kidney damage (see Chapter 17). Birds dislike eating medicated feed or pellets, and therapeutic blood levels are reached only within ten days. Because infected birds will continue to shed, the delayed induction of proper blood levels poses an additional risk for caretakers and for other birds. No other food components can be fed during the treatment period.

Oxytetracycline

Intramuscular injections of oxytetracycline (OTC) at a dosage level of 100 mg/kg have been suggested. The birds listed in Table 34.3 should be given 75 mg/kg. Oxytetracycline (LA 200) produces a long-lasting blood level at a dose of 75-100 mg/kg body weight. Injections induce effective blood levels within hours, and the shedding of *Chlamydia psittaci* will stop 24 hours post-injection. This treatment regime also allows a bird to remain on its normal diet while being treated (see Chapter 18). OTC has the same side effects as CTC. In addition, severe muscle necrosis may occur at the site of injection.

Table 34.3 Birds that Respond to Lower Food Concentrations of CTC

Large macaws	Eastern Rosella
Genus *Agapornis*	Pale-headed Rosella
Grey-cheeked Parakeet	Red-fronted Parakeet
Canary-winged Parakeet	Turquoise Parakeet
Red-winged Parrot	Scarlet-crested Parrot
Mulga Parrot	Bourke's Parrot
Western Rosella	Cockatiel

Doxycycline

Doxycycline is a preparation that has been developed for intravenous administration in humans. The solvents are different in doxycycline products manufactured in the United States and Europe. Intravenous preparations available in the United States cause severe local necrosis of the muscles when given intramuscularly. European preparations may be safely given intramuscularly and induce blood levels of 1 mg/ml that last approximately seven days when administered at a dose of 75-100 mg/kg body weight. The quantity of drug to be injected is rather large, and several injection sites should be used.

During long-term treatment, which is still legally stipulated in many countries, the drug is increasingly eliminated from the blood so that injection intervals decrease. Some countries have regulations controlling the injection intervals, although these should vary according to the species. Doxycycline is excreted mainly extrarenally (feces, bile), and the metabolites are microbiologically almost inert. This treatment reduces the destruction of autogenous intestinal flora seen with other tetracyclines. A doxycycline-medicated food was found to provide >1 μg/ml plasma concentration in a group of psittacine birds (Table 34.4).

Table 34.4   Doxycycline-medicated Food Diet

29% canned cooked kidney beans
29% canned whole corn
29% cooked white rice
13% dry oatmeal cereal (by weight)
1000 mg doxycycline hyclate (from capsules) per kg of seed

Medicated diets have been found to maintain acceptable plasma doxycycline concentrations in Goffin's Cockatoos, African Grey Parrots, Blue-fronted Amazon Parrots and Orange-winged Amazon Parrots.

An antimicrobial that can be added to the drinking water and effectively treat chlamydia in Psittaciformes remains elusive, but enrofloxacin has shown some potential. Birds in the USA with severe, acute chlamydiosis can be initially treated with an IV injection of Vibramycin, followed by oral doxycycline when the bird is stabilized (generally in 24 hours).

A micronized suspension of doxycycline has shown moderate promise in the treatment of chlamydia. In one study involving pigeons, IM administration of micronized doxycycline (100 mg/kg body weight) three times at weekly intervals maintained a plasma level about 1 μg/ml for 43 days.

Apart from specific treatment with tetracyclines, symptomatic therapy in acutely sick birds is frequently necessary. Birds should be kept isolated in warm rooms, and intravenous fluids, hepatoprotective therapy and paramunity inducers should be administered according to the clinical signs. Chicks should be fed frequently with small amounts of a liquid formula. [*Editor's Note: Often, secondary bacterial pathogens must be addressed separately as most will not respond to the tetracyclines.*]

Enrofloxacin

Enrofloxacin inhibits the *in vitro* growth of *C. psittaci*, but only a few avian strains have been tested. The MIC of enrofloxacin for *C. psittaci* was found to be 0.125 mg/L; the minimum bactericidal concentration is much higher: 50-75 mg/L. Concentrations between 0.5 and 1.0 mg/L evoked irreversible damage to the majority of the chlamydia particles.

Preliminary results indicate that treatment with enrofloxacin-medicated food for three weeks was effective in eliminating chlamydia from parakeets. Seven groups of experimentally infected budgerigars and other psittaciforme birds (Alexander Ringnecked Parakeet, Senegal Parrot, Canary-winged Parakeet) were effectively treated for 14 days with medicated food containing 500 ppm (budgerigars=250 ppm) enrofloxacin. From seven days after the beginning of treatment until four to five weeks after the end of treatment, no chlamydia could be isolated. Complete elimination of chlamydia from a quarantined group of 196 Senegal Parrots was reached only after substituting their normal mixed food with medicated corn containing 1000 ppm enrofloxacin. A minimum blood level of 0.5 mg/L for enrofloxacin for at least 14 days was considered necessary to control chlamydiosis.

Control

Persistent, probably lifelong, infections require new ideas on control. Legal regulations should be reformulated and concentrate on clinically sick and seropositive birds. Seronegative birds should not be treated. During treatment and in clinically healthy but infected flocks, regular cleaning and disinfecting programs will minimize the chlamydial contamination in the environment and reduce the occurrence of reinfection or transmission. Birds that recover from chlamydiosis are fully susceptible to future infections. Ideally, breeding birds would be seronegative for chlamydia but, given the prevalence of the organism as detected by antibody titers in the companion bird population, it seems unlikely that a seronegative population could be established. Free-ranging birds that may transmit chlamydia should not have access to aviary birds.

Zoonotic Potential

C. psittaci strains from Psittaciformes, domesticated ducks (in Europe) and turkeys (in USA) appear to cause the most severe disease in humans.

Human infections are characterized by flu-like clinical signs including a high fever, severe headaches, chills, shortness of breath and general debilitation. If untreated, atypical pneumonia or CNS signs mainly caused by meningitis can develop, in addition to liver and kidney lesions due to the presence of toxicity.

In rare cases, neuritis with severe pain is described. Chronic manifestations can be arteritis, cardiovascular insufficiencies and thrombophlebitis including insufficiency of the venal valves. Treatment with doxycycline is recommended for three weeks.

Chlamydiosis is a reportable disease in the United States because of its potential as a zoonotic agent. Current regulations dictate closing a business or aviary, a forced quarantine period and treatment of all exposed birds with chlortetracycline-medicated foods. These recommendations do not effectively address the problems associated with treating or controlling chlamydiosis and should be evaluated and modified accordingly.

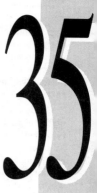

MYCOSES

Louise Bauck

Common Fungal Diseases

Candidiasis

Candida albicans is an opportunistic yeast that can cause a variety of problems associated with the avian digestive tract. *Candida* sp. can apparently be a primary cause of crop-related infections or can be a secondary pathogen that takes advantage of an already damaged esophageal mucosa or of a slowed crop-emptying time.

Transmission and Predisposing Factors

The loss of normal bacterial flora (eg, through the use of antibiotics) can cause an increase in the number of candida organisms. Immature animals are thought to develop spontaneous primary candidiasis possibly because of an immature immune system or incompletely developed gastrointestinal (GI) defenses. Neonatal cockatiels are thought to be especially prone to primary candidiasis.

Pathogenesis and Incubation

The magnitude and outcome of the infection may depend on the age of the bird and status of the immune system. Chronic or systemic infections may result in septate hyphae and reproductive chlamydospores that can be demonstrated by histologic examination. *Candida* sp. infections are characterized by necrosis with minimal inflammation.

Systemic candidiasis is rare but has been reported in companion birds. In these cases, yeast may be present in the blood, bone marrow and parenchymous organs. Severe stress or immunosuppression may be necessary to potentiate systemic infections.

Clinical Disease and Pathology

In most young birds, the crop is the principal site of a candida infection. In many cases, the crop may be the only portion of the digestive tract affected. However, several reports also indicate that in some young birds, the proventriculus or ventriculus can be the primary site of yeast replication in the absence of crop lesions. The characteristic *Candida* lesion is a catarrhal-to-mucoid exudate consisting of raised, white mucosal plaques and whitish-to-clear mucus that may or may not be associated with a foul odor. Chronic cases may develop a "turkish towel" appearance produced by multiple tag-like plaques of mucosa and inflammatory cells.

Clinical signs associated with candida-induced ingluvitis in neonates include regurgitation or vomiting, increased crop-emptying time, depression, anorexia and occasional crop impactions. In older birds, the crop may be distended with mucus, and crop emptying may be hindered by necrotic mucosal debris. Candida lesions in the oral cavity are recognized by the appearance of white plaques covered by a tenacious mucus. Candida has been associated with impacted food, beak abnormalities and tongue necrosis in a variety of adult birds. Yeast infections in ratites have been associated with extensive necrosis of the upper beak.

Yeast infections affecting the cloaca and vent of turkeys and geese have been reported. Skin lesions, particularly on the head and neck, have been described in companion birds and pigeons. Primary candida infections have also been associated with foot lesions in waterfowl. Respiratory infections caused by candida occasionally have been reported in psittacine birds.

Diagnosis and Differential Diagnosis

A Gram's stain of material collected from the site of suspected infection is helpful in confirming a diagnosis. Identifying yeast with a Gram's stain suggests only that the organism is present. Histologic evaluation of biopsy samples is necessary to confirm that the yeast are causing pathologic changes. However, identifying large numbers of budding organisms is suggestive of a prolific population of yeast. Negative cytologic results do not rule out candidiasis, because deep mucosal scrapings are necessary to achieve adequate samples in some cases.

Gram's stains usually provide adequate visualization of yeast but dry smears can also be stained with Diff-Quik and new methylene blue. Lactophenol cotton blue is recommended for wet mounts. The yeast organism, which is often budding, is small (3-6 μm diameter), and has been compared to the size of an avian red blood cell nucleus. Hyphal forms are considered more diagnostic of a primary yeast infection but are less commonly found in a live patient.

Because candida is frequently a secondary pathogen, the clinician should attempt to determine the predisposing factors that lead to a candida infection. Oral and upper gastrointestinal candidiasis may show signs similar to those of trichomoniasis, hypovitaminosis A, avian poxviruses, bacterial infections, psittacine beak and feather disease, neonatal gastrointestinal viruses, ingested foreign bodies and toxicities. Culturing the organism may be helpful, especially in cases involving beak abnormalities or systemic problems. Sabouraud's or cornmeal agar are the recommended culture media.

Treatment

Nystatin is the most frequently used medication for initially treating upper gastrointestinal candidiasis in the avian patient, although some of the azole antifungals are undoubtedly more effective. Nystatin has few side effects and is not absorbed from the gastrointestinal tract following oral administration. It is readily accepted by most birds and can be mixed with a neonate's feeding formula (Table 35.1). Ocular candidiasis is usually responsive to amphotericin B ointment or amphotericin B injected subconjunctivally.

Ketoconazole is recommended for severe or refractory candidiasis. Ketoconazole is normally mixed with a slightly acidic liquid (eg, orange juice, pineapple juice) to facilitate its dilution.

Strains of *Candida* spp. resistant to ketoconazole have been reported, and fluconazole has been suggested as a treatment of choice for these strains.

Itraconazole has also been used to treat candidiasis, but may offer no real advantage over other azoles. Azole antifungals may cause depression, anorexia, vomiting and hepatic toxicity.

Table 35.1	Some Antifungal Agents Used in Companion Species
Amphotericin B (injectable)	1.5 mg/kg IV q8h x 3 days 1 mg/ml saline intratracheal q12h 1 mg/kg saline nebulized for 15 min. q12h
Flucytosine (capsules)	250 mg/kg PO q12h x 21 days
Ketoconazole suspension (tablets)	10-30 mg/kg q12h x 21 days
Itraconazole (beads in capsules)	5-10 mg/kg q12h in food x 7-21 days
Fluconazole (tablets)	5 mg/kg q24h x 7 days
Nystatin suspension	100,000 units (1 ml) per 400 g bird PO q12h x 7 days

Aspergillosis

Aspergillosis is a frequent cause of respiratory disease in companion, aviary and free-ranging birds. *Aspergillus fumigatus* is the most common etiologic agent, followed in frequency by *A. flavus* and *A. niger*. Aspergillosis may be chronic and insidious, or it may cause peracute death. Established aspergillosis infections are clinically challenging to resolve.

Transmission and Predisposing Factors

Among companion birds, a high prevalence of aspergillosis has been reported in African Grey Parrots, Blue-fronted Amazon Parrots and mynah birds.

Gallinaceous birds (particularly quail) often become infected as chicks following inhalation of spores from contaminated brooders. Hand-raised psittacine birds could be infected in a similar manner. Older gallinaceous birds, and presumably aviary birds as well, can be exposed when maintained on moist contaminated bedding.

Pathogenesis and Incubation

Aspergillus is ubiquitous, and infections should always be considered to occur secondarily to an immunosuppressive event. It has been suggested that healthy birds exposed to high concentrations of spores are generally resistant to infections, while immunocompromised hosts exposed to small concentrations of spores are frequently infected.

Clinical Disease and Pathology

Clinical signs associated with aspergillus infections of the respiratory tract may include dyspnea, depression and emaciation (Table 35.2). Open-mouthed breathing, pronounced excursions of the keel, tail "bobs" and respiratory distress after exercise are typical. Biliverdinuria is common. Wheezing, squeaking or stertor and a voice change are also sometimes present. Posterior paresis and lameness were the presenting signs in a Black Palm Cockatoo with *Aspergillus* spp. air sacculitis that spread to the kidney and pelvic nerve roots.

Table 35.2 Clinical Findings in Companion Birds with Aspergillosis

Emaciation	64%
Respiratory distress	26%
Neuromuscular disease	18%
Abnormal droppings	11%
Regurgitation	9%
Vocalization changes	7%
Poor appetite	7%
Nasal discharge	4%
Gout	4%
Hemoptysis	2%

Destruction of adjacent tissue, including bone or beak, may be substantial. Nasal aspergillosis typically presents as a dry, granulomatous, destructive swelling within one nostril. Tracheal or syringeal aspergillosis lesions usually occur as plugs of creamy white necrotic debris at or near the tracheal bifurcation. Ocular aspergillosis in chicks may be recognized as a white exudate within the conjunctival sac.

Diagnosis and Differential Diagnosis

Fungal culture, hematology, serology, cytology, radiology and endoscopy or exploratory surgery are among the methods used to diagnose infections. It should be noted that culture of *Aspergillus* spp. in the absence of lesions is not diagnostic, because the organism is ubiquitous in the environment. Radiographic findings can be negative or may show hyperinflation (enlargement) of the abdominal air sacs, focal densities in lungs or air sacs, reduced coelomic cavity details, loss of definition of air sac walls and asymmetrical opacity of abdominal air sacs. Cytology of air sac washes or endoscopic-guided biopsy is useful in diagnosing lower respiratory infections.

Table 35.4 Typical Clinical Pathology Changes with Aspergillosis

Leukocytosis - heterophilia	Monocytosis
Lymphopenia	Nonregenerative anemia
Hyperproteinemia	Hypergammaglobulinemia

For definitive antemortem diagnosis, cytologic samples from granulomas with associated mycelial areas (wet mounts with lactophenol cotton blue, new methylene blue and culture on Sabouraud dextrose agar or blood agar) may be diagnostic. The presence of branching septate hyphae, sometimes with spores and sporulating areas, is highly suggestive. If access to a suggestive lesion is not available, then serology may be helpful. Although not widely available, aspergillosis titers using ELISA systems show promise in diagnosing infections.

The differential diagnosis for a mature bird with weight loss and severe heterophilia might include chlamydiosis and mycobacteriosis. Neoplastic disease may sometimes cause weight loss and heterophilia.

Treatment

Treatment of aspergillosis often depends on the location and extent of the lesion. Resolving advanced cases of aspergillosis is difficult, especially in anatomic areas where surgical removal of affected tissues is not possible. Correction of underlying stress factors is a mandatory component of successful therapy. Surgical debridement of plaques and granulomas should be employed when feasible. Flushing lesions with amphotericin B or chlorhexidine solutions may be helpful, although caution should be exercised in certain anatomic areas. A severe granulomatous sinusitis occurred in an African Grey Parrot following the accidental use of amphotericin B suspension rather than a solution as a nasal flush.

Intratracheal administration of amphotericin B has been used in treating tracheal and pulmonary aspergillosis. The medication is given via the glottis during inspiration and the patient is positioned to distribute the drug to the affected anatomic area. Nebulization with antifungals may be helpful in early cases of upper respiratory aspergillosis.

Systemic therapy is difficult because amphotericin B must normally be administered intravenously q8h for three days. Intraosseous administration should be possible, but has not been documented. Amphotericin B is potentially nephrotoxic.

Flucytosine is also frequently used to treat aspergillosis, especially in combination with amphotericin B (Table 35.5). The advantage to this drug is that it can be administered orally; however, bone marrow toxicity has been reported in some cases. Monitoring for hematologic changes suggestive of bone marrow damage is recommended when this drug is used.

Table 35.5 Suggested Concurrent Therapy for Advanced Aspergillosis

Amphotericin B - IV and/or IT or in the affected air sac - q12h x 5 days
Ketoconazole - orally - q8h x 10 days
Flucytosine - orally - q8h x 20-30 days
Kapracydin A - orally - q8h x 5 days

Ketoconazole has been used to successfully treat aspergillosis in some avian species. This drug preparation has an advantage over other antifungals in having a wide therapeutic index.

Current information suggests that itraconazole may have greater efficacy against *Aspergillus* spp. than amphotericin B or any other azole antifungal. Itraconazole is thought to be less toxic than amphotericin B, but its safety in most companion bird species has not been established. Itraconazole has been used in waterfowl, shorebirds, poultry and penguins without serious side effects. Anorexia, vomiting and depression have been reported in an African Grey Parrot being treated with itraconazole.

Cryptococcosis

Cryptococcus neoformans is an imperfect, saprophytic yeast that has been reported as a cause of disease in psittacine birds and pigeons. In companion birds, a diagnosis of cryptococcosis is usually made at postmortem.

Antemortem diagnosis of cryptococcosis may be challenging. An impression smear of any accessible gelatinous material may reveal the characteristic encapsulated yeast-like organism. A latex agglutination antibody titer may be elevated in an exposed or infected bird.

Dyspnea, weight loss and anemia are frequent clinical signs, and heterophilia may or may not be present. The clinician should exercise caution when being exposed to clinical material that may contain *C. neoformans* spores.

The prognosis for disseminated cryptococcosis is poor. Amphotericin B and ketoconazole have been suggested as possible therapies. Cryptococcosis is a potentially serious zoonosis and may occur when humans inhale dust from the dried droppings of pigeons, starlings or other avian species. Treating cryptococcus cases should be carefully considered given the zoonotic potential for this organism.

Histoplasmosis

Histoplasmosis is similar to cryptococcosis in many ways but is less commonly reported in birds. *Histoplasma capsulatum* is an infectious but not contagious disease of the reticuloendothelial system. This fungus could potentially proliferate in enclosed aviaries with dirt floors.

Diagnosis of histoplasmosis is based on culture of the organism (mycelial phase may sometimes be recovered on Sabouraud's agar) and histopathology (periodic acid-Schiff, Bauer's and Gridley stains).

Histoplasma sp. has zoonotic potential and may cause pneumonitis that progresses to a disseminated disease of the reticuloendothelial system.

PARASITES

Ellis C. Greiner
Branson W. Ritchie

It should be stressed that identifying a parasite (or parasite egg) does not imply clinical disease. Many parasites coexist with their avian hosts without causing pathologic changes. Long-term symbiotic parasite-host relationships are usually characterized by benign infections compared with parasites that have been recently introduced to a new host. The fact that companion and aviary birds from widely varying geographic regions are combined creates an opportunity for exposure of a naive host to parasitic organisms that may cause few problems in their natural host. Parasites that are apathogenic in endemic avifauna can cause chronic disease or rapid death in unnatural hosts.

With companion and aviary bird species, parasitic infections are most common in birds that are recently imported or that have access to the ground. Some parasites are host-specific, while others can infect a wide range of avian species. Free-ranging birds should be restricted from an aviary to prevent them from serving as sources for parasites. Parasitic problems are best managed by designing facilities that restrict a bird's access to infectious stages of a parasite and by practicing sound hygiene. Birds maintained indoors or in suspended welded wire enclosures are unlikely to have parasites that have an indirect transmission cycle. In contrast, parasitic infections are common in countries where birds are maintained in walk-in type aviaries with access to the ground.

Diagnosis of Parasites

Diagnosis in the Living Bird

Depending on the parasite, appropriate antemortem diagnostic samples could include feces, blood, tissue biopsies or integument for the detection of intact parasites, eggs or intermediate life forms.

The diagnostic stage of most avian helminths is an egg that is detected in the feces by either flotation or sedimentation. The most generally used flotation medium is saturated sodium nitrate (568 g sodium nitrate/1000 ml water). Sheather's sugar solution (500 g table sugar, 320 ml water and 6.5 g phenol crystals) is most commonly used to detect coccidian oocysts. Saturated zinc sulfate (336 g zinc sulfate/ 1000 ml water) is best for concentrating cysts of *Giardia* and may be better for detecting spiruroid eggs than sodium nitrate.

Fecal sedimentation is used primarily for the detection of fluke eggs that do not float in commonly used media. Feces is mixed in a liquid soap-in-water solution (0.1-1%) and allowed to stand for five minutes without centrifugation. The supernatant is gently removed and the tube is refilled with soapy water and allowed to stand for another five minutes. This procedure removes particulate material and concentrates the fluke eggs. It can also be used in place of flotation to detect eggs and cysts but is more time-consuming and may not be as sensitive as a flotation method.

Greiner's Tenets for Fecal Examination

1. Examine an adequate quantity (1-2 grams) of fresh feces. Some nematode eggs will larvate if allowed to age, producing atypical eggs or larvae that are difficult to identify. Some parasitic forms (trophozoites of *Giardia* for example) are fragile and will perish if the sample is not examined immediately.

2. Collect feces per cloaca or from nonabsorbent cage lining such as waxed paper or aluminum foil. Using nonabsorbent material to collect feces provides a moist sample of greater volume when compared to scraping a sample off newsprint or paper toweling. Samples collected from corn cob, wood shavings or cat litter should not be considered diagnostic.

3. Conduct the test that specifically demonstrates the parasite that is most likely to be causing the clinical changes. Fluke eggs cannot be demonstrated by flotation. Trophozoites of *Giardia* and *Trichomonas* will be destroyed if placed into saturated salt or sugar flotation solutions. *Giardia* trophozoites die in tap water and are best identified by using warm saline or lactated Ringer's solution as a diluent.

4. Examine each prepared sample completely and systematically. The low power objective (10x) should be used for scanning. The high dry objective can be used to magnify and examine a particular structure. Scan the coverslip beginning at one corner and traversing the length of the coverslip, then move the slide to the next field of view and reverse the field of movement. Repeating this procedure until the entire coverslip has been viewed will provide a systematic examination of the total preparation and reduce the likelihood of missing a parasite. Examine the entire slide and do not stop when eggs of one kind have been identified. Some helminths produce very few eggs that may not be detected unless the entire slide is examined.

5. Standardize procedures so that results are repeatable and comparable. If a diagnostic technique is not standardized, the results are of limited value. Egg counts are of little value because there is no direct correlation between the number of eggs per gram of feces and the number of adult parasites present. Comparing egg counts between treated and untreated birds may provide some information on the effect of an anthelmintic.

A direct smear is best for detecting motile protozoan trophozoites (*Giardia, Trichomonas* or *Hexamita*). Samples are not diagnostic if they are more than 15 minutes old. Feces or tissue swabs are mixed with LRS or normal saline (0.85% sodium chloride), not tap water. The proper density of the preparation is achieved when newsprint can be easily read through the preparation. The microscope light should be adjusted to provide maximum contrast. The morphology of the parasites may be confirmed by fixing feces in polyvinyl alcohol and staining a slide preparation with trichrome.

Blood films are used to detect avian hematozoa, including microfilariae of filarial worms. Commonly identified blood parasites include intracellular stages of *Plasmodium, Haemoproteus, Leucocytozoon* and *"Atoxoplasma,"* and extracellular stages of *Trypanosoma* and microfilariae from various filarial worms.

Arthropods collected for identification should be fixed and stored in 70% ethanol. Mites, ticks, fleas and lice can be placed directly into 70% alcohol. Arthropods may be removed from the skin or feathers with forceps, or those living under crusting skin can be collected by scraping the encrusted area with a dull scalpel and allowing the crusts to fall into a petri dish containing 70% ethanol.

Feather mites can be collected by placing the affected feather in 70% ethanol. Quill mites (ones living in the shaft of the feather) may be detected by microscopically examining the transparent portion of plucked primary feathers or coverts. These parasites can be recovered by slitting the shaft lengthwise and placing it in alcohol. The use of a pyrethrin-based flea spray, designed for puppies and kittens, is a safe and easy way to collect topical parasites from birds. A minimal dose (one drop under each wing of a cockatiel) is effective.

Diagnosis in Dead Birds

Any bird that dies should be necropsied and tissues should be collected for histopathology. If parasites are identified, they should be collected for classification. Gross and histologic lesions should be correlated with any recovered parasite to determine if the organism is contributing to a specific set of clinical changes.

It is always a good policy to contact the parasitologist and request special submission instructions.

The complete gastrointestinal tract should be opened lengthwise, section by section. In small birds, each section of bowel may be opened in a series of petri dishes containing water. In large birds, the bowel contents should be washed through #40 and #100 standard sieves. The mucosa should be scraped to free attached helminths, and the residue on the sieve should be back-flushed into a dish and evaluated for the presence of parasites. Detection and recovery of helminths can also be accomplished by placing the gut contents into one-liter flasks and allowing a sediment to form. This procedure is repeated until the water remains clear. Parenchymous organs should be sequentially sliced and evaluated for the presence of helminths. The body cavities, air sacs and orbits of the eyes should be examined grossly for worms. Skin over swellings on the feet or legs should be excised, and the area should be examined for the presence of adult filarial worms. All recoverable parasites should be collected to maximize the information that can be ascertained from the infection.

Nematodes should be placed briefly in full-strength glacial acetic acid or hot 70% ethanol. This process should kill and fix the nematodes in a straight, uncoiled manner. They should then be transferred into glycerin alcohol (9.0 parts 70% ethanol and 1.0 part glycerin) for storage.

Cestodes should be relaxed in tap water in a refrigerator for two to four hours and then fixed in AFA (8.5 parts 70% ethanol,

1.0 part full strength formalin and 0.5 part glacial acetic acid). The parasites collected should have an intact scolex (holdfast), which is important in tapeworm identification.

Trematodes should be relaxed by placing them in tap water in the refrigerator for 30-60 minutes. Thin-bodied flukes should be placed into AFA. Thick-bodied flukes should be gently held in place between two glass microscope slides while AFA is instilled between the slides. After a few minutes, the top slide is removed.

Acanthocephalans should be gently removed from the gut wall to prevent rupture of the parasite, which will destroy the hydraulic system that extends the proboscis (making identification of the parasite nearly impossible). Acanthocephalans may lose their torpor and detach from the gut wall when the host dies. They may then resemble a yellowish to whitish, short, wrinkled tapeworm. Placing the parasite into tap water overnight in a refrigerator may cause the proboscis to extend, at which point the parasite is fixed in AFA.

A fecal examination should be performed at necropsy so that eggs detected by fecal flotation or sedimentation can be compared to the eggs in the adult worms.

Clinically Significant Parasites

Protozoa

Gastrointestinal Flagellates

Trichomonas: Trichomonads do not require an intermediate host or vector and are transmitted through direct contact or through ingestion of contaminated water or food. Infected adults can transmit the parasite to their chicks during feeding activities. Parental feeding of young is an effective method of parasite transmission. There is no resistant cyst form, and only the motile trophozoite has been described. This extracellular parasite measures 8-14 mm in length (may vary in different host species), has four free anterior flagella and possesses an undulating membrane that creates a wave-like appearance along the cell surface. It moves in a jerky manner and the body diameter remains constant as it moves.

Depending on the species, infections may be localized in the mouth, oropharynx, esophagus, crop and trachea, or the pulmonary and hepatic tissues can be invaded. Infections in young birds are generally associated with poor growth and high mortality. In adult birds, infections are usually characterized by emaciation, dyspnea or vomiting. Blue-fronted Amazon Parrots, cockatiels and budgerigars are known to be susceptible. Trichomoniasis is particularly common in pigeons and raptors (frounce) (see Chapter 8). Pathogenic and non-pathogenic strains of *T. gallinae* have been described in pigeons; thus, not all infections may be a threat to the host. Feeding pigeons to captive raptors (especially species that do not normally eat pigeons such as eagles and large hawks) may result in the transmission of *Trichomonas*. Advanced cases with large necrotic masses are difficult to treat and generally have a poor prognosis (see Chapter 19).

Giardia: The *Giardia* sp. recovered from budgerigars appears to be morphologically distinct from those found in other animals and has been identified as *G. psittaci*. Most reports of giardiasis in psittacine birds involve budgerigars, cockatiels, lovebirds and Grey-cheeked Parakeets. Rarely, infections may be detected in Amazon parrots, conures, cockatoos, macaws, toucans, Galliformes and Anseriformes. Giardia has not been reported in finches or canaries.

Giardia sp. is commonly found in the feces of asymptomatic adult budgerigars and cockatiels, suggesting an asymptomatic carrier state.

Psittacine birds with giardiasis may be asymptomatic, or the birds may exhibit signs of loose, malodorous stools, mucoid diarrhea, debilitation, gram-negative enteritis, anorexia, depression, recurrent yeast infections, eosinophilia and hypoproteinemia. Dry skin and feather picking, particularly in the carpal-metacarpal, flank, axilla and lower leg areas, have been described as clinical signs of giardiasis in budgerigars and cockatiels (see Chapter 24). Giardiasis can cause poor growth and high mortality in budgerigar and cockatiel neonates. Mortality rates of 20-50% have been described in some infected budgerigar flocks.

Birds that recover from an infection are susceptible to reinfection indicating that a long-lasting protective immune response does not occur with infection.

Direct transmission occurs following the ingestion of food contaminated with feces from infected birds. The environmentally stable cysts can serve as a source of infection to other hosts.

Cytologic preparations must be examined within ten minutes of collection or trophozoites may not be recognized. False-negative results are common if the feces is over ten minutes old when it is examined. Trophozoites are flat and move in a smooth rolling manner. If a fecal sample cannot be examined immediately, it should be fixed in polyvinyl alcohol for trichrome staining.

Multiple, fresh, direct fecal smears stained with carbol fuchsin (one minute) or iodine may help in detecting trophozoites. Flotation techniques with zinc sulfate may improve the accuracy of a diagnosis. Trophozoites can range from 10-20 μm in length and 5-15 μm in width, depending on the host or type of fixation. The trophozoites have eight paired flagella (including an anterior and trailing posterior pair), two nuclei and a sucking disc that occupies most of the rounded end. The sucking disc may be seen if the light is adjusted to maximize contrast. The cysts measure 10-14 μm x 8-10 μm and contain four nuclei and fibrillar structures.

Keeping the aviary as clean and dry as possible will reduce the viability and number of cysts available for transmission. Relapses are common after treatment either from endogenous parasites that are not destroyed or from reinfection from exposure to environmental reservoirs. *Giardia* appear to be limited in host range, and species isolated from birds have not been found to be infectious in mammals.

Hexamita: *Hexamita* sp. has been detected in emaciated Splendid Grass Parakeets and cockatiels and can cause loose stool and weight loss. This genus has a trophozoite with eight flagella and two nuclei as does *Giardia*, but it lacks the sucking disc and is often truncated in appearance. Cysts are probably the infectious form. Generally, *Hexamita* is smaller than *Giardia,* swims in a smooth linear fashion and may be associated with chronic diarrhea. *Hexamita* has been described as a cause of disease in lories.

Histomonas: Histomoniasis is common in gallinaceous birds. The induced disease is called blackhead and is caused by a flagellated protozoan parasite (*Histomonas meleagridis*). When lesions occur, they generally include hepatomegaly (with necrosis) and ascites. Most infections occur following the ingestion of infected embryonated eggs of the cecal worm *Heterakis gallinarum.* The histomonas are released from the larvae and invade the wall of the cecum where they may cause ulceration or small nodules. Parasites in the liver can cause severe hepatocellular necrosis.

Coccidia

Coccidian parasites include a variety of life styles and means of transmission. Oocysts of most genera are passed unsporulated. They are typically less than 45 μm in length, contain a granular-appearing spherical body (sporoblast) and may be round, ellipsoid or ovoid. There may be a thinning of the wall (the micropyle), and if the micropyle is present, it may have a cap. The wall may be smooth, mammillated or pitted and colorless to dark brown. Coccidia are common in mynahs, toucans, pigeons, canaries, finches and lories.

Eimeria and Isospora: Two species of *Eimeria* and one of *Isospora* have been described in psittacines. *Eimeria dunsingi* oocysts are ovoid, lack a micropyle and are 26-39 x 22-28 μm. *E. haematodi* has broad ovoid oocysts with a large micropyle and measures 25-40 x 21-35 μm. *Isospora psittaculae* are round to broadly elliptical and measure 29-33 x 24-29 μm. Sporulated oocysts of *Eimeria* are subdivided into four sporocysts each with two sporozoites, whereas with *Isospora*, the oocysts have two sporocysts each with four sporozoites.

Isospora is most common in Passeriformes, Psittaciformes and Piciformes, and *Eimeria* is most common in Galliformes and Columbiformes. Infected birds may be asymptomatic or develop clinical signs of melena, depression, diarrhea, anorexia and death. Direct transmission occurs through ingestion of fecal-contaminated food or water.

Atoxoplasma: *Atoxoplasma* spp. may cause disease in canaries and other Passeriformes. Adults are generally asymptomatic carriers that shed oocysts in the feces. Prevalence can be high in young birds during fledging. The *Atoxoplasma* sp. found in House Sparrows was not found to be infectious to canaries, indicating a degree of host specificity.

Mortality can approach 80% in juvenile birds between two and nine months of age. Clinical signs are nonspecific including depression, anorexia and diarrhea. An enlarged liver and dilated bowel loops can occasionally be observed through the transparent skin.

Atoxoplasma serini has an asexual reproductive cycle in the mononuclear cells, and spreads through the blood to parenchymal organs where it infects reticuloendothelial and intestinal epithelial cells. *Atoxoplasma* spp. may be diagnosed by finding 20.1 x 19.2 μm oocysts in the feces or by demonstrating reddish intracytoplasmic inclusion bodies in mononuclear cells (Giemsa stain). Staining a buffy coat may improve the diagnostic sensitivity of blood smears. Transmission is direct through ingestion of contaminated feces. Coccidial oocysts are environmentally stable and are not killed by most disinfectants.

No effective therapy for atoxoplasmosis has been described, but primaquine has been suggested to suppress the tissue form of the parasite, and sulfachlor-pyrazine may decrease oocyst shedding. *Atoxoplasma* infections may persist for over four months, while *Isospora* infections are usually resolved within several weeks.

[*Editor's Note: Placing perches to eliminate defecation in food and water bowls and using wire cage bottoms to limit chick access to feces helps prevent infection of young birds.*]

Cryptosporidium: *Cryptosporidium* are spheroid-to-ovoid protozoa that infect and may cause disease in the mucosal epithelial cells lining the gastrointestinal, respiratory and urinary tracts of birds. *Cryptosporidium* develop intracellularly at an extracytoplasmic location on the apical surface of epithelial cells. This is in contrast to other coccidia, which replicate in the cytoplasm. *Cryptosporidium* oocysts are the smallest of any coccidia, usually measure 4-8 μm in diameter and contain four naked sporozoites.

Cryptosporidiosis has been documented in Galliformes, Anseriformes, Psittaciformes, ostriches, canaries and finches (Table 36.4). Limited data suggest that cryptosporidial infections may be transmitted among closely related species, which should be considered when managing this coccidia in a collection.

TABLE 36.4 Location of Cryptosporidiosis Lesions by Species

Chickens	Respiratory tract, gastrointestinal tract, urinary tract
Ducks	Respiratory tract
Turkeys	Respiratory tract, gastrointestinal tract
Peafowl	Respiratory tract
Pheasants	Respiratory tract
Quail	Respiratory tract, gastrointestinal tract
Junglefowl	Respiratory tract, urinary tract
Geese	Gastrointestinal tract
Psittaciformes	Gastrointestinal tract
Finches	Urinary tract

This coccidian parasite can be transmitted through the ingestion or inhalation of sporulated oocysts. The life cycle is direct. *Cryptosporidium* undergoes endogenous sporulation resulting in autoinfection in the parasitized host.

Cryptosporidium spp. are sporulated when shed in the feces so the frequent cleaning regimes that are used to control other coccidia are ineffective in preventing exposure to cryptosporidial oocysts. It is resistant to many disinfectants. Formal saline (10%), ammonia (5%) and heating to 65°C for 30 minutes have been suggested as effective control measures for *Cryptosporidium*.

The small size of the organism (4-6 μm) and low shedding rate make diagnosis of infection difficult. Diagnosis can be improved by centrifuging diluted feces in a high-concentration salt solution or using Sheather's flotation. *Cryptosporidium* spp. that infect birds are different from the species that infect mammals and there is no known zoonotic potential.

Toxoplasma: *Toxoplasma* is a coccidian parasite with an indirect life cycle. Toxoplasmosis, causing fatal infections in most species, has been documented in the Red Lory, Swainson's Lorikeet, Regent Parrot, Superb Parrot and Crimson Rosella. *Toxoplasma gondii* is considered a ubiquitous organism with a broad host range, and probably could infect any mammalian or avian host. Oocysts produced and passed in the feces of infected cats would be the only source of infection to psittacine birds. Infections may cause congestion and consolidation of the lungs, hepatomegaly, vasculitis and necrotic foci in the lungs, liver and heart.

Sarcocystis: Sarcocystis is a coccidian parasite that undergoes sexual multiplication in the intestine of a definitive host. *Sarcocystis falcatula* appears to be restricted to North America and has been associated with acute deaths in a variety of psittacine species. The pathogenicity of sarcocystosis in psittacine birds appears to depend on the species of bird and the infective dose of the parasite. Severe life-threatening infections are most common in Old World Psittaciformes although neonates of New World species may also die following infection. Adult New World Psittaciformes appear to be relatively resistant.

Infections are usually peracute; birds may appear normal and healthy one day and be dead the next.

Pulmonary edema with hemorrhage is the most consistent sign in birds that die acutely. Splenomegaly and hepatomegaly also are common. Generally, psittacine birds die before sarcocysts develop in the muscles.

The two-host replication cycle of *S. falcatula* involves sexual reproduction and sporogony in the intestines of the definitive host (opossum) with passage of infectious sporulated oocysts or sporocysts in the feces. Following ingestion of the sporocysts, asexual reproduction with schizogony and sarcocyst formation occur in the intermediate host (psittacine birds). The ingested sporozoites invade intestinal mucosa followed by infection of numerous tissues and schizogony in the reticuloendothelial cells, particularly in the lungs. Asexual reproduction then occurs in the walls of arterioles (first cycle) and capillary and venule walls (second cycle). These replication cycles can cause occlusion of the affected vessels resulting in the fatal lesions characteristic of infections in Old World Psittaciformes.

Psittacine birds in outdoor facilities throughout the range of the opossum are at risk. Infected opossums can shed sporocysts in the feces for 100 days. Cockroaches can serve as transport hosts by eating infected opossum feces and being consumed by susceptible birds. Prevention requires fencing to prevent access of opossums to the aviary. Flightless chickens have been suggested as a method of controlling cockroaches within a compound (see Chapter 2).

In a zoologic collection, five Eclectus Parrots and four Hispaniolan Amazon Parrots were diagnosed with sarcocystosis over a six-month period. Four of the Eclectus and two of the Amazon parrots died. Elevations in CPK, AST and LDH enzyme activities were noted in all the affected birds. Clinical signs included weakness, dyspnea and blood in the oral cavity. Affected birds died one to 36 hours after presentation. Radiographic findings indicated an increased lung field density, hepatomegaly, splenomegaly and renomegaly. Some birds that were only slightly lethargic and had no other clinical signs survived following treatment with 0.5 mg/kg pyrimethanamine PO q12h and 30 mg/kg trimethoprim-sulfadiazine IM q12h for 30 days. The surviving birds responded to therapy with improved attitude, appetite and decreased serum enzyme activity. Muscle biopsies after treatment revealed multifocal myositis and sarcocysts, indicating that the birds had survived the schizogony phase of the infection allowing muscle cysts to form.

Encephalitozoon sp. is a microsporidian parasite with a broad host range that includes mammals and birds. This parasite has complex spores measuring 1.5 x 1.0 μm and containing a coiled polar filament. The latter will be seen only with the aid of electron microscopy. Lovebirds of the genus *Agapornis* are frequently infected, but an Amazon parrot with a microsporidian infection has also been reported. The spores were documented in kidney tubules, lung, liver and the lamina propria of the small intestine.

Few birds have been reported with this parasite and all cases were detected at necropsy. One report gave the details of a die-off of 140 lovebirds in Great Britain in which the birds were moved to a different facility, stopped eating and lost condition.

An infected Amazon parrot developed progressive anorexia, weight loss, respiratory disease and diarrhea over a one-month period. Postmortem findings included pale, swollen kidneys and an enlarged, mottled liver.

Hemoparasites

Haemoproteus: Under normal circumstances, species of *Haemoproteus* are considered nonpathogenic and a few species of *Leucocytozoon* and *Plasmodium* are considered pathogenic. If clinical signs occur, they are associated with anemia, splenomegaly, hepatomegaly and pulmonary edema. The lymphoid-macrophage system becomes hyperplastic. High parasitemias of apathogenic *Haemoproteus* and *Leucocytozoon* can cause clinical problems if a bird is stressed or immunosuppressed. Racing pigeons infected with *H. columbae* are frequently discussed as performing poorly in comparison to uninfected birds.

Haemoproteus spp. are the most commonly occurring avian blood parasite; they use *Culicoides* (biting midges or punkies) or louse flies as vectors. In some studies, up to 50% of recently imported cockatoos were found to be positive. In contrast, only 5% of long-term captive cockatoos were found to have *Haemoproteus*. In a survey of 81 African Grey Parrots, 5.7% had *Haemoproteus*. Most infected birds are subclinical but severe infections in stressed birds may lead to life-threatening anemia. Infections may be potentiated by concurrent disease or stress.

H. handai gametocytes completely encircle the red blood cell nucleus. Initial parasite development occurs in endothelial or skeletal muscle cells followed by the production of pigmented gametocytes in RBCs.

Leucocytozoon: *Leucocytozoon* spp. use Simuliidae (black flies) as vectors. Initial development occurs in the liver and spleen followed by the development of unpigmented gametocytes in white blood cells or RBCs, depending upon the species. Infected host cells are distorted beyond recognition.

The parasite produces an anti-erythrocytic factor, which causes intravascular hemolysis and anemia, the principal clinical sign. *Leucocytozoon* is highly pathogenic in young Anseriformes and Galliformes. Fatal infections have been described in budgerigars. Hepatomegaly, splenomegaly, pulmonary congestion and pericardial effusion are the most characteristic gross findings. Pyrimethamine has been suggested for treatment.

Plasmodium: *Plasmodium* spp. use mosquitoes as vectors. Initial parasite development occurs in the avian reticuloendothelial system followed by the development of pigmented schizonts and gametocytes in the erythrocytes (RBCs). Schizogony occurs in the erythrocytes, which means that blood-to-blood transfer, without an intermediate host, can result in an infection.

Some strains of *Plasmodium* are highly pathogenic in canaries, penguins, Galliformes, Anseriformes, Columbiformes and falcons. Clinical signs are most common in recently infected birds and are characterized by anorexia, depression, vomiting and dyspnea for a few hours or days prior to death. In penguins, depression, anemia, vomiting, seizures and high levels of mortality may be noted. Nonpathogenic strains of *Plasmodium* have also been described in many of these same avian orders.

Trypanosoma: *Trypanosoma johnbakeri* is an extracellular, flagellated blood parasite that is transmitted by a biting midge and has been demonstrated in Roseate Parakeets, but has not been associated with clinical signs. In one study, trypanosomes were identified in 14% of imported Hyacinth Macaws, and 20% of imported Green-winged Macaws examined.

Helminths

Flatworms

Flukes: Flukes living in the bile ducts are members of the family Dicrocoelidae. All of the cases reported in North America have probably occurred in imported birds (Old World species) that were infected by endemic species in their country of origin. Birds may be infected by eating an arthropod, which serves as a second intermediate host. Liver flukes have rarely been demonstrated in New World Psittaciformes, even though there are a number of genera that occur in North American avifauna. Clinical changes associated with liver fluke infections include hepatomegaly, depression, anorexia, mild anemia, weight loss, diarrhea, hepatic necrosis, elevated liver enzymes and death.

Hepatic trematodiasis has been reported in cockatoos. Numerous trematode eggs were seen on direct smears of the feces.

Necropsy findings were primarily limited to the liver and were characterized by hepatomegaly, increased firmness, numerous streaks, brown and yellow mottling and fibrosis. In some birds, trematodes were found in dilated bile ducts. Clinical improvement following treatment with fenbendazole and praziquantel was minimal; however, the number of eggs per gram of feces did decrease dramatically following therapy.

Tapeworms: Tapeworms infecting psittacine birds can be asymptomatic or the parasite may steal nutrients from the host causing a bird to appear unthrifty and have diarrhea. Infections are most common in finches, African Grey Parrots (15-20% of imported birds), cockatoos (10-20% of imported birds) and Eclectus Parrots. Infections occasionally occur in South American Psittaciformes. In general, infections are nonpathogenic although large numbers of worms can cause impaction. With severe infections, birds may die following a period of weight loss and diarrhea.

Tapeworms require intermediate hosts, and infections are uncommon in birds that do not have access to the ground. Either proglottids or whole worms may be noted in the feces. Focusing through the individual rounded eggs to see the hooks on the hexacanth larva may be necessary to demonstrate that these are tapeworm eggs.

Roundworms

Roundworms (nematodes) are more diversified than flatworms and live in the small intestine (*Ascaridia, Ascarops* and *Capillaria*), proventriculus and ventriculus (*Microtetrameres, Procyrnea* and *Ascarops*), the surface of the eye (*Thelazia, Oxyspirura, Ceratospira* and *Annulospira*) and in subcutaneous regions, body cavity and air sacs (*Eulimdana, Pelecitus, Cardiofilaria* and *Cyathospira*).

Ascarids: Ascarids are the most common parasite found in birds that are maintained in enclosures with access to ground. Infections are particularly common in budgerigars and cockatiels.

The direct life cycle requires a two- to three-week period for embryonated larva to form within the egg, which is viable for extended periods in moist warm environments. The ingested larvae infect the intestinal mucosa. Mild infections can cause malabsorption, weight loss, anorexia, growth abnormalities and diarrhea. Heavier parasite loads may cause intussusception, bowel occlusion or death.

Providing a dry clean environment will decrease the possibility that eggs will survive to embryonate. Piperazine, pyrantel pamoate and fenbendazole may be effective in resolving infections.

Cerebrospinal nematodiasis caused by larvae from *Baylisascaris procyonis* (raccoon ascarids) has been reported in gallinaceous birds, cockatiels, ratites and several Passeriformes. When they enter the central nervous system, the larvae induce considerable damage leading to ataxia, torticollis, depression and death.

Because no diagnostic stages of the parasite are released to the environment, and no commercially available serological diagnostic kit is available, this parasite is normally diagnosed histologically at necropsy. The best means of control is to prevent access of free-ranging raccoons to aviaries, and thus prevent contamination of the environment by these thick-walled, long-lived eggs.

Capillaria: Species of *Capillaria* are tiny thread-like nematodes that may infect the gastrointestinal tract of most species of companion and aviary birds. Infections appear to be most common in macaws, budgerigars, canaries, pigeons and gallinaceous birds. Severe infections can cause diarrhea (which may contain blood), weight loss, anorexia, vomiting and anemia. The life cycle of *Capillaria* is direct.

Embryonation requires approximately two weeks, and eggs can remain infectious in the environment for several months. The adults can burrow into the mucosa of the esophagus, crop or intestinal tract causing depression, dysphagia, regurgitation, diarrhea, melena and weight loss. *Capillaria* that infect the crop, esophagus and oral cavity burrow into the mucosa, creating tracts that may fill with blood, producing hyperemic streaks. Frank hemorrhage may occur in the upper intestinal tract in heavily parasitized animals. Diphtheritic lesions may occur in the mouth, pharynx, esophagus and crop of some infected species.

Scrapings of suspect lesions or fecal flotation can be used to detect the characteristic bipolar eggs.

Spiruroidea: The superfamily Spiruroidea represents the most diversified group of nematodes in birds. The life cycle probably involves an insect intermediate host. *Ascarops* sp. has been recovered from the intestines of a Greater Sulphur-crested Cockatoo and *A. psittaculai* was described in a Rose-ringed Parakeet. *Procyrnea kea* was described from the New Zealand Kea where it lives under the koilin of the ventriculus. *Microtetrameres nestoris* was found in the proventriculus of the North Island Kaka where it caused hyperplasia and metaplasia of the duct epithelium, glandular atrophy and limited necrosis and hemorrhage.

Four genera of eyeworms (*Thelazia* and *Ceratospira*) have been reported. The intermediate host is considered to be the fly. Eyelid spasms and mild conjunctival hyperemia were evident in a Senegal Parrot with *Thelazia* even though only three adults were recovered. In contrast, no pathology was associated with numerous *Ceratospira* infecting a Moluccan Cockatoo.

Oxyspirura sp. is common in the eye of cockatoos where it resides beneath the nictitating membrane or in the conjunctival sac. Severe infections may cause conjunctivitis, chemosis and scratching at the eye. The parasite has an indirect life cycle that involves an arthropod (cockroach) intermediate host. Ivermectin can be used to kill the worms, which are then removed by flushing.

Streptocara spp. are pathogenic spiruroids that burrow into the mucosa of the esophagus, crop, proventriculus and ventriculus, principally in Anseriformes. Crustaceans serve as an intermediate host.

Spiroptera incerta and *Dyspharynx nasuata* have been reported in association with thickening of the proventricular mucosa in a number of Psittaciformes. The adult worms burrow into the proventriculus causing ulcers, inflammation and nodule formation. The proliferative mucosa may prevent the passage of ingesta resulting in chronic vomiting and weight loss.

A large-mouthed worm (*Cyathostoma cacatua*) related to gapeworms has been reported from the air sacs of a Sulphur-crested Cockatoo.

Syngamus: *Syngamus trachea* (gapeworm) has been diagnosed in many species of companion birds. Infections are rare in companion birds but are common in Galliformes and Anseriformes. The red Y-shaped adult parasite can be visualized on the mucosa of the trachea and primary bronchi. Coughing, open-mouthed breathing, dried blood at the beak commissure, dyspnea and head shaking are common. With severe infections, death can occur secondary to tracheal ulceration, anemia and asphyxiation. The eggs of the parasite can be detected in the feces. The life cycle is direct but earthworms can serve as a transport host. Thiabendazole has been recommended for treatment. Ivermectin can be used to kill the parasites and they can be mechanically removed by repeated transtracheal washes.

Filariidea: The filariid nematodes have indirect life cycles and are transmitted to birds by blood-feeding diptera. The diagnostic stage of these worms is the microfilaria and in most cases, the microfilariae have not been matched to the adults. The adults live in the body cavity, chambers of the eyes, heart or air sacs.

In most situations, the adults and microfilariae are considered apathogenic; however, filarial worms in the joints and subcutaneous tissues can cause severe problems and should be removed.

Adult filarial worms filling the pericardial sac of a Red-vented Cockatoo caused death. An Umbrella Cockatoo with a one-week history of anorexia, ataxia, diarrhea and increased vocalization was found at necropsy to have microfilariae in the small vessels of the brain, lungs, kidneys, spleen, heart and liver. Adult filariae were identified in the vena cava. Adult filariae were found in the heart of a recently imported Ducorp's Cockatoo with PBFD.

Arthropods

Hematophagous diptera including mosquitoes, black flies and biting midges can feed on psittacine birds and transmit blood parasites. Direct effects of these parasites may include anemia.

Biting lice known to occur on psittacines include *Neopsittaconirmus*, *Psittaconirmus*, *Eomenopon* and *Pacifimenopon*. Lice may cause pruritus and poor feather condition. The parasites can be observed directly, or the nits (eggs) can be seen attached to the feathers. Most species are host specific and die quickly when they leave a host. Dusting with pyrethrin can control infections.

Mites and Fleas: Numerous mites have been detected on and in psittacine birds. The scaly leg and face mite, *Knemidokoptes pilae*, is the most frequently diagnosed and causes prominent and disfiguring lesions. Infections are most common in budgerigars, but they may also occur in other Psittaciformes and Passeriformes. Typically, there is a proliferation of tissue on the beak. Lesions may also occur on the feet, legs and cloaca in some birds. Tunnels in the proliferative tissue create a characteristic honey-combed appearance. The mites can be detected by examining skin scrapings.

Young birds are commonly affected, but adults may be infected in some situations. A genetic predisposition to develop *Knemidokoptes* infections has been suggested because only a few birds in a group may be infected. A selective immunosuppression may also be a predisposing factor, but has not been documented. In canaries, *Knemidokoptes* infections on the feet and legs may cause large proliferative masses frequently referred to as "tasselfoot."

Sternostoma tracheacolum can infect the trachea of canaries, finches (especially Lady Gouldians), parakeets and cockatiels. The larva, nymph and adult forms of the parasite can be found in the respiratory tract of affected birds, suggesting that the entire life cycle occurs in the infected host. Clinical signs include dyspnea, coughing and sneezing. Nasal discharge and open-mouthed breathing may also be noted. Infections can be mild to severe with resulting death by asphyxiation. These small black mites can be identified by transillumination of the trachea, or the eggs can be identified in the feces or following a transtracheal wash. Young birds may be infected when being fed by infected parents. The incubation period in Gouldian Finches is three weeks but may be months in other species. Mite-free Society Finches can be used to cross-foster Gouldian Finches to produce mite-free flocks.

Numerous feather mites have been described in birds. Feather mites have highly specific microhabitats, infecting specific portions of the feathers. In general, feather mites are apathogenic in their host-adapted species, but can cause clinical problems in non-host adapted species, or with heavy infestations when the mites move from the feathers to the skin.

Myialges (*Metamicrolichus nudus*) were demonstrated in a Grey-cheeked Parakeet with sinusitis, weight loss, pruritic dermatitis and feather loss of the head. The skin was hyperkeratotic (several millimeters thick), and the parasite was demonstrated in pits within the stratum corneum and feather cavity.

Myialges was diagnosed by finding eggs in a skin scraping taken from an Amazon parrot with a one-week history of scratching around the eyes. The skin around the lores was dry and flaky and the head, cere and lore area appeared to be pruritic. Ivermectin was effective in controlling the infection.

Nonhost-specific fleas are occasionally noted in companion and aviary birds. If they cause clinical problems (eg, pruritus, anemia, poor feather condition) they can be controlled with a light dusting of pyrethrin powder. The mite protectors sold in most pet supply stores have no effect on common external avian parasites and may cause liver disease. The use of these products is discouraged.

Other mites have been associated with occasional skin or feather disease in birds. *Dermanyssus* feed on blood and may cause anemia, pruritus and poor growth in young birds. They infect the bird only at night and spend the daytime in crevices within the aviary. Under magnification, they can be recognized as rapidly moving dark brown spots. Free-ranging birds can serve as a source of infestation and should not be allowed to nest or roost in the aviary. *Ornithonyssus* can cause problems similar to those seen with *Dermanyssus*. This parasite completes its life cycle on the bird. Dusting with pyrethrin should be effective for controlling the mites.

Table 36.1 Suggested Parasite Treatments

Parasites	Therapy
Haemoproteus	Not recommended in asymptomatic birds
Leucocytozoon	Pyrimethamine, Clopidol (0.0215-0.025%) in food as preventative
Plasmodium	Chloroquine phosphate, Primaquine
Giardia	Metronidazole
Histomonas	Ipronidazole, Dimetrodazole
Atoxoplasma	See text
Cryptosporidium	No effective therapy
Sarcocystis	Pyrimethamine, Trimethoprim, Sulfadiazine
Cestodes	Praziquantel
Ascarids	Pyrantel pamoate, Piperazine
Oxyspirura	Ivermectin
Capillaria	Mebendazole, Fenbendazole, Ivermectin (resistant strains occur)
Syngamus	Ivermectin, Physical removal
Knemidokoptes	Topical ivermectin
Sternostoma	Ivermectin, Physical removal
Gapeworms	Thiabendazole, Mebendazole
Trichomonads	Dimetronidazole, Metronidazole
Coccidia	Metronidazole

Table 36.2 Common Parasites in Companion Birds

African Grey Parrots	Tapeworms (common), blood parasites* (occasional)
Australian Parakeets	Proventricular worms (common), nematodes (frequent)
Budgerigars	*Trichomonas* (common), *Giardia* (common)
Canaries	Air sac mites
Cockatiels	Ascarids* (common), *Giardia* (frequent)
Cockatoos	Tapeworms (common), *Haemoproteus*,* microfilaria,* liver flukes*
Finches	Air sac mites, tapeworms (common), *Trichomonas**
Lorikeets	Coccidia, roundworms* (frequent)
Macaws	*Capillaria* (frequent, imports), ascarids* (common)
Toucans	*Giardia* (common), coccidia (frequent)

* Relatively uncommon in captive-bred birds in the United States

Table 36.3 Best Tests for Detecting Avian Parasites

Parasite	Test
Hexamita, Giardia, Trichomonas	Fresh direct mount with warm LRS (not H_2O)
Coccidia oocyst	Flotation - Sheather's sugar
Giardia, spiruroid eggs	Flotation - Zinc sulfate
Nematodes, cestodes, acanthocephala	Flotation - Sodium nitrate
Flukes	Sedimentation
Plasmodium, Haemoproteus, Leucocytozoon, Atoxoplasma, Trypanosoma, microfilaria	Blood smear - Wright's stain
Microfilaria, *Trypanosoma*	PCV tube, inspect at blood plasma interface using microscope

TOXINS

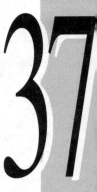

Genevieve Dumonceaux
Greg J. Harrison

Birds are curious pets and frequently investigate unusual textures, containers and locations throughout the home. Many of the items that birds may encounter during these quests can be dangerous.

Most compounds considered toxic to mammals should also be considered toxic to birds. Table 37.1 offers a guide for treatment of intoxication from some common household products. Based on their size and physiology, birds are more prone than mammals to intoxication by some compounds, such as volatile chemicals and fumes.

Birds should be supervised at all times when out of their enclosures. It has been suggested that the consumption of foreign bodies (eg, metal, wood, jewelry), overconsumption of grit and coprophagy may all be mediated by malnutrition. Therefore, birds on a formulated diet would be expected to chew less on plants, perches and toys than birds on a seed-based diet.

Birds are generally more susceptible to inhaled toxins than mammals because of their rapid metabolic rate, small size, highly efficient respiratory system and low body fat content. In comparison, many compounds that cause intoxication following ingestion by mammals are relatively nontoxic in companion birds; however, birds should be restricted from access to compounds known to be toxic in mammals.

Information on products and chemicals as well as assistance with poisonings is available from the National Animal Poison Control Center, University of Illinois, College of Veterinary Medicine, Urbana, IL 61801, 1-800-548-2423 (credit cards only, $30 per case) or 1-900-680-0000 ($20 for the first 5 minutes, plus $2.95 for each additional minute [$20 minimum]). This center's experience is limited when dealing with companion birds and they often refer calls to experienced practitioners.

A useful conversion in toxicology analysis is 1 ppm = 100 μg/dL.

Table 37.1 Normal Household Compounds That May Be Toxic to Birds

Agent	Toxic Components	Clinical Effects	Therapy
Bleaches, pool chemicals	Chlorine	Photophobia, epiphora, coughing, sneezing, hyperventilation, GI irritation or ulceration	Dilution with water or milk orally. Irrigate skin with cool water. GI protectant, demulcent
Cleaning agents, accumulated excrement	Ammonia	Respiratory tract irritation, immune suppression	Fresh air, antibiotics, supportive care
Combustion exhaust (autos, furnaces)	Carbon monoxide	Somnolence, depression, cyanosis, death	Fresh air, oxygen, warmth, support
Denture cleaners	Sodium perborate	Direct irritation, salivation, lacrimation, vomiting, sometimes CNS depression	Irrigate with water, GI protectant, demulcent
Deodorants	Aluminum chloride, aluminum chlorhydrate	Oral irritation and necrosis, hemorrhagic gastroenteritis, incoordination and nephrosis	Careful lavage of crop and proventriculus
Detergents (anionic)	Sulfonated or phosphorylated forms, alkaline product	Dermal irritation, vomiting, diarrhea, GI distension, usually not fatal	Lavage with water
Detergents (cationic)	Quaternary ammonium with alkyl or any substituent groups	Vomiting, depression, collapse, coma, may cause corrosive esophageal damage	Oral milk or activated charcoal. Soap for surface areas. Treat seizures and shock as needed.
Drain cleaners	Sodium hydroxide, sodium hypochlorite	Caustic to skin and mucous membranes, irritation, inflammation, edema, necrosis, burns in mouth, tongue, pharynx	Flush affected areas with water or milk. Do not use emetics or lavage. Treat for shock and pain.

Table 37.1 Normal Household Compounds That May Be Toxic to Birds

Agent	Toxic Components	Clinical Effects	Therapy
Fireworks	Nitrates, chlorates, mercury, antimony, copper, strontium, barium, phosphorous	Abdominal pain, vomiting, bloody feces, rapid shallow respiration, chlorates may cause methemoglobinemia	Crop or gastric lavae. Use methylene blue or ascorbic acid for methemoglobinemia. Treat for specific metal(s) ingested.
Furniture polish	Petroleum, hydrocarbons, mineral spirits	Early CNS depression, disorientation, necrosis, mucosal irritation, aspiration or hydrocarbon pneumonia, hepatorenal damage	Prevent aspiration pneumonia. Avoid gastric lavage or proceed with caution. Monitor and treat for pneumonia.
Gasoline, crude oil	Petroleum and petroleum distillates	GI irritation, skin and feather damage, aspiration pneumonia	Wash feathers and skin with mild soap and water. Vegetable or mineral oil gavage. Antibiotics and supportive care.
Matches	Potassium chloride	Gastroenteritis, vomiting, chlorates may induce methemoglobinemia with cyanosis and hemolysis	Treat symptomatically. Use methylene blue or ascorbic acid for methemoglobinemia.
Paint/varnish removers	Benzene, methanol, toluene, acetone	Dermal irritation, depression, narcosis, pneumonia, hepatorenal damage	See "furniture polish." Rinse contact areas thoroughly with warm water.
Pencils	Graphite	GI irritation	Demulcent
Perfumes	Volatile oils	Local irritation of skin and mucous membranes, pneumonitis, hepatorenal damage with albuminuria, hematuria, glycosuria, excitement, ataxia, coma	If ingested, gastric or crop lavage with weak bicarbonate solution. Prevent aspiration. Demulcents. Provide plenty of ventilation.

Table 37.1 Normal Household Compounds That May Be Toxic to Birds

Agent	Toxic Components	Clinical Effects	Therapy
Pine oil disinfectants	Pine oil 5-10%, phenols 2-6%	Gastritis, vomiting, diarrhea, followed by CNS depression, occasional mild seizures, phenols may induce nephrosis	If ingested, gastric lavage with caution to prevent aspiration. Mineral oil. Monitor pulmonary and renal function. Provide fresh air if strong fumes are present.
Overheated non-stick cookware, drip pans, heat lamps, irons, ironing board covers	Polytetrafluoroethylene	Sudden death, dyspnea, depression, pulmonary hemorrhage	Fresh air or oxygen, fluids, steroids for pulmonary edema, antibiotics, supportive care
Poor grade peanuts, peanut waste, moldy grains, corn and corn screenings, moldy cheeses, meats	Mycotoxins: aflatoxin, ochratoxin, trichothecenes	Gastrointestinal irritation, dermal irritation, oral necrosis, secondary infections due to immunosuppression	Clean feed, antibiotics for secondary infections. Treatment as indicated for clinical syndromes.
Rodenticides	Anticoagulants	Weakness, dyspnea, hemorrhage, petechiation, anemia	Vitamin K_1 (2.5-5 mg/kg) IM or PO q24h. Minimize stress. Warfarin, treat for 10-14 days. Chlorophacinone, treat for 21-28 days. Brodifacoum, treat for 28-30 days.
Rodenticides	Cholecalciferol	Causes hypercalcemia and renal failure, vomiting, diarrhea, depression, anorexia, polyuria, polydipsia	Activated charcoal, fluid therapy. If hypercalcemic, saline diuresis, prednisolone PO 2 mg/kg q12h, furosemide 2-5 mg/kg q8-12h, salmon calcitonin SC 4-6 IU/kg q2-3h until calcium stable (mammalian protocol)

Table 37.1   Normal Household Compounds That May Be Toxic to Birds

Agent	Toxic Components	Clinical Effects	Therapy
Rubbing alcohol	Ethyl alcohol	Impaired motor coordination, cutaneous hyperemia, vomiting, progress to peripheral vascular collapse, hypothermia	Gastric or crop lavage. Monitor temperature, cardiac and pulmonary function.
Shampoo	Laurel sulfates and triethanolamine dodecyl sulfate	Ocular irritation, stimulation of mucous production, ingestion causes diarrhea	Activated charcoal or kaolin orally
Salt, crackers, chips, prepared foods, salt water, sea sand (as grit)	Sodium chloride	Gastrointestinal irritation, dehydration, depression, weakness, PU/PD, death	Rehydration, offer small amounts of water frequently. SC, IV or IO fluids, supportive care
Styptic pencil	Potassium aluminum sulfate	Corrosive due to release of sulfuric acid during hydrolysis of the salt, oral necrosis from chewing pencils	Oral neutralizer such as magnesium oxide or hydroxide. Do not give bicarbonate orally for acid poisonings.

Many of the therapeutic recommendations for the above products have been taken from small animal sources.

Ingested Toxins

Lead (Pb)

Table 37.3 offers some examples of possible household sources of lead.

A simple lead testing kit is available for the detection of lead in environmental samples. This rapid, in-home test is less reliable than tests performed by commercial laboratories.

Table 37.3   Potential Sources of Lead

- Weights (curtains, penguin bird toys, fishing and diving, sailing and boating accessories, wheel balances)
- Bells with lead clappers
- Batteries
- Solder
- Lead pellets from shotgun shells
- Air rifle pellets
- Lead-based paints (varnishes, lacquers)
- Hardware cloth
- Galvanized wire (lead and zinc)
- Champagne and wine bottle foils (some)
- Base of light bulbs
- Linoleum
- Contaminated bone meal and dolomite products
- Leaded gasoline fumes
- Glazed ceramics (especially imported products)
- Costume jewelry
- Contaminated cuttlefish bone
- Plaster
- Stained glass (decorative glass) - lead seam
- Seeds for planting (coated with lead arsenate)
- Some lubricants (lead naphthalate)

Clinical Signs

Chronic leadintoxications are most common in Anseriformes and other free-ranging birds. The most commonly reported effect in free-ranging birds is a decrease in population densities. Because companion birds are carefully observed on a daily basis, the non-specific signs of acute lead toxicosis are frequently recognized and birds are presented for medical evaluation.

The presence and severity of clinical signs depends on the amount of lead ingested, the surface area of the particles and the length of time the lead is in the gastrointestinal tract. The type and amount of abrasive material in the ventriculus alters the speed of lead digestion and may affect the type of clinical presentation.

Once in the bloodstream, lead causes pansystemic damage, particularly to the gastrointestinal, nervous, renal and hematopoietic systems. Clinical signs of lead intoxication in psittacine birds may include lethargy, depression, anorexia, weakness (wing droop, leg paresis), regurgitation, polyuria, diarrhea, emaciation, ataxia, head tilt, blindness, circling, paresis, paralysis, head tremors, convulsions and death. Some birds may die with no clinical signs and in others, the only noted abnormalities may be weakness and chronic weight loss. Hemoglobinuria has been reported as a clinical sign of lead poisoning in Amazons and African Grey Parrots, but it may not occur in all cases. Lead poisoning in waterfowl, cranes and pigeons may cause ileus of the crop, esophagus, proventriculus and ventriculus. In waterfowl and poultry, lead poisoning can cause clinical signs similar to those that occur with botulism. Response to chelation therapy (lead or zinc) or antitoxin (botulism) is suggestive of a diagnosis (see Chapters 28, 33, 46).

Pathology

In some cases, hematologic parameters may provide an indication of lead intoxication. A hypochromic, regenerative anemia occurs in some affected birds. Basophilic stippling and cytoplasmic vacuolization of red blood cells reported in mammalian lead poisoning cases are not recognized in avian patients.

Elevations of LDH, AST and CPK have been reported. Increased LDH and AST are primarily related to liver damage in birds. High CPK activities may be a result of lead-induced neuronal damage.

The functional capacity of the renal system should be carefully evaluated in birds suspected of having lead poisoning. Most commonly used chelating agents have potentially nephrotoxic side effects, and therapy for heavy metal intoxication should be instituted with caution in birds with impaired renal function.

Radiography

The identification of metallic densities in the gastrointestinal tract of birds with clinical signs of heavy metal intoxication is suggestive. However, the absence of metal densities in the presence of clinical signs does not rule out heavy metal intoxication.

Toxicologic Analysis

Whole, unclotted blood is the sample of choice for determining lead concentrations because 90% of circulating lead is in red blood cells. Lithium heparin is a suitable anticoagulant. EDTA should not be used because this anticoagulant may interfere with testing.

Whole blood lead levels greater than 20 μg/dL (0.2 ppm; 1.25 μmol/dL) are suggestive, and levels greater than 40-60 μg/dL (0.4-0.6 ppm; 2.5 μmol/dL) are diagnostic of lead intoxication in psittacine birds when accompanied by appropriate clinical signs (Table 37.4). Some birds may have clinical signs and respond to therapy with levels as low as 10 μg/dL. Higher levels of blood lead have been reported in many avian species with no clinical signs of intoxication.

Table 37.4	Suggested Normal Blood Lead Levels
Swan	6 μg/dL
Mallard	5-39 μg/dL
Canada Goose	10-37 μg/dL
Pigeon	17-81 μg/dL
Cockatiel	5 μg/dL
Most Psittaciformes	<20 μg/dL

With a strong suspicion of lead intoxication, therapy should be initiated while awaiting laboratory results. A rapid response to therapy lends evidence to a diagnosis of lead (or other similar heavy metal) poisoning.

A decrease in delta-aminolevulinic acid dehydratase (ALAD) activity has been used as a reliable and sensitive indicator of exposure to lead in ducks. It also has been recommended as a diagnostic tool in other avian species. In cockatiels, ALAD activities less than 86 units were considered indicative of lead poisoning.

Lead interferes with ALAD activity, which reduces heme synthase activity and causes an increase in protoporphyrin IX concentrations in the blood. Free erythrocytic protoporphyrin (FEPP) and zinc protoporphyrin (ZPP) levels are considered accurate methods of detecting lead intoxication in birds. FEPP levels were found to be suggestive of acute toxicity, while ZPP levels were of more value in documenting chronic lead poisoning.

Treatment

Supportive care for heavy metal poisoning may include chelation therapy (both oral and IM), intravenous lactated Ringer's, 5% dextrose solution, multicomplex B vitamins, iron dextran, antibiotics, assisted alimentation and prophylactic treatment for aspergillosis (waterfowl).

The prognosis for lead intoxication is guarded if chronic exposure has occurred or if the bird has severe CNS signs. In other cases, the response to therapy is dramatic, with most patients responding to chelation therapy within six hours of administration. Many hematuric birds can die in this same time period. Gastrointestinal stasis and impaction of the proventriculus is a complicating factor in waterfowl.

The recommended dosage of CaEDTA is 10-40 mg/kg twice daily intramuscularly. CaEDTA is poorly absorbed from the gastrointestinal tract and must be used parenterally to remove circulating lead in critically ill patients. Chelation therapy should be used for the least amount of time that is necessary to resolve the intoxication. In general, therapy should not persist for over ten days without a break in drug administration; however, some clinicians have used CaEDTA until there is no radiographic evidence of lead in the gastrointestinal tract (up to 30 days) with no clinically apparent side effects. CaEDTA may be administered orally at twice the injectable dose two to three times daily in asymptomatic birds to prevent lead from being absorbed. CaEDTA must be used carefully as it may cause gastrointestinal and renal toxicosis. If evidence of chelation toxicosis is seen (eg, polydipsia, polyuria, proteinuria, hematuria), CaEDTA should be discontinued for a period of five to seven days. Therapy can then resume if the patient is stable.

D-penicillamine (PA) is an effective lead chelator that can be used orally (55 mg/kg twice daily). Recent reports suggest that PA is a superior chelating agent to CaEDTA and does not increase absorption. Combining CaEDTA and PA for several days until a bird is asymptomatic followed by the use of PA for three to six weeks may prove to be the best therapeutic regime for lead poisoning. Birds should be monitored for clinical signs of copper depletion including lethargy, anemia and weight loss.

Dimercaprol (British Anti-Lewisite - BAL) is the best agent for removing lead from the CNS; however, this agent is rarely used because of its low therapeutic index and the positive response of most birds to PA or CaEDTA. The recommended treatment regime is 2.5 mg/kg IM every four hours for two days, then twice daily for up to ten days or until clinical signs resolve.

Lead-induced seizures can be controlled with diazepam at 0.5-1 mg/kg intramuscularly two to three times daily as needed.

Emollient cathartics (mineral oil or peanut butter) can be administered to aid in the passage of small particles of heavy metal out of the gastrointestinal tract. Other substances that have been used to aid in the passage of heavy metal particles include barium sulfate, psyllium and corn oil. The comparative effectiveness of these agents has not been determined. The use of sodium sulfate (Glauber's salts) has also been recommended for the removal of lead. Additionally, this agent can be mixed with activated charcoal and used following the ingestion of unknown toxins for its cathartic and absorptive effects. The sodium sulfate is given as a slurry for up to two doses (in large birds) or until lead is gone from the gut.

The administration of three to five appropriately sized pieces of grit may help in the removal of metal particles from the ventriculus by reducing their size and facilitating passage, particularly when used in conjunction with psyllium (hemicellulose).

Activated charcoal is recommended to bind small lead particles in the gastrointestinal tract and make them unavailable for absorption. The small animal dose for activated charcoal is 200-800 mg/kg body weight. This should be gavaged as a slurry with water according to manufacturer's instructions. Activated charcoal will be inactivated if administered with mineral oil. Activated charcoal may be administered one to two hours before administration of a cathartic. This allows sufficient time for free heavy metals to be bound to the charcoal before the system is purged.

Endoscopic removal of heavy metal particles using appropriate forceps or gastric lavage can be attempted in stable patients that are of sufficient size to tolerate this procedure. Occasionally, a proventriculotomy may be necessary if other attempts to remove metal particles fail (see Chapter 41).

Zinc (Zn)

Zinc is another frequently encountered heavy metal that causes toxicity when ingested by birds. Zinc toxicosis should be included in the differential list when heavy metal intoxication is suspected. Galvanized wire and the clips used to construct enclosures are common sources of zinc. The clinical syndrome described in birds that ingest zinc from a wire enclosure is frequently referred to as "new wire disease." The occurrence of "new wire disease" can be reduced (but not eliminated) by scrubbing the wire with a brush and mild acidic solution (vinegar). Galvanized wire may also contain lead. Galvanized containers and dishes are other sources of zinc contamination. Pennies minted in the USA since 1982 contain from 96-98% zinc that is coated with copper. Monopoly™ game pieces are made of 98% zinc.

Common signs reported in zinc-intoxicated birds include polyuria, polydipsia, gastrointestinal problems, weight loss, weakness, anemia, cyanosis, hyperglycemia and seizures. Systemic effects are related to hypoproteinemia-induced damage in the kidneys, gastrointestinal system and pancreas. There are two cases of zinc depressing fertility, one in a male Mallard and one in a female Black Bustard.

Only glass or all-plastic syringes and tubes should be used for samples intended for zinc analysis. Rubber stoppers on serum tubes and the grommets on most plastic syringes can be a source of zinc contamination. Serum tubes with royal blue-colored stoppers are free of zinc and are best for sample handling. In general, blood zinc levels of greater than 200 μg/dL (2 ppm) are considered diagnostic for zinc toxicosis. The pancreas proved to be the best tissue for postmortem zinc level determination.

Calcium EDTA is recommended as an effective chelating agent. D-penicillamine is also useful. Radiographically and clinically, zinc toxicosis cannot be differentiated from lead intoxication. Fortunately, the therapy is the same for poisonings caused by either of these heavy metals. If a bird has ingested galvanized wire, this zinc-coated ferrous metal can be removed using a powerful neo-dymium-ferro-barium alloy magnet attached to a small diameter catheter with a removable, flexible steel grid wire.

Copper (Cu)

Factors that have been shown to affect the toxicity of copper in mammals include dietary zinc and molybdenum concentrations. There are wide differences in how various animal species maintain copper hemostasis in the body, and birds appear to tolerate higher levels of copper than many mammals.

Clinical abnormalities associated with copper intoxication have rarely been reported in birds. A Mute Swan with inanition, anemia and generalized weakness showed signs of toxicity with liver copper levels in excess of 3000 mg/kg and over 50 mg/kg copper in the kidneys. Postmortem findings following copper intoxication include anemia and coal-black discoloration of the liver.

D-penicillamine increases the renal excretion of copper and is the chelating agent of choice for copper toxicosis in mammals. High-quality nutritional support is necessary to prevent chelation and removal of other vital minerals. Supportive care with fluids, warmth and minimal stress may aid in recovery. In severely anemic birds, blood transfusions may be necessary. In advanced cases the prognosis is poor.

Mercury (Hg)

Fish accumulate mercury, which is then further concentrated in fish-eating birds. An Amazon parrot that consumed the back of a mirror died following a period of profuse hematuria. BAL (and presumably DMSA) and d-penicillamine chelate mercury.

Arsenic (Ar)

Polyuria, polydipsia, feather picking, pruritus, weight loss, dyspnea (air sacculitis), egg binding, poor feathering and death occurred in a group of aviary birds, presumably secondary to the consumption of arsenic-contaminated mineral block. Necropsy findings included cystic ovaries and adrenal gland enlargement. Clinical changes started when a new group of mineral blocks was used in the aviary. These blocks were found to contain 0.5% arsenic, and all clinical problems in the birds resolved when the mineral blocks were removed.

Oil

Crude oil is extremely toxic.

Selenium

A dog shampoo containing selenium sulfide caused the death of a budgerigar.

Nitrates

Nitrates are common components of fertilizers and may cause polydipsia, dyspnea, cyanosis and death following ingestion. The pelletized forms of nitrate-containing fertilizers are particularly hazardous because they resemble seeds and may be readily consumed by birds.

Plants

Plant intoxications are rare (Table 37.6). It has been proposed that parrots can consume toxic plants because they carefully remove the outer covering, which frequently contains the highest concentration of toxins.

Birds have been reported to die as soon as 9-15 hours after consuming avocado. Some birds died within 10-15 minutes after developing signs of respiratory distress without prior clinical signs.

Table 37.6 Poisonous Plant Cases Documented in Birds

Avocado	Psittaciformes (C,E)
Black Locust	Budgerigars (E)
Clematis	Budgerigars (E)
Diffenbachia	Canaries (E)
Foxglove	Canaries (E)
Lily of the Valley	Pigeons (C,E)
Lupine	Canaries (E)
Crown Vetch	Budgerigars, cockatiels, lovebirds (C)
Oleander	Budgerigars, canaries (E)
Parsley	Ostriches (C), ducks (E)
Philodendron	Budgerigars (E)
Poinsettia	Budgerigars (E)
Rhododendron	Budgerigars (E)
Virginia Creeper	Budgerigars (E)
Yew	Pheasants (C), canaries (E)

C = clinical report; E = experimental

The state of an animal's health should be expected to have an impact on its response to ingested plants. The experimental doses used to demonstrate that some of these plants were toxic are not likely to occur in natural settings.

Oak toxicosis (coast live oak - *Quercus agrifola*) was confirmed in a cassowary that consumed the leaves. Clinical changes included anorexia, ataxia, diarrhea, severe polydipsia and death.

Mycotoxins

Mycotoxins are chemical metabolites produced by various species of fungi that grow on grains and foodstuffs.

Toxins can enter an avian host through surface-to-skin contact. The effects of mycotoxin exposure can vary based on the type of toxin and on the species, nutritional state and physiologic status of the patient. A stressed bird or one on a poor diet is more likely to be poisoned by a lower dose of mycotoxin than is a healthy, well-fed bird.

There are no specific antidotes for mycotoxicoses. It is easier to prevent exposure to mycotoxins than to attempt treatment following their ingestion. All foods and seeds available to birds should be clean and fresh. Particular caution should be exercised with poor quality corn and peanuts, as these are common sources of toxin-producing molds. Some high-quality formulated diets are certified free of mycotoxins. Treatment involves providing clean food free of molds, supportive care, broad-spectrum antibiotics and specific therapies for clinical signs.

Diagnosis is based on clinical signs, postmortem and histopathologic findings, and detecting high quantities of the toxin in the gastrointestinal contents or the food. However, it is difficult to establish a diagnosis of mycotoxicosis in birds.

Aflatoxin B_1 is a known hepatotoxin. It is produced by *Aspergillus* spp. and may cause depression, poor growth, anorexia and other signs related to liver disease. Postmortem changes include an enlarged, pale liver (probably the result of fatty infiltration), an enlarged spleen, an enlarged pancreas, atrophy of the cloacal bursa and less-than-normal body fat deposits.

Aflatoxins inhibit protein and nucleic acid synthesis. Microscopic examination shows hepatic cell degeneration and bile duct hyperplasia. The kidneys may have swollen proximal convoluted tubules. Anticoagulant activity is altered, and a bird with a prolonged whole blood clotting time and prothrombin time may be suffering from aflatoxicosis. Gastrointestinal hemorrhage is also common. Immunosuppression through a reduction in alpha and beta globulins has also been linked to aflatoxin exposure. Serum electrophoresis to detect this IgG pattern may be useful in diagnosing aflatoxicosis.

The trichothecenes, including T_2 toxin, are produced by *Fusarium* spp., which commonly grow on crops in the field. This toxin has corrosive effects on the mucous membranes of the oropharynx, and occasionally the gastrointestinal tract, causing necrotic lesions of the hard palate and other oral areas. Lesions can appear within 48 hours of ingestion.

Trichothecene T_2 toxin may also cause contact dermatitis (from contaminated litter), poor growth and feathering, constrictive lesions of the digits (dry gangrene) and occasionally neurologic disorders.

Ochratoxin is produced by species of *Aspergillus* and *Penicillium* fungi. The toxin has an immunosuppressive effect and has been associated with air sacculitis, nephrotoxicity, CNS signs, hepatotoxicity and bone marrow suppression. It has been shown to cause depression of the immunoglobulin-containing cells in the lymphoid organs. Clinical changes are commonly related to secondary infections that take advantage of a depressed immune system.

Ethylene Glycol

Free-ranging birds may consume ethylene glycol. In gallinaceous birds, consumption of antifreeze has been associated with lethargy, ataxia and polyuria. Characteristic calcium oxalate crystals form in the kidneys.

Harmful Foods

Chocolate is contraindicated as a treat for any pet, including birds. Consumption of small quantities of chocolate can result in hyperactivity, vomiting, diarrhea, cardiac arrhythmias, seizures, dark-colored feces and death.

Excessive consumption of sodium chloride can cause polydipsia, polyuria, depression, neurologic excitement, tremors, opisthotonos, ataxia and death.

Consumption of alcoholic beverages can lead to severe ataxia and death. Additionally, birds may become intoxicated if compounds containing high levels of ethanol (STA) are used to clean open wounds.

Iatrogenic Intoxications

The most common cause of iatrogenic drug toxicosis is a failure to base the dose on an accurate weight.

Administering drugs at the proper dose, at an appropriate time interval, through a recommended route of administration and with consideration for patient-specific contraindications will minimize the potential for iatrogenic intoxications.

Some drugs given parenterally at the appropriate dosage (especially IM) can cause various degrees of local tissue damage. Many of these reactions can be attributed to the carrier in the formulation. Injectable products that contain propylene glycol (PG) or oil as a carrier may cause an abscess or toxic reaction.

Anthelmintics

Ivermectin in a PG base may cause toxic reactions when administered IM to budgerigars. Oral or topical administration is safer and equally efficacious. Ivermectin that is diluted in PG and allowed to stand should be mixed thoroughly before administration. Oral administration of a product that was not shaken caused seizures in several canaries and budgerigars. High-dose steroids reversed the clinical signs in these cases. Ivermectin persists in the environment and is excreted unchanged in the urine. Low concentrations that accumulate in water are extremely toxic to crustaceans, and whales may be particularly sensitive to this drug.

Dimetridazole was shown to have a low therapeutic index when added to the drinking water of cockatiel chicks. In nestlings (one to eight days old), the recommended concentration of 0.1% dimetridazole in the drinking water caused signs of toxicity including weakness, depressed growth rates, tremors and death. Older nestlings (over eight days old) showed no signs of toxicity at 0.1% concentrations.

Treatment of adult cockatiels at the recommended dose appears to be safe. Dimetridazole should not be used in the drinking water during the breeding season when males may consume excess quantities of the drug and feed it to nestlings, causing toxicosis and death.

Vetisulid and some other sulfa-containing antibiotics have been reported to cause hypersensitivity reactions leading to a hemorrhagic syndrome in gallinaceous birds. They may also interfere with renal tubular excretion and are contraindicated in dehydrated or uricemic patients. These antimicrobial agents should be limited in use to sensitive bacteria and the treatment of coccidiosis.

Levamisole hydrochloride (oral) and levamisole phosphate (injectable) have been used to treat intestinal parasites in birds. Side effects associated with these agents in Psittaciformes and Galliformes include regurgitation, ataxia, recumbency, catatonia, dyspnea and death. The dosage range used to study toxic effects in birds was 22-100 mg/kg. A dose rate of 22 mg/kg was considered effective for some parasites and was well tolerated by many genera of aviary birds.

The parasiticides praziquantel and fenbendazole have been reported to cause problems in finches and pigeons ranging from feather malformations to vomiting and death.

Antibiotics

Aminoglycosides have a narrow therapeutic index and are nephrotoxic. Gentamicin causes severe renal tubular necrosis and is the most frequently discussed member of the group. Systemic, topical and ophthalmic canine products can cause nephritis and are generally contraindicated in all companion birds. Amikacin is a safer alternative when an aminoglycoside is indicated. Renal function should be monitored during treatment. If an intoxication is suspected, the antibiotic should be discontinued and diuresis with physiologic saline should be initiated immediately.

Tetracyclines, cephalosporins (especially cephaloridine) and amphotericin B may also cause nephrotoxicosis in patients with impaired renal function. Procaine penicillins have been associated with some toxic reactions in birds (see Chapter 18).

The popularity of enrofloxacin has been increasing in avian medicine because of its broad spectrum of activity and its good tissue penetration. Abnormalities in articular cartilage have been reported in squabs dosed at 800 ppm. Only one chick was affected at a dose of 200 ppm. Enrofloxacin was not shown to cause clinically recognizable joint abnormalities in a group of psittacine birds from a large aviary.

Chloramphenicol, penicillin, tetracycline, oxytetracycline and sulfa drugs may cause deformities in embryos and should not be used in hens near or during the breeding season.

Antifungals

Antifungal agents can have serious side effects, particularly with prolonged use. Amphotericin B has been associated with acidosis, azotemia, vomiting, seizures, hypokalemia, hepatic dysfunction, anemia, anaphylaxis and nephrotoxicosis. Flucytosine may cause bone marrow depression, anemia, thrombocytopenia and leukopenia. A severe granulomatous sinusitis occurred in an African Grey Parrot following the accidental use of of amphotericin B suspension rather than a solution as a nasal flush.

Hypervitaminosis

Of particular concern are vitamins A, D_3 (cholecalciferol) and calcium. Many formulated diets contain excess quantities of these nutrients, and further supplementation of these diets with vitamin and mineral products can result in life-threatening toxicities.

Hypervitaminosis A can cause osteodystrophy characterized by thickening of the proliferative-maturation zone, metaphyseal sclerosis, hyperosteoidosis and decreased numbers of osteoclasts. Parathyroid gland hyperplasia can also occur. Hypervitaminosis D_3 can cause mineralization of parenchymal organs including the liver, kidneys, stomach, intestines, heart and blood vessels. High levels of vitamin D_3 cause an increase in serum calcium levels, which may affect cardiac conduction and smooth muscle contractions. Renal calcification in macaws and African Grey Parrots suggests that they may be particularly sensitive to hypervitaminosis D and excess calcium consumption.

Vitamin injections are often used in debilitated birds. If the patient has been on a formulated diet or over-supplemented previously, parenteral administration of a multivitamin preparation may cause or exacerbate a vitamin intoxication problem.

Airborne Toxins

Administering 100% oxygen to birds for more than 12 hours was found to be fatal with death occurring in four to eight days; exposed birds appeared stressed and uncomfortable as early as three days post-exposure.

Polytetrafluoroethylene Gas

Polytetrafluoroethylene (PTFE) gas, released when various non-stick surfaces such as Teflon® overheat or burn, is a common respiratory toxin in birds.

The lungs are the target organ for PTFE poisoning in birds. Clinical signs are usually limited to sudden death, but depending on the degree of exposure may include somnolence, dyspnea, wheezing, incoordination, weakness, respiratory distress and terminal convulsions. Death usually occurs too rapidly for treatment to be initiated.

With minimal exposure, birds may respond to immediate transfer to fresh air, coupled with the administration of intratracheal and systemic steroids, broad-spectrum antibiotics, fluids and a warm environment to prevent shock, pulmonary edema and bronchopneumonia.

Tobacco Products

Birds should never be allowed to consume tobacco products. Ingestion of small quantities of nicotine can cause hyperexcitability, vomiting, diarrhea, seizures and rapid death. Treatment is supportive and symptomatic.

Passive inhalation of cigarette, cigar and pipe smoke can cause chronic ocular, dermatologic and respiratory disease in companion birds (see Chapter 22). Birds that live in homes with smokers will often present with clinical signs including coughing, sneezing, sinusitis and conjunctivitis due to continuous irritation of the respiratory system. Secondary bacterial invasion of the damaged respiratory epithelium is common and requires therapy; however, therapy for these infections will be of little value if the bird is continuously exposed to smoke.

Exposure to secondary smoke from marijuana can cause severe depression and regurgitation and should be strictly avoided.

Pododermatitis has been observed in some birds handled by people who smoke routinely. Macaws may suffer a similar dermatitis on the bare cheek patches following repeated contact with a smoker's hands. Many birds with severe feather picking problems will resume normal preening behavior when removed from exposure to cigarette smoke.

Disinfectants

Disinfecting agents used to clean enclosures and food dishes should be used cautiously in aviaries and where companion birds are housed.

All enclosures, nest boxes or aviary tools that are placed in disinfectants should be thoroughly rinsed with clean water before they are in contact with a bird.

Direct contact between the bird and cleaning solutions should be avoided. When ingestion of cleaning products or disinfectants occurs, the manufacturer's recommendations for therapy should be followed. If recommendations are not available, then birds ingesting noncaustic materials should be treated with a mild laxative to speed passage of the solution out of the body. Gentle gavaging or flushing is indicated if corrosive material has been ingested to prevent perforation of the esophagus or crop. Corrosive materials require immediate dilution with water. Eyes or skin areas exposed to corrosives must be rinsed with clean water for at least twenty minutes.

Ammonia and bleach are frequently used in household cleaning. Ammonia can be absorbed into the circulation by inhalation. One study showed that blood ammonia concentration in excess of 1 mg/dL was an indication of toxicity.

Ammonia and chlorine vapors can also irritate the epithelial linings of the eyes, conjunctiva, nares and respiratory tract. The resulting inflammation and damage can predispose these surfaces to secondary bacterial and fungal infections. Severe inflammation from exposure to strong concentrations of ammonia may impair respiration. Treatment consists of oxygen therapy, steroids to reduce inflammation and broad-spectrum antibiotics to combat secondary bacterial infections.

Miscellaneous Aerosols

Common household aerosol products such as perfumes, deodorants and cleaning agents may cause respiratory problems in birds. These problems arise from direct irritation of the respiratory tract by the fluorocarbons and particulates in these aerosols. The most common effect is inflammation and edema of the respiratory tract leading to dyspnea. In severe cases, death may occur shortly after a large or direct exposure. Formaldehyde fumes have been associated with epiphora, dyspnea and death in canaries. An ozone generator caused the deaths of some birds in a pet shop. A cockatoo that was in the same room where a suede protector was used developed dyspnea within two hours, and died five hours after being exposed to the fumes from this product.

Leaks in natural gas lines may cause subtle respiratory signs in birds, even when no odors are detected by the clients. With more serious leaks, sudden death can occur. When birds are presented with respiratory problems or weakness of unknown etiology, careful questioning concerning the home environment may help determine if a leaking gas line could be a contributing factor. Kerosene fumes may also be toxic to birds, and combustible space heaters should not be used in homes containing companion birds.

Carbon monoxide (CO) is an odorless, colorless, tasteless gas produced by combustion engines and some furnaces. Birds maintained in poorly ventilated, heated areas, or transported in poorly ventilated vehicles (especially in car trunks) are at high risk of CO poisoning.

Birds suffering from CO poisoning may die acutely and have bright red, apparently well oxygenated blood and pink- or red-colored tissues. Other signs of CO poisoning include depression, somnolence and dyspnea.

If CO poisoning is suspected, fresh air should be provided immediately, and emergency care should include the administration of 90-95% oxygen in a cool, dark, stress-free environment.

Pulmonary silicosis caused chronic dyspnea and death in a Blue and Gold Macaw. The bird was exposed to the silicone through peat moss used as nesting material.

Insecticides

Exposure to high concentrations of pesticides can lead to nonspecific signs of poisoning including gastrointestinal problems, tremors, weakness, dyspnea, seizures or sudden death. Chronic low-grade exposure to pesticides may induce more subtle clinical signs that are more difficult to attribute to a toxin exposure. These exposures may cause immunosuppression and increased susceptibility to disease, decreased reproductive activity or generalized unthriftiness.

While pyrethrins and carbamates are occasionally used as pesticides in association with birds, these agents are nonetheless toxic, especially following inhalation or contact with high concentrations. All grain products, fruits and vegetables that are not certified organic have levels of pesticides that have been determined to be acceptable ("safe" is a relative term) for human consumption. The effects of constant exposure of birds to these toxins has not been determined.

If absolutely necessary, dusting powders containing pyrethrins or carbamates (eg, 5% Sevin) can be used with some margin of safety on birds. These compounds are not absorbed through the skin and are more likely to penetrate the feathers than sprays; however, excessive preening (ingestion) or inhalation of the dusts can lead to systemic intoxication that is dose-related.

Organochlorines

Migratory birds may be exposed in other countries that still use DDT produced in the United States. Poisoned birds may develop signs of convulsions, blindness (pupils may or may not respond to light), ataxia, anemia and hypoproteinemia.

Organophosphates

Clinical signs of organophosphate toxicity are caused by inhibition of acetylcholinesterase. Organophosphate poisoning in raptors appears clinically different than is typically described for mammals. Raptors are frequently contaminated by consuming poisoned starlings or grackles. Clinical signs include ataxia, spastic nictitans, a detached attitude, inability to fly and occasionally convulsions. If present, convulsions are characterized by rigid paralysis, tightly clinched talons, rapid respiration, salivation, twitching of muscles and anisocoria.

Dichlorvos (DDVP, Vapona) is a commonly used organophosphate that is impregnated in insect repellent strips. It is best for birds not to be exposed to any inhaled toxins; however, if a dichlorvos insecticide must be used, it should be placed in a well ventilated room of appropriate size. Other sources of avian exposure to organophosphates include flea collars, contaminated fruit limbs and frequently treated baseboards.

Pyrethrins have perhaps the lowest degree of toxicity in birds and warm-blooded mammals. They are often combined with the synergist piperonal butoxide to enhance insecticidal activity.

General Considerations

While taking a history, clients should always be questioned about their use of insecticides in and around (outside open windows) the home.

A tentative diagnosis of insecticide poisoning is usually possible with a history of recent exposure and appropriate clinical signs. Whole blood acetylcholinesterase activity can be used to confirm a diagnosis of organophosphate intoxication.

A definitive postmortem diagnosis can be made by tissue analysis of the liver, kidneys, body fat and gastrointestinal contents for insecticide residues. Brain cholinesterase activity can be used to determine if the bird's death was due to an organophosphate intoxication; clinical analysis of tissues may not always be reliable due to the rapid metabolism of these insecticides. Any tissues to be analyzed for insecticide residues or acetylcholinesterase activity should be submitted frozen in separate containers.

Treatment for organophosphate toxicosis includes supportive care (supplemental heat, fluids and diazepam to control seizures). Atropine is indicated for cholinergic signs (0.2-0.5 mg/kg one-fourth dose IV or IM every three to four hours). Pralidoxime hydrochloride (2-PAM) is antidotal for organophosphate intoxications. 2-PAM was administered to King Pigeons with good results at 10 mg/kg IM. Steroids may be beneficial for the treatment of pulmonary edema or shock. For maximum effectiveness, antidotal therapy must be initiated within 24 hours of exposure. Organophosphates irreversibly bind to acetylcholinesterase. The more binding that is allowed to occur, the less effective the antidote will be.

Carbamates

Carbamates' mode of action, induced clinical signs and methods of diagnosis and treatment are the same as for organophosphates, although 2-PAM is contraindicated.

Rodenticides

Most rodenticides are of the anticoagulant variety. Clinical signs of toxicity include depression, anorexia, petechiation, epistaxis and subcutaneous hemorrhage. The antidote is vitamin K_1. Some rodenticides contain cholecalciferol or bromethalin and are potentially more difficult to treat than the anticoagulant types.

MYCOPLASMA AND RICKETTSIA

Helga Gerlach

The mycoplasmatales consist of three genera, which can be distinguished roughly by the following properties:

Mycoplasma need cholesterol for growth (production of the cellular membrane).

Acholeplasma do not need cholesterol for growth, but many strains can be inhibited by the thallium acetate that is commonly used for inhibiting gram-negative bacteria in media used for the isolation of mycoplasma.

Ureaplasma were formerly called T-strains because of their tiny colony sizes. They require urea for their energy metabolism and also cholesterol for growth.

Mycoplasmatales

Transmission

Mycoplasmatales are relatively low in infectivity. Close contact between individuals is necessary for transmission, and infections are most common in dense populations. The respiratory and genital tracts are the primary portals of entrance. The organism is spread by respiratory excretions and by the gonads of both sexes as well as hematologically through the body. Infected air sacs can lead to contact transmission of the ovary (and developing follicle). Transovarian transmission is epornitically important, although in clinically healthy breeders, the egg transmission rate is low (between 0.1 and 1.0 %); however, there are some exceptions. Close contact is the primary mode of transmission in neonates. Offspring feeding on contaminated crop regurgitations (eg, crop milk in pigeons) may also become infected.

Pathogenesis

Mycoplasmatales preferably colonize the mucosa of the respiratory and the genital tracts. Strains capable of inducing systemic infections can be found in the brain and joints. Because the agent may be hidden in the recesses of the host cell membrane, it can remain rather inaccessible by therapeutics and the host defense mechanisms. As a consequence, only negligible amounts of humoral antibodies, if any, are produced.

Depending on the virulence of the strain in question, cellular damage may be caused at the site of colonization. The host reacts with a serofibrinous inflammation and activation of the cell-mediated defense system. The excessive response of the latter (which is genetically determined) governs the type and magnitude of pathologic changes.

Many mycoplasmatales cause transformation of the host lymphoblasts (mainly T-cells) by excreting a mutagenic substance. Affected cells function improperly and there is a severe proliferation of immature lymphocytes in local lymph follicles with invasion of the lymphoid cells into the infected area. These altered lymph follicles can appear similar to those described for lymphoma.

Pathology

At necropsy, lesions caused by various mycoplasmatales in respective hosts vary in degree but not in presentation. Serous to serofibrinous conjunctivitis, rhinitis, sinusitis, tracheitis, air sacculitis and focal bronchopneumonia have all been described. The nasal cavity and the infraorbital sinus frequently display a unilateral, seromucoid (later fibrinous) exudate that also fills the choanal fissure. In ducks and turkeys, the exudate is often semigelatinous, fibrinous or caseous, and leads to distention of the infraorbital sinus. The mucous membranes are swollen and may show petechiation. The tenacious exudate can be mixed with fibrinous debris.

Differential Diagnosis

The rule-out list includes many viral, bacterial and fungal diseases. In Psittaciformes, pigeons, ducks and geese, chlamydiosis is the main rule-out. The genital tract can be infected by other microorganisms as well. Embryopathologic lesions and embryonal death are suggestive. With mycoplasmatales, infected embryos generally die late in incubation. Embryos that die after pipping frequently have air sacculitis of the left thoracic air sac group (exceptions are geese that have air sacculitis bilaterally). After hatching, chronic lymphofollicular proliferation can be so severe that lymphoma must be considered in the rule-out list.

Diagnosis

A tentative diagnosis can be made by histopathologic examination. Isolation of the agent is necessary for identification and biologic assays. Because of the fastidious nature of this organism and the difficulties in identifying the agent, specialized laboratories are necessary to isolate *Mycoplasma*. In addition, the mycoplasmatales need to be differentiated from bacterial L-forms. Swabs from the upper respiratory tract, or the phallus in males, can be taken from live birds. Endoscopic biopsies of affected air sacs are useful diagnostic aids. Samples from air sacs, salpinx, lungs and spleen should be collected for postmortem evaluation. Transport media are necessary for shipping samples.

Indirect diagnosis of mycoplasmatales by serology is hampered by false-positive (cross-reactions) and false-negative tests. The most frequently used tests are: serum slide agglutination (SSA), HI test (for the hemagglutinating species), growth- or metabolic-inhibition test, immunodiffusion test, immunofluorescence test, ELISA, and recently the polymerase chain reaction.

Treatment

Clinical infections can be treated with tylosin, spiramycin and erythromycin or spectinomycin in combination with clindamycin or pleuromutilin. The efficacy of tetracyclines against avian mycoplasmatales has yet to be proven. However, in Psittaciformes, the tetracyclines are recommended because of the clinical similarities between mycoplasmosis and chlamydiosis. The pigeon strains are highly resistant to erythromycin and, to a lesser extent, tylosin. Only pleuromutilin was able to inhibit 57 of 65 strains recovered from pigeons. The LD_{50} for pleuromutilin in pigeons is 440 mg/kg, considerably less than for chickens and turkeys. This drug must be carefully used when treating pigeons that are feeding offspring or if used in the water during hot weather.

Spiramycin given parenterally to Ploceidae, Estrildae and even canaries may lead to sudden death from unknown causes. The same dose given via drinking water is well tolerated. Spiramycin is one of the macrolid antibiotics and is given at a dose of 100 mg/kg body weight IM, or 100-200 mg/kg body weight orally. Since the primary patent has expired, several manufacturers produce it. Enrofloxacin has been used to treat mycoplasmosis in poultry. There have been no reports of success in treating mycoplasmosis with enrofloxacin in other birds. Treatment is designed to allow clinically affected birds to recover. The organism is difficult to eliminate.

Rickettsia

Little information is available on rickettsial infections in birds. Rickettsia form a group of microorganisms, the taxonomy of which has still not been fully determined. They are obligatory cellular parasites, and can be differentiated from chlamydia by the absence of a developmental cycle and the capacity to synthesize energy-rich compounds (ATP). Rickettsia are small rods or coccoids with an average size of 0.3-0.5 μm in diameter and 0.8-2.0 μm in length. They may also be pleomorphic, and are generally nonmotile. Multiplication takes place by binary fission. The organism parasitizes reticuloendothelial cells, vascular endothelial cells or erythrocytes. Infections may occur in arthropods, which can serve as vectors or as primary hosts.

Rocky Mountain Spotted Fever (RMSF)

RMSF is a mammalian disease caused by *Rickettsia rickettsii*. RMSF is transmitted by ticks (mainly *Dermacentor* spp.) and rodents. Dogs and opossum are thought to be reservoirs. Birds, including chickens, several Columbiformes, pheasants, Falconiformes and the Magpie, are susceptible to experimental infection and may also serve as reservoirs. Pigeons may be particularly important reservoirs. Clinical abnormalities have not been described in infected birds.

Q-Fever

Q-fever, caused by *Coxiella burnetti*, is an aerosol-borne disease in humans with worldwide distribution. Direct and indirect transmission (arthropods) can occur in humans and other host species. This agent differs considerably from other members of the Rickettsiaceae. The cells are smaller (0.2-0.4 μm by 0.4-1.0 μm) and replicate in vacuoles of the host cells. In contrast to chlamydia, *C. burnetti* infections result in the formation of phagolysosomes.

The host spectrum of *C. burnetti* is wide, and includes arthropods (particularly ticks), birds and mammals. Avian susceptibility to *C. burnetti* seems to be high, and this organism has been demonstrated in at least 49 avian species. No clinical disease has been observed in any susceptible avian species.

C. burnetti can be identified in tissues using various staining methods (Giemsa, Macchiavello's, Castañeda) as for chlamydia. Antibodies can be demonstrated using the CF test or the ELISA.

Therapy with tetracyclines is effective for the clinical disease, but elimination of the organism is not possible. Treatment for infected birds is not encouraged because of the high immunosuppressive side effect of the tetracyclines.

Aegyptianella (Ae.)

Ae. pullorum is the causative agent of anemia and hepatitis in chickens and other birds. It is an erythrocytic parasite that produces endocytoplasmic inclusions, which stain using the Giemsa or Pappenheim procedures. The inclusions measure 0.3 by 4.0 μm, and each can contain up to 26 initial bodies (reproducing form up to 0.8 μm in diameter).

The organism is most common in tropical and subtropical regions including the Mediterranean.

Clinical signs in young birds are characterized by an acute onset of anemia, anorexia, weakness, weight loss, greenish diarrhea and death. Chronic infections in older birds are characterized by icterus, which may not be clinically recognizable.

The rule-out list includes internal bleeding, chlamydiosis and chronic diseases of various etiology. For diagnosis, a blood smear stained according to Giemsa or Pappenheim shows the parasites in the erythrocytes. Tetracyclines are effective for treatment. Tick control is mandatory to prevent reinfection and epizootics.

ANESTHESIOLOGY

Leslie C. Sinn

With the refractory attitudes of many birds toward even mild restraint, sedatives and local anesthetics are of little use in most avian species. General anesthesia, however, with appropriate agents, can enable clinicians to safely and rapidly perform fluid administration, emergency procedures, blood collection and radiography, or to perform prolonged invasive surgical procedures in avian patients.

As in other animal species, general anesthesia in birds can be accomplished with either injectable or inhalant anesthetic agents. Injectable anesthetics are far inferior to gas anesthetics for use in avian patients, and for private avian practice, isoflurane is the only recommended anesthetic.

Anesthetic Agents and Equipment

Contraindications for anesthetizing an avian patient should include severe obesity, fatty liver, liver or kidney failure, dehydration, shock, anemia, dyspnea and fluid in the crop. Unfortunately, patients presented with many of these problems are those that require anesthesia for proper resolution of the case. In all situations, the anesthetic of choice is isoflurane.

Because of the anatomy and structure of the avian respiratory system, even healthy birds may not be properly oxygenated when anesthetized and placed in dorsal recumbency. It may be impossible for some species that have a large pectoral muscle mass (eg, Galliformes and Anseriformes) to adequately ventilate. Because of their unique respiratory anatomy, intubation and the use of gentle intermittent positive pressure ventilation (IPPV) (20-40 per minute at 15 mm H_2O) is strongly recommended in anesthetized patients.

Isoflurane

Isoflurane is rapidly replacing halothane and methoxyflurane as the gas anesthetic of choice for small animal patients. This surge in popularity is based on isoflurane's rapid induction time, rapid and smooth recoveries, rapid change in anesthetic level, high margin of safety for both the patient and hospital staff, reduced arrhythmogenic properties, reduced cardiovascular depression and reduced respiratory depression. The drug can also be safely used to obtain diagnostic information from high-risk and critically ill birds. Recovery from even long surgical procedures requires only minutes.

Isoflurane can have a dose-related depressant effect on the respiratory and cardiovascular system. Fortunately, there is a substantial interval between respiratory and cardiac arrest. The hypotensive effects of isoflurane have been shown to be severe in cranes. The effect was dose-dependent and was potentiated by spontaneous respiration when compared to assisted ventilation (IPPV). Isoflurane is only 0.3% metabolized compared to 15% for halothane and 50% for methoxyflurane; thus, isoflurane does not produce the hepatic damage induced by halothane and methoxyflurane. Isoflurane has a blood solubility of 1.4 compared to 13 for methoxyflurane and 2.4 for halothane. Minimum alveolar concentration (MAC) has been found to be approximately 1.3 (cranes and ducks).

Oxygen

The oxygen flow should be high enough to ensure that a precision vaporizer is accurate in its delivery of the anesthetic gas. For most precision vaporizers, the minimum flow rate is 500 ml/min. Some vaporizers function adequately at low settings but the manufacturer's recommendations should always be followed. If a semi-open system is used, the oxygen flow should be three times the respiratory minute volume, which for a 450 g bird is about 275 ml/min. As a general guideline, this ratio can be used to determine the respiratory minute volume of any avian species. For most psittacine birds, the oxygen flow rate during induction is 1 L/min and maintenance is 0.5 to 1 L/min depending on the size of the patient.

Nitrous Oxide

Nitrous oxide (N_2O) has successfully been used in birds in combination with isoflurane anesthesia. N_2O is not potent enough to induce anesthesia on its own; however, it does allow for the reduction in the percentage of isoflurane necessary for anesthetic maintenance. Because cardiovascular and respiratory depression caused by isoflurane are dose-dependent, N_2O is an important addition to the anesthetic regime. N_2O does have the characteristic of diffusing into closed gas spaces faster than nitrogen (room air) can diffuse out. This means that N_2O is contraindicated in situations where dead gas spaces are present. Because the avian respiratory system including the air sacs freely intercommunicate, the use of N_2O is not contraindicated. Some species differences do exist. For instance, diving birds have naturally occurring subcutaneous air pockets, and the use of N_2O in these birds may lead to subcutaneous emphysema.

Pre-anesthetics

The routine use of atropine as a pre-anesthetic has been avoided in avian patients because it thickens respiratory secretions, slows gastrointestinal motility and increases the heart rate. The thickening of respiratory secretions could contribute to a life-threatening occlusion in patients intubated with small-diameter endotracheal tubes. Additional elevation of the heart rate is not desirable in patients that already have a rapid rate. Glycopyrrolate does not have as marked effect on the heart, but it too causes thickening of respiratory secretions. Consequently, these drugs are used only as specific therapy for bradycardia.

Injectable Anesthetics

With most commonly used injectable agents, the anesthetic level cannot be rapidly decreased, and the recovery is prolonged because the drug must be totally removed by metabolic pathways. Increased recovery times create excessive stress, increase the period of hypothermia and prolong the deviation from a physiologically normal state.

The most commonly reported injectable anesthetics used in birds are combinations of ketamine and xylazine and, less frequently, ketamine and diazepam. Etorphine, methoxymol, propafol, midazolam, tiletamine/ zolezapam and barbiturates have all been used in birds. Initial data are promising for some of these drugs, but in many cases actual clinical trials are not available. In general, phenobarbital, methohexital, thiobarbiturates and barbital should not be used in companion birds.

Ketamine anesthesia is typified by cardiac and respiratory depression, increased blood pressure, reduced body temperature, slow violent recoveries and prolonged physiologic changes.

Ketamine is rarely used alone. Because of the muscle rigidity produced by this drug and the inadequacy of the analgesia achieved, ketamine is most often used in combination with either xylazine or diazepam. The ratio for both ketamine/diazepam or ketamine/xylazine combination is 10:1 on a mg/kg basis. Either combination provides for more rapid induction, smoother maintenance and less violent recovery than when ketamine is used alone.

Xylazine produces good muscle relaxation and transient analgesia. It can cause bradycardia and heart blocks.

Diazepam is an excellent sedative and provides some muscle relaxation. Ketamine/diazepam combinations can be useful when mild restraint is required.

The dosages for the drugs to be administered in combination are calculated based on a ketamine dosage of 5-30 mg/kg IM (or 2.5-5.0 mg IV) mixed with xylazine 1.0-4.0 mg IM (or 0.25-0.50 mg IV). Alternatively, diazepam (0.5-2.0 mg/kg IM or IV) may be substituted for the xylazine. The two drugs chosen are mixed together and administered either intramuscularly or intravenously. Reduced doses are necessary in seriously ill, pediatric and geriatric patients and for intravenous administration. Ratites require only 3 mg/kg of ketamine. Because these drugs have a narrow therapeutic index and the species and individual dose responses vary widely, clinicians are advised to start at the lower end of the dosage range. The intravenous route is preferred, as the dose can be titrated to effect.

Both xylazine and diazepam can be mixed in the same syringe with ketamine. Care must be taken, especially with smaller doses, to eliminate all air pockets from the syringe and to thoroughly mix the two drugs. Recovery from intravenous administration of these injectable anesthetic combinations may take 15-45 minutes, while recovery from intramuscular administration, especially if additional dosages have been necessary, may take hours. Recovery may be violent. Yohimbine has been shown to be an effective reversal agent for ketamine/xylazine anesthesia in raptors. A dosage of 0.1 mg/kg yohimbine was effective in reversing anesthesia caused by the administration of intravenous ketamine (4.4 mg/kg)/xylazine (2.2 mg/kg). Tolazoline (15 mg/kg IV) has been used to successfully reverse ketamine/xylazine anesthesia in turkey vultures.

Etorphine has been successfully used in large birds such as ostriches and cassowaries. A dosage of 0.02-0.03 mg/kg IM is utilized for restraint. This can then be reversed with 0.04-0.06 mg/kg IV of diprenorphine.

Midazolam (same group as diazepam) (15 mg/kg IM) was successfully used to reduce the percentage of isoflurane necessary for general anesthesia in racing pigeons. It was then effectively reversed with the drug flumazenil (0.1 mg/kg IM).

Gas Anesthetic Equipment and Delivery

Anesthetic Machines and Vaporizers

Most of the available models of anesthetic machines are adequate for an avian practice. What is required is an out-of-circuit, precision vaporizer for the administration of isoflurane. The vapor pressure of isoflurane (261 mm Hg) is so close to halothane (243 mm Hg) that the same type precision vaporizer can be used for both agents. However, once converted to isoflurane, a machine should no longer be used for halothane. A vaporizer can be purchased that is manufactured specifically for use with isoflurane, or a halothane vaporizer can be cleaned with ether and recalibrated for use with isoflurane. A vaporizer cannot be used for halothane and isoflurane at the same time. Calibration of the vaporizer is necessary after a conversion has occurred from halothane to isoflurane. Once isoflurane is in use, the vaporizer should be cleaned and recalibrated on a yearly basis.

Breathing Systems

Tank systems used to induce anesthesia in small mammals should not be used in birds. These chambers prevent monitoring of the patient, create a potential for beak, head, neck or spinal trauma and release high concentrations of gas into the environment when the top is opened.

Semi-open systems rely on an Ayres T-piece, Y-piece, Norman elbow or Kuhn circuit that prevents the rebreathing of expired gases. Because of the relatively low resistance to air flow present in these systems, they are ideal for avian patients.

Semi-closed systems rely on the complete rebreathing of expired gases. The resistance inherent in the circuit makes them impractical for birds.

A non-rebreathing anesthetic system is recommended for patients under seven to eight kilograms (most birds). This reduces dead space and decreases the effort that the patient must exert in order to breathe. This is especially important in birds, because both expiration and inspiration involve active use of the trunk muscles. Either an Ayer's T-piece or Bain's circuit can be effectively used with most birds. Some clinicians prefer the Bain's circuit because in theory, the patient's expired gases warm the in-flowing gases and reduce the loss of body heat. This can be critical in birds because their small size predisposes them to hypothermia, and respiration is one of the major routes through which body heat is lost. In patients over seven to eight kilograms, conventional human pediatric supplies are adaptable, easy to obtain and easy to maintain. In larger avian patients (eg, ostriches), standard small animal anesthetic equipment and supplies are applicable.

A standard 0.5 liter reservoir bag can be used in some larger avian patients, but better control and monitoring of respiration can be achieved with a smaller volume bag specifically designed for birds. These can be handmade from plastic bags, or an inexpensive, disposable avian anesthesia bag is commercially available.

An appropriate scavenging system is the best protection for operating room personnel from secondary gas exposure.

Endotracheal Tubes

Non-cuffed infant, Magill or Cole (smallest size = 2 mm) endotracheal tubes can be used in medium- to large-sized birds. Cuffless tubes are used because birds have complete tracheal rings that cannot expand if excessive amounts of air are introduced into a cuffed tube. Alternatively, some clinicians choose to make their own endotracheal tubes out of red rubber feeding tubes. The end of the tube is snipped off and small holes are cut in the surface of the tube to allow for air exchange. The tip of the tube should be blunted by heating it with a flame and pressing it on a hard surface.

Face Masks

The delivery of inhalant gases from a precision vaporizer can best be achieved by manually restraining the patient and placing the nostrils and mouth in a face mask connected to an Ayres T-piece anesthetic circuit. Common canine or feline anesthetic masks, while not ideal, can be used for induction. To avoid nosocomial infections, a disposable plastic drinking cup, with soft paper products placed between the cup and the patient's neck to prevent gas leaks, is used as a face mask. In birds less than 150 g, an effective mask is made by covering the end of a 12 ml syringe case with a section of latex glove.

Care of Equipment

With the large number of infectious bacterial, fungal and viral agents encountered in avian patients, any equipment used during anesthesia, including tubing and endotracheal tubes, should be thoroughly disinfected to reduce the chance of nosocomial infections. Equipment should not be used for other companion animals and then used for birds without sterilization. While the face mask and Ayres T-piece can be easily disinfected in cold sterilization solutions, anesthetic bags are much more difficult to disinfect.

Delivery of Inhalant Anesthetics

Two methods of anesthetic induction with isoflurane have been discussed. One method is to place the bird in a face mask and slowly increase the gas to a level of 2.5-3%. However, the editors believe that the rapid induction achieved by using a 5% setting initially, followed by a decrease to maintenance levels of 1-2% is a better method.

After induction, any patient that will be anesthetized for more than ten minutes should be intubated with an appropriately sized endotracheal tube.

Following intubation, the endotracheal tube can be connected directly to the semi-open system. If there is a possibility of regurgitation, the tongue and glottis should be pulled cranially, and the esophagus should be packed with moistened cotton to prevent aspiration.

Air Sac Administration

For surgery of the head, trachea or syrinx, anesthesia can be delivered by placing a short endotracheal or red rubber tube into the clavicular or caudal thoracic air sacs. The placement procedure is rapid and may be indicated as an emergency tactic when an animal is presented with respiratory arrest or when severe dyspnea has been induced by foreign body aspiration. To place an air sac tube, the animal is positioned with the leg extended to the rear as for a surgical sexing procedure. An alternative to this site is behind the last rib or between the last two ribs, at the same site used for standard lateral laparoscopy. A small skin incision is made over the sternal notch, and hemostats are used to produce an entrance through the body wall and into the left abdominal air sac (see Chapter 13). A shortened endotracheal tube can then be inserted into the air sacs and the Ayres T-piece connected directly to the tracheal tube.

Management of the Anesthetic Patient

Patient Evaluation

The goal of a preanesthetic evaluation is to detect and correct any underlying pathology prior to inducing anesthesia. In some cases, several days or weeks of supportive care may be needed in order to adequately stabilize a compromised patient before anesthesia can be safely administered. In other cases, eliminating abnormalities may not be possible, and consequently, adjustments must be made in inducing and monitoring anesthesia to ensure a successful outcome.

The patient evaluation associated with the use of isoflurane for short-duration procedures (five to ten minutes) is generally limited to a thorough history and physical examination. The theory in using isoflurane for short-term procedures with a limited database is that this drug has a wide therapeutic index and has consistently been shown to be relatively safe even in severely compromised patients.

If a bird is going to undergo anesthesia for more than ten minutes, then in addition to the history and physical examination, a minimum database ideally should include a fecal parasite check, Gram's stain of feces and choana, PCV, TP, WBC with differential, a platelet estimate, estimated clotting time, bile acids, AST, LDH and UA. Additional tests may be indicated depending on the initial assessment and the type of procedure requiring anesthesia.

Risk Classification

Successful risk classification depends on conservative evaluation of the minimum database. Practically, risk assessment allows one to estimate the duration of safe anesthesia, the intensity of monitoring required and the supportive care and technical assistance needed to ensure patient safety.

Table 39.2 Risk Classification of Potential Anesthesia Patients	
Class I (minimal risk)	Young, healthy patient undergoing an elective procedure.
Class II (some risk)	Young, healthy patient undergoing a non-elective procedure, or a healthy patient undergoing an elective procedure.
Class III (risky)	Patient with an ongoing health problem undergoing a procedure for this or another problem.
Class IV (very risky)	Patient with a major health problem (unstable in nature) undergoing a procedure.
Class V (moribund)	Last ditch effort to save bird's life.

A commonly encountered complication of anesthesia in birds is liver dysfunction. Hepatopathies may be suspected when performing the initial physical examination and confirmed with findings of lowered protein levels, elevated or depressed bile acids and tissue enzyme values, and radiographic findings of hepatomegaly, or conversely, a loss of liver mass. Liver dysfunction may reduce a patient's ability to metabolize anesthetic agents and may also be associated with coagulopathy. The use in these patients of any anesthetic drug that is dependent on the liver for metabolism is contraindicated (most injectables, halothane, methoxyflurane). If anesthesia cannot be postponed to allow sufficient stabilization, then anesthetic agents that are minimally metabolized by the liver (eg, isoflurane) and vitamin K injections to help promote clotting are suggested.

Obesity is common in companion birds. Excess fat deposits interfere with the patient's ability to ventilate. Respiratory effort is further compromised when a bird is anesthetized and placed in abnormal body positions for surgery. With elective procedures, dietary changes and treatment for underlying metabolic disorders are indicated before general anesthesia is performed.

Surgery is frequently required for egg-related peritonitis, especially in small species (eg, cockatiels, lovebirds, budgerigars). These patients should be carefully stabilized prior to anesthesia. This stabilization process may take weeks and in some cases render surgical intervention unnecessary. An abdominal tap and diuretic therapy are indicated prior to anesthesia to reduce the volume of fluid in the abdomen and to improve the patient's ability to breathe.

These patients should be maintained in an upright position to prevent abdominal fluid and debris from entering the lungs through rents in the air sacs. The surgery table should be tilted so that the patient's head is slanted up.

In non-elective procedures on obese patients or those with an abdominal fluid accumulation, proper intubation is mandatory to ensure a patent airway. Gentle IPPV will help maintain adequate oxygenation. Keep in mind when providing IPPV that the avian lungs inflate minimally, and pressure placed on a breathing bag should be less than 15 mm H_2O to prevent rupture of the air capillaries.

Preanesthetic Stabilization and Preparation

Nutritional Therapy

For elective procedures, inadequate diets should be corrected three to four weeks before surgery.

Fluid Therapy

Correcting dehydration will dramatically improve the patient's ability to physiologically cope with anesthesia.

It has been suggested that all birds suffering from trauma and disease can be assumed to be at least ten percent dehydrated, and that the following formula should be used to calculate their fluid requirements: normal body weight (grams) x 0.1 (10%) = fluid deficit in ml. The dose for maintenance fluid is estimated at 50 ml/kg/day.

Calculated fluid requirements can be administered in severely dehydrated patients by an intravenous or intraosseous route (see Chapter 15). Fluids administered by oral or subcutaneous routes are not as effective in restoring or maintaining circulating volume.

A non-lactated solution is the fluid of choice. A balanced electrolyte solution protects renal function better than sugar solutions. Five percent dextrose is not a satisfactory replacement solution because the dextrose is metabolized, leaving free water. Fluids administered to anesthetized birds should be heated (96°F) to prevent hypothermia.

Fluids must be carefully administered to birds to prevent volume overload. The maximum acute fluid load that can be tolerated by healthy patients is 90 ml/kg/hr. In a cockatiel this would be a maximum of 9 ml in an hour or 0.15 ml per minute. Most avian patients, however, are unstable and cannot tolerate such a high rate and volume of fluid administration.

If no means of determining the bicarbonate deficit is available and the patient is dehydrated or critically ill, the administration of 1 mEq/kg of bicarbonate at 15-30 minute intervals to a maximum of 4 mEq is suggested.

Fasting

Practically speaking, the patient should be kept off food long enough for the upper gastrointestinal system to become empty. This process takes overnight in large birds and four to six hours in smaller birds. One should palpate the crop and postpone surgery if it is not empty. In an emergency, a patient with food in the crop should be held upright during the induction procedure, with a finger blocking the esophagus just below the mandible. Once the animal is anesthetized, the crop can be emptied by placing a finger covered with cotton or gauze over the choanal slit to prevent food entering the nasal cavity, turning the bird upside down and manually emptying the crop and esophagus. The esophagus can then be packed with gauze, and the head and neck positioned on an upward slant to minimize the chances of passive regurgitation. The trachea should be intubated using an appropriately sized tube.

Patient Monitoring

Depth should be monitored by combining information obtained from heart rate monitored by either an ECG or Doppler, respiratory rate and effort, toe pinch, palpebral and corneal reflexes and wing tone.

In a light plane of anesthesia, the patient has a palpebral, corneal and pedal reflex but has lost voluntary motion. The ideal anesthetic level, as described in one study, was when the bird's eyelids were completely closed and mydriatic, the pupillary light reflex (pupillary response to light) was delayed and the nictitating membrane moved slowly over the entire cornea. The muscles were relaxed and all pain reflexes were absent. The loss of a corneal reflex (no reflex closure of the lid after touching the peripheral cornea with a dry swab) was considered to indicate deep anesthesia.

The respiratory rate should be slow and deep. If a patient becomes too deep, all reflexes will be lost and the respiratory rate will be slow and irregular. Wing flutter is often an early indicator that an animal is becoming light. An excellent plane of anesthesia for most procedures can be accomplished by reaching a depth of anesthesia where wing tone has just disappeared.

Body Temperature

Loss of heat during surgical anesthesia is a very important factor in anesthetic survival and in the rate of return to a physiologic normal state following anesthesia. Even with supplemental heat, it is not unusual to have rapid reductions in core temperature during anesthesia.

All patients undergoing long surgical procedures should be placed on water circulating heating pads. Keep in mind that these devices need at least a 20-minute warm-up period before they reach the pre-set temperature. The clinician may choose to minimize the amount of alcohol used in the surgical scrub and instead use chlorhexidine or povidone iodine to minimize heat loss through evaporation.

Body temperature (normal=105-107°F) can be constantly monitored during anesthesia to properly evaluate the degree of heat loss. A patient under anesthesia will experience a time-related reduction in body temperature (maybe as much as 10°F), which can predispose to cardiac arrhythmias and increased recovery times.

Heart Monitoring

Esophageal stethoscopes equipped with pediatric tubing can be used for auscultation of the heart in avian patients the size of Amazon parrots and larger. Dopplers can be used, but are extremely positional in nature and difficult to maintain in birds. Some oximetry units provide pulse rates up to 250 bpm; these units are easy to use and are not positional like the Doppler. In a group of cockatiels maintained in a surgical plane of anesthesia, the heart rate remained above 450 bpm. An ECG is an excellent way to monitor the depth of avian anesthesia. As a bird gets deeper, the T-waves become smaller and may totally disappear. As the depth further increases, the R-wave will increase in magnitude and the S-wave is reduced.

Respiratory Rate

Respiratory rates during anesthesia should be slow and regular (see Table 39.3). An increase in the respiratory rate may indicate that a bird is entering a lighter plane of anesthesia, that the bird is having difficulty breathing (occluded tracheal tube) or that the bird has an elevated $paCO_2$. Direct visualization of chest movement as an indication of respiration can be facilitated by using clear sterile surgical drapes.

When using halothane or methoxyflurane, apnea and cardiac arrest may develop at the same time without prior warning. With isoflurane, apnea usually proceeds cardiac arrest by several minutes.

Apnea monitors do work in birds; however, less expensive units may not be sensitive enough to detect the respirations of smaller patients.

Table 39.3   Heart Rate and Respiratory Rates in Birds Anesthetized with Isoflurane

	Beats per Minute	Breaths per Minute
Budgerigar	600-750	55-75
Cockatiel	450-604	30-40
Pigeon	93.1 ± 5.4	15-25
Parrot	120-780	10-20
Ostriches	60-72	2-20

Anesthetic Emergencies

Respiratory Arrest

If respiratory arrest occurs, the anesthetic system should be disconnected from the bird and the chest should be lightly pressed and released to induce air intake, or fresh air can be gently delivered into the tracheal tube. If the patient is not intubated, an air sac tube should be placed or the animal should be immediately intubated. The practitioner must keep mind that air sac intubation may result in apnea while the paO_2 is increasing and the $paCO_2$ is decreasing.

If respiratory arrest occurs in response to injectable anesthetics, the reversal agent should be administered intravenously. The administration of doxapram HCl on the tongue may help stimulate respiration. The pulse rate should be carefully monitored and resuscitation should continue until the bird is breathing unassisted. Birds that show respiratory arrest should be rescheduled for the procedure; a second or third episode of apnea in these cases is often followed by cardiac arrest.

Cardiac Arrest

Cardiac arrest represents a poor prognosis. Resuscitation efforts are often unsuccessful. If success is to be achieved and cardiac arrest truly does exist, the clinician should be aggressive and utilize open heart massage. The rate should be 60 or more compressions per minute and they should be accompanied by coordinated artificial ventilation. These efforts should be continued for up to five minutes. Although rare, some birds may recover following cardiac arrest.

Hemorrhage

If hemorrhage occurs during surgery, a significant portion of that loss can be replaced via fluid therapy using isotonic solutions. If hemorrhage is severe, a transfusion will be necessary (see Chapter 15).

Postanesthetic Monitoring and Recovery

Anesthetic recovery should occur in a pre-heated environment, preferably a pediatric or avian incubator.

Anesthetic recovery is best accomplished by wrapping the bird in a towel to prevent wing-flapping and self-inflicted trauma. The lights should be dimmed and the noise level kept to a minimum to prevent violent reactions. The patient should be rolled over every few minutes, and the pharynx should be monitored for the accumulation of mucus or vomit. In severely depressed birds, IPPV can be continued until the patient is no longer willing to tolerate the tracheal tube.

SURGICAL CONSIDERATIONS

R. Avery Bennett

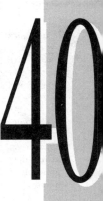

When possible, a clinical database acquired prior to surgery should include a complete history, physical examination and laboratory data. A minimum database for any preoperative evaluation should include hematocrit, total serum solids and WBC. If possible, a complete blood chemistry profile, whole body radiographs, electrocardiogram and cultures, if indicated, should be obtained. A blood glucose is useful in Anseriformes and raptors.

Patients with blood glucose of <200 mg/dL should receive 5% dextrose IV intraoperatively. Patients with total serum solids of <2 mg/dL are usually severely debilitated and are poor candidates for surgical recovery. A hematocrit >60% is indicative of dehydration, and fluid therapy should be instituted. If the hematocrit is <20%, surgery should be delayed or a whole blood transfusion should be administered. Blood transfusions are best made from donors of the same species; however, heterologous transfusions appear to be safe and efficacious. A serum uric acid of >30 mg/dL indicates dehydration (prerenal) or renal disease. Surgery should always be postponed until a patient is adequately hydrated. The hematocrit and total serum solids can be used to determine whether primary renal disease is a factor.

Serum cholesterol, AST and LDH activities may be helpful in evaluating the preoperative condition of a patient. Of 54 birds used to evaluate various anesthetic agents, three deaths occurred, two of which had preanesthetic serum parameters: AST=>650 IU/L, LDH=>600 IU/L and cholesterol=>700 mg/dL. Many of the birds that survived had high AST and LDH activities but not in combination with a high serum cholesterol level.

Respiratory recovery time is determined by the time it takes a bird to return to a prestressed respiratory rate following two minutes of handling. A return to normal respiratory rate within 3-5 minutes indicates respiratory stability adequate for most anesthetic and surgical procedures. Periods longer than five minutes indicate severe respiratory compromise.

The bird's nitrogen balance should be addressed, especially in birds that have been anorectic for several days. In a properly hydrated bird, an increase in body weight is a good indicator of a positive nitrogen balance.

Birds have relatively little glycogen stored in the liver. A decrease in blood glucose and insulin combined with an increase in glucagon stimulate hepatic glycogenolysis. Liver glycogen stores may decrease as much as 90% during a 24- to 36-hour fast and potentially quicker in smaller birds. Vomiting and regurgitation may occur if the patient is not fasted, and can result in aspiration pneumonia (see Chapter 39). A short fast of five to eight hours will help decrease the probability of aspiration pneumonia and will have minimal effects on blood glucose. In emergency situations when the digestive tract is full, it should be partially emptied before the bird is placed in dorsal recumbency (see Chapter 39).

When significant hemorrhage is anticipated, intraoperative IV fluid therapy should be provided. A patient may be suspected to have a clotting disorder if perifollicular bleeding occurs during surgical preparation. When a mature feather is removed, there should be virtually no hemorrhage around the follicle.

Nutritional Support

Carbohydrates (not fats) are nitrogen-sparing energy sources that best correct a stress-related negative nitrogen balance. The postoperative surgical patient must have a positive nitrogen balance to facilitate tissue repair, and a source of nonprotein energy to meet increased caloric requirements.

[*Ed. note: See Chapter 15 for determination of energy and fluid needs.*]

Patient Preparation

Feather Control

In preparing the skin for surgery, feathers surrounding the proposed surgical site should be gently plucked for a distance of two to three centimeters. The large flight feathers (remiges and retrices) are attached to the periosteum of the underlying bone and have highly developed feather muscles and ligaments. Removing these feathers is painful and is best accomplished while the patient is anesthetized. When flight feathers must be removed, they should be removed individually by holding the feather at its base and pulling in the direction of feather growth. To avoid injury to the skin, muscles and periosteal attachments, the other hand is used to carefully secure the tissues at the base of the feather while it is being removed.

Small feathers should be pulled in groups of three or four in a direction opposite their growth. If the skin has been damaged or torn, the feathers in this area can be cut to avoid further damage to the skin.

If primary or secondary feathers are removed, the bird will not be able to fly until they regrow. The removal of primary and secondary feathers should be avoided because it is easy to damage the follicle, resulting in the growth of malformed replacement feathers. Feathers in adjacent pterylae can be retracted using a stockinette, masking tape or water-soluble gel.

Creating a Sterile Field

Standard aseptic technique must be adhered to when performing surgery on avian patients.

Concentrations of chlorhexidine diacetate (0.05%) and povidone iodine (1.0%) are effective for skin preparation. Chlorhexidine gluconate (4%) is equally effective when rinsed with saline or alcohol.

Chlorhexidine is generally preferred over povidone iodine solution as a patient preparation because it has a broader spectrum of antimicrobial activity, longer residual antimicrobial activity, is efficacious in the presence of blood and organic matter and is nontoxic and hypoallergenic.

Patient drapes are currently available in a variety of sizes, shapes and materials. With avian patients clear drapes are recommended, as they allow the surgeon and anesthetist to visually monitor the patient during the procedure. Clear plastic drapes are commercially available with or without povidone iodine impregnation. These drapes have an adhesive that will stick to dry avian skin and create a sterile field, but must be removed with care to prevent damaging the tissue. As an alternative, a clear plastic drape can be made from plastic kitchen wrap. The border of the plastic should be edged with masking tape, making it easy to find the edges and open the drape.

In most cases, the plastic drape is small and does not allow the surgeon to create a sterile field incorporating the entire surgery table and instrument stand. In order create such a field, the clear plastic drape is placed over the patient and a large drape sheet with a central fenestration large enough to allow the draped patient to be exposed, is placed over the entire field. This will prevent accidental contamination of the arms and elbows by touching them to an undraped table.

Perioperative antibiotic therapy involves the use of antibiotics such that there are therapeutic tissue levels of the agent present at the time of exposure to bacteria. With most antibiotics, parenteral administration one to two hours preoperatively, and maintaining therapeutic doses for 8-16 hours postoperatively, will accomplish this goal. Unless there is infection or significant contamination, use of antibiotics beyond this period is not indicated and has been shown not to decrease the incidence of surgical wound infections.

Wound Healing

Wound healing has been thoroughly studied in mammals, and five phases have been described: the inflammatory stage, the fibroblastic phase, the epithelialization phase, the contraction phase and the remodeling phase.

Freshly created (within eight hours), uncomplicated wounds should be treated by primary closure with anticipated first intention healing; however, this is not appropriate for the treatment of open, contaminated wounds.

Instrumentation

In many cases, ophthalmic instruments are suitable and should be included in the standard avian surgery pack. Iris scissors (curved and straight), forceps with fine teeth, micro Halstead mosquito forceps, jeweler's forceps (curved and straight), iris hooks, eyelid retractors for abdominal retractors, retinal forceps, adventitia scissors, spring handled scissors and Castroviejo needle holders are particularly useful. Because avian tissues are delicate, the use of toothed forceps is seldom appropriate. Debakey-type forceps are relatively atraumatic and serve well in avian surgery. Penrose drains or other sterile rubber materials may be used to wrap around structures for elevation or retraction, and eyelid retractors work well as wound retractors. A sterile gavage or feeding tube can be used for irrigation or for flushing out hollow viscera (such as the proventriculus during proventriculotomy). Various sizes of bone curettes are useful to retrieve foreign bodies from the ventriculus or proventriculus. A tuberculin syringe with an attached 25 ga needle can be fashioned into a tissue hook by bending the tip of the needle 45-90° under the operating microscope.

A mini-Frazier suction tip is well suited for avian surgery because of its small, delicate size. This type of suction tip also has a small hole at the finger rest, which the surgeon may use to adjust the amount of suction created at the tip. Red rubber urinary catheters and infant feeding tubes are available in varying sizes and may be cut off and adapted for use as a suction tip. The strength of suction can be controlled on most suction units and should be adjusted so that fluids can be evacuated without damaging tissues. A Poole-type suction tip can be fashioned from a catheter by cutting multiple fenestrations along the terminal two to three centimeters of the catheter. By having many fenestrations, the suction force is distributed among the inlets, decreasing the force at any one hole. Additionally, if some of the holes are occluded by tissue, the remaining inlets continue to evacuate the celomic cavity.

A one- to three-millimeter rigid endoscope is helpful for visualizing areas that the surgeon may not be able to access with the operating microscope (eg, lumen of hollow viscera). Abdominal retractors appropriate for small avian patients should maintain retraction but not have blades that extend deep into the body cavity. Mini-Balfour retractors are useful in large patients such as macaws and cockatoos, Alm retractors are appropriate for medium-sized patients like Amazons and conures, and Heiss retractors work well in small avian patients including cockatiels and budgerigars.

In many situations, the placement of ligatures in deep surgical sites is unachievable or results in unacceptable tissue damage due to the relative inaccessibility and delicate nature of avian tissues. Hemostatic clips are best for controlling bleeding in these cases. The appliers are available either straight or with a 45° bend. The bent-tipped applier is useful for deep clip placement; however, the bent-tipped instruments are about twice the size of the equivalent straight-tipped applier, making them more cumbersome to use. Generally, the small and medium clips are used most frequently.

Number 15 and No. 11 scalpel blades are most appropriate for avian surgery. Small gauze pads (2 x 2) and sterile cotton-tipped applicators should also be available. Surgical spears are small, wedge-shaped, highly absorbent, synthetic sponges attached to a stick. The point of the spear provides critical control when working under magnification. Absorbable gelatin sponges are valuable for controlling hemorrhage, as is oxidized regenerated cellulose.

With avian patients it is best to place the patient on a restraint board, which is then placed on the operating table. This allows the surgical assistant to move the patient intraoperatively to achieve proper visualization of structures. This is especially important when using the operating microscope as it is much easier to move the patient than to move and refocus the microscope. Such boards are commercially available or can be easily constructed from a plastic container lid, a piece of styrofoam or section of cardboard. Tape restraints are preferred over velcro restraints because they are disposable and minimize the risk of disease transmission.

An ideal monitor for the surgical patient would be easy to apply, unaffected by the surgical environment, economically priced and provide data on the patient's heart rate, respiration, body temperature and hemoglobin oxygen saturation. The high heart rate and small tidal volume of small avian patients are not easily detected by traditional monitors. Pulse oximeters have become standard in human anesthesia but may be unable to detect the high pulse rate of some smaller patients. Sensitive respiratory monitors that have a thermistor that extends to the end of an endotracheal tube are effective in intubated patients but do not function properly if the patient is maintained using a face mask (see Chapter 39). Remote thermometers are available at a reasonable price. The best monitor for surgical anesthesia is still a well trained and experienced surgical technician.

Radiosurgery (Electrosurgery)

When set for monopolar operation, a radiosurgery unit employs two electrodes (an active electrode and an indifferent electrode or ground plate). Monopolar radiosurgical techniques are acceptable for gross tissue manipulations in avian patients weighing more than two kilograms. The ground (indifferent electrode) should be large and placed as close as possible to the surgical area, and the contact with the patient should be improved using an electrode paste. It is important to keep the active electrode clean and free of char and debris. A dirty electrode will drag through the tissue, inhibiting the cutting action and increasing tissue coagulation, which can delay healing and predispose the wound to dehiscence. Many types of active electrode tips are commercially available. Ball-type electrodes create a lot of tissue destruction and are used for fulguration and coagulation of large vessels. Loop electrodes are used to contour tissues, obtain organ biopsies and remove large masses in a piecemeal fashion. Skin incisions and incisions into other fine tissues are best accomplished with fine wire electrodes.

Bipolar Forceps

Bipolar radiosurgical forceps are superior to monopolar forceps in patients weighing less than two kilograms and when manipulating tissues in the realm of microsurgery. With bipolar forceps a ground plate is not needed as one of the tips serves as the active electrode and the other as the indifferent electrode. Compared with the fine-needle or wire monopolar electrodes, the tips of the bipolar forceps are broader, allowing the current to be dispersed just enough to accomplish the tissue welding that is critical for hemostasis.

Forceps with the active electrode slightly bent are commercially available and are best for avian surgery. A lower energy setting can be used with these forceps. With the Surgitron, the fully filtered wave pattern of the cutting settings are used most commonly. The unit set at 1 for vessel coagulation, 2 for muscle transection, and 3 for incision of dry skin. For vessels that are difficult to coagulate, the *cutting/coagulation* settings may occasionally be indicated. The *coagulation* setting is used primarily for tissue fulguration (such as the destruction of cloacal papillomas).

Incision Techniques

The Harrison modified bipolar forceps may be used to make primary skin incisions, coagulate cutaneous vessels prior to blade incision and coagulate individual vessels. These forceps may also be used with or without current for tissue dissection. Skin incisions should be planned in a manner to minimize the effect on feathers and feather tracts and to avoid the major blood supply to feathers. The skin is tented with thumb forceps and grasped with the bipolar forceps at the location of the proposed incision.

The current is activated (using a foot switch) precisely as the grasp on the tissue is relaxed slightly, and with a smooth, rapid motion, the forceps are pulled off the tissue. When correctly applied, fine, white blanching of the tissues occurs with barely discernible separation of the skin that can be seen under magnification. This will create a small incision in the tissue that may then be parted to allow introduction of the indifferent electrode of the bipolar forceps (non-bent tip). The electrode is inserted subcutaneously to the extent of the proposed incision. The electrodes of the bipolar forceps are lightly apposed, the current is activated and the forceps withdrawn. This creates a skin incision with minimal damage. If properly performed, the skin should remain a normal color except immediately adjacent to the incision (which should be white), and there should be no hemorrhage.

When thicker tissue is to be transected, small bites of tissue are grasped with the bipolar forceps, the current is activated and the forceps are withdrawn through the tissue, creating a small nick. This process is repeated until the tissue is completely transected, stroke by stroke.

Coagulation Techniques

If hemorrhage is encountered, a sterile cotton-tipped applicator is used to dry the area for radiocoagulation, which cannot be achieved in a wet field. The swab is rolled toward the source of blood flow with gentle pressure to serve as a tourniquet. The pressure is relaxed slightly to identify the source of hemorrhage. Once the vessel is identified, the slightly broader, flat indifferent electrode is placed under the vessel, and the bent-tipped, active electrode is loosely apposed to occlude the vessel. The current is activated as the forceps are relaxed, sealing the vessel. At high current or coagulation settings, the vessel frequently retracts within the tissue due to vasospasm. This results in temporary hemostasis only. As the vessel relaxes, the hemorrhage recurs.

When using monopolar radiosurgery, the power settings vary with the type and size of the electrode, the area of electrode surface in contact with tissue, the nature of the tissue, the operation performed (cut or coagulation) and the depth of the incision desired. Higher settings are necessary with tough tissues, deep incisions and large electrodes. Healing after radioincision is by first intention. When used correctly for creating an incision, the current should be activated *before* touching tissue, and the electrode should glide effortlessly, producing only a slight color change in the tissue. When used for coagulation, the electrode should be activated after contacting the tissue and should produce a white spot at the site of energy transfer. Current applied repeatedly to the same area will cause excessive heating and damage to underlying tissues.

The fine-tipped monopolar electrode requires a higher setting when used on avian tissues than when used on thicker mammalian skin. When a vessel is encountered at these high settings, the electrode has a tendency to cut rather than coagulate the vessel, resulting in hemorrhage. A second effort must then be made to locate the vessel and coagulate it separately, creating the potential to induce more damage to the vessel and surrounding tissues. In mammals, the tissues surrounding vessels will heat slightly with the application of radiocurrent, which helps seal any transected vessels.

Magnification

Some form of magnification is recommended for avian surgery and is an integral part of an avian specialty practice.

Operating Microscope

In patients weighing less than a kilogram, an operating microscope and microsurgical instrumentation are mandatory and would be considered advantageous in larger birds. Binocular magnification loupes of 2.5x to 8x are adequate for many procedures. Attaching a fiberoptic lamp to the loupe facilitates vision. With the use of magnification, individual vessels are more easily identified for coagulation, minimizing the degree of hemorrhage associated with a procedure. The major disadvantage of performing surgery under an operating microscope is that it generally requires more time to complete a procedure than when a magnification loupe is used.

The operating microscope should have a lens objective of approximately 150 mm with 12.5 mm ocular lenses. An electronic zoom is advantageous. A fiberoptic ring light can be attached to the lens for improved illumination of the surgical field.

Microsurgical Instruments

There are four requirements for microsurgical instruments: they should be long, be counterbalanced, have round handles and have miniaturized tips. It is important that only the tips of microsurgical instruments are miniaturized. The handles should be of normal length to help provide stability to the tips and diminish the effect of hand tremors. The handles should be long enough to rest comfortably in the hand between the thumb and index finger. The instrument should be held like a fine writing instrument and be manipulated with minimal pressure.

It is important to note that totally miniaturized instruments (older generation of ophthalmic instruments) are not appropriate for microsurgery. These instruments have short shanks and handles, and their use under the operating microscope results in loss of balance and control leading to fast, jerky movements.

The microsurgical pack should include micro-scissors, micro-needle holders and a variety of micro-forceps. Needle holders should not have a clasp or box lock, as the motion that occurs when the lock is set and released is enough to cause the needle to tear tissues. Inexpensive forceps can be fashioned by placing vulcanized silicone on the handles of jewelry forceps. Layers of liquid plastic (dispensed from a hot glue gun) may be applied to the handles to achieve the necessary round shape. An ophthalmic Castroviejo needle holder can be modified for microsurgery by grinding the tip narrower, removing the box lock and making the handle round.

For microvascular work, specialized clips are used to maintain the severed ends of the vessel in approximation. A colored background is placed under the vessel to improve contrast and make identification of the vessel easier. These backgrounds are commercially available or can be made from pieces of balloon appropriately sterilized. Vessel dilators are also necessary. A vascular irrigation system can be made using a 27 or 30 ga needle, the tip of which has been cut off and polished smooth so it will not damage the vascular intima. A motorized rotary tool and the operating microscope are used to modify the needle. Heparinized irrigation solution in a hand syringe with the modified needle attached is used to clear the vessel of clots and debris. Suture material for small avian patients usually is of 6-0 to 10-0 size, while for microvascular work, 10-0 nylon suture on a 75 micron needle is routinely used.

Suture Materials

The goals of incision repair are to limit the adverse effects of the repair technique and to restrict the loss of tissue function. In routine avian surgery, suture sizes of 3-0 to 6-0 are most commonly used. For small patients and microsurgery, sutures of 10-0 may be necessary.

Suture is a foreign material in a surgical wound and may potentiate infection. Where there is contamination or infection, a monofilament, nonreactive material such as nylon is indicated, as it will not allow bacterial wicking and will retain its tensile strength long enough for resolution of the infection and completion of tissue healing. In a study of the ability of bacteria to adhere to suture material it was found that monofilament, nonabsorbable materials have the least capacity for adherence while polyglycolic acid and polyglactin 910 have the most.

Sutures should be placed with a minimum amount of both intrinsic (tension on tissue within the loop of suture material) and extrinsic (tension on surrounding tissues) tension. Knots must be securely tied, yet the surgeon must attempt to use the least amount of suture material to decrease the foreign body reaction. It is important to use the fewest throws to create a secure knot, which will fail by suture breakage and not by knot failure. For chromic catgut, polyglactin 910, polyglycolic acid and polypropylene, three throws are required and four are required for polydioxanone and nylon. When starting and finishing a continuous pattern, a different number of throws is required to create a secure knot. To start a continuous pattern with polygycolic acid, polyglactin 910 and polypropylene three throws are required. Four are required for chromic catgut and five for polydioxanone. When ending a continuous pattern, it takes five throws for polypropylene, chromic catgut and polyglycolic acid, six for nylon and polyglactin 910, and seven for polydioxanone to create a secure knot. (The editors have experienced some adverse reactions with Polyglactin 910 in psittacine birds; therefore they personally use nylon for subcutaneous sutures and stainless steel wire for skin.)

Tissue Adhesives

Tissue adhesives of cyanoacrylate have many applications in avian medicine and surgery. The cyanoacrylate monomer is a liquid that polymerizes in the presence of the small amount of water present in tissues. The time required for the liquid to become solid and bond tissues depends on the amount of water (more water present will delay curing) and the thickness of the acrylic applied (thicker will delay curing). Medical grade adhesives are biologically inert and cause minimal tissue reaction.

These materials hold tissues in approximation to allow healing to progress; however, cells cannot penetrate the adhesive. It is important not to allow the adhesive to run between the tissues to be apposed as the presence of the acrylic will delay healing by creating a physical barrier. In some cases, especially with water birds, the acrylic may be applied in a thin layer over the apposed incision to create a seal yet allow epithelial cells to migrate under the acrylic during the healing process. These adhesives may also be used to secure IV catheters in place, to attach the limbs or digits of tiny patients to splints for orthopedic problems and various other purposes. Caution should be exercised when using these materials in the presence of anesthetic gases with which they are synergistic and may cause ocular irritation and vomiting in avian patients.

Postoperative Care

The patient should be placed in an incubator at 85°F with supplemental oxygen during recovery from surgery. It is best to continue maintaining the postsurgical patient in a small, controlled environment during the convalescent period (see Chapter 39). The patient's activity level should be kept to a minimum to allow proper tissue healing. A square, box-type enclosure is preferred and in most circumstances perches should be removed or lowered to decrease the likelihood of falling. Food and water should be placed where they are easily accessed by the patient. Toys and extraneous objects within the enclosure should be removed.

Postoperative antibiotic therapy should be instituted when there is a specific indication, such as with open, contaminated wounds or where there has been intraoperative contamination of the surgical field. IM perioperative antibiotic therapy is recommended for general prophylaxis in these cases.

In general, avian patients do not traumatize their surgical incisions, and they poorly tolerate bandages and other devices. Elizabethan collars or neck braces should be reserved for the most desperate cases. If an Elizabethan collar is considered necessary, the patient's neck should first be wrapped so the collar will be held in position against the mandible. Using this technique, a smaller, looser collar may be utilized.

In some patients, the center core of cardboard from a roll of bathroom tissue may be padded and used as a neck brace alone or in conjunction with an Elizabethan collar. The first day, the Elizabethan collar should open rostrally in the traditional manner. This will allow the patient time to become accustomed to the collar, and it will not damage the wings while the patient is struggling to escape the device. The second day, the collar should be reversed such that the cone opens caudally. This will allow the patient more ready access to food and water. The patient should be kept in a plain box with nothing to trap and hold the collar. Food and water should be placed on a pedestal for easy access. The patient's weight should be closely monitored to assure that an adequate amount of food and water is being consumed. The collar should be regularly evaluated for evidence of pressure or esophageal obstruction.

Analgesics

Historically, it has been considered that birds have a remarkable capacity to deal with pain, although the assessment of what animals perceive as pain is difficult. Research in the area of avian pain perception has been minimal. Companion birds have a well developed sense of touch and react by loud vocalization and withdrawal when potentially painful stimuli are applied. Clients expect that analgesia will be provided for their pet, and it is the responsibility of the entire staff to relieve a patient's postoperative pain and suffering.

Doses of 3- 4 mg/kg of butorphanol given to budgerigars had no statistically significant effect on heart rate or respiratory rate; however, some treated birds lost motor control. This effect was considered minor and all birds remained alert. Return to normal motor coordination occurred within two to four hours post-administration. No gastrointestinal effects were observed with this agent. This study did not evaluate the minimum and maximum effective doses. It would be advisable to start with a standard dose of 0.2-0.4 mg/kg of butorphanol, recognizing that doses up to ten times this dose are safe in birds.

Buprenorphine hydrochloride is another opioid with agonist/antagonist activity that appears to be effective in controlling pain in avian patients. A dose of 0.01-0.05 mg/kg IM appears to provide adequate postoperative analgesia.

Flunixin meglumine is a nonsteroidal anti-inflammatory agent that is a potent analgesic for certain types of pain; however, surgical pain is rarely responsive to this class of analgesic, and it is more appropriate for use in the treatment of inflammatory conditions. It has been recommended for use as an analgesic in companion birds at 1-10 mg/kg q24h IM or IV. Flunixin at 10 mg/kg had no effect on respiratory or heart rates in budgerigars. Additionally, motor function remained normal following IM administration of flunixin. Regurgitation or vomiting occurred within two to five minutes after administration in five of six patients. Tenesmus was also observed several minutes after administration of flunixin. Aspirin has been recommended at a dose of one 5 gr tablet dissolved in 250 ml drinking water. These nonsteroidal agents have the potential to cause serious gastrointestinal side effects and may prolong clotting time. They should be used with caution until their benefits and limitations are better understood.

SOFT TISSUE SURGERY

R. Avery Bennett
Greg J. Harrison

The most substantial limitation to soft tissue surgery of the abdomen is the small size (<100 grams) of many avian patients. Some of these problems can be overcome with the use of magnification, but others are a result of having limited surgical access to an area, and are difficult to overcome. Surgery of the thoracic area, even in large companion birds, presents a similar problem, in that the organs of interest are covered by the sternum and heavy musculature. Continued improvements in the endoscopic surgical equipment available in human medicine will undoubtedly improve the surgeon's ability to perform surgery in difficult-to-reach areas of the avian body.

When necropsies are necessary, the clinician should approach this procedure from the perspective of a surgeon rather than of a pathologist, by dissecting and reviewing anatomy from a regional approach rather than by performing the necropsy strictly from the traditional ventrodorsal approach.

Surgery of the Skin

Passerine Leg Scales

Passerine leg scale syndrome is characterized by the development of abnormally large scales of the legs and feet, possibly as a result of mite infection or malnutrition (see Chapter 43). These scales can coalesce and act as a constricting band. They also predispose the bird to bacterial pododermatitis (usually *Staphylococcus* spp). If present, the shiny, convex carapace of the female *Knemidocoptes* mite can usually be visualized, with the aid of an operating microscope, inside the created burrows. In most instances, lesions resolve after treatment with ivermectin or correction of nutritional deficiencies. In severe cases, it may be necessary to surgically debride the proliferative scales to prevent vascular compromise. A 22 or 25 ga needle with the point bent to a 90° angle can be used to lift the scales and scabs, which then can be grasped with the microforceps. Skin softeners may also be beneficial.

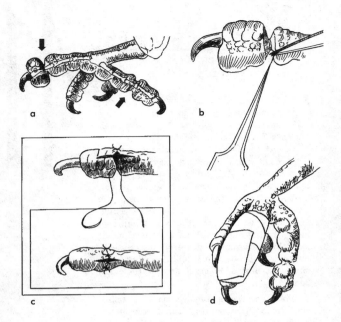

FIG 41.1 a) Constriction of the digits (arrows) is common in some macaw and Eclectus Parrot neonates. **b)** The lesion is repaired by using an operating microscope to remove the circumferential scab and create a fresh tissue margin. **c)** The wound edges are then apposed with shallowly placed sutures, and longitudinal incisions are made through the constriction on the medial and lateral sides of the digit to compensate for swelling and growth. **d)** The wound is covered with a hydroactive dressing to keep it clean and prevent dehydration.

Toe Necrosis (Constricted Toe Syndrome)

Avascular necrosis of digits may occur secondary to circumferential constriction caused by fibers, scabs or necrotic tissue. Removal of the offending tissue or fibers and supportive care are frequently successful. Avascular necrosis of the digits has been described in passerine birds and Amazon parrots. Scabs should be debrided or incised to prevent vascular compromise, and hydroactive dressings should be applied to the affected digits to prevent the formation of additional scabs. Complete healing may require weeks to months.

In small birds (eg, Passeriformes), constricting fibers may be visualized using the operating microscope. A bent 25 ga needle is helpful for removing constricting fibers. The tip can be used to elevate the fiber, which can then be cut by gently rolling the needle such that the beveled edge severs the fiber. Microsurgical forceps may be used to untangle the fibers. Even severely swollen digits with exposed tendons may heal without incident once the fibers are removed. A hydroactive dressing should be placed on any wounds created by the fibers to prevent desiccation and the formation of a constricting scab.

Neonates (especially macaws and Eclectus Parrots) may develop constrictive toe lesions that can result in avascular necrosis of the digit. Increasing the environmental humidity or providing hot moist compresses and massage may be effective in resolving lesions in the early stages. More advanced lesions require surgical intervention. The circumferential indentation is treated using magnification to remove the constricting tissue.

A tourniquet fashioned from a rubber band held tightly with a mosquito hemostat may be used to control hemorrhage for short periods until the injury is properly treated. Hemostatic agents including radiocoagulation should be avoided. The blood supply to the digits is minimal, and anything that interferes with proper blood flow may predispose the digit to postoperative necrosis.

Feather Cysts

Feather cysts on the wing that are treated by lancing and curettage frequently recur. Fulguration with a radiosurgical unit has been reported to be successful in some cases; however, the depth of destruction is difficult to control, resulting in damage to adjacent follicles.

Blade excision appears to be the treatment of choice. A tourniquet can be applied to aid in hemostasis. The entire follicle, including any bony attachments, should be excised. Adjacent follicles and their blood supply should be carefully avoided. In the postoperative period, the wing should be bandaged to prevent movement at the site of follicle excision while healing occurs by second intention. As adjacent feathers begin to regrow, debris should be gently removed by flushing with warm sterile saline several times daily.

With a single cyst or a large feather, the follicle may be saved by marsupializing the lining of the cyst with the skin surrounding the follicle. An incision is made centered on the cyst, parallel to the direction of feather growth. Hemorrhage is controlled with 6-0 ligatures, not with radiocautery. The lining of the cyst is cultured and the debris is removed. Redundant tissue is excised and the follicle is thoroughly lavaged with sterile saline. The margin of the cyst is then sutured to the skin using a simple continuous pattern of fine suture. New feather growth must be closely monitored.

Feather cysts of the tail may be severe and disfiguring, requiring amputation of the pygostyle. Blunt dissection to the coccygeal vertebrae allows disarticulation at the sacrococcygeal junction without entering the cloaca. Soft tissues are closed routinely.

Feather cysts on the body are easily removed using elliptical or fusiform excision followed by primary skin closure. Treatment of individual feathers is generally unrewarding in cases where an entire feather tract is involved. A technique for radical excision of an entire pteryla of affected feathers in canaries has been described. A fusiform incision is made from the flank to the thoracic inlet around the affected pteryla. The main vascular supply to the tract is located centrally at the cranial third of the pteryla. Large cysts may be supplied by relatively large individual vessels that should be coagulated or ligated.

Xanthomas of the Wing Tip

Probucola (25 mg/day for an Amazon parrot) and dietary management should be used in combination with surgical excision of the mass. Serum cholesterol levels should be closely monitored because they are usually elevated in birds with xanthomatosis and should be medically reduced to a normal level prior to surgery. The diet should be low in protein (13%) and fat (5.5%).

A monopolar, wire electrode functions well for removal of xanthomatous masses. The wound is left to heal by second intention. The wound may be protected with tissue adhesive or a hydroactive dressing, which should be changed every three to five days. Complete healing often requires several weeks. If subcutaneous tissues are involved (especially bone), the affected wing may require amputation.

Excision of the Uropygial Gland

Excision of the gland should be considered in cases where impaction recurs, the gland has ruptured, a tumor is present or chronic infection of the gland is not responsive to medical management.

A fusiform incision is made along the dorsal midline to incorporate the papillae of the gland. The skin is reflected with the aid of blunt dissection and radiocoagulation of damaged vessels. The gland is bilobed, and each lobe receives its blood supply from a vessel that branches at the cranial, middle and caudal portions of the gland. The gland may extend deeply to the synsacrum and caudally to the insertion point of the tail feathers. The vessels are identified and coagulated or ligated. Bipolar coagulation should be used to minimize damage to the follicles of the rectrices. Dissection is continued, beginning at the cranial extent of the gland proceeding circumferentially until its removal is possible.

Extensive dissection and debridement are necessary if the gland has ruptured. An additional caudal incision perpendicular to the dorsal midline incision may be necessary. In these cases, extensive tissue trauma increases the likelihood of postoperative dehiscence and damage to the follicles of the rectrices. Dehiscence usually occurs at the junction of the two perpendicular incisions. If possible, it is preferable to remove a diseased uropygial gland prior to its rupture.

Surgery of the Eye

Lateral Canthoplasty for Inferior Ectropion

Idiopathic paralysis of the inferior eyelid occurs with some degree of frequency in cockatiels and occasionally in Umbrella Cockatoos. A lateral canthoplasty will create a smaller aperture, reducing the risk of exposure keratitis and associated conditions.

Indolent Corneal Ulcers

Successful treatment of indolent corneal ulcers in birds appears to require debridement of the entire superficial layer of the cornea. Under the operating microscope, a cotton-tipped applicator moistened with 10% acetylcysteine is used to gently debride the edge of the ulcer toward the limbus. Once the affected epithelium has been debrided, it should be excised using a #11 scalpel blade or a corneal knife. Standard ulcer treatment is instituted postoperatively. The corneal surface will reepithelialize from the limbus.

Lens Removal

In a study of older macaws, immature cataracts were present in at least one eye of most birds over the age of 35. Those birds with rapidly developing cataracts frequently became blind due to phacolytic uveitis.

For lens removal in these macaws, no attempt was made to dilate the pupil preoperatively. The macaw cornea is approximately seven millimeters in diameter, which is too small for phacoemulsification instrumentation, and the cataracts were removed using standard surgical technique. In the immediate postoperative period, the eyes were treated with a topical steroid-antibiotic ointment, followed by weekly subconjunctival injections of triamcinolone for up to a total treatment period of four weeks.

Enucleation

The technique is similar to that described for mammals, except that birds have a very short optic nerve, and excessive traction on the globe can result in pressure trauma to the brain. Visualization of the muscles and blood vessels is enhanced by collapsing the globe at the start of the procedure. After the cornea is incised, the lens and vitreous are expressed through the incision. The lid margins must be excised to eliminate glandular tissue and provide a cut edge for the blepharoplasty. It is also important to remove all conjunctival tissues and any secretory tissue.

One enucleation technique involves suturing the eyelids together to improve the precision of the incision of the skin, which needs to be made a few millimeters from the lid margin circumferentially. The dissection is continued subcutaneously around the globe such that the palpebral conjunctiva will be excised with the globe. Hemorrhage is controlled with the bipolar radiosurgical forceps. Once all attachments have been transected except for the optic nerve and associated vessels, hemostatic clips are placed on this neurovascular bundle. Two clips should be applied to assure hemostasis. Curved appliers facilitate placement of the clips caudal to the globe and minimize traction on the optic nerve. The optic nerve is severed and the globe is removed. Any remaining hemorrhage is controlled using radiosurgery.

Surgery of the Respiratory System

Rhinoliths

Rhinoliths may occur secondary to chronic malnutrition and rhinitis. Clinical signs include sneezing, upper respiratory sounds and inflation of the infraorbital air sac during expiration.

Removal of rhinoliths requires magnification. Nasal tissues are friable and bleed easily when traumatized, which also predisposes the mucosa to infection. A 3-0 to #1-sized blunt ear curettes work well to loosen and remove the mass.

Once the rhinolith is removed, the lining of the nasal cavity should be swabbed and evaluated cytologically and by culture for mycotic and bacterial pathogens. The nares should be flushed with dilute chlorhexidine, and any fungal or bacterial component should be treated systemically with appropriate antimicrobial medications.

Infraorbital Sinusitis

Infraorbital sinusitis in birds may lead to secondary lacrimal and conjunctival infections, chronic rhinorrhea and other upper respiratory problems. Effective treatment requires a definitive diagnosis. Frequently, nutritional problems such as hypovitaminosis A predispose a bird to secondary infections with bacteria, yeast and fungi. A sinus flush technique can be used to obtain samples for cytology and cultures (see Chapters 10 and 22).

The infraorbital sinus is initially opened in the same location described for sinus flushing (see Chapter 10). This area is highly vascular, and laser, if available, is best for providing hemostasis. Bipolar radiosurgical units on higher coagulation settings may also be effective. Pressure may be applied to the area with a cotton-tipped applicator to allow visualization of the vessels. The sinus must be thoroughly and deeply explored, as purulent debris may be located within the nasal cavity, the recesses of the beak and even between the sinus and the nasal cavity caudal to the turbinates. It may be necessary to remove affected portions of the periorbital bone.

Supraorbital sinus trephination may be used to gain access to the dorsal and caudal-most areas of the sinus that cannot be accessed using nasal flushes and sinus injections. The purpose of sinus trephination is to create an opening in the sinus through which irrigation and antimicrobial solutions may be instilled over a long period of time. Its major disadvantage is the risk of ocular injury. The site for trephination varies with the species, and the anatomy should be carefully studied prior to attempting this procedure.

To create an opening in the supraorbital sinus, the skin is incised exposing the frontal bone. Holes are made in the bone with a sterile rotary tool about one-half to two-fifths the distance between the rostral-most plane of the eye and the naris. The hole is angled toward the midline. Cortical bone is removed until the cancellous bone above the supraorbital sinus is visualized. Drilling proceeds into the supraorbital sinus and may then be widened to an appropriate diameter. Samples for cytology and culture are obtained, and the sinus is flushed with irrigation solution. The passage of irrigation solution through the choana and into the oral cavity confirms that the hole is properly placed. The periorbital tissue will bulge when fluids are introduced, and these tissues should not be over-distended. If indicated, this procedure may be performed bilaterally in some Passeriformes, whereas a single trephination site is sufficient in Psittaciformes in which the infraorbital sinuses communicate (see Chapter 22).

Hyperinflation of the Cervicocephalic Air Sac

This condition is thought to occur secondary to trauma, but the location of leakage of air into the subcutaneous space is generally not identifiable. A procedure for surgically implanting a cutaneous stent at the poll of the head to allow the air to escape (in a location where the bird cannot remove the device) has been described. A Teflon stent, with a 5 mm outer rim that allows the skin to be placed under its edge to prevent the dermis from closing over the opening, is used for the procedure.

Thoracic Surgery

Tracheal/Syringeal Obstruction

Seed or other foreign body aspiration, fungal granulomas resulting from aspergillosis or candidiasis or concretions of epithelial cells and mucus may occlude the trachea or syrinx resulting in respiratory distress. Some birds present with no premonitory signs, while others have a history of voice change and a more gradual onset of dyspnea.

Therapy depends upon the size of the patient and the configuration of the trachea.

Establishment of a patent airway is crucial. Placement of an air sac cannula will allow the patient to ventilate through an alternate airway until the obstruction can be removed. It may be beneficial to place the bird in an oxygen-enriched environment prior to manipulating the patient for placement of the air sac cannula.

In small birds (cockatiels and smaller), the tracheal diameter (approximately 1.5 mm for cockatiels) precludes use of an endoscope to retrieve a foreign body or granuloma. If the obstruction is the result of a granuloma or inspissated cells and mucus, a suction tube (urinary catheter) slightly smaller than the diameter of the trachea may be utilized to remove material from the trachea and syrinx (see Chapter 22). By maintaining anesthesia with an air sac cannula, the trachea may be occluded with the suction tube without compromising respiration. If squamous metaplasia secondary to hypovitaminosis A is suspected, dietary modification and vitamin A supplementation should be instituted.

In medium to large birds, a rigid or flexible endoscope can be used to evaluate the cause of an obstruction and potentially aid in its removal. In some cases, the endoscope may allow visualization of the object, but the tracheal diameter may be too small to use a wire basket or grasping forceps to remove the object. In these cases, the endoscope can be used to brush off plaques or physically alter lesions sufficiently to open the airway, and the loosened plaques can be removed with a suction tube.

In some cases, tracheal foreign bodies may be retrieved using grasping forceps, a Foley catheter or a Fogarty catheter with the aid of an endoscope. The size of the patient's tracheal diameter will determine which catheter is most appropriate. The catheter is passed beyond the foreign body and the balloon is inflated sufficiently to occlude the airway but not to prevent it from being withdrawn. With the balloon inflated, the catheter is withdrawn, resulting in removal of the foreign body.

As a last ditch effort in medium- to large-sized birds (parrots, raptors, doves, pheasants and peafowl), the thoracic inlet may be approached surgically for removal of tracheal or syringeal foreign bodies (Figure 41.9). The patient is positioned in dorsal recum-

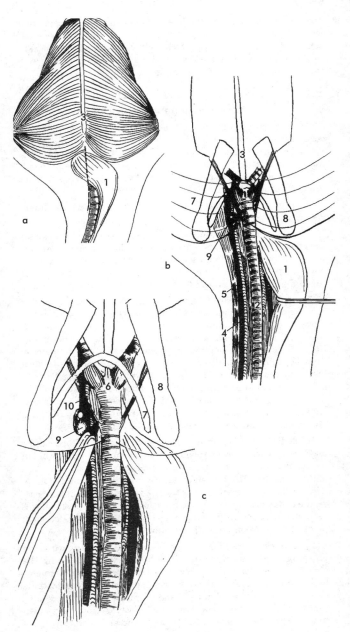

FIG 41.9 If all other techniques for removal fail, some foreign bodies and granulomatous plaques can be removed from the trachea and syrinx using a tracheotomy. **a)** An incision is made over the crop on the ventral midline. **b)** The crop is retracted laterally to the right. **c)** The tracheal muscles are transected using bipolar radiosurgery. *(continued on next page)*

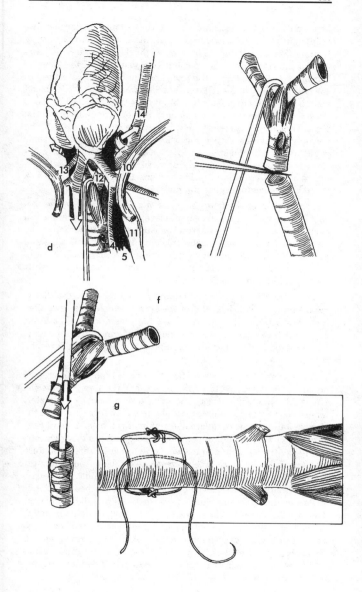

d) A spay hook is used to gently pull the syrinx into the thoracic inlet. **e)** The trachea is transected. **f)** A blunt probang or suction device can be used to remove debris. **g)** Closure is completed by apposing the tracheal rings. 1) crop 2) trachea 3) sternum 4) internal carotid artery 5) jugular vein 6) syrinx 7) clavicle 8) coracoid 9) thyroid 10) sternotracheal muscle 11) esophagus 12) primary bronchi 13) pulmonary artery and 14) aorta; lateral arrows show primary bronchi to lungs.

bency on a surgical restraint board. A tube should be placed in the esophagus to allow for its easy identification to prevent iatrogenic trauma. The skin is incised from the right clavicular/sternal junction to the clavicular/ coracoid junction just cranial to the crop. The skin is elevated from the crop, and the right lateral aspect of the crop is gently dissected from surrounding tissues. Major blood vessels are easily avoided using blunt dissection. Once the crop is freed from its clavicular attachments, it should be reflected to the right. The trachea is identified by its complete cartilage rings. The sternotracheal muscles are identified traversing obliquely to their caudolateral attachments, and both sets of sternotracheal muscles are transected. A large blood vessel between the muscle bellies should be coagulated prior to transection of the muscles. A small canine vaginal speculum may aid in visualization.

At this point, the use of the operating microscope becomes essential. The restraint board should be elevated at the cranial end such that the operating microscope can be used to visualize the structures deep in the thoracic inlet. It may take some time and patience to achieve proper positioning and focus, but this technique allows the surgeon to visualize critical structures while having both hands free for manipulations.

The interclavicular air sac is bluntly dissected to expose the syrinx. A blunt hook is looped over the syrinx, which is gently pulled into view. In Amazon parrots, small macaws and smaller birds, this procedure may result in avulsion of the bronchi from the lung. For these patients, a left lateral approach to the syrinx is recommended as a last desperate attempt.

A transverse tracheotomy (50% of diameter) can also be created on the ventral surface to allow retrieval of the foreign material. Unless absolutely mandatory, the trachea should not be completely transected in order to maintain its alignment, reduce tension on the closure and prevent complete disruption of the blood supply. Stay sutures placed around the tracheal rings adjacent to the tracheotomy allow atraumatic manipulation of the trachea. Foreign materials located cranial to the tracheotomy site can be pushed out of the trachea with a sterile probang. Those located caudal to the tracheotomy site can be removed by suction. If the trachea completely separates during manipulations, anastomosis may be performed. The incision should be closed with a small-sized, monofilament, absorbable suture material encompassing at least one tracheal ring on each side of the tracheotomy incision. A simple interrupted pattern is best performed by pre-placing the encircling sutures. Knots should be placed external to the tracheal lumen. Intraluminal granuloma formation at the sutures is common.

A lateral thoracic approach to the trachea can be used in very small birds where there is no other means to approach and evaluate the syringeal area. Practice and microsurgical techniques are essential for this procedure. The patient is positioned in right lateral recumbency. An incision is made over the second and third ribs. These ribs are exposed using blunt dissection, and they are transected at both ends to allow their complete removal. This will expose the cranial portion of the lung. Using a moistened cotton-tipped applicator, the cranial extent of the lung is gently dissected and reflected from its attachments. The jugular vein, pulmonary artery and branches of the subclavian artery may be identified and should be avoided. Dissecting between these vessels allows visualization of the syrinx, which is incised (2 to 3 mm) using bipolar radiosurgical forceps at its junction with the left primary bronchus. A foreign body may then be removed using a combination of tracheal endoscopy, visualization and suction through the syringeal incision.

The syringeal incision is allowed to close by second intention. The ribs are not replaced. The lung is repositioned in its normal location. Soft tissues are apposed and the remainder of the closure is routine. This is a difficult procedure that should be used only as a life-saving technique when all other methods for foreign body removal have failed.

Pneumonectomy

Removal of lung tissue may be indicated in the treatment of abscesses or granulomas. In some instances, a surgical lung biopsy may be required instead of an endoscope-guided biopsy for diagnosis of a respiratory disease.

The lungs can be approached through the caudal thoracic air sac or the intercostal space by removing one or more ribs as described for the lateral approach to the syrinx. The affected lung tissue is elevated from the ribs and surrounding structures using a moistened cotton-tipped applicator or a spatula. The affected area is isolated using vascular clips, and the tissue to be removed is incised such that the clips remain with the viable portion of lung. No studies have been conducted to determine the amount of lung that may be removed or the physiologic effects of partial pneumonectomy; however, clinically, partial pneumonectomy patients appear to function normally.

Surgery of the Gastrointestinal System

Pharyngostomy Feeding Tube

The right side of the neck at the caudal extent of the lower mandible is prepared for surgery. A small incision is made through the skin, and the esophagus is identified. A moistened cotton-tipped applicator is inserted per os into the esophagus to aid in identification and to prevent the incision from penetrating the opposite side of the esophagus. A small (1-2 mm) stab incision is made into the esophagus to allow passage of a feeding tube. The tube is advanced into the crop or lower esophageal sphincter and sutured in place. A bandage is used to protect the site and to direct the tube to the dorsal cervical area away from the patient's field of vision. When it is no longer needed, the tube is removed, and the esophagus and skin defects are allowed to heal by second intention.

Oropharyngeal Abscesses

Oropharyngeal abscesses in birds frequently occur secondary to hypovitaminosis A. Abscessation occurs following squamous metaplasia and the development of a bacterial infection. These may be located at the base of the tongue, the intermandibular space, the choana, the pharynx or the larynx. These abscesses are often highly vascular necessitating careful dissection and hemostasis for removal.

Surgical management of an oral abscess involves pretreatment with antibiotics and vitamin A (if indicated). A fine-needle aspirate may be used for culture and sensitivity. In cases of hypovitaminosis A, parenteral vitamin A administration will help encapsulate the abscess and reduce inflammation and vascularization. In some cases, beta carotene therapy has resulted in complete resolution of the abscess without the need for surgical intervention.

Abscesses that are lanced and curetted frequently recur because minute fragments of material may be located within the tissue surrounding the abscess. The abscess will reform when the mucosa heals over the trapped necrotic debris. Removing the tissue surrounding the abscess is preferable. In some locations, such as with intermandibular abscesses, the abscess and its capsule may be removed intact. Dissection is meticulous and time-consuming, and accurate hemostasis is imperative.

Choanal abscesses must be lanced to remove necrotic material followed by surgical removal of the abscess. Laser or radiosurgery is best for controlling hemorrhage in this highly vascular area. Invasive abscesses may erode the palatine artery and result in severe hemorrhage.

Oropharyngeal Papillomas

Oral papillomas are uncommon except in some macaw species. These masses can be removed using cryosurgery, radiosurgery or chemical cautery (silver nitrate). Papillomatous growths that extend into the crop and proventriculus are currently considered untreatable, and are eventually fatal.

Esophageal Perforation

Esophageal perforation may occur from using a rigid feeding tube for supportive alimentation in a struggling bird, in enthusiastic, violently bobbing neonates or from feeding overheated formula. As the tube penetrates the esophagus, food or medication may be deposited in the subcutaneous tissues. A proventricular feeding tube should be placed to bypass the damaged esophageal tissue. Fasciotomy, copious irrigation, debridement, topical antiseptics and systemic antimicrobials are indicated. Surgical debridement and closure may be possible in three to five days when the affected tissues begin to granulate and appear healthy. Extensive fasciotomy and copious irrigation are probably the most important portions of the initial treatment.

Esophageal Strictures

A case of esophageal stricture of undetermined etiology in a Hyacinth Macaw was successfully treated by bougienage. The stricture was located in the thoracic esophagus and was believed to be obstructing the flow of ingesta to the proventriculus. Initially a 5 Fr rubber feeding tube was the largest bougie that could be inserted. Three sessions of bougienage separated by a few months produced an increase in lumen size to accommodate an 11 Fr bougie.

Crop Fistula Repair

Crop fistulae occur most commonly in neonates being hand-fed. One source of injury to the neonatal crop is penetration resulting from improper or careless gavage tube-feeding. Crop burns most frequently occur when food is warmed in a microwave oven and not thoroughly mixed.

Chronic crop fistulae are generally easier to deal with than acute crop burns. Because a fistula has developed, the serosa of the ingluvies and the skin have healed together as one tissue. These must be separated using scissors to circumferentially excise the edge of the fistula. Using meticulous dissection, the tissue plane between the ingluvies and the skin is identified and separated. The skin is normally adherent to the crop, being attached by two layers of striated muscle that form a sling-like support for the diverticulum of the crop. Once the two tissues are separated, closure is as described for ingluviotomy. It is important to repair the crop as a separate structure from the skin to minimize the chance of dehiscence, which is more likely to occur if the two are closed as one tissue. Placement of a tube from the mouth through the crop into the distal esophagus or into the proventriculus will aid in identifying the crop lumen.

Cases of acute crop burn are significantly more challenging than chronic crop injuries. Severe cases of crop burn may be fatal as a result of metabolic changes, sepsis and absorption of toxins from necrotic tissues. Initial treatment should be supportive and should include shock therapy, broad spectrum antibiotic therapy and antifungal medication. In cases of severe burns with significant edema, fasciotomy may be beneficial. The affected area should be liberally opened, copiously irrigated and left to heal by second intention or a delayed closure performed at a later date.

The feeding regimen will need to be changed in order to bypass the damaged tissues. This can be accomplished using a needle catheter, intestinal feeding tube, or by tube-feeding directly into the proventriculus. It is important to instruct the owner on proper methods for tube-feeding, and it must be stressed that the proventriculus cannot hold the same volume of food as the ingluvies; therefore, feedings will be more frequent and of smaller volume.

In most cases, it will be three to five days before the delineation between healthy and devitalized tissues becomes apparent, and it may take as long as 7-14 days. Prior to this, it will be difficult to determine what tissue should be removed and what is viable and should remain. Burned tissue becomes pale and edematous and then becomes dry, dark and leathery. Eventually, the devitalized tissue will separate from viable tissue and the edges of the crop and skin will heal together, forming a fistula.

Any tissue that is obviously necrotic should be debrided to reduce the body's burden of necrotic tissue. If a skin and crop defect result from this debridement, this defect can be used to intubate the proventriculus for nutritional support and also to cleanse and apply topical antiseptics to reduce the chances of developing fungal or bacterial infections.

The definitive correction should be postponed until approximately five days after the injury when the demarcation between healthy and devitalized tissue is apparent. It is often beneficial to endoscopically examine the crop prior to planning the surgery. A small catheter can be used to inject air and dilate the crop, and an endoscope can be used to detect avascular, darkened areas. It is important to evaluate the entire crop, because devitalized mucosa may occur away from the primary burn. The aboral extent of the crop at the thoracic inlet is a location where devitalized areas are often missed.

At surgery, all necrotic tissue must be removed and the tubular structure of the esophagus and ingluvies reestablished. In some cases this may be very challenging, as major portions of crop may be devitalized. If possible, the length of the crop should be maintained even if only a thin strip of esophageal tissue remains. Esophageal strictures are more likely to occur if a resection and anastomosis have been performed than if a thin strip of normal esophagus is preserved and allowed to granulate over a stent. If enough viable tissue remains, it may be sutured around a pharyngostomy feeding tube, through which the patient can receive alimentation while the crop is healing.

Ingluviotomy

Indications for ingluviotomy include foreign body removal, placement of a feeding tube and gaining endoscopic access to the proventriculus and ventriculus. To perform an ingluviotomy, the patient is positioned in dorsal recumbency with the head elevated and the esophagus occluded with moist cotton to prevent fluids from refluxing into the oral cavity. An incision is made through the skin, only over the cranial edge of the left lateral sac of the crop. The skin incision can be made using a radiosurgical unit. Because of the ability of the ingluvies to stretch, the incision should be made only about half the size necessary to accomplish the procedure; however, having adequate exposure is more important than having a small incision, and retrieval of large foreign bodies through small ingluviotomy incisions should not be attempted. The crop incision should be made with a blade in an avascular area. Radiosurgery should be used to seal only specific vessels. Use of the radiosurgical forceps will result in unnecessary tissue trauma. The incision is closed using an inverting technique with an absorbable material swaged on an atraumatic needle. Two-layer inverting patterns are frequently recommended; however, one layer of simple continuous appositional sutures oversewn with an inverting pattern is effective and is less compromising on the size of the crop lumen.

Celiotomy

Surgical approaches to the abdomen involve invasion of the air sac, allowing anesthetic gas to escape through the celiotomy site. This effect can be minimized by packing the borders of the incision with saline-moistened gauze sponges. Additionally, an air sac cannula may be introduced into the abdominal air sac on the side contralateral to the surgical incision. This will allow anesthetic gas to enter an intact air sac, pass through the lung and out the trachea. Using this technique, anesthetic gas does not escape from the surgery site, and waste gas can be scavenged from the trachea. For any celiotomy, the patient should be positioned with the cranial part of the body elevated 30-40° to prevent irrigation fluids from flowing craniad and entering the lungs following incision of the air sacs. Similarly, patients with ascites should have the fluid removed from the coelomic cavity prior to opening the air sacs. Moistened cotton may be placed in the caudal pharynx to occlude the esophagus and prevent proventricular reflux from entering the oral cavity and causing aspiration pneumonia.

Left Lateral Celiotomy

A left lateral celiotomy provides the best exposure of the proventriculus, the ventriculus, the female reproductive tract and the left kidney.

With the patient in right lateral recumbency, the left leg should be retracted as far caudally as possible, creating a fold of skin (knee web) in the flank extending from the stifle to the lateral margin of the sternum. The skin incision will extend from the cranial extent of the pubis to just dorsal to the uncinate process of the fifth or sixth rib. The incision is started in the knee web and continued ventral and caudal following the boundaries of the postventer and postlateral regions, passing through the groove of the groin web caudally to the region of the pubic bone. Care should be taken to incise only the skin, which is easily accomplished using the modified bipolar radiosurgical forceps. Once the skin is incised, the left leg may be further retracted caudally and somewhat dorsally to expose the abdominal wall. A branch of the superficial medial femoral artery and vein should be identified passing over the lumbar fossa toward the pubis. These vessels should be sealed or ligated prior to incising the musculature. The radiosurgical body wall incision is initiated in the external abdominal oblique muscle, just caudal to the last rib. The incision is extended caudally through the internal abdominal oblique and transversus abdominis muscles to the cranial extent of the pubis.

The intercostal vessels coursing along the cranial border of the last two or three ribs should be ligated or coagulated. In small birds, these vessels may be sealed by inserting the indifferent electrode inside the thoracic wall, lightly opposing the electrodes, withdrawing the electrodes until the cranial aspect of the rib is encountered, then activating the electrodes. In larger birds, it is best to cut the rib, clamp the vessel cranial to the rib to achieve hemostasis, then identify the vessel visually and apply a hemostatic clip. In larger birds, the caudal-most two or three ribs will need to be transected at their dorsal and ventral extents and removed to achieve adequate visualization of the viscera. In small birds, excision of the ribs may not be required. They may be fractured and retracted dorsally to provide proper exposure. This method is preferred, because closure of the incision is easier. Once the incision is made through the musculature, the shiny surface of the caudal thoracic or the abdominal air sac is visualized. In some patients, the lung extends caudally as far as the seventh rib. Care must be taken to prevent lacerating the lung, which can be gently elevated using a moistened cotton-tipped applicator if necessary.

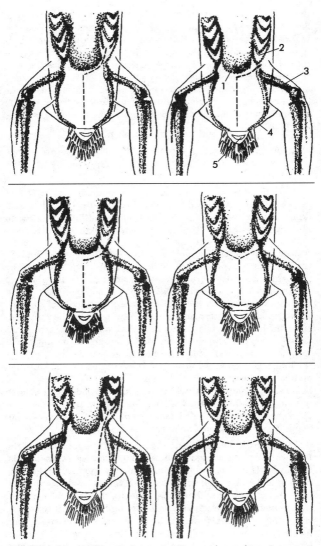

FIG 41.14 Several different celiotomy incisions can be used to gain access to the abdomen of birds. 1) sternum 2) eighth rib 3) femur 4) pubis and 5) vent.

A Heiss, Alm or mini-Balfour retractor should be positioned to maintain retraction of the body wall. Often the intestines are the first structures encountered. They can be gently retracted using a cotton-tipped applicator. The intestines are fragile and should not be manipulated with toothed forceps, which will create severe bruising and potential perforation. Once the intestines are retracted caudally, the kidney may be identified at the dorsomedial aspect of the coelom. The ovary or left testicle should be encountered at the cranial division of the kidney. The adrenal gland is located between the gonad and the cranial division of the kidney, but may be obscured if the gonad is large.

If the seventh and eighth ribs have been removed, closure will require the placement of tension sutures from the abdominal musculature to the sixth rib. Sutures passed around the pubic bone may be necessary when closing large incisions.

Ventral Midline Celiotomy

A ventral midline celiotomy is used primarily for surgery of the small intestines, liver biopsy, egg-related peritonitis, abdominal masses, egg binding and repair of a cloacal prolapse. This approach provides access to both sides of the coelomic cavity.

The skin is incised in the midpostventer region from the sternum to the interpubic space (see Figure 41.14). The linea alba is usually broad and easily identified. It must be incised carefully because the duodenum crosses from left to right just inside the body wall. It is best to initiate the incision between the pubic bones over the cloaca. Once a two millimeter incision is initiated, it may be extended craniad to the level of the sternum. If exposure is limited, the incision may be extended to one or both sides approximately two millimeters from the sternal border creating a muscular flap. Further exposure is achieved by extending the incision along one or both sides of the pubic bones in a similar fashion. This approach provides the best exposure to mid-abdominal masses, uterine masses and generalized abdominal disease (peritonitis). The size of the incision should be sufficient to allow a procedure to be performed, but as small as possible to minimize tissue damage and air sac disruption, and to make it easier to maintain anesthesia. If it is necessary to approach a large area of the abdomen, it is often best to open and close each area before proceeding on to another area.

Transverse Celiotomy

Transverse celiotomy provides exposure to a large area of the abdomen. The bird is positioned in dorsal recumbency and the postventer region is prepared. A transverse skin incision is made midway between the sternum and the vent (see Figure 41.14). The abdominal wall is lifted and incised with care to avoid lacerating the underlying intestines. The ventriculus and duodenum are the first organs encountered, but may be reflected to expose the cranial aspect of the cloaca, the middle and caudal lobes of the kidneys and the lower reproductive tract of hens.

Proventriculotomy and Ventriculotomy

The proventriculus tears easily when excessive tension is applied. The ventriculus is composed of dense muscle and fascia and holds sutures well, but is more difficult to seal with suture and cannot be inverted.

Proventriculotomy is most often indicated for the removal of foreign objects or toxic materials (such as lead or zinc-containing coins) from the proventriculus or ventriculus that cannot be retrieved using rigid or flexible endoscopes. A definitive diagnosis of neuropathic gastric dilatation may require a ventricular biopsy, although there are some discussions that biopsies of the crop may provide similar information.

A left lateral celiotomy approach will provide exposure of the ventriculus and proventriculus. The ventral suspensory structures are bluntly dissected to allow the proventriculus to be retracted caudally. The proventriculus in some birds is quite fragile and toothed forceps should be avoided. Stay sutures may be placed in the ventriculus to aid with exteriorization and manipulation of the proventriculus. Stay sutures should not be placed in the proventriculus. The coelomic cavity should be packed off with moist gauze sponges to prevent contamination of the abdominal cavity with gastric contents.

The isthmus or intermediate zone is identified as a constriction between the ventriculus and the proventriculus. The vessels on the surface of the proventriculus are easily identified and avoided. The proventriculotomy incision is initiated at the isthmus and extends orad into the body of the proventriculus. Hemorrhage from the cut edge of the proventriculus may be controlled using radiocoagulation. Thumb forceps may be used to gently clamp the cut edge to occlude the vessel, allowing it to be identified and appropriately coagulated. Proventricular contents should be removed using suction. Small spoons or curettes may be used to remove solid contents. A combination of irrigation and suction is useful to completely evacuate the proventriculus and ventriculus. A small diameter flexible endoscope may be used per os, or through the proventriculotomy to assure that all foreign objects have been removed.

The proventriculotomy is closed using a simple continuous appositional pattern of a fine, synthetic, monofilament, absorbable material over-sewn with a continuous or interrupted inverting pattern such as a Cushing or Lembert pattern. The inverting pattern should extend beyond the actual incision to ensure an adequate seal. The closure may be evaluated for leakage using an orogastric tube to insufflate the proventriculus with air or sterile saline.

Food and water should be offered in the immediate postoperative period. The wound strength immediately following suture placement is stronger than during the debridement phase of wound healing, which occurs three to five days postoperatively. Unless one intends to withhold food until wound strength begins to increase again (the phase of fibroplasia), fasting for one to two days postoperatively is not indicated. Incisional leakage of gastric contents occurs with some frequency in birds. If the proventricular wall appears thin and friable, the potential for postoperative incisional leakage may warrant placement of a duodenal feeding tube. This will allow enteral alimentation of the patient while bypassing the gastric incision.

The ventriculus is best approached through a proventriculotomy incision. The incision in the isthmus is extended aborad toward the ventriculus. The opening into the ventriculus can be gently dilated to allow the introduction of instruments appropriate for removal of ventricular contents. Some surgeons suggest that a ventriculotomy (transverse abdominal approach) is easier than a proventriculotomy (left lateral approach). The lighter-colored, elliptical area of the ventriculus, where the muscle is thin and the fibers can be seen to course in a different direction from the remainder of the ventriculus, is the location where the incision is made.

The incision is made transversely across the muscle fibers into the lumen. At closure, sutures must be placed close together to prevent leakage, because a serosal seal cannot be created by using an inverting suture pattern.

Intestinal Surgery

Surgery on the intestines may be necessary to repair an accidental enterotomy created during a ventral midline celiotomy or to debride necrotic bowel secondary to constrictions caused by adhesions. These cases generally carry a poor-to-grave prognosis. A midline, flap or transverse celiotomy may be appropriate, depending on the location of the lesion. In most circumstances, microsurgical technique is indicated due to the extremely thin nature of the avian intestine. The technique used to anastomose the bowel requires microsurgical manipulation of 6-0 to 10-0 monofilament suture on a one-fourth circle atraumatic needle. Typically, six to eight sutures are used for an end-to-end anastomosis in a simple interrupted appositional pattern. Side-to-side anastomosis may prove to be more appropriate in birds and is easier to perform.

Intestinal Feeding Tubes

The catheter is placed through a ventral midline incision. The ascending duodenum is easily identified by its close association with the pancreas. A "through-the-needle" catheter (indwelling jugular catheter) is used with the needle passing first through the left abdominal wall, then into the descending loop of duodenum. The catheter diameter should be less than one-third the diameter of the intestine. The catheter is advanced through the descending and ascending loops of duodenum (4-6 cm), and the needle is withdrawn from the intestine and body wall. One or two sutures are placed between the left body wall and the duodenum at the entry site of the catheter to secure the intestine to the body wall and allow a seal to form (monofilament 5-0 prolene). The midline celiotomy is closed routinely.

The catheter is secured to the outside left abdominal wall using a "finger trap" technique. The needle is protected within its "snapguard," and the snapguard is bent to conform to the contour of the bird's body. The snapguard is then sutured to the skin to secure it in place. The catheter is brought caudal to the leg and under the wing. The excess is coiled and the catheter is secured to the lateral and dorsal body wall using two sutures. The catheter is flushed with saline to assure patency, and an injection cap is placed to create a sealed system for alimentation.

Once the caloric need is calculated (see Chapter 40), the amount of liquid diet required is calculated based on the caloric density of the diet. The amount should be divided into equal volumes and injected four to six times daily at a rate of approximately 1 ml/15 seconds to allow the intestine to accommodate the volume. The catheter should be flushed with water or LRS (1-2 ml) before and after injection of the diet to prevent plugging.

The catheter should be maintained a minimum of five days to allow a seal to form between the intestine and the body wall. If the catheter is dislodged prematurely, leakage of intestinal contents may occur. Once the catheter is no longer needed, the finger trap suture is cut, the catheter removed and the defect left to heal by second intention.

Cloacal Prolapse

Cloacopexy is indicated to correct problems with chronic cloacal prolapsing. This condition appears to be most common in Old World psittacine birds, especially cockatoos, and is associated with reduced sphincter tone. Chronic gram-negative enteritis may be an initiating factor, underscoring the need for cloacal cultures as part of the patient evaluation process. Minor prolapses may respond to placement of a mattress suture on either side of the cloaca. These must be placed close enough together to prevent recurrence of the prolapse, but far enough apart to allow the normal passage of droppings. These sutures may be left in place from a few days to several weeks depending on the clinical situation. Purse-string sutures are contraindicated due to frequent postsurgical cloacal atony secondary to nerve damage.

A percutaneous cloacopexy may be performed as a temporary or definitive treatment for cloacal prolapse. The prolapse is reduced using a moistened cotton-tipped applicator. The applicator is maintained within the cloaca to help identify its limits, and two or three sutures are placed percutaneously through the skin, body wall and urodeum. The sutures should be removed in two to four weeks. This procedure carries the risk of inadvertently entrapping or perforating the ureters, rectum, duodenum and pancreas.

In some cases, prolapse is due to atony of the vent sphincter. This condition may be treated by surgically narrowing the vent opening. One-half to three-fourths of the margin of the circumference of the vent is incised to provide a cut surface for healing. Simple interrupted sutures are placed from one side of the vent to the other in order to partially close the opening. This will decrease the size of the vent opening permanently, preventing prolapse of the cloaca.

A rib cloacopexy is an effective treatment for severe cloacal prolapse. A ventral midline celiotomy is performed and the cloaca is identified (Figure 41.17). This approach provides exposure to the entire cloaca and its associated structures. It may be necessary to use a moistened cotton-tipped applicator or the finger of a gloved assistant to reduce the prolapse and define its limits intraoperatively. Fat on the ventral surface of the cloaca should be excised. This appears to be crucial for a successful surgery. A suture is placed around the last rib on each side of the bird and passed through the full thickness of the ventral aspect of the craniolateral extent of the urodeum. The suture should be tied with enough tension to slightly invert the vent. Large sections of tissue must be used for suture placement, and it appears to be important to penetrate the cloacal lumen. Several other sutures are then placed between the body wall and the wall of the cloaca. The cloaca may be sutured to the caudal border of the sternum instead of the ribs, if

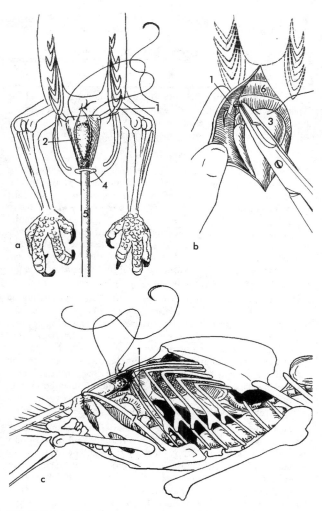

FIG 41.17 A rib cloacopexy is indicated to permanently correct chronic cloacal prolapse. **a)** The cloaca is pushed cranially with a moistened cotton-tipped applicator and sutures are placed between the cranio-lateral border of the cloaca and the eighth rib. **b)** Pushing the eighth rib caudally with a finger will help in the placement of sutures. **c)** Lateral view of the cloacopexy procedure showing the placement of the suture between the cloaca and the eighth rib, and the suturing of the cloaca to the abdominal wall during closure. 1) eighth rib 2) skin incision 3) cloaca 4) vent 5) swab 6) intestines and 7) pubis.

the rib sutures place excessive inverting tension on the cloaca. This procedure may not be effective in birds with a thin-walled cloaca.

Surgery of the Reproductive Tract

Egg Binding

Any bird presenting for egg binding should be evaluated for hypocalcemia prior to planning surgery, and any abnormalities should be addressed. Medical management including ovocentesis should be attempted prior to considering surgical intervention.

Ovocentesis

If medical management of egg binding fails, ovocentesis and collapsing the egg may be successful. Under general anesthesia, the opening of the vagina into the cloaca is identified. A blunt probe is used to dilate the opening. Once the egg is visualized, a needle can be inserted into the egg to aspirate its contents. Following ovocentesis, the egg can be collapsed and the shell fragments removed (see Chapter 29). The vagina and uterus should be flushed repeatedly to verify that all egg material has been evacuated. A radiograph may be valuable to rule out the presence of another egg or remaining fragments.

If the egg is near or within the pelvic canal, it may be delivered using an episiotomy-type incision. The incision is made on the ventral midline through the cloacal sphincter extending craniad through the urodeum. If necessary, the incision may extend into the uterus. After the egg is removed, the uterus and cloaca are closed with a simple interrupted or simple continuous pattern of a slowly absorbable material. Closure of the body wall and skin are routine. This is a radical procedure and is indicated only in critical cases in which the hen is likely to die or the egg is of major importance for species propagational purposes.

In cases where the egg is lodged farther cranial in the oviduct, it may be best to perform a midline celiotomy, and hysterotomy may be the best technique for removing the egg. The hysterotomy incision should be closed with a simple appositional continuous or inverting pattern of a fine monofilament synthetic absorbable material. Postoperatively, hormone therapy or photoperiod regulation should be used to prevent subsequent laying until the hysterotomy has healed. If hysterectomy is indicated, a left lateral approach is preferred to gain access to the entire oviduct.

Salpingohysterectomy

Salpingohysterectomy is indicated to terminate pathologic egg laying, alleviate egg binding, remove an infected or ruptured oviduct and to treat a prolapsed oviduct and recurring egg-related peritonitis.

Salpingohysterectomy carries a significant degree of risk and is generally not recommended as a preventive measure.

Salpingohysterectomy may be accomplished through a left lateral celiotomy. The ovary may be visualized following lateral and ventral retraction of the proventriculus. The oviduct is identified and elevated away from the large caudal vena cava. Minor damage to this vessel will result in life-threatening hemorrhage. The ventral ligament causes the convolutions in the uterus and oviduct. The ligament courses caudally and collects as a muscular cord at the vagina. There are no vessels in this ligament, and it should be dissected to allow the oviduct and uterus to be stretched into a linear configuration.

At the base of the infundibulum and coursing caudally along the uterus, the dorsal ligament suspends the uterus and a branch of the ovarian artery. A small blood vessel can be identified coursing from the ovary through the infundibulum. This vessel should be coagulated or a hemostatic clip should be applied to control hemorrhage. If it is inadvertently transected or broken, it will retract under the ovary in a virtually unretrievable location. A small piece of absorbent gelatin sponge may be packed against the ovary to achieve hemostasis. The remainder of this suspensory structure may then be dissected with the bipolar radiosurgical forceps.

Once the infundibulum is free, the oviduct is retracted ventrally and caudally, exposing the dorsal suspensory ligament. Several small blood vessels, branches of the ovarian artery, can be seen in this structure perpendicular to the oviduct and uterus. These should be identified and coagulated. Each vascular stump should be inspected for residual hemorrhage before closure. As this dissection is continued caudally toward the cloaca, the ureter can be identified as a white tubular structure extending from the kidney to the cloaca. This structure should be avoided. As the dissection approaches the cloaca, the uterus courses along with the terminal colon and enters the cloaca. The uterus should be ligated at its junction with the vagina by placing one or two hemostatic clips a short distance from the cloaca. In cases where the vaginal tissue has been damaged, the clips may be applied at the cloaca, being careful not to entrap the ureter.

Egg-related Peritonitis

Mild cases may respond to antibiotic therapy and supportive care (see Chapter 29). Surgical intervention is usually necessary to resolve severe cases. In some cases, surgery should be postponed and the patient treated medically until the condition stabilizes. A ventral midline celiotomy is preferred because fluids are easily drained out the incision rather than down into the air sacs, and potentially into the lungs. Once the celiotomy is performed, the intestines should be retracted using moistened cotton-tipped applicators or other suitable atraumatic instruments. Any yolk or tissue debris should be removed. The cavity should be copiously irrigated prior to closure. Implantation of Penrose drains may be indicated in some cases, but do not generally provide adequate coelomic drainage. This condition warrants a guarded-to-poor prognosis. Birds that recover frequently have abdominal adhesions, distention and muscular dysfunction.

Removal of the Gonads

The vascular supply to the ovary may be destroyed using vascular clips, but this is a difficult procedure, performed without being able to visualize vital structures. Microsurgical equipment is essential. Clients should be informed that this procedure is extremely difficult and the possibility of complications is high. The patient should be treated medically to reduce the size of the ovary and improve visualization. Through a left lateral celiotomy, the ovary is identified. A hemostatic clip is applied dorsal to (under) the ovary to occlude all ovarian vessels. In small birds, one clip applied from a caudal to cranial direction is adequate. Two clips, one from a cranial direction and the other from a caudal direction, may be required for large birds. Angled appliers should be used to place the clips under the ovary parallel to the spine, which reduces the possibility of inadvertently entrapping the aorta or peripheral nerves.

Orchidectomy

Neutering a male is theoretically easier than neutering a female because the testicles are not as adherent to deeper structures as the ovary, making clip application easier and safer. However, orchidectomy must be performed bilaterally, making a ventral approach more applicable than a left lateral approach. The placement of vascular clips is similar to that described for the ovary. Orchidectomy in companion birds is extremely difficult and many birds do not survive the surgery.

A technique for orchidectomy in ostriches has been described. The procedure is indicated to control aggressive behavior in birds that present a danger to keepers, handlers, the public or other birds. The surgical approach is through the costal notch and lumbar fossa on each side. The skin and body wall are incised adequately to allow introduction of a gloved hand. The testicle on the corresponding side is palpated, grasped and twisted until it is torn from any attachments. It is recommended that the procedure be performed at the onset of breeding season when the testicles have begun to increase in size so they can be easily located.

Miscellaneous Surgical Procedures

Abdominal Hernias

Abdominal hernias in birds may be congenital or acquired. In most cases, the hernia is of little clinical consequence. Herniorrhaphy is necessary if secondary clinical problems such as cloacal urolithiasis or egg binding occur.

Lipomas

Lipomas are frequently the expression of obesity. Central necrosis and ulceration may occur. Some lipomas are covered by xanthomatous skin. Efforts should be made to reduce the size of the mass medically before attempting surgical extirpation. Diet and exercise are effective over a period of several months. Lipomas are generally well encapsulated and shell out easily.

Leg Amputation

When a leg must be amputated, it is best performed at midfemur. If the stump is too long, the bird may continue to use it for ambulation, causing trauma and granuloma formation to the stump. A mid-femoral amputation allows adequate soft tissue coverage of the end of the bone and prevents the patient from traumatizing the surgical site. Most companion birds with one leg are able to function normally. Psittacine birds compensate particularly well because they use their beak as an aid to ambulation. Pododermatitis of the contralateral foot, as occurs commonly in raptor amputees, is rarely a problem in companion birds on a formulated diet.

A semicircular incision is created both medially and laterally at about the level of the stifle. The muscles should be transected at the stifle. Use of the radioscalpel will aid in hemostasis. The muscles are elevated from the femur to the mid-diaphyseal region using a periosteal elevator. The ischiatic nerve should be injected with lidocaine or bupivacaine prior to transection for temporary postoperative analgesia. The femur may be cut with a bone cutter, an osteotome, a gigli wire, a sagittal saw or other suitable instruments appropriate for the patient's size. Following the osteotomy, the muscles are sutured over the end of the bone to provide padding.

Toe Amputation

Hemostasis is aided by the use of a tourniquet. Hemostatic agents should be avoided. The heavily keratinized scale surfaces may be gently debrided exposing the more supple epidermis below. The site of amputation should be at the joint proximal to the affected area. The skin should be incised distal to the joint to provide adequate skin for closure.

Wing Amputation

Amputation of the humerus at the junction of the middle and proximal thirds of the bone provides adequate soft tissue coverage and creates a stump short enough to prevent self trauma. The skin incision should be made at the distal humerus, just proximal to the elbow. If additional skin is needed for closure, the patagium may be utilized. The muscles are transected at their musculotendinous junctions near the elbow. The radial and medianoulnar nerves should be injected with lidocaine or bupivacaine for short-term postoperative analgesia prior to their transection. Brachial musculature is mobilized by blunt dissection to remove attachments from the humerus. The humerus should be transected at the proximal third, to provide sufficient muscle distally to be sutured over the stump. Subcutaneous and skin closure are routine.

Vascular Access Devices

Vascular access devices are subcutaneously implanted devices with a reservoir that is accessed through surgically prepared skin using a non-coring needle (Huber point needle). These have been maintained in humans for years and in birds for up to 12 weeks.

The right jugular vein is the preferred site for implantation. The skin is moved dorsally and an incision is made over the jugular vein. When the skin is released, the incision site will be ventral to the jugular vein and not over the reservoir. The jugular vein is identified and isolated for a distance of approximately 15 mm. Dissection must proceed cautiously as the vein is very fragile. Two ligatures are placed around the vein, one at the cranial extent and the other at the caudal extent of the isolated area. The caudal suture is elevated to occlude blood flow. The jugular vein will distend and the cranial suture is then tied off permanently occluding jugular flow. This does not seem to affect cerebral hemodynamics.

At this point, a small segment of the jugular vein remains distended. Using fine iris scissors and magnification, a transverse venotomy is created in the distended portion of the vein. This incision will not transect the vein but will allow the catheter to be inserted. After the blood from the distended segment is cleared, the end of the catheter is inserted into the venotomy site. The tension on the caudal ligature will have to be loosened to allow the catheter to pass, but enough tension should be maintained to prevent reflux hemorrhage. The venotomy may be widened using fine forceps or a vascular introducer. The catheter is advanced to the right atrium and secured in place by suturing above and below the retention ring at the venotomy site to prevent the catheter from advancing or backing out.

A Huber needle attached to a three-way stopcock and a saline-filled syringe is used to test the ease of injection and withdrawal of a sample. The position of the catheter tip should be evaluated using contrast radiography. Some catheters are radiopaque. With those that are radiolucent, the position can be evaluated by injecting a vascular contrast medium.

A subcutaneous pocket is created dorsal to the jugular vein large enough to accommodate the reservoir, which is placed into the pocket and sutured in place to the fascia of the neck musculature. A 2-4 cm loop of catheter is left to allow for neck movements. Subcutaneous and skin closure are routine. During recovery, feathers over the reservoir should be removed and the skin aseptically prepared. The device should then be filled with heparin at 100 IU/ml. Only non-coring needles should be used with these devices. With a minimal amount of practice, these devices can be implanted in 10-15 minutes.

The skin area above the port must be aseptically prepared before each use. Chlorhexidine has been shown to be three to four times more effective at preventing bacterial colonization of the catheter than povidone iodine. The individual administering the therapy should wear sterile gloves and use sterile equipment. The non-coring needle is inserted into the reservoir until it hits the base plate and the injection can then be made.

When catheters are used daily or several times daily, there is no need for heparin locks, which eliminates the potential for heparinizing the patient. However, there is a higher potential for thrombus formation with small gauge catheters, and a heparin lock may still be necessary.

Perinatal Surgery

With practice and management, fine suture (8-0 to 10-0) and an atraumatic needle can be used for closure of the umbilicus. However, hemostatic clips are more appropriate for application to the umbilicus than suture ligatures. Featherless neonates are highly prone to developing hypothermia. Anesthesia and surgery time should be less than 15 minutes, and the operating room temperature should be elevated to 75-85°F. Supplemental glucose should be provided through an intraosseous cannula as necessary.

Because of their small blood volume, perinatal patients are more likely to require transfusion if major blood loss occurs or if the hematocrit is below 20-25%. Respiratory movements may be difficult to observe in perinatal patients, making the use of clear drapes and small nonrebreathing bags essential. The crop of altricial avian neonatal patients is usually full, increasing the risk of regurgitation and aspiration. The patient may be fasted until the crop volume has diminished or the contents may be removed by aspiration. Elevating the head and packing the thoracic esophagus with moist cotton will also help prevent reflux of crop contents.

Yolk Sac Removal

The yolk sac is a diverticulum from the small intestine attached by the yolk stalk. It is normally internalized prior to hatching. After the yolk has been completely absorbed, the remnant of the yolk sac becomes the vitelline or Meckel's diverticulum.

A procedure for removal of unabsorbed yolk sacs has been successful in decreasing mortality in affected chicks (see Chapter 48). Candidates for surgery demonstrate one or more of the following clinical signs: abdominal distention, exercise intolerance or dyspnea, weight loss and anorexia, failure to grow or inability to stand or walk. Abdominal palpation and radiography support the diagnosis of unabsorbed yolk sac. Percutaneous aspiration of the yolk should not be attempted as the yolk sac is very thin and will leak yolk into the coelomic cavity resulting in peritonitis. Injecting antibiotics directly into the yolk sac carries the same risk. Systemic antibiotics are not effective alone.

ORTHOPEDIC SURGICAL TECHNIQUES

Howard Martin
Branson W. Ritchie

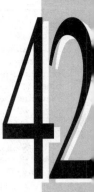

Regardless of the specific techniques employed in fracture repair, it is important to:

- Treat contaminated and infected wounds.
- Preserve soft tissue structures.
- Appose, align and control rotation of fractures and reduce luxations.
- Rigidly immobilize the fracture site.
- Maintain range of motion in all joints affected by the fracture or fixation technique.
- Return the affected limb to "normal function" as soon as possible.

The presence of a fracture certainly suggests major trauma, and a thorough physical examination should be performed to determine other injuries.

In many cases, birds may require several days of stabilization with fluids, steroids, antibiotics or supportive alimentation before anesthesia and surgery can be safely performed (see Chapter 40).

It is common for subtle injuries to occur that are difficult to detect by physical examination. Survey radiographs of affected skeletal areas as well as the abdomen and thorax are needed to assess any bony or soft tissue changes that may have occurred during a traumatic episode.

Fracture stabilization techniques used in free-ranging birds must be designed to increase the likelihood that a rehabilitated bird can be released. Repair of a wing fracture, particularly near a joint, must be nearly perfect with no ankylosis and minimal soft tissue damage to ensure return to full flight.

Prognosis

Companion and aviary birds rarely require full mobility following fracture repair, and the post-fracture prognosis for return to function with these birds is generally excellent. By comparison, free-ranging birds (particularly raptors), which can be viewed as finely tuned athletes, must have near perfect wing function in order to survive in the wild.

Postoperative Care

Postoperative radiographs should be taken at two- to four-week intervals to assess bone healing. The radiographic changes associated with bone healing can appear similar to those that occur with osteomyelitis including periosteal reaction, sclerosis and increased radiodensities in the medullary canal (Figure 42.2).

To improve vascular supply to damaged tissue and to speed the bone healing process, active and passive rehabilitative techniques should be instigated as soon as possible after an orthopedic surgery.

Bone Healing

Stable, properly aligned fractures appear to heal more rapidly in birds than in mammals. Clinical stability of a fracture (two to three weeks) may precede radiographic evidence that the bone is healed (three to six weeks). Devitalized, uninfected fragments should be left in place to provide structural support for callus formation.

Osteomyelitis

Avian heterophils lack the proteinase necessary to liquify necrotic tissue, and birds tend to form granulomas that wall off infectious agents and necrotic material. Consequently, osteomyelitis is characterized by caseous, dry, nondraining lesions that are frequently restricted to the site of infection and rarely induce secondary systemic infections. With mild infections, it is common for the host defense mechanism to wall off the necrotic debris and form callus around the infected tissue.

Debridement and flushing should be used to remove necrotic tissue and debris from all open fractures to reduce the chances of postoperative osteomyelitis. Samples for culture and sensitivity should be collected from the fracture site at the time of surgery. The use of intraoperative, broad-spectrum antibiotics with good tissue penetration (trimethoprim-sulfa, cephalosporins, chloramphenicol, tetracyclines) should be considered in these cases.

Bone Grafts

Bone grafts promote fracture healing through osteogenesis (production of new bone), osteoinduction (recruitment of mesenchymal cells that differentiate into chondroblasts and osteoblasts) and osteoconduction (osteoblast ingrowth from the host into the graft providing structural and mechanical support). In general, cancellous bone is better than cortical bone for grafting because the former has a larger surface area and a large number of viable cells for stimulating new bone production.

Autogenous medullary bone (collected from the tibiotarsus), corticocancellous bone (collected from the sternum or ribs) and cortical bone (devitalized fragments from the fracture site) have been shown to augment bone healing in birds.

Fracture Repair Techniques

It is best to have a command of a variety of fracture fixation techniques and to be ready with alternative plans at the time of surgery. Reassessment of the injury intraoperatively may necessitate a change in the surgical procedure.

Many closed fractures may heal without any type of coaptation or fixation. However, with unsupported long bone fractures, excessive callus formation, malalignment of the bone ends and shortening of the limb (overridden fractures) will dramatically reduce normal function. Nondisplaced fractures of the pelvic girdle, coracoid, clavicle and scapula will generally heal with minimal support. Displaced fractures of the coracoid must be surgically repaired or the fracture will usually result in an inability to fly. Fractures of the radius or ulna, in which the other bone is intact, can generally be repaired with external coaptation and forced rest.

External Coaptation: Bandages and Splints

Bandages and splints should be made of the lightest weight materials with the minimal amount of padding needed to compensate for swelling of damaged soft tissue. External coaptation is acceptable as a primary stabilization technique only when a limited postfracture range of motion is satisfactory, a patient is too small to facilitate surgical repair, a fracture is minimally displaced or anesthesia and surgery would jeopardize the patient's life (eg, liver failure, kidney failure, heart disease, head trauma).

In general, external coaptation should be considered an emergency method of stabilizing fractures until surgery can be performed.

Some companion birds may not require full return to flight; in these patients, some wing fractures can be effectively managed with external coaptation.

External Fixators

External fixators are generally considered the best stabilization technique for immobilizing fractures in birds that require a full return to function.

When properly used, external fixators provide rigid stabilization and preserve joint and periarticular structure, while neutralizing rotational, bending and shear forces. In many cases, external fixators allow a bird to use a repaired limb within several days of surgery.

Type II (through-and-through) fixators are more stable and stronger than Type I fixators, which tend to loosen rapidly. The use of positive-profile threaded pins in a Type I fixator configuration is particularly useful in repairing fractures of the proximal humerus and femur, where interference with the body wall makes it difficult or impossible to place a Type II fixator.

Application of an External Fixator

External fixator pins should be placed by making a small incision in the skin, and should not be placed through a primary incision site or open wound. This placement technique will decrease the likelihood that the pins will promote an infection at the surgical site. Pins should be inserted so that they avoid large muscle masses (minimizes loosening) and should be passed through predrilled holes to decrease wobble (improperly increases the size of the hole) and increase pin purchase on the cortices. It is best to place from three to four pins on each side of a fracture to decrease the stresses on any one pin. A minimum of two pins must be placed in each bone segment to ensure that the fixator will provide adequate fixation without rotation.

Positive-profile threaded pins inserted through predrilled holes have been found to maintain solid bone-to-pin interfaces for prolonged periods (up to three months) in some birds. By comparison, other types of threaded or unthreaded pins are frequently loose in the cortex within three to six weeks of insertion. The diameter of positive-profile threaded pins is not reduced by the threading process and these pins are less likely to fail from the stress-riser effect than other types of threaded pins. Placing unthreaded pins at an angle (35-55°) perpendicular to the bone will decrease the chance that the fixator will slip from side to side, but would not be expected to be as effective as positive-profile threaded pins.

In addition to KE clamps, stabilization pins can be connected with polymethylmethacrylate, cast material and dental acrylic. In comparison to KE clamps, these materials are inexpensive, lightweight and are malleable so that pins that are not in perfect alignment can be easily connected. The tips of the stabilizing pins can be carefully bent parallel to the long axis of the bone to increase their holding strength in the connecting material.

Polymethylmethacrylate (PMM) can be attached to the stabilizing pins by mixing the material until it is the consistency of dough and then molding it around the stabilizing pins. The material can also be used by passing the stabilizing pins through a hole in a clear plastic tube (eg, clear straw). The plastic tubes used for a mold should be thin-walled to ensure that the methylmethacrylate column is of adequate diameter (approximately equal to that of the bone). When the pins are properly positioned (fracture site reduced and in proper alignment), the PMM is placed in a syringe and injected into the straw while it is still liquid. The fracture is held in place until the PMM hardens (generally ten minutes).

In birds that weigh less than 200 g, hypodermic needles can be used as stabilizing pins and these can be attached with cyanoacrylate glue (SuperGlue) to other needles or tooth picks that function as temporary connecting rods. An index card can be fashioned into a V-shaped trough and placed over the pins. Five-minute epoxy cement is then poured into the trough to firmly bind the stabilization pins and connecting bars.

Intramedullary Fixation

Intramedullary Pins

Generally, intramedullary pins neutralize bending forces and provide adequate fracture alignment, but they do not protect the fracture from rotational or shear forces. Minimal rotational deformities in the wing bones can inhibit flight by altering the dynamics of the wing aerofoil. Techniques that use IM pins in combination with external coaptation have been frequently discussed in the literature; however, the combination of these two fixation techniques should be avoided to prevent ankylosis of the associated joints. Because of the relatively thin cortices of birds, the use of threaded IM pins has been suggested to provide better bone purchase than nonthreaded pins. However, IM pins are primarily used to counter bending force which would not be influenced by the degree of purchase in the cortex.

(RHH Editors' note: Intramedullary pins have several disadvantages when compared to external fixators. They have the inherent potential to cause articular and periarticular damage resulting in ankylosis of the joints. Even properly placed pins that exit near a joint can cause sufficient tendon or ligament damage, resulting in a partially dysfunctional limb. Unless an IM pin can be placed so that it does not exit through or near a joint, it is best not to use this method of internal fixation in birds that require full post-fixation use of a limb. Even pins that do not exit near a joint can still injure the vasculature and significantly alter the growth pattern of the bone.

Retrograde placement of pins through the distal humerus, normograde placement from the lateral or medial epicondyle of the humerus, placement through the distal ulna or retrograde placement from the elbow can cause severe periarticular fibrosis and wing dysfunction.)

The use of IM pins, with or without interfragmentary wires, is effective for stabilizing some fractures in companion birds when clients are not concerned with postsurgical return of flight. When IM pins are used, they should be of sufficient size to fill about one-half to two-thirds of the medullary canal. Excessively large pins can interfere with endosteal blood supply, which may cause avascular necrosis or iatrogenic fractures.

Cerclage, hemicerclage and interfragmentary wires can be used as an adjunct to internal or external coaptation to neutralize rotational and shear forces. They are most useful for adding stability to long oblique and spiral fractures and for holding fragments of bone in apposition during the application of other fixation devices.

Doyle Technique

A fracture fixation method has been developed by J.E. Doyle that combines intramedullary pinning concepts with those of external fixation. In both the distal and proximal fracture segments, a pin is placed through one cortex and angled to bounce off the opposite cortex and remain in the medullary canal. Hooks are fashioned on the external end of each pin, and the fracture site is then compressed and stabilized by stretching a dental impact type rubber band over the hooks of each pin. The technique requires that the smallest fracture segment be of sufficient size for the safe placement of a stabilizing pin. Kirschner wires (0.028, 0.035, 0.045 or 0.062 cm) are adequate for most avian fractures. In small birds, various-sized catheter needles or hypodermic needles can be used in place of the K wires.

As with any pin that is placed through the cortex, the stabilizing pins used in this technique should be inserted through predrilled, appropriately sized holes (smaller than the pin size). The pin is inserted as far away from the fracture as possible without

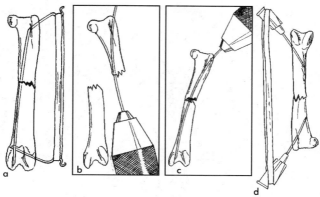

FIG 42.15 a) Doyle technique to repair long bone fractures. This technique allows for the use of intramedullary pins while reducing the degree of perivascular and trabecular damage and providing the maximum compression of the fracture site. Note that the longest pin does not penetrate the cortex of the bone, and that the shortest pin is placed into the cortex. **b,c)** A battery- or air-driven drill is used to place the pins. A dental rubber band attaches the cupped ends of the pins. **d)** In small birds, side cutters are used to notch the hubs of hypodermic needles, which are used in place of intramedullary pins.

compromising the periarticular tissues. Once the pin has entered the cortex, the angle is changed so that the pin bounces off the opposite cortex and can be threaded into the medullary canal, past the fracture site and as deep as possible into the smaller fracture segment (the long pin should not penetrate through the cortex in the smaller segment) (Figure 42.15).

The exterior portion of the pin is bent in two places using locking pliers. A right angle bend is placed in the pin as it exits the skin so that the pin is relatively perpendicular to the bone. A semicircle (hook) is fashioned in the end of the pin about 1 cm from the skin. A second pin is placed in the smaller fracture segment. This pin is inserted at a 45° angle to the long axis of the bone and parallel to the initial pin. This pin should penetrate but not exit the opposite cortex. A rubber band is placed around the hooks to compress the fracture. Postoperatively, several opened gauze pads are placed between the skin and the rubber band to prevent irritation. The affected appendage is placed in an appropriate bandage (leg: Robert Jones; wing: figure-of-eight body wrap). The rubber bands can generally be removed within 10-21 days, and the pins between 21 and 40 days after surgery.

Either cerclage wires or fracture transversing staples can be used to minimize overriding or rotation in oblique and comminuted fractures (Figure 42.16).

The Doyle technique can be used in combination with cleaning, calcium hydroxide and acrylics to repair the beak and fractures of the mandible. Pins are placed into the fracture segments and connected with rubber bands. The fracture site and beak defect are covered with calcium hydroxide paste to prevent dental acrylic from entering the defect and causing a malunion. The fracture is

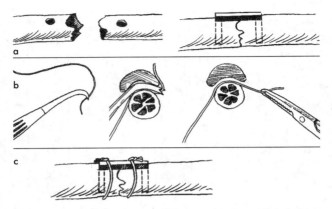

FIG 42.16 Doyle staple technique: **a)** To prevent fracture rotation, the bone ends are notched, and a section of IM pin wire is bent and placed into pre-drilled holes. **b)** The wire is passed around the bone using a slotted periosteal elevator and **c)** is tied over both sides of the staple.

then covered with dental acrylic or a hydroactive dressing. The defect and fracture will generally require six weeks to heal.

Surgical Approaches

The Wing

The Carpometacarpus

If the single artery and vein located between the third and fourth metacarpal bones are damaged, avascular necrosis to the distal portion of the wing can occur. The most direct approach to fractures of the carpometacarpus is the dorsal approach. The bone can be visualized immediately beneath a dorsal skin incision. Minimally displaced closed fractures of the carpometacarpus may be repaired with a figure-of-eight bandage (see Chapter 16).

Fractures of the carpometacarpus are ideally suited for small, lightweight external fixators that allow freedom of movement in the carpal joint. These are usually applied using small K wires or hypodermic needles and then attached by a connecting bar composed of plastic tubing filled with methylmethacrylate cement. IM pins may be added to help with alignment; these are usually placed through the fracture site and normograded distally and then retrograded back to the proximal fragment. Passing IM pins normograde from the carpus reduces the damage to the carpal joint.

The Radius and Ulna

Occasionally, birds are presented with fractures of the radius alone. Given the larger size of the ulna, radial fractures are often anatomically stabilized and splinted by the larger ulna. Bandages or simple enclosure rest may result in adequate fixation of minimally displaced radial fractures. If displaced, IM pins introduced through the fracture site and normograded out the wall of the distal radius (avoiding the joint) and then retrograded back through the proximal fragment may be useful in reducing the fracture.

Traumatic injuries frequently cause fracture of both the ulna and radius. For minimally displaced mid-shaft fractures, bandaging or external coaptation (figure-of-eight to immobilize the elbow and carpus) may be adequate. However, given the resulting decrease in range of motion of the elbow and carpal joints, it is preferable to repair these fractures with external fixators.

The dorsal approach to the radius and ulna is preferred. An incision is made on the dorsocranial aspect of the ulna just cranial to the insertion point of the secondary feathers. In some cases in which both bones are broken, repair of the ulna alone is sufficient. However, with severely displaced fractures, the surgeon may need to stabilize the radius to allow proper healing. The same incision may be useful for stabilizing both bones depending on the location of the radial fracture. The intraosseous space between the radius and ulna houses the radial nerve and the radial artery, both of which should be avoided. The ulna can be easily identified and exteriorized for debridement and repair through the dorsal incision. If intramedullary pins are used, they are introduced through the fracture site and retrograded out the olecranon (avoiding the elbow) and then normograded into the distal fragment.

To approach the radius separately, an incision is made over the dorsal aspect of the radius between the extensor metacarpi radialis muscle anteriorly and the extensor digitorum communicans over the intraosseous space. IM pins placed in the radius can be retrograded out through the distal radius and then normograded back into the proximal fragment.

The Humerus

A dorsal approach is recommended for most fractures of the humerus. However, the surgeon must cautiously incise dorsally over the midsection of the humerus to avoid the radial nerve. Once the incision is made through the skin, the radial nerve should be immediately identified and retracted. The humerus is exposed immediately beneath the skin. Proximally, the muscles of the biceps and deltoids will overlie the humerus.

A variety of methods may be used to repair fractures of the humerus. The choice of fixation technique is based on the nature of the fracture, the type of patient and the surgeon's experience. External fixators in combination with shuttle pins or intramedullary pins are preferred for free-ranging birds. Type II external fixators should be carefully applied to prevent pins and connecting bars from inducing soft tissue trauma medially on the trunk of the animal. Threaded pins in a Type I or biplanar Type I external fixator will reduce the chances of fixation-induced injuries to the animal. Stabilizing splints and bandages must immobilize the shoulder joint as well as the elbow and, therefore, must be wrapped around the body of the bird. Some birds may be highly intolerant of this type of bandaging.

The Coracoid

Minimally displaced fractures may be stabilized successfully by bandaging the wing to the body. Surgical correction is necessary if the fracture is markedly displaced. A skin incision is made along the caudal edge of the furcula starting laterally and then continuing medially along the lateral edge of the keel for the first one-fifth or one-sixth of the length of the keel bone.

The superficial pectoral muscle is encountered, and an incision is made through the superficial pectoral muscle along the caudal edge of the furcula. This muscle can then be elevated from the keel bone medially. Radiosurgery is necessary to control hemorrhage from the clavicular artery, which supplies part of the pectoral muscle. This vessel is usually encountered at the caudal midpoint of the furcula. An incision or blunt dissection is used to penetrate the deep pectoral muscle. The coracoid is located immediately beneath the deep pectoral muscle and runs from the point of the shoulder at approximately a 45° angle to the cranial aspect of the sternum. Trauma associated with a fractured coracoid can be significant, resulting in massive soft tissue damage and hematoma formation. Because of the location of the coracoid, the surgeon works in a small, deep hole, and radiosurgery as well as irrigation are mandatory to keep the surgical field clean.

The proximal fragment of the coracoid should be grasped and rotated into the incision. Following cleaning and debridement, multiple small intramedullary pins are introduced at the fracture site and exteriorized through the point of the shoulder. The distal fragment is rotated up into view and cleaned, and the fracture is aligned. Intramedullary pins must be carefully normograded back into the distal fragment. If the pins are advanced too far caudally and penetrate the sternum, the pins may perforate the pericardium and the heart. This problem can be prevented by carefully measuring the length of the distal fragment and using this distance to advance the pins. Muscle bellies are reapposed using a simple continuous pattern and absorbable suture material. The superficial pectoral muscle may also be secured to the furcula. The wing should be wrapped to the body for five to ten days following surgery.

The Leg

The Tarsometatarsus

A lateral dorsal or medial dorsal approach may be used. A straight dorsal approach is generally not used because of the scutes overlying this area and the extensor tendons beneath. The surgeon should be aware of the concave nature of the caudal aspect of the tarsometatarsus (Figure 42.25). A groove, which houses the flexor tendons of the foot as well as the dorsal metatarsal artery, runs dorsomedially along with the vein and should be avoided when approaching the tarsometatarsus.

Any number of fixation methods may be utilized for fractures in this area. However, external fixators are ideally suited, and Type II configurations are easy to apply and provide excellent stability. If IM pins must be used, they are generally introduced through the

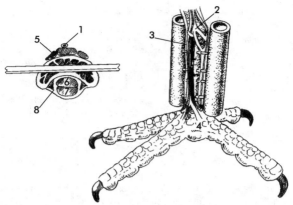

FIG 42.25 Type II external fixators are ideal for repairing tarsometatarsal fractures. The clinician should be aware of the concave nature of the tarsometatarsal bone. 1) dorsal metatarsal artery 2) M. fibularis longus 3) M. extensor digitorum longus 4) M. extensor brevis digiti IV 5) M. extensor hallicus longus 6,7) M. flexor digiti II, III, IV and 8) M. gastrocnemius.

fracture and exteriorized in a retrograde fashion laterally or medially to the joint, then normograded back into the distal fragment.

The Tibiotarsus

A skin incision over the craniomedial aspect of the tibiotarsus provides access to the distal two-thirds of the underlying bone. The medial belly of the gastrocnemius muscle may have to be retracted from the cranial tibial muscle and fibularis longus craniolaterally to achieve access to some fractures. The cranial tibial artery, which runs over the mid to distal tibiotarsus in a craniolateral position, should be avoided when making this approach.

External fixators are ideally suited and easy to apply in this area. IM pins may be introduced from the tibial crest and normograded down through the proximal and then into the distal fragments. This positioning prevents the pin from penetrating the stifle. External fixation can be used to repair metaphyseal fractures by placing stabilizing pins on both sides of the affected joint.

The Femur

The lateral approach to the femur is initiated by making a craniolateral skin incision. The cranial and caudal bellies of the iliotibialis muscle are separated using blunt and sharp dissection. The iliofibularis muscle is located caudally. With this approach, the femorotibialis medialis muscle will be located craniolateral and ventral to the pubo-ischio-femoralis muscle which will be located caudally. Distally, a branch of the lateral genicular artery may require attention when working around the epicondyles and condyles.

The femur is generally easy to approach except in those species that have a well developed femorotibialis medialis muscle that originates on the lateral aspect of the femur (eg, Anseriformes). In these species, the muscle is transected and elevated cranially and caudally to expose the femur.

A variety of fixation methods may be used for femoral fractures. Plates provide excellent stabilization especially in closed fractures. Type I or biplanar external fixators may be used alone or in combination with intramedullary pins. IM pins are passed through the fracture site and retrograded out through the greater trochanter laterally and then normograded back through the distal fragments. Shuttle pins are also ideally suited for this area.

Dome Osteotomy

Dome osteotomies have been successfully used to correct angular limb deformities in Psittaciformes, Falconiformes and Strigiformes, and offer several advantages over other osteotomy techniques.

The procedure is planned from a tracing of a radiograph of the affected limb. The radiographic view that indicates the most severe angular deformity should be used for planning the procedure. Lines are drawn sagittally through the center of the distal and proximal ends of the bone. The point where the two lines intersect is the location for the dome osteotomy. The osteotomy is performed by using a drill to make a series of small holes in a half-circle fashion at the osteotomy site. The holes are then connected using high-speed air drill and a side cutting bit. The distal bone segment can then be rotated freely in the proximal segment to allow proper bone alignment. Appropriate fixation, generally an external fixator, then used to stabilize the fracture during healing. Radiographic findings in birds suggest that when properly applied, a dome osteotomy site will undergo primary bone healing with minimal to no callus formation.

Repair of Luxations

Femoral head luxations are generally craniodorsal to the acetabulum. Open reduction may be successful in repairing acute cases. A femoral head osteotomy has been recommended for repair of chronic luxations of the hip. Coxofemoral luxations may be approached laterally or medially for stabilization. Spica-type splints are recommended, as well as supporting sutures, which are placed from the greater trochanter to the ilium and to the ischium. These sutures, usually of nonabsorbable materials, support the reduced hip in its normal location and are recommended in those avian species with a gliding hinge-type coxofemoral joint (noncursorial species such as most psittacine birds and raptors). It is important to remember that some cursorial species of birds (eg, ratites), have a ball and socket-type coxofemoral joint and these sutures would not be appropriate.

Elbow luxations in raptors usually result in a straight caudal or dorsocaudal displacement of the ulna. If treated early, closed reduction of these luxations can be made and then supported with external fixators or bandages. In one report, five of nine raptors with elbow luxations were successfully returned to the wild following closed reduction and support with external fixators or bandages for seven to ten days.

Luxations of the shoulder have also been reported in raptors. These are usually accompanied by an avulsion fracture of the ventral tubercle of the proximal humerus. These can be stabilized by application of a figure-of-eight bandage to immobilize the wing to the body for 10-14 days. A surgical approach may be warranted to reduce and reattach the ventral tubercle with wires or lag screws. It is important to note that luxations do not necessarily suggest a hopeless prognosis for return to complete function, particularly if addressed soon after the injury occurs.

The collateral ligaments of the knee may be damaged following many traumatic events. A positive drawer sign is characteristic. Techniques used to repair collateral ligament damage in mammals can also be used for birds.

Repair of the Beak

Initially, therapy for any beak injury should be provided to control hemorrhage, maintain nutritional support and prevent secondary infection. Birds with beak injuries that result in defects can also readily adapt to soft diets. Prosthetic beak devices require continuous replacement as the beak grows, and must be carefully monitored to prevent bacterial or fungal infections.

Fractures

Mandibular fractures are the most common injury and should be addressed in two stages: repair of the bone, and repair and re-alignment of the keratinized beak. Fractures through the beak will not heal side-to-side. Forces encountered by the beak must be neutralized or they will be transferred to the underlying bone and interfere with healing.

Depending upon patient size and the location of the fracture, pins, wires, cements, screws and plates may be useful in repairing mandibular fractures. For most smaller birds, hypodermic needles and cerclage wires are useful. The primary goals are re-alignment and stabilization of the fracture site. Pins and hypodermic needles may be inserted into the body of the mandible, antegraded across the fracture site from the rostral point of the beak, and stabilized with cerclage wires (plus or minus cements).

Once the fracture is repaired, soft tissue injuries must be treated. If the injury is of a degloving type, every attempt should be made to reappose the displaced skin. Tissue glues are useful for facilitating this repair. If glues are not applicable, the fracture site should be dressed with a self-adherent wet/dry type dressing.

Fractures of the upper beak are generally more difficult to manage due to the presence of small bones and the kinetic nature of the maxilla. These fractures frequently involve the quadrate and jugal bones, which are thin structures that are difficult to immobilize. The use of small hypodermic needles is usually necessary to facilitate repair, but their effectiveness is limited. Healed fractures often result in beak abnormalities such as lateral deviation of the maxillary beak.

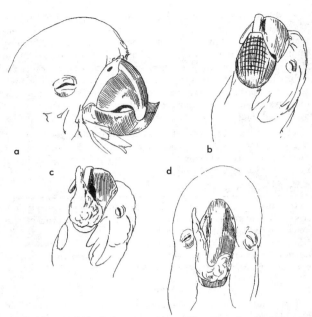

FIG 42.34 a) Scissors beak can be corrected by using pins placed through the frontal bone or by using a prosthetic device attached to the gnathotheca. **b)** The gnathotheca is scarified with a dental burr and cleaned and covered with a light coat of dental acrylic. **c)** Nylon dental mesh is covered with dental acrylic to create a ramp that pushes the tip of the beak into proper alignment. **d)** The prosthesis after being shaped with a Dremel tool.

Beak Deformities

Two common defects in psittacine neonates are scissors beak (lateral deviation of the upper beak) and mandibular prognathism. The etiology of these problems is only speculative. If mandibular prognathism is recognized early, it can be corrected by applying gentle outward pressure to the beak for ten minutes, six to eight times daily. The same technique can be used to correct some early cases of scissors beak. If cases are allowed to progress, they must be corrected using various beak prostheses or surgical techniques to redirect the forces applied to the beak and its underlying bones.

Scissors Beak

Correction procedures are designed to change the forces that direct the anterior growth of the rhinotheca (Figure 42.34). Redirected growth is achieved by applying a prosthesis to the lower beak on the affected side or by placing pins in the calvarium and using rubber bands to apply pressure to the tip of the beak (similar to orthodontic techniques used in humans).

Scissors beak is easiest to repair in a young bird because the bones and beak are actively remodeling. The prosthetic device must be sufficiently anchored to the lower beak to prevent normal beak occlusion from dislocating the prosthesis. The keratin of the gnathotheca on the affected side is grooved with a Dremel tool.

The grooves should be deep enough to increase the surface area for prosthetic attachment but should not be so deep as to induce hemorrhage.

The scored gnathotheca is cleaned and disinfected, and a light coat of cyanomethacrylate is applied to the area and allowed to dry. Stainless steel or nylon dental screen mesh is molded to the gnathotheca. The mesh should be extended to create a ramp that redirects the beak tip to the midline with each bite. The ramp is covered with cyanoacrylate and smoothed with a Dremel tool. When the defect is corrected, the implant is removed.

Bragnathism

Bragnathism can be repaired by placing a KE wire into the frontal bone just caudal to the maxilla joint and caudal to the nares. A caudally directed hook is bent into the external portion of the pin. A second pin is placed in the maxilla midway down the beak at the point at which the internal rotation of the maxilla is most severe. Acrylic is applied to the area, incorporating the pins to supply extra support. A rubber band placed between the two pins will pull the beak tip into proper apposition. When the rhinotheca is properly positioned on the outer surface of the gnathotheca, the rubber band can be removed. The pins can remain in place for several more days until it is apparent that the bragnathism will not recur. When it is apparent that the problem is permanently corrected, the acrylic and pins can be removed.

PASSERIFORMES

Patricia Macwhirter

Passeriformes (perching and songbirds) is the largest order of birds. It contains nearly 60% of all bird species ranging in size from the tiny Weebill (80 mm in length) to the Superb Lyrebird (130 cm long, including a 72 cm tail). Canaries, finches, starlings and mynahs are examples of passerine birds that are common in captivity. Passerines are widely distributed throughout the world, and all passerines share a common anisodactyl foot structure with three unwebbed toes pointed cranially and one caudally. The altricial young are usually naked when hatched and are reared in a nest.

Anatomy and Physiology

Digestive System

The basal metabolic rate (BMR) of passerine birds is generally about 65% greater than that of non-passerines, and their body temperature is about two degrees Centigrade higher (around 42°C). While some desert passerines such as the Zebra Finch have been known to survive months without drinking water, most small passerine birds drink from 250-300 ml/kg body weight of water each day and may eat up to 30% of their body weight daily. These figures are higher than those for most non-passerines, which tend to be larger birds.

Most passerine species have a narrow, triangular tongue compared with the thick blunt tongue of parrots. The tongue is rarely involved in clinical problems. The tongue of passerines may become hyperkeratotic at the tip and extend rostrally through the beak. The syndrome appears to cause few clinical problems, but the hyperkeratotic tissue can be slowly trimmed back with a pair of strabismus scissors, taking care not to cut healthy mucosa. A ventriculus is present in granivorous and insectivorous species such as finches, but not in species such as honeyeaters that consume nectar and soft foods. If present, cecae are generally small and vestigial.

Some finches will regurgitate crop contents to feed their young. Pathogens can be transmitted from parent to offspring during this process, particularly with foster-raised chicks that probably did not receive yolk-derived antibodies against microorganisms from their foster parents' digestive system. For example, although *Cochlosoma* sp. may cause inapparent infections in adult Bengalese (Society) Finches, significant mortality may occur in juvenile Gouldian Finches being fostered by Bengalese parents.

The spleen in most passerines is oblong, not spherical, as it is in Psittaciformes.

Respiratory System

In non-insectivorous Passeriformes, unlike in Psittaciformes, the right and left nasal sinuses do not communicate. In these passerine birds, separate samples for rhinal disease (bacterial, viral, chlamydial) cytology examination should be taken from each sinus if a bilateral nasal discharge occurs.

Like psittacine birds but unlike ratites and penguins, passerine birds have a highly developed neopulmonic and paleopulmonic parabronchi. This allows for highly efficient oxygen exchange. In most passerines, the cranial thoracic air sacs are fused to the single median clavicular sac, making a total of seven air sacs as opposed to the nine air sacs of psittacine species.

Reproductive System

In general, only the left ovary and oviduct develop in normal female passerines. Both testicles develop in males and during the breeding season these may reach enormous proportions in relation to the size of the bird. These physiologically enlarged testicles should not be mistaken for pathologic conditions.

Role of Light in Reproduction

Stimulation of the reproductive cycle is best accomplished by a progressive increase (four-week period) of exposure to light. In general, the maximum effect of increasing day length will occur when a passerine individual is exposed to 10-14 hours of light. In males, the release of testosterone may occur in less than 24 hours following exposure to appropriately increased daylight hours. This in turn can result in rapid development of secondary sexual characteristics and breeding display (territorial calling, testicular and cloacal enlargement, courtship behavior).

Response of females to increased photoperiod is less dramatic, and it may require the presence of a male in breeding condition to trigger appropriate nesting and egg laying responses. By gradually increasing the light exposure, a more natural reproductive cycling occurs, and a male is less likely to brutalize a slowly responsive hen. This also accounts for the common aviculture practice of separating males and females during the nonbreeding season.

Many aviculturists use a "breeder" cage with a removable partition that allows the male to feed the female through an opening. At various intervals, the partition separating the two sexes is removed, and if the female "accepts" the male, they are left together. The nest is put in the male's side of the cage along with a source of nest material, which he collects in the nest as part of the courtship activity. An experienced canary breeder can remove the partition at precisely the right time for the female to accept the male.

After a period of long daylight hours, birds become refractory to photostimulation, and plasma concentrations of both LH and FSH begin to fall. Following the molt and period of decreasing daylight hours (fall), the breeding season starts again with the increasing daylight hours in the late winter and early spring.

Testosterone-induced Singing

Male canaries will usually sing best in the spring in response to the endogenous testosterone "surge." If a bird becomes ill, it may stop singing and may not recommence vocalizations until the following spring, even though the initial illness has resolved. In contrast, some canaries (even some females) sing year round and birds that stop singing because of illness recommence singing as soon as their general condition improves. Injectable testosterone has been suggested as a method of inducing singing in birds that have stopped after a period of illness. This is a practice that should be discouraged because the testosterone has a negative feedback that causes shrinking of the testes and reduced fertility.

Avicultural Considerations

Housing

Aviaries for Passeriformes should provide adequate protection from the elements, with tropical species requiring the greatest degree of protection. In mild climates, hardy species of Passeriformes do well in carefully planned, planted aviaries that provide adequate protection as well as visually attractive surroundings. Indoor, temperature-controlled rooms may be necessary to raise finches in harsher climates or when artificial lighting control is necessary to increase production.

Some passerine birds require special materials for nesting or to stimulate display behavior. Care must be taken that the type of objects provided for these birds are safe. Any contact with fine synthetic fibers should be avoided because these may become entangled around the birds' feet, toes or other body areas and cause damage, loss of limb or death. Burlap (hessian) cut into small squares, torn strips of facial tissue or coconut fiber make suitable, safe nesting materials.

Disease Control

Disease control in planted aviaries can be challenging because of the difficulties involved in controlling microorganisms and in medicating individual birds. Because it is difficult to eliminate infectious agents once they are introduced into a planted aviary, it is critical that any new birds be quarantined, tested and treated for parasites and infectious diseases prior to introduction.

Free-ranging birds should be excluded from aviaries to prevent the transmission of microorganisms. Sparrows, for example, may transmit poxvirus, *Plasmodium*, feather lice, mites and *Haemoproteus* to canaries.

Nutrition

Passeriformes may be granivorous, nectivorous, fructivorous, insectivorous, omnivorous or carnivorous. Some species adapt readily to commercially available diets, while others may require live food and are thus difficult to maintain in captivity. Some free-ranging species have specific dietary preferences (Gouldian Finches prefer sorghum) but may adapt to diets provided in captivity. Even finches that are considered omnivorous or carnivorous can be successfully raised on properly balanced vegetable-based diets.

Finches may consume up to 30% of their body weight daily in food compared with 10% for larger parrots. If dietary supplementation is based on a percentage of particular ingredients in the diet, finches may be consuming greater amounts on a per gram body weight basis than larger species. Overdosage of vitamins and minerals may occur, resulting in infertility, renal calcification, gout and general poor condition; thus, only diets specifically formulated for finches should be used.

Feather color is dietary-dependent in species with carotenoid pigmentation. Red factor and new color canaries have genotypes that require exogenous sources of carotenoids or related compounds to enable full development of yellow, orange and red pigments in feathers. Foods for these birds contain carotenoids and xanthophylls to enable proper color development. Reduced or absent carotenoids during feather formation produces pale or whitish feathers while excess carotenoids will cause a deepening of yellow and red pigments. Commercial diets that contain algae (spirulina) should have sufficient levels of naturally occurring carotenoids to maintain proper feather coloration. In the United States, "colored" foods generally contain carotene-soaked stale bakery products and should be avoided in favor of more natural sources of carotenoids.

Vitamin A lacks color even though it is related to carotenoid pigments.

Seasonal Feeding Practices

Most successful breeders of these species mimic natural conditions by lowering the caloric, protein and fat content of diets and maximizing the birds' physical condition by allowing free flight in open aviaries during the nonbreeding season. At the beginning of the breeding season, the birds are "flushed," or encouraged to come into a breeding condition by increasing the plane of nutrition. Misting some species with water (to mimic rainfall) and providing green, fresh foods and foliage may stimulate breeding, particularly those species from desert environments such as the Australian grass finches.

Sexing Passerines

In some passerines, there are obvious or subtle morphologic differences between the genders. Males are generally brightly colored or elaborately marked, particularly during the breeding season. Differences in singing, courtship or nesting behavior may also provide clues as to gender.

In males of many species, the caudal end of the ductus deferens forms a mass of convolutions called the seminal glomerulus.

During the culmination phase of the breeding cycle, the seminal glomerula pushes the cloacal wall into a prominent projection, the cloacal promontory. This can be observed by blowing the feathers on the bird's vent cranially.

Laparoscopy can be used to determine gender in monomorphic passerine birds, but the small size of many species may increase the risk of this procedure. Newer methods of gender determination using DNA technology are proving useful and will probably be used more extensively in the future.

Combating Aggression

While passerine species may be small, some are quite territorial and others have well developed pecking orders.

Appropriate measures to prevent combat aggression will vary depending on individual circumstances. Suggestive control measures include:

- prevent overcrowding; the fewer birds, the better
- keep stocking densities low
- clip the wings or remove particularly aggressive individuals
- provide extra vegetation or visual barriers (burlap sheets) to provide less dominant birds with an escape area
- provide multiple perches, feeding locations and nesting sites
- maintain subdued lighting in indoor areas
- simultaneously introduce all birds into a new environment.

Parents that become aggressive toward their chicks are preparing to lay a second clutch of eggs and the chicks should be removed.

Sick or injured birds should be housed separately from other birds to prevent them from being injured by their healthier companions.

Parrots from the genera *Neophema* (Bourke's or Scarlet-chested Parrots) or *Polytelis* (Princess Parrots) are usually sedate and will mix well with finches. In contrast, rosellas (except for the Western Rosella) or *Psephotus* parrots (Hooded or Blue Bonnet Parrots) are usually aggressive and will kill other birds that are in their space.

Cross-fostering Techniques

Species with long histories of domestication, such as Bengalese (Society) Finches, will usually breed freely in captivity without the use of specialized techniques. Members of this species are sometimes used as foster parents to incubate and raise other finches. Similarly, Border Canaries may be used as foster parents for other canary varieties.

One of the inherent problems in cross-fostering is that it does not enable selection for good parenting ability in the offspring. Some organisms such as *Campylobacter* spp. and *Cochlosoma* spp. may cause inapparent infections in foster parent birds but be transmitted to cross-fostered juveniles where disease may result. By comparison, using foster parents may prevent some infectious diseases that are transmitted from infected parent to offspring. For example, colonies of Gouldian Finches that are air sac mite-free have been established by using Society Finches, which are not susceptible to air sac mites, as foster parents.

Imprinting

One of the major disadvantages of fostered birds is that they imprint on the foster parents and may be less likely to breed with their own species. For species-specific imprinting to occur, a finch should be exposed to its own species from the 15th to 40th days of life.

Breeding Parasitic Species of Passerines

Some finch enthusiasts relish the challenge of breeding parasitic species (birds that lay their eggs in the nests of other species) such as Paradise Whydahs (parasitize various species of the *Pytilia* family) and Broad-tailed Whydahs (parasitize Aurora Finches). Whydahs are generally bred in large planted aviaries where the parasitized finch species has first been firmly established and is breeding freely.

Special Considerations in Managing Passerine Patients

Difficulties in collecting samples from small birds may limit diagnostic and treatment options. Veterinary care in these species is frequently directed toward appropriate preventive husbandry measures and approaching medical problems from a flock perspective.

Restraint and Handling

A "lights out/perches out" approach to capture is often useful for small active birds. Birds will generally not move in a dark room and can easily be removed from an enclosure with minimal stress. Once out of the enclosure, the bird can be restrained by placing the head between two fingers so that the body rests in the palm of the hand, or it can be restrained by holding the head gently between the thumb and first finger.

Blood Collection Techniques

The right jugular vein is generally the best site for collecting blood or giving intravenous fluids.

The lymphocyte is the predominant white cell in most passerine species, and lymphocytes rather than heterophils tend to increase in stress-related conditions.

Treatment Techniques

Therapeutics

Although the right jugular vein can be used for administering intravenous fluids, intraosseous catheterization using a 26 ga needle is a practical means of fluid administration in a finch.

Hemorrhage may be a problem following intramuscular injections into the pectoral muscles in small birds. To minimize risk, the injection site should be located in the caudal third of the chest muscles, and a fine gauge needle should be used (25 ga or less).

Drug dosing in small patients must be based on an exact weight (as determined by a gram scale) and should be delivered with precise microliter or insulin syringes to avoid overdose. There is little room for a dosing error in a small bird.

Fiber Removal

It is common to see canaries and finches with fine fibers (cotton or synthetics) wrapped around their feet or legs.

If numerous fibers are present, it is best to cut through all the fibers down to the skin, keeping the incision parallel to the long axis of the leg or digit. The incision should be made on the lateral side of the appendage or wherever the fibers are least imbedded. Pulling on deeply imbedded fibers can cause them to further constrict vascular structures. Once all the fibers have been severed, they may be removed with reduced risk of iatrogenic damage.

Splinting

In small birds, lower limb fractures can often be repaired with a sandwich adhesive or masking tape splint. The limb should be positioned in moderate flexion to enable the bird to move and to prevent bending that may occur if the leg is splinted straight. Several layers of tape may be needed. This type of splint is also used to provide support to weakened or damaged bones following the removal of tight leg bands.

Diseases

Mutations and Genetic Diseases

Feather Cysts (Hypopteronosis Cystica)

Heavily feathered canaries, particularly those with "double buff" soft feathers, may develop feather cysts. The condition is believed to be hereditary but the mode of inheritance is not simple. The possibility of a vertically transmitted virus infection causing folliculitis with secondary cyst formation has been suggested.

Some canary breeders believe that iodine given at 0.1-50 ml drinking water will hasten the maturation of feather cysts and allow some to desiccate and slough naturally. Controlled trials to verify this mode of therapy have not been performed, and some feather cysts will heal without treatment. Once mature, the material can be expressed from small cysts but the problem will recur with the subsequent molt.

Surgical options for feather cysts include excision of individual cysts, removal of complete feather tracts or lancing and curetting individual cysts.

The author's preference for treating feather cysts is to place hemostats at the base of the cyst and remove all tissue to the base of the hemostats with a radiosurgical unit. With this technique, the contents of the cyst are removed along with the skin that forms the wall of the cyst but the cyst is not totally excised. The hemostats are removed, and any remaining keratinous material is curetted from the base of the cyst. The small remaining part of the interior lining is cauterized with the radiosurgical unit.

Birds with feather cysts should not be used for breeding. Unfortunately, cysts may not develop in a bird until after it is reproductively active.

Crested Canaries

The desirable crested phenotype is heterozygous for the autosomal crested gene. Birds that are homozygous for the crested gene die. Crested canaries are produced by breeding crested birds (coronas) with non-crested (consorts or crest-bred) canaries. This mating will result in 50% crested birds (Cc) and 50% non-crested birds (CC). If crested birds are mated to crested birds, normal Mendelian genetics will result in 25% non-crested, 50% crested and 25% dead chicks.

Dominant White Lethal Factor

Two dominant white birds should not be mated.

Straw Feathers

Canaries and Zebra Finches occasionally show retention of the feather sheath and incomplete development of the barbs and barbules. The disease may affect first-molt fledglings or adult birds in a symmetrical fashion; it is believed to be genetically determined.

Cataracts

Cataracts are occasionally seen in canaries, particularly in Norwich and Yorkshires. Affected birds will often be found on the bottom of the cage or aviary, possibly avoiding flight after a previously misjudged landing. Histologically, there may be disorganization of lens cortex, fragmentation of fibers, globule formation and lens resorption. Cataracts are reported to be caused by a recessive gene in Yorkshire and Norwich canaries. They may be removed surgically.

Viral Diseases

Poxvirus

Clinical Presentation: Canaries and House Sparrows are particularly susceptible and may show the cutaneous, septicemic or diphtheroid forms of the disease. The cutaneous form of poxvirus has also been reported in a variety of free-ranging Passeriformes, eg, starlings, juncos, silvereyes and Australian magpies.

Mortalities of up to 100% have occurred in some outbreaks of canary pox. Acutely affected birds may show lethargy, ruffled feathers, open-mouthed breathing and death in two to three days. In less acute cases, birds may show conjunctivitis, blepharitis and lacrimation before the appearance of characteristic proliferative lesions around the eyes and mouth. Death may result if these lesions cause pharyngeal obstruction. The skin lesions should be differentiated from mosquito bite abscesses, which result in discrete lumps that contain caseous material when lanced. An uncomplicated pox lesion is a contained fibrous reaction without a necrotic, expressible center.

While birds affected with poxvirus will typically show intracytoplasmic Bollinger bodies, intranuclear inclusions have been demonstrated in the junco.

Treatment and Control: There is no specific treatment for poxvirus. Antibiotics may be useful to control secondary infections, and vitamin A or its natural precursor may aid in the healing process. Scarifying individual pox lesions may result in spontaneous remission. Topical application of astringent solutions such as mercurochrome or alcohol may be useful. Adenine arabinoside ointment a has also been recommended. Mild baby shampoo may be gently applied to any lesions around the eyes to remove scabs. Immune stimulants such as PEP-E and echinacea may be of possible value.

Avian poxviruses can be transmitted by mosquitoes, mites or by contact through damaged epithelial surfaces. Bird rooms should be mosquito-proofed and treated with insecticides to eliminate vectors, and affected birds should be isolated until fully recovered. Recovered birds generally have lasting immunity to the disease but may become carriers and shed the virus. A modified live virus canary pox vaccine is available in some countries.

Herpesvirus

Herpesviruses have been isolated from Estrildid finches, Ploceid finches (weavers and whydahs) and canaries, but in most cases they have not been associated with disease.

Cytomegalovirus

An epidemic of conjunctivitis with respiratory distress and a 70% mortality rate was reported in Australian grass finches maintained in Europe.

Polyomavirus

Polyomavirus-like infections have been associated with several clinical presentations in passerine birds. Sporadic deaths have occurred in adult finches of various species, particularly in birds that have been stressed by transport or other factors.

In color mutation Gouldian Finches, polyomavirus-like infections have been reported to cause acute mortality in two- to three-day-old babies, and poor growth, dirty feathering and late fledging in older nestlings. Many affected birds had an abnormal lower mandible that was long and tubular.

In a separate report, deaths in fledgling and immature Gouldian Finches occurred without any concurrent feathering or beak defects. The most consistent gross lesion was a swollen, pale liver. Currently there is no effective treatment for polyomavirus. Controversy exists as to whether it is best to depopulate, rest breeding stock or to continue to breed with the expectation that birds will develop immunity (see Chapter 32). Diagnosis is based on the histologic presence of large, clear-to-amphophilic, intranuclear inclusion bodies in one or more organs.

Papillomavirus

Avian papillomavirus has been demonstrated in association with papillomas on the legs of wild European chaffinches. Viral papillomatosis has also been described in canaries from Argentina.

Paramyxovirus

Group 1 (Newcastle Disease Virus): Many weaver finches are susceptible and show conjunctivitis, pseudomembrane formation in the larynx and death. Neurologic signs are rare. Canaries rarely develop clinical signs, and infected birds should be considered asymptomatic carriers.

Group 2: Free-ranging passerines, particularly weaver finches in North Africa, are considered to be carriers of this virus. Many infected birds are asymptomatic but others may die following a period of emaciation and pneumonia.

Group 3: This virus has been isolated from a variety of passerines including canaries, Gouldian Finches and weaver finches. It is generally associated with an overall poor condition and central nervous system signs (tremor, paralysis or torticollis).

Leukosis

Sporadic deaths associated with enlarged pale livers and spleens and histopathologic lesions suggestive of leukosis have been reported in canaries in Europe, Australia and North America. A viral etiology has been proposed but has not been confirmed. Treatment with prednisolone may slow the progression of the disease.

Chlamydia Infections

Passeriformes are less susceptible to chlamydiosis than Psittaciformes. Chlamydiosis should be suspected in passerines with recurrent respiratory disease especially if they are exposed to psittacine birds.

Mycoplasma

Mycoplasma spp. have been isolated from canaries with wheezing, respiratory signs including tail-bobbing and conjunctivitis. Many cases of conjunctivitis and upper respiratory disease in canaries are responsive to tylosin. However, there has been no conclusive experimental work proving that mycoplasma is associated with this syndrome.

Tetracyclines are believed to be effective against many mycoplasma isolates as well as chlamydia. A therapeutic trial with tetracyclines may be appropriate if they are suspected of being part of a disease complex.

Bacterial Infections

Some investigators believe that bacteria and other microorganisms should seldom be found in stained fecal smears from normal canaries and finches. Others believe that low levels of gram-positive rods or cocci are considered normal. There is generally no bacterial growth on routine aerobic microbiological cultures taken from passerine birds.

If a decision is made to use water-based medication, frequently used drugs include trimethoprim and sulfamethoxale, amoxicillin, chloramphenicol, tetracyclines and enrofloxacin. Some passerines are particularly sensitive to certain antimicrobial agents (dimetridazole, furacin) and care should be exercised when administering any medication to a finch or canary (see Chapter 18).

Gram-positive Flora

Staphylococcus spp. are normal inhabitants of the gastrointestinal tract and the skin but occasionally virulent strains may cause disease in susceptible hosts (see Chapter 33). Staphylococcal infections are commonly associated with the occurrence of thrombi in arterioles. Digit necrosis, gangrenous dermatitis and pododermatitis are likely outcomes. Other clinical syndromes that have been associated with staphylococcus infections in passerines include high embryonic mortality, omphalitis, septicemia and arthritis.

Streptococcal infections have also been associated with embryonic mortality, omphalitis, septicemia and arthritis in passerines.

Enterococcus fecalis (formerly *Streptococcus fecalis*) has been associated with chronic tracheitis, pneumonia and air sac infections in canaries. These changes are similar to those caused by the tracheal mite *Sternostoma tracheacolum*. Concurrent infections are possible.

Mycobacterium avium: Passerines are susceptible to *Mycobacterium avium* and may show nonspecific signs similar to those seen in other avian species: chronic wasting, diarrhea, polyuria, anemia, dull plumage and leukocytosis.

Red-hooded Siskins may be particularly susceptible to tuberculosis. Treatment of companion birds for *Mycobacterium* spp. is not recommended because of the public health concerns.

Listeria monocytogenes is a ubiquitous organism that may be transmitted by the oral route. Canaries are particularly susceptible to listeriosis and flock outbreaks may occur. Clinical signs include torticollis, tremors, stupor, paresis or paralysis. A marked monocytosis may occur. Tetracyclines may be useful therapy in the early stages of the disease but treatment is usually ineffective in birds with CNS signs.

Megabacterium: A large, rod-shaped, gram-positive bacteria that was difficult to culture and was associated with a proliferative, inflammatory reaction in the proventriculus of canaries was described in Europe.

Enterobacteriaceae and Other Gram-negative Bacteria

Enterobacteriaceae are generally considered secondary pathogens. Oral neomycin or spectinomycin may be useful for infections localized to the gastrointestinal tract.

Escherichia coli has been associated with a variety of disease problems in passerine birds including diarrhea, septicemia and ascending oviduct infections.

Salmonella typhimurium var copenhagen is commonly isolated from finches in Europe that develop a characteristic granulomatous ingluvitis, which can be confused with crop candidiasis or capillariasis. *Salmonella* spp. have also been isolated from cases of osteomyelitis and subcutaneous granulomas in canaries.

***Citrobacter* sp.** is commonly found as a secondary invader in weaver finches and waxbills. It has also been associated with acute septicemia and death.

Yersinia pseudotuberculosis is a common cause of peracute mortality in finch and canary aviaries as well as causing general ill health, diarrhea and dyspnea. Enteritis and pinpoint or large abscesses throughout the liver and spleen are characteristic gross findings. Affected birds are often too sick to respond to therapy but treatment of exposed birds with antibiotics based on sensitivity testing will usually stop an outbreak. Decontaminating the aviary and rodent-proofing food and water supplies should accompany any antibiotic therapy.

***Klebsiella, Pasteurella* and *Haemophilus* spp.** are occasionally isolated from Passeriformes. Pasteurella is often associated with fatal septicemias following cat bite wounds. Even if injuries seem minor, birds that have been bitten or scratched by cats should receive antibiotics immediately.

Campylobacter fetus var. jejuni has been associated with pale, voluminous droppings ("popcorn poohs") in canaries and finches of a variety of species (particularly Gouldian Finches). European investigators have suggested that adding animal protein, minerals and vitamins (soft food) to the diet may strengthen the bird's immune system and protect against repeated infections. Antibiotics (particularly erythromycin and tetracyclines) may also be useful.

***Pseudomonas* sp.** infections may originate from the consumption of contaminated drinking water, misting bottles or inappropriately prepared soaked seed. The organism may cause foul-smelling diarrhea or mucopurulent pneumonia and air sacculitis. Treatment should be based on sensitivity testing, as the bacteria is often resistant to routinely used antibiotics. Steps should be taken to identify and remove environmental sources of contamination.

Fungal Infections

Candida albicans

Identifying candida in fecal swabs from passerines should be evaluated with caution. Many passerine species are fed bread products that are made with yeast.

Candida albicans is occasionally associated with upper gastrointestinal tract infections in passerines, particularly in immunosuppressed or hand-fed neonates. Vomiting, anorexia, weight loss and diarrhea are characteristic findings. The lining of the crop may be thickened and covered with whitish "turkish towel" coating. Yeast blastospores or hyphae may be identified on Gram's stain of material from a crop wash. Systemic candidiasis has also been reported in canaries. Nystatin or ketoconazole may be useful in infections confined to the gastrointestinal tract (see Chapter 15).

Aspergillus spp.

Aspergillosis may cause weight loss, respiratory distress, anorexia, vomiting or diarrhea in infected passerines. Immunosuppression, usually from malnutrition, along with contaminated environmental conditions are primary factors in the development of the disease.

Superficial Mycoses

Dermatomycoses are occasionally reported in passerines and generally cause feather loss (especially of the head and neck) or hyperkeratosis. *Microsporum gallinae* and *Trichophyton* spp. are the most common etiologic agents.

Protozoa

Cochlosoma

Cochlosoma spp. are flagellates that inhabit the gastrointestinal tract of some finches. Bengalese Finches may be inapparent carriers of this organism; when they are used to foster species of Australian finches (such as Gouldians), they may pass the organism on to juveniles, causing high mortality in nestlings. Typical clinical signs include debility, dehydration and passing whole seeds in the droppings. At necropsy the intestine may be filled with a yellow suspension or whole undigested seeds. Most affected birds are six to twelve weeks of age.

The organism may be identified by direct wet preparation of fresh warm droppings or at necropsy using intestinal contents. Cochlosoma has six anterior flagella with a helicoidal, anterior ventral sucker.

Treatment with ronidazole at 400 mg/kg in egg food and 400 mg/liter of drinking water for five days has been suggested. After a two-day rest period, the treatment is repeated. Dimetridazole may also be used at no more than 100 mg of active ingredient per liter of water for five days. Water containers should be disinfected and rinsed clean (the organism is sensitive to most common disinfectants) and the aviary should be kept clean and dry.

Trichomonas

Trichomonas spp. infections are occasionally seen in finches, particularly those housed near infected budgerigars. Clinical symptoms include gagging, neck stretching, regurgitation, respiratory distress, nasal discharge, green diarrhea and emaciation. Diagnosis is made by identifying the flagellate on a wet smear prepared from a crop wash.

Giardia

Giardia sp. has also been reported to be associated occasionally with gastrointestinal tract infections in finches. Treatment is the same as for cochlosomiasis.

Coccidiosis

Coccidia infections in passerine birds may be asymptomatic or associated with diarrheal syndromes (sometimes with blood in the droppings), emaciation, general ill health and systemic disease.

Coccidia in the Eimeriidae family have a single host. Sporulation of oocysts usually takes place outside the host and oocysts of different genera have a characteristic number of sporocysts, each with one or more sporozoites (see Chapter 36).

When examining fresh fecal material, it is often not possible to classify coccidial oocysts because sporulation may take several days to occur (see Chapter 36).

Atoxoplasmatidae are single-host coccidia with merogony in the blood and intestinal cells, gametogeny in the intestinal cells of the same individual and sporulation outside the host. This family contains a single genus, *Atoxoplasma*. The parasite is transmitted directly via oocysts in the feces and is host-specific.

Coccidia in Canaries

Oocysts from *Atoxoplasma* or *Isospora* spp. may be found in the feces of infected canaries. Isospora is less pathogenic and completes its life cycle within the intestines while atoxoplasma develops asexually in mononuclear blood cells and spreads hematogenously to other organs including the liver, spleen and lungs.

Canaries with atoxoplasmosis may be defined as having "black spot," referring to the enlarged, dark liver that is visible beneath the skin. Diarrhea, nonspecific illness and death sometimes occur. The organism can be diagnosed by identifying sporozoites on Giemsa-stained impression smears of the spleen, liver or buffy coat. The sporozoites are found in the cytoplasm of lymphoid-macrophage cells and appear as oval structures containing pink-staining chromatin. Indentation of the host nucleus often occurs (see Chapter 36).

Sulpha drugs or amprolium are usually effective for *Isospora* sp. but *Atoxoplasma* sp. is resistant to treatment. Maintaining clean surroundings to reduce the birds' exposure to the infective oocysts may help control infections, but will probably not eradicate the organism from an aviary.

Eimeria spp. generally follow the same pattern as *Isospora* and complete their life cycle in the intestinal tract.

Sarcocystis

Sarcocysts are common in the skeletal muscles of passerines from many geographic regions. North American cowbirds, grackles and other Passeriformes have been shown to be the intermediate hosts of *Sarcocystis falcatula*, for which opossums are the definitive host. Cysts can sometimes be observed through the skin.

Toxoplasmosis

Toxoplasma gondii is occasionally identified in passerines and in isolated cases may cause death.

Cats and other members of the Felidae family are definitive hosts for *Toxoplasma gondii*, and birds must ingest oocysts from cat droppings or visceral cysts from other animals in order to be infected. Birds infected with toxoplasmosis may be asymptomatic or show neurologic symptoms, ophthalmitis or sudden death.

Cryptosporidiosis

Cryptosporidium sp. has a direct life cycle but oocysts have not been identified in the droppings of clinically affected passerines. The true clinical significance of the organism is not known, as it is often associated with other disease entities.

Blood Parasites

Plasmodium

Plasmodium spp., the cause of avian malaria, are mosquito-borne protozoa of the family Plasmodiide that occur worldwide. Sporogony occurs in the invertebrate host, schizogony occurs in erythrocytes and pigment is formed from the host cell hemoglobin. Each of the avian plasmodia has a limited host range but they do not appear to be particularly host-specific.

Treatment with chloroquine or pyrimethamine was successful in some cases but the birds did not have any lasting immunity.

Avian malaria has been reported to cause deaths in canaries and other species.

Haemoproteus

Like *Plasmodium* sp., *Haemoproteus* spp. are found worldwide and are capable of infecting a variety of birds. Each species appears to have a limited host range but they are not particularly host-specific and generally cause only mild or inapparent clinical symptoms. Diagnosis is based on identification of typical pigment containing gamonts in erythrocytes. For most species of *Haemoproteus* the intermediate hosts are hippoboscid flies, biting midges (*Culicoides* spp.) or tabanids.

Extensive myopathy and myonecrosis may be associated with intramuscular megaloschizonts. These birds show multiple, yellow streaks in pectoral and other muscles, and most are presented thin, weak and unable to fly. Treatment with antimalarial drugs (chloroquine at 250 mg/120 ml drinking water for one to two weeks) may be useful. Orange juice may be added to the drinking water to make the drug more palatable.

Leucocytozoon

Leucocytozoon spp. occur worldwide except for South America (where appropriate simuliid vectors are absent). These parasites may infect either erythrocytes or leukocytes. Parasitized cells are so distorted by the organism that it may be difficult to determine their origin. Pigment is not produced by leucocytozoon and schizonts do not appear in peripheral blood. Megaloschizonts can be found in brain, liver, lung, kidney, intestinal tissue and lymphoid tissue. Most leucocytozoon infections are subclinical.

Trypanosoma

Trypanosomes are found worldwide but their incidence is low and they may only be found during summer months in temperate climates. Vectors are thought to include hippoboscid flies (*Ornithomyia avicularia*), red mites (*Dermanyssus gallinae*), simuliids and mosquitoes. Evidence suggests that the parasites may be transmitted by contamination rather than inoculative routes. Diagnosis is by finding the parasites on stained blood smears.

Trypanosomes have been identified in over 14 passerine families, including Fringillid finches and canaries, swallows, tits and pipits.

Avian Piroplasmosis

Aegyptianella sp. is a rickettsial organism that appears as a small, signet ring-shaped structure in the cytoplasm of infected erythrocytes. Clinical signs of infection may include anemia, fever, lethargy and occasionally jaundice. Treatment with doxycycline or antimalarial drugs may be useful.

Filarial Worms

Most infections have not been associated with any disease and the parasites have been found incidentally in blood smears (microfilaria) or at necropsy (adults).

Internal Parasites

Acanthocephalans

Both adult and intermediate stages of acanthocephalan parasites may be found in free-ranging passerines. Adult worms are generally susceptible to benzimidazole anthelmintics.

Cestodes

Because tapeworms require arthropods as intermediate hosts, they are predominately a problem in softbill and insectivorous finches. They are normally not seen in canaries or exclusively seed-eating birds (such as Gouldian Finches), except in situations where parent birds feed insects to their offspring or the insects are accidentally consumed with the seeds.

Many different tapeworms have been described in passerines but in most cases, infectivity levels are low, and the parasites cause no clinical disease. Emaciation, diarrhea, general debilitation and death may occur in birds that are stressed and are continuously exposed to infected intermediate hosts.

Tapeworms can be avoided by limiting access to intermediate hosts and by using insect-proof screening. Other sources of protein (such as commercially available formulated diets, insectivore mixes, egg food or grated cheese) may replace live invertebrates as food items. However, some birds may not accept these alternative foods and may die or be left susceptible to disease because of poor nutrition. Others will be reluctant to breed without live food or may desert their nestlings.

Effective anthelmintics for passerines include praziquantel and oxfendazole. In cases where it is not appropriate to prevent access to intermediate hosts, a regular deworming program will lower the infection rate.

Trematodes

These parasites have complicated life cycles that typically involve snails as initial intermediate hosts and other invertebrates as secondary intermediate hosts. It is unlikely that appropriate conditions for completion of the life cycle will be found, except possibly in planted aviaries.

Schistosomes are trematodes that live in blood vessels. Gigantobilharzia huronensis is a blood fluke that has been reported in North American goldfinches and cardinals. It has also been experimentally transmitted to canaries.

Nematodes

Ascaridia: Two main types of roundworms affect passerines: *Ascaridia* spp., which have direct life cycles, and *Porrocecum* spp., which have indirect life cycles with invertebrates such as earthworms as the intermediate host. Both types of roundworms may be associated with weight loss, diarrhea, general debility and sometimes neurologic symptoms.

Capillaria: Capillaria spp. are cosmopolitan in their distribution and affect a range of passerine species. The life cycle is direct or may involve earthworms as paratenic hosts.

Birds with low numbers of capillaria may be subclinical. Higher parasite loads may lead to weight loss, diarrhea, general ill health and death. These worms may localize to a variety of sites along the gastrointestinal tract. Ova with typical bipolar plugs may be found by directly swabbing lesions or by fecal flotation.

Capillaria are often more difficult to treat than ascarids. Aviary hygiene and removal of earthworms are important control measures. Levamisole, fenbendazole and oxfendazole may be effective in some cases.

Spiruroid: Acuaria skrjabini has been associated with significant mortalities in Australian aviaries housing both native and imported finches. This ventricular and proventricular worm parasite does not affect psittacine birds. The parasite lives under the koilin lining of the ventriculus, and characteristic embryonated eggs are passed in the feces. The parasite is resistant to treatment with many common anthelmintics, but oxfendazole may be effective.

Eye Nematodes: *Oxyspirura mansoni* has been reported in mynahs, sparrows and other passerines. The parasite is found behind the nictitating membrane or in the conjunctival sac or the nasolacrimal duct. The intermediate host is the cockroach. Worms should be mechanically removed and any inflammation treated symptomatically. Ivermectin is effective.

Respiratory Nematodes: Syngamus trachea (gapeworm) affects a range of passerine species as well as birds from other orders. Earthworms may act as transport hosts. Levamisole, ivermectin and fenbendazole are effective in treating this parasite, but caution should be exercised when treating birds with heavy infections. Tracheal obstruction may occur when the parasites are killed. Mechanical removal of worms and treatment with low doses of anthelmintics over several days is an effective therapeutic plan.

Arthropod Parasites

Respiratory Mites: Respiratory acariasis ("air sac mite infection") caused by *Sternostoma tracheacolum* is a common cause of dyspnea, open-mouthed breathing and wheezing respiration in canaries and Gouldian Finches. "Air sac mites" is a misnomer given that these parasites are frequently found in the trachea, particularly near the syrinx. Occasionally, the mites may be visualized by wetting the feathers of the bird's neck with alcohol and transilluminating the trachea with a bright source of light.

There are several options for treating this mite. Ivermectin may be used orally or topically. A dichlorvos pest strip may be placed (according to manufacturer's directions) near but out of reach of the birds. Birds may also be sprayed with pyrethrin synergized with piperonyl-butoxide insecticide spray.

A nasal rhynonyssid mite *Speleognathus sturni*, which occasionally causes nasal discharge, has been recorded in starlings.

Cytodites nudus is another mite that has been associated with respiratory disease in free-ranging passerines.

External Parasites

Skin and Feather Mites

Scaly Mites: *Knemidokoptes pilae* (and several other less common species) tend to cause hyperkeratotic lesions on the feet in passerines. Hyperkeratosis caused by scaly mite needs to be differentiated from generalized hyperkeratosis of the feet and legs that occurs with malnutrition and age in some canaries and other passerines. Scaly mite lesions in passerines are sometimes referred to as "tasselfoot" because of this characteristic appearance.

Knemidokoptes spp. may be treated with topical ivermectin. A single dose may be effective in mild cases. A repeat dose three weeks later may be needed in more severe cases.

Feather Mites: *Dermanyssus* sp. (red mites) and *Ornithonyssus* sp. (fowl mites) are not host-specific and may be found on a variety of Passeriformes including canaries, starlings and mynahs. These mites commonly cause irritation and anemia. Deaths have been reported with heavy infections in small birds. Nonpathogenic feather mites of a variety of genera (*Anlages, Megninia* and *Rivoltasia*) may also occur. Lightly dusting birds with pyrethrin or carbaryl powders may be effective. Placing the powder in a salt shaker and "lightly salting" is sufficient.

Quill mites are not particularly species-specific and may attack both passerine and nonpasserine species. *Dermoglyphus, Syringophilus, Picobia* and *Harpyhynchus* are genera that have been reported on Passeriformes. Hanging a dichlorvos pest strip near birds affected with quill mites has eliminated the parasite in some cases. Treating the bird with ivermectin should be effective.

Epidermoptic Mites, which may be carried mechanically by hippoboscid flies, cause a depluming dermatitis followed by scale formation. Epidermoptic mites may be easily identified on microscopic examination of skin scrapings. Treatment options are like those described for quill mites.

Lice

Lice are more common on Passeriformes than they are on Psittaciformes. Some of the genera of biting lice (*Amblycera*) that occur on passerines include *Colpocephalum, Menacanthus, Machaerilaemus, Mysidea* and *Rininus*. These lice are not specialized for life on particular feathers and are able to move quickly. Chewing lice (*Ischnocera*) are often specifically adapted to a particular part of the bird's body and are generally more sluggish than biting lice. Signs of the presence of lice include restlessness and biting, excessive preening and damage to plumage. Some cases of baldness in canaries are caused by lice.

Lice undergo a complete life cycle on the bird, and a weekly dusting with pyrethrin is an effective method of control.

Metabolic Diseases

Iron Storage Disease and Related Entities

Various Passeriformes species including Indian Hill Mynahs, Rothschild's Mynahs, quetzals, Birds of Paradise, Green Cat Birds and tanagers have been reported to be susceptible to excessive accumulation of iron in the liver. In a group of 11 mynah birds that varied from five to ten years in age, clinical signs associated with hepatomegaly and ascites included a three-day to three-month history of listlessness, regurgitation, dyspnea, weight loss, diarrhea, coughing, wheezing and syncope. Most of the birds died within several days of presentation.

Radiographs may reveal hepatic enlargement and ascites in affected birds. Liver enzymes are typically elevated while total serum protein is low. Diagnosis using biopsy is discussed in Chapters 13 and 20.

Neoplasia including lymphosarcoma, hepatocellular carcinoma and erythroblastosis has been associated with iron storage disease. The neoplastic cells do not contain iron.

Susceptible species should be kept on low-iron diets such as fresh fruit and commercially available formulated rations that are low in iron (less than 60 parts per million) (see Chapter 20).

Amyloidosis

Amyloidosis is common in Gouldian Finches and is occasionally seen in other Passeriformes species.

Hepatic Lipidosis

Fatty livers are occasionally seen in Estrilid finches (Zebra Finches, parrot finches and Star Finches) and may be associated with inadequate exercise and high-energy diets such as soft foods and mealworms.

Toxicosis

Canaries and finches are particularly susceptible to inhalant toxins because they breathe more air per gram of body weight than larger birds, and they have a highly efficient gas exchange system (see Chapter 22). Carbon monoxide exposure from any source (car exhaust, gas furnace leaks, kerosene stoves) can be rapidly fatal. Passerines, like psittacines, are very susceptible to the gases released from overheated polytetrafluoroethylene (see Chapter 37).

Certain varieties of avocado may be toxic to some Passeriformes.

Ethanol toxicity has been reported in free-ranging passerines (especially Cedar Waxwings) following the ingestion of hawthorn pommes or other fruits that have frozen and then thawed allowing yeast fermentation of sugars to produce ethanol.

Heavy metal toxicities caused by the consumption of wire are uncommon in passerines because they have limited capacity to damage metal objects. Lead or zinc toxicosis has occasionally been seen when galvanized wire has been use in the construction or repair of enclosures (see Chapter 37).

Neoplastic Diseases

Passeriformes have one of the lowest incidence of tumors of any order of birds or mammals. Neoplasms that have been regularly reported include leukosis in canaries, adenomas associated with poxvirus, papillomas in finches and neoplasia associated with iron storage disease.

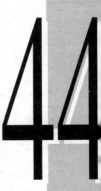

COLUMBIFORMES

Curt Vogel
Helga Gerlach
Mait Löffler

Columbiformes are among the most ancient domesticated animals in the world. Of special interest and importance is the Rock Pigeon, from which a whole variety of domestic breeds and color variations has been developed via mutations and recombinations throughout the millennia.

Selected Anatomy and Physiology

Integument

The plumage of the pigeon does not have the powder down (plumae) found in many other avian groups. The powder found in pigeons is produced by modified semiplumes as well as downs (semiplumae), which can be generally called pulviplumes.

The powder is derived from cells that surround the differentiating cells of the barbules of a growing feather. They are not a fragment of the sheath or the feather itself. Powder is shed only while the feathers are emerging from their sheaths.

The feather powder is composed entirely of keratin. The keratin particles inhibit abrasion of the feathers, provide the plumage its silky gray gleam and keep the ends smooth and pliable.

Frequent exposure to feather powder has been associated with allergic alveolitis (pigeon breeder's lung) in some susceptible, genetically predisposed humans. The same pathogenesis has been determined for the feather powder coryza.

The uropygial gland is absent or poorly developed in many species and in some breeds of the domesticated pigeon.

Vascular Plexus

The Columbiformes have an anatomic characteristic called the plexus arteriosus et venosus intracutaneous seu subcutaneous collaris. This plexus of anastomosing vessels extends from the cranium to the crop and base of the neck.

The plexus is used for sexual and territorial display and regulates circulation and body temperature in both genders. Injections in or

Table 44.1	Nine Distinguishing Characteristics of Groups of Domesticated Pigeons

- Colored pigeons, eg, German toys (These birds are selectively bred for coloration and plumage morphology.)
- Medium-sized varieties (with a body mass of up to 500-700 g)
- Heavy-sized varieties (with a body length of up to 55 cm, a wing spread of up to 105 cm, and body weight of over 700 g)
- Trumpeters (with their characteristic vocal expressions)
- Frillbacks, Fantails, Jacobins and Monks, Owls, Dewlaps and Swifts (each with a particular feather structure and design)
- Tumblers (These birds are considered flight sports breeds and represent the largest group with several hundred varieties worldwide.)
- Wattled Pigeons (They have a characteristic bulged, distended or wart-like cere, as well as more or less prominently developed naked or wart-like rings around the eyes.)
- Pouters (including the ringbeaters) with a singularly developed round, egg-shaped, pear-shaped or sac-like crop area, which varies according to the breed.
- Hen Pigeons (with their fowl-like body morphology and body posture.)

damage of this plexus, especially during display and in hot weather, can cause fatal hemorrhage.

The heart rate of Rock and domesticated pigeons ranges from 180-250 beats per minute; the respiratory rate is 20-35 breaths per minute. During sustained flight, the heart rate may reach 5.2-6.2 beats per second with a high of 9.4 beats per second at the time of take off.

The blood volume of pigeons is approximately 0.1 ml/g body weight. The prothrombin time, which is a sensitive indicator of hepatopathies, is 15.1 minutes (range of 11.5-18.7) for undiluted pigeon plasma. Pigeons generally have a lymphocytic blood differential. Hematologic and clinical chemistry values are listed in the Appendix. Electrocardiographic data are provided in Chapter 27.

In contrast to most avian species (except hummingbirds and some finches), pigeons and doves drink water by placing the beak up to the nares in water and sucking it up like a vacuum pump. With each drinking cycle, domesticated pigeons ingest approximately 0.6 ml of water.

Behavior

Columbiformes are rather aggressive, particularly during the reproductive cycle, and have no behavioral inhibitions against killing members of their own species or their offspring. Birds should always have a place that they can use to escape from an aggressive male.

Homing Abilities of Racing Pigeons

Only racing pigeons have an innate homing ability that has been enhanced through selective breeding and continuous training. Their capacity to return home is based on special senses that enable them to determine the direction of home as soon as they are released.

According to recent findings, racing pigeons obviously do not rely on any one single sense to find their way home, but are assumed to use a combination of orientation factors.

Husbandry

Nutrition

Diets for pigeons should be rich in concentrated nutrients but should not contain high amounts of water or fiber. Effective formulated diets are readily available for domesticated pigeons (nutritional requirements are listed in Tables 44.2-44.5). Commercially available mixed seeds used for many pigeon and dove species can be enriched by adding brewer's yeast, vegetables and vitamin preparations.

The daily feed consumption of pigeons and doves is approximately 1/5 to 1/20 of their body weight. The feed intake of squabs ranges from 10-100% of their body weight, depending on their age. The daily amount of drinking water varies between 5 and 8% of the body weight.

The feed quality is of the utmost importance. Grains, seeds or formulated diets should be stored in a dry, clean, pest-free location. Fungi, particular mycotoxins, feed mites and toxic seeds from weeds should be avoided.

Housing

The housing (lofts, dovecotes, aviaries, pens and flypens) criteria for pigeons are listed in Table 44.6. Pigeons must be protected

Table 44.2 Suggested Mineral Mixture for Pigeons (%)

Components	Breeding Pairs	Squabs
$CaCl_3$	84.79	61.32
Ca_2PO_4	9.21	31.58
NaCl containing iodine	4.80	4.80
$FeSO_4$	0.75	1.50
$MnSO_4$	0.15	0.30
$CuSO_4$	0.10	0.10
$ZnSO_4$	0.20	0.40

Table 44.3 Vitamin Requirements for Pigeons

Vitamins (Unit)	Per kg BW*	Per Adult Pigeon**	Per kg Feed
A (IU)	200	100	7,500
D_3 (IU)	20	10	750
E (mg)	2	1	15
K_3 (mg)	0.2	0.1	3
B_1 (mg)	0.3	0.15	3.5
B_2 (mg)	0.3	0.15	3.5
B_6 (mg)	0.3	0.15	3.5
B_{12} (mg)	1	0.5	15
Biotin (mg)	6	3	300
Choline (mg)	70	35	1000
Folic acid (mg)	0.05	0.025	1
Nicotinic acid (niacin) (mg)	3	1.5	35
Pantothenic acid (mg)	0.70	0.35	15

*Body weight
**Body weight approximately 500 g for a racing pigeon

Table 44.4   Recommended Diet for Pigeons*

Component	Quantity per kg feed
Crude protein	30-150 g
Crude fat	20-35 g
Crude fiber	50 g
Metabolizable energy	12 ME
Methionine	3.5 g
Methionine and cystine	6.5 g
Lysine	8 g
Calcium	10 g
Phosphorus	6 g
Sodium	1.5 g
Zinc	50 mg
Iodine	1 mg
Copper	2 mg
Manganese	50 mg
Vitamin A	7,500 IU
Vitamin D_3	750 IU
Vitamin E	15 mg
Vitamin K_3	3 mg
Vitamin B_1	3.5 mg
Vitamin B_2	3.5 mg
Vitamin B_6	3.5 mg
Vitamin B_{12}	15 mg
Biotin	300 mg
Choline	1000 mg
Folic acid	1 mg
Niacin	15 mg
Pantothenic acid	15 mg

* Recommendations during breeding, racing and main molting period

Table 44.5   Composition of Homemade Pigeon Stones

Component	Percentage
Clay	40
Vitamin/mineral mix (see Table 44.2)	30
$CaCO_3$ granules	20
Grit or gravel (2-3 mm in diameter)	10

from raptors, cats, dogs, foxes, opossums, raccoons, skunks, martens, weasels and rats.

For tumblers and other flight sport breeds, room should be provided for the bird's flight training (the exact specifications can be requested from local breeder associations for those breeds). Each loft should have compartments for newly weaned birds. Excrement should be removed on a routine basis or the birds should be placed on gratings (steel bar, metal lattice or rip-wire frames) so that the feces can drop through the grate.

Preventive Medicine

Each bird in the loft should be visually examined daily to determine its overall state of health. Pigeons that appear abnormal should be isolated, observed and evaluated by an experienced

Table 44.6   Design Criteria for Pigeon Lofts

Floor area/kg body weight	0.25-0.5 m²
Air space/kg body mass	0.25-0.5 m³
Hourly air exchange/kg body weight	270-320 ml
Maximum content of dust	10 mg/m³ air
Maximum content of toxic gases:	
CO_2	2000 ppm
NH_3	20 ppm
H_2S	10 ppm
Room temperature	5-28°C

avian veterinarian. Birds that cannot be treated are euthanatized immediately and submitted for a complete veterinary and laboratory examination.

Good hygiene demands that excrement and discarded food be removed from the loft and flypens daily. Drinking containers, hoppers, cafeteria troughs and gutters should be thoroughly cleaned at least three times per week or better, daily.

Lofts should be designed with well drained concrete floors to facilitate proper cleaning and disinfection. The concrete floor can be covered with clean litter, sand, gravel or grasses planted in removable flat boxes. If natural soil is used as a floor, excrement should be removed regularly. The upper layer should be removed and replaced with sand or gravel once a year. Flypen floors covered with grass should be cut regularly and the clippings discarded. The lawn should be chalked with unslaked lime, and holes in the surface should be reseeded.

Recently purchased birds must be placed into quarantine before being added to the flock. This includes birds with veterinary certificates stating that they are free of the most important pathogenic agents. Sentinel birds, preferably very young birds, are placed together with the new ones in the quarantine room. If the sentinel and quarantined birds remain healthy for eight weeks, they can be introduced to the flock.

Any free-ranging pigeons that appear in the loft should be isolated immediately, provided food and water and then released. Birds that do not leave should either be treated according to legal regulations or, if these do not exist, euthanatized or placed into quarantine.

Special Management Considerations

During the Racing Season

During the racing season (May to September in the northern hemisphere), active racing pigeons should have a veterinary certificate indicating that they are clinically free of salmonella, helminths and other contagious agents. The veterinary certificate should be based on clinical examinations and laboratory testing. Many organizations in Europe request that pigeons be vaccinated against paramyxovirus-1-pigeon.

Racing pigeons that return very late to the loft or appear weak without any obvious reason should be isolated and may be reintroduced to the flock only after successfully passing through quarantine. Birds involved in races should be considered exposed to infectious agents.

The transport baskets and boxes should always be cleaned and disinfected following each transportation. Birds being shipped long distances should be provided food and water and should have at least a three hours' rest before being released.

Prior to the Breeding Season

Fecal samples should be collected from pigeons in all lofts, compartments or flypens and evaluated for bacteria (salmonella) and parasites (coccidia, helminthic eggs) prior to the breeding season (January and February in the northern hemisphere). Groups in which salmonella, protozoa or helminths are identified should be treated. Between treatments, the loft, flypens and all equipment should be cleaned and disinfected as dictated by the respective agent.

Vaccination with avian paramyxovirus-1-pigeon is recommended, and in appropriate regions, vaccination with pigeon poxvirus should also be considered. The latter is usually administered in the late summer but should be available on all appropriate occasions. There is still no efficacious vaccine for *Salmonella typhimurium var. cop.*

During the Breeding Season

Approximately two weeks before the first clutch of eggs hatches, all breeding pigeons should be treated with carnidazole, dimetridazole, metridazole or ronidazole to control trichomoniasis. One tablet of carnidazole might be an effective treatment. The tablet should be administered into an empty crop to reduce the chances of regurgitation. For large flocks, a second prophylactic treatment for trichomonas is recommended from mid-April to the beginning of May. A breeding pair with massive trichomonas should be retreated two weeks before the subsequent clutch hatches. Trichomoniasis should be considered a secondary disease, and the initiating factors that allow an infection to occur should be identified (see Chapter 36).

During the warm season, it is especially important to observe pigeons and their environment for ectoparasites, in particular the red mites, northern feather mites, pigeon ticks, bed bugs, pigeon bugs, pigeon flies and chicken and pigeon fleas. Many of these parasites are found on the birds only at night. If necessary, the animals and their environment should be treated with carbaryl powder or pyrethrin.

Squabs should be placed together in compartments immediately after separation from their parents. If necessary, the weaned squabs should be tested for bacteria (particularly salmonella) and parasites as well as for antibodies against paramyxovirus-1-pigeon. If necessary, the youngsters should be vaccinated.

In the northern hemisphere, all young racing pigeons should be vaccinated for pigeon pox around the end of July. The breeding pairs should be separated from each other at the end of the breeding season.

During the Nonbreeding Season

Pigeons that will be involved in exhibition should be removed from the nesting area at the beginning of September to induce an undisturbed molt. During the main molt period, pigeons should be provided food that is high in energy, essential amino acids, minerals, trace elements and vitamins.

Until the middle of October, pigeons for exhibition are separated by gender and are allowed to fly free in segregated groups. Most exhibitors require a veterinary certificate indicating that the birds are free of salmonella and parasites; some also require vaccination again for paramyxovirus-1-pigeon.

A complete physical examination should be performed on each breeding pair and their offspring. Any bird that does not meet breeding target or that is determined to be abnormal should be removed from the flock.

Reproduction

All Columbiformes are monogamous. Pigeons generally are sexually mature by four to six months of age and will select a mate for the breeding season.

The females of large species lay a single egg; medium-sized species, two and small species occasionally three. Domestic female pigeons lay two eggs, the first at about 5:00 p.m. on one day, and the second approximately 40 hours later (ie, at 2:00 p.m. two days later). Incubation periods and weaning ages are listed in Table 44.7. The hen and cock share incubation duties and two eggs hatch after 17-19 days of incubation.

Production of Crop Milk

Columbiformes feed their offspring exclusively "crop milk" for the first days of life and as a supplemental food until they are 16 days of age. Crop milk is a holocrine secretion of the epithelium of the crop and consists of 75% water, 12.5% protein, 2.5% non-protein, 8.5% lipids and 1.5% minerals. In addition, it contains all essential amino acids, fatty acids, gammaglobulins (IgA), vitamins, minerals and trace minerals. Carbohydrates are present only in small amounts, if at all. Recent research has shown that crop milk is essential for squabs and cannot be replaced by other material, at least not during the first six days of life. Artificial incubation of pigeon eggs is simple; successful hand-feeding remains difficult.

Gender Determination

With most Columbiformes, including the domesticated pigeons, there are few differences between the secondary sexual signs in the male and female. The sexes cannot always be distinguished with certainty by body size or morphology, the shape of the head, cere or neck, or by differences in specific behavior. Endoscopy might be necessary for definitive determination of gender (see Chapter 13).

Gender can be determined in most Columbiformes using a modified nose speculum to examine the inside of the cloaca. The lateral part of the speculum is ground off and smoothed so that the ends are only 17-25 mm long and 3-5 mm wide. To perform this procedure, the bird is held in a vertical restraint position with the head upside down and the feet toward the examiner. The speculum is inserted carefully about 1 cm into the cloaca (de-

Table 44.7   Incubation Period and Fledging Age for Pigeons (days)

Common name	Incubation Period	Fledging Age
Nicobar Pigeon	28-30	90
Blue-crowned Pigeon	28-30	28
Domestic Pigeon	17-18	21-28
Stock Dove	17	28
Wood Pigeon	16	20-25
Band-tailed Pigeon	15-18	28
Turtle Dove	15-17	14-16
Zebra Dove	12	11-12
Peaceful Dove	13	11-12
Diamond Dove	12-13	11-12
Picui Ground Dove	14	12-14
Plain-breasted Ground Dove	12	14-18
Emerald Dove	12	12-13
Common Bronze-wing	12-14	16-20
Crested Pigeon	14	12
Plumed Pigeon	17	14-17
Squatter Pigeon	17	14-17
Cinnamon Dove	15	12-21
Grey-fronted Dove	17	14-17
Ruddy Quail Dove	10-12	8-11
Luzon Bleeding Heart	15-17	12-14
Pintailed Green Pigeon	16	13-15
Nepal Thick-billed Green Pigeon	14	12
Lilac-capped Fruit Dove	18	9-12
Seychelle Blue Pigeon	28	14-16
Banded Imperial Pigeon	18	14-16

pending on the size of the bird), then opened and slowly advanced dorsally and cranially. The cloacal lips widen and some of the internal cloacal structures become visible. The female is identified by visualization of the orifice of the oviduct on the left side, while the male has bilateral papillae where the vas deferens open into the cloaca. This method of gender determination is reliable for adult birds, but less so for younger pigeons.

Artificial Insemination

Managing the Male

The best males to use for semen donors are mature birds that are with hens eight days before, or up to four days after, egg laying. Two people are required for collecting the semen. One person restrains the bird upside down with the tail toward the examiner. The other person holds a Pasteur pipette in one hand, and the tail is lifted up and held between the thumb and index finger of the same hand. The opening of the cloaca is literally pressed together to push the spermatozoa out of the papilla of the ductus deferens.

This pressure also causes blood plasma to pass from the capillaries under the cloacal epithelium. This blood plasma collects in the median part of the cloaca and combines with the spermatozoa to produce 0.1-0.2 ml of semen.

Managing the Female

The most suitable females for artificial insemination are those that have been sexually stimulated by a sterile male. Males are sterilized by transecting the ductus deferens, which are visible as meandering whitish cords between connective tissue folds of the peritoneum (cave ureters).

The collected semen is used to directly inseminate the female. The oviductal mucosa contains glands that store sperm and keep it viable for several days. Insemination is best performed around 8:00 p.m. four days before the first egg of a clutch would be laid. This method maximizes the chance that any eggs produced will be fertilized. Insemination is achieved by restraining the hen in the same manner as described for semen collection. An assistant opens the proctodeum with a short vaginal speculum. The orifice of the oviduct is identified on the left side of the urodeum, and should not be confused with the opening of the cloacal bursa or the entrance to the coprodeum.

Insemination is most successful if performed with undiluted ejaculate immediately or shortly after collection.

Clinical Examination

A bird's feathers should be carefully protected during the examination procedure. Damage to the feathers of a racing or exhibition bird can substantially affect their performance.

Therapeutic Methods

The subcutaneous connective tissue of the caudal third of the neck is most suitable for subcutaneous injections. The skin near the base of the neck should be gently lifted to create a fold, and the needle should be directed strictly dorsomedian with a relatively flat cranial orientation. The plexus arteriosus et venosus intracutaneous collaris must be avoided. Large volumes of fluid can be administered into the subcutaneous connective tissue on the side of the thoracic wall and behind the wings.

Pigeon poxvirus vaccines can be administered by feather follicle or wing web method. A feather follicle vaccine is applied by removing approximately ten feathers on the lateral thigh and rubbing the vaccine into the follicles using a brush provided by the manufacturer. This method should not be used for emergency vaccination because field virus can infect the traumatized skin. The wing web method employs a puncture through the propatagium with a special needle provided by the manufacturer. Both methods should be used only as recommended by the manufacturer.

The iliotibialis muscle of the thigh is a good site for intramuscular injections in some pigeons or doves. The injection is administered at the middle of the femur, and the needle runs distally. The pectoralis muscle is used for IM injections in larger Columbiformes that require a higher injection volume.

For intravenous injections, the ulnar vein or medial metatarsal veins can be used.

Anesthesia

General Anesthesia

Isoflurane is the anesthetic of choice for use in pigeons (see Chapter 39).

The use of injectable anesthetics in pigeons is fraught with problems that include widely variable responses and levels of safety among patients.

Local Anesthesia

Columbiformes are sensitive to many local anesthetic agents and may develop adverse drug reactions or die following the administration of 0.5 ml/kg of 2% procaine or lidocaine hydrochloride. Local anesthesia can be achieved with 1% procaine or 2% lidocaine hydrochloride with the addition of adrenalin 1:20,000. The addition of adrenalin increases safety, decreases absorption and prolongs anesthetic duration. Local anesthesia is achieved within two to ten minutes of application.

Diseases

The primary disease problems are due to infectious agents. Table 44.8 provides a checklist of infectious diseases.

Pigeons frequently have trichomoniasis (canker) of the oropharynx and the crop as well as occasional systemic infections, which cause lesions in the liver, base of the heart and lungs. With cooling down of samples or cadavers, the agent becomes invisible. Therefore, sending samples to a diagnostic laboratory is of no benefit.

In pouters, so-called sour crop (ingluveitis) is a common problem. Sour crops have to be emptied and rinsed with saline at body temperature, possibly with some added antibiotic.

Table 44.8   Check List of Infectious Agents in Pigeons

VIRUS
Pigeonpox
Herpesvirus
– Inclusion body hepatitis in pigeons (syn. infectious esophagitis)
– Contagious paralysis (syn. pigeon herpes encephalomyelitis)
Avian adenovirus
Avian parvovirus
Avian reovirus
Eastern and western equine encephalomyelitis
Venezuelan equine encephalomyelitis
Rubivirus
St. Louis encephalitis
West-Nil-Virus
Avian paramyxovirus, serotype 1
Newcastle disease, serotype 1 pigeon, serotype 7
Avian influenzavirus A
Avian retrovirus
– Type C retrovirus group (avian leukosis-related viruses) including avian sarcoma and leukemia viruses
– Avian reticuloendotheliosis virus

CHLAMYDIA
Chlamydia psittaci

MOLLECUTES
Mycoplasma spp.
Acholoplasma spp.

RICKETTSIA
Coxiella burnetii
Aegyptianella pullorum

BACTERIA
Staphylococcus spp.
Streptococcus spp.
Mycobacterium avium-intracellulare
Erysipelothrix rhusiopathiae
Listeria spp.
Clostridium spp.
Enterobacteriaceae
Pseudomonas aeruginosa
Aeromonas hydrophila
Alcaligenes faecalis
Bordetella spp.
Campylobacter spp.
Vibrio spp.
Borrelia anserina
Pasteurella spp.
Actinobacillus spp.
Haemophilus spp.

Cytophaga anatipestifer (*syn.*
Pfeifferella, Moraxella,
Pasteurella)
Acinetobacter calcoaceticus
Salmonella spp.

FUNGI
Microsporum spp.
Candida albicans
Cryptococcus neoformans
Histoplasma capsulatum
Aspergillus spp.

ECTOPARASITES
Argas spp.
– (*A. reflexus* = Pigeon tick)
Ixodes spp.
Dermanyssus gallinae
– Roost mite syn. chicken mite
Ornithonyssus
– Northern fowl mite
Syringophilus columbae
– Quill mite
Sarcopterinus nidulans
Cytodytes nudus
– Air sac mite
Laminosioptes cysticola
– Forms nodules within the subcutis
Neonyssus spp.
– In nasal and sinus cavities
Speleognathus striatus
– As above
Cheyletiella heteropalpa
– Feather mite
Falculifer spp.
– Feather mite
Megninia spp.
– Feather mite
Analges bifidus
– Feather mite
Hemialges anacentros
– Feather mite
Knemidocoptes mutans
– Scaly-leg mite
Neoknemidocoptes laevis
– Depluming scabies

FLUKES (Trematodes)
Echinoparyphium spp.
Echinostoma spp.
Hypoderaeum conoideum
Cotylurus cornutus
Ribeiroia ondatrae
Apatemon gracilis
Brachylaema spp.
Harmostomum spp.
Postharmostomum spp.
Cryptocotyle concavum
Amphimerus elongatus
Tanaisia bragai

ROUNDWORMS (Nematodes)
Ascaridia columbae and
   other *A.* spp.
– Common or large roundworm
Ornithostrongylus quadriradiatus
Trichostrongylus tenuis
Tetrameres spp.
Dispharynx nasuta
– Spiral stomach worm
Pelucitus spp.
– Filaria in the subcutis of the neck
Capillaria spp.
– Thread worms
Syngamus trachea
– Red worm syn. forked worm

INSECTS
Columbicola columbae
– Slender pigeon louse
Campanyulotes bidentatus
– Golden feather louse
Colocera spp.
– Little feather louse
Hohorstiella spp.
– Large body louse
Neocolpocephalum spp.
– Narrow body louse
Bonomiella columbae
Physconelloides spp.
Cimex spp.
– Bedbugs
Haematosiphon inodora
– Adobe bug
Oeciacus vicarius
Triatoma spp.
– Assassin bug
Ceratophyllus spp.
– Fleas
Echidnophaga gallinacea
– Stick-tight flea
Tenebrio molitor
– Yellow mealworm
Dermestes lardarius
–Larder beetle
Neocrophorus vestigator
Silpha spp.
– Carrion or Sexton beetle
Pseudolynchia canariensis
– Pigeon louse fly
Ornithomyia spp.
– Louse fly
Ortholfersia spp.
– Louse fly
Stribometapa podostyla
– Louse fly
Lynchia spp.
– Louse fly
Microlynchia pusilla
– Louse fly

TAPEWORMS (Cestodes)
Aporina delafondi
Choanotaenia infundibulum
Hymenolepis spp.
Raillietina spp.
Cotugnia spp.
Diphyllobothrium mansoni
(only larvae)

PROTOZOA
Eimeria spp.
Toxoplasma gondii
Sarcosporidia spp.
Haemoproteus spp.
Plasmodium spp.
Leucocytozoon spp.
Trypanosoma hannai
Spironucleus columbae
Trichomonas gallinae

GALLIFORMES

Christian Schales
Kerstin Schales

45

Members of the order Galliformes occur on every continent except Antarctica. The Red Junglefowl, Common Turkey and Helmeted Guineafowl have been domesticated for centuries and are of considerable economic importance. Some varieties reach monstrous proportions and some members of the order, like the Japanese Quail and various pheasants, are approaching a level of complete domestication.

Anatomy and Physiology

Integument

Many gallinaceous species develop a durable, vascularized thickening of the corium in the ventral thoracic region called a brooding spot. The feathers in this region are temporarily lost, and body heat is transferred directly from the brooding bird to the eggs.

Some gallinaceous birds have unique skin appendages. Junglefowl possess marked unpaired carneous combs. The paired wattles of the throat are similar in structure to the comb. Like the comb, the size of the wattles is influenced by hormones, and both are better developed in cocks than in hens. Paired cheek or ear lobes are located ventral to the auditory canal and are red or white if subepithelial capillary sinusoids are absent.

The structure of the skin appendages on the head and neck of turkeys varies from those described in junglefowl. The dewlaps of turkeys are smooth, can increase and decrease in size and can change color. Turkeys have a single snood on the forehead that can increase or decrease in length. Numerous red caruncles are located on the poorly feathered skin of the head. A beard consisting of tough dark bristles is present at the border between the neck and chest.

The cocks of many gallinaceous birds have spurs, which are osseous eminences originating from the tarsometatarsus and are covered by keratinized epidermis. The cocks' spurs are frequently sharp and can easily injure rivals, females, clients or veterinarians.

Locomotor System

The furcula (wishbone) of the domestic fowl is V-shaped and has a ventral process. In the Crested and Plumed Guineafowl, an indentation exists at the junction of the two clavicles. This indentation holds the U-shaped loop of the elongated trachea. The medial notch of the sternum extends far cranially, and the lateral and medial notches are connected by fibrous membranes. In this region, the liver is not protected by the sternum, and injections, abdominocentesis or handling procedures must be carefully performed.

The first digit of the gallinaceous birds is oriented mediocaudally and the three other digits are directed cranially.

Respiratory System

Desert-dwelling gallinaceous birds such as sand partridges, possess well developed salt glands situated in an osseous indentation above the eyes. The cocks or both genders of some gallinaceous birds have elongated tracheas. The additional length produces a U-shaped or circular loop in the trachea that lies between the skin and the muscle layer in the ventral thoracic or cranial abdominal region. In Helmeted Curassows, the loop extends to the cloaca, and in some other cracids, it extends to the caudal end of the sternum.

The neopulmo, which is the phylogenetically younger portion of the lung, is well developed in Galliformes. A phylogenetic increase in the size of the neopulmo is accompanied by a decrease in the size of the caudal thoracic air sacs. The Common Turkey has a well developed neopulmo and has no caudal thoracic air sacs.

Alimentary Tract

The tongue of gallinaceous birds is shaped like an acute triangle, is stabilized by a bone and has no intrinsic musculature. Most gallinaceous birds have a crop.

The ventriculus and its associated musculature are well developed in most gallinaceous birds. Gallinaceous birds have a gall bladder and two bile ducts. All gallinaceous birds have well developed ceca. In some species, bacterial digestion of cellulose occurs in the ceca. The cecal flora probably plays an important role in the synthesis of vitamins and the metabolism of nitrogen. The ceca are usually emptied once a day, typically in the morning.

Husbandry

Most gallinaceous birds are best maintained in combination indoor and outdoor aviaries and can live to 6-20 years depending on the species.

A pair of pheasants can be maintained and bred in an aviary with a floor space 4 by 6 meters with an additional 4 square meter shelter. A Common Pheasant cock with 5-6 hens needs 30-40 square meters. An aviary for peafowl should be at least 3 meters wide, 3 meters deep and 3 meters high. These species are best maintained in open-air enclosures or big gardens. One pair of Bobwhite or California Quail needs a minimum of 1.5 m x 1.5 m floor space. For grouse, small aviaries measuring 4 meters in depth and 8 meters in width are recommended, because these birds may injure themselves if they fly into netting at the high speeds attained in larger flights.

Many Galliformes prefer to roost in elevated positions, making the height of an aviary important. Tropical or subtropical species maintained in cold climates require an indoor aviary or, if kept outdoors in winter, a heated shelter. The mesh size of netting should be small enough to prevent a bird from placing its head through the mesh. It should also prevent the smallest predators from entering the aviary. Some gallinaceous birds, especially the Common Pheasant, fly straight up when panicked. For this species, the top netting in an enclosure should be loose to provide some give and reduce the chances of head and neck injuries. An opaque barrier can be placed at the back of the aviary, extending up to one-half of the height, to provide extra visual security for the birds.

Ground-dwellers like some quail, some partridges and some francolins do not need elevated perches. Perches should be placed far enough from walls or wire netting to prevent the tail or wing feathers from contacting these surfaces. Peafowl, Reeve's Pheasant, argus pheasants and Phoenix Fowl require especially high perches, three to four meters above the ground, to accommodate their long tail feathers. Sharp corners should be avoided in designing the aviary. Curved corners or dense bushes planted in the corners reduce the possibility of trauma.

Shrubs also help to landscape an aviary and provide shelter for the birds; however, the aviary should not be overplanted. Too many plants will make an aviary difficult to clean. Natural turfs are attractive, but are not recommended when keeping birds that are highly susceptible to infectious diseases. An aviary with a concrete floor that is covered with an exchangeable layer of sand meets the needs of sensitive species (like grouse or the Cheer Pheasant) and is better than natural soil. Plants may be grown in containers that are removed when the aviary needs cleaning.

Snowcocks need large rocks for perching and shaping their bills. Some species like monals, eared pheasants and the Cheer Pheasant use their upper bill to search the soil for roots and insects. If these birds are maintained on artificial substrate, natural abrasion of the bill will not occur and manual trimming will be necessary. Gallinaceous birds do not bathe in water. Most gallinaceous birds like to take dust or sand baths. The placement of abrasive materials on the plumage may function to lightly abraid and polish the edges of the feathers, and may help reduce the number of external parasites as long as the sand itself is not contaminated. Insect powders should be used only if they are known to be nontoxic for the species concerned and only if the birds in fact have parasites. In the winter, Willow Ptarmigan bathe in the snow.

Various bird species should generally not be mixed in one aviary because of possible interspecific aggression and the potential transmission of infectious agents. If species are combined, it is best to mix birds that do not compete for the same food or biotope. Ground-dwelling gallinaceous birds can be combined with bush- or tree-living species like thrushes, babblers, starlings, bulbuls and doves (with the exception of the Ground Pigeon); however, mixing of species is not recommended.

Losses to predators can occur in open-topped facilities, particularly with respect to chicks. Rare species should not be maintained in an open-topped enclosure. A breeder who uses open-topped enclosures should expect that the loss of a bird to a predator is the responsibility of the breeder and not the fault of the predator. Some gallinaceous birds are noisy, especially the Indian peafowl and guineafowl during the breeding season, and should be maintained in secluded areas to avoid complaints from neighbors.

Nutrition

"Easy" Birds

Many gallinaceous birds are omnivorous. The nutritional requirements of Common Pheasant, Golden Pheasant, Lady Amherst's Pheasant, Silver Pheasant, peafowl, guineafowl, turkeys, partridges and New World quail are relatively easy to provide. Commercial diets for domestic fowl, domestic turkey, Common Pheasant and Japanese Quail are available in many countries. Pellets designed for turkeys can be used in species without special requirements. Adding fresh green plants to the diet provides the birds with nutritional diversity. Grass or corn silage can also be offered in small quantities. During the breeding season, the diet should contain 20-25% crude protein. Outside the breeding season, a maintenance diet containing less than 20% crude protein is best. Commercial diets for domestic turkey are usually better suited for pheasants than diets developed for domestic fowl. Feeding is best accomplished by providing small portions of the diet several times a day in the nonbreeding season and offering food ad libitum during the breeding season.

Most New World quail are primarily seed-eaters and are easy to feed. Forest-adapted species may be largely insectivorous and have higher and more specific protein requirements in comparison to other gallinaceous birds. Cracids are mainly, but not exclusively, vegetarians. They can be sustained on pellets containing 21% crude protein supplemented with fruits but no grains. During the breeding season, they are fed soybean paste, chopped hard-cooked eggs, chopped meat or mealworms (larvae of the meal beetle). Megapodes can be fed a commercial poultry diet.

Birds with a High Protein Requirement

Some gallinaceous birds like peacock pheasants, argus pheasants and the Roulroul (Crested Wood Partridge) do best with high-protein diets. In addition to high-protein turkey or pheasant diets, adult peacock pheasants should be fed mealworms, chopped meat, fruits and a small quantity of grain. Green plants are rarely consumed by these species. The Roulroul is fed a commercial soft feed for insectivorous birds mixed with live insects, chopped hard-cooked eggs and chopped meat. The primarily meat diet of these birds results in an odoriferous feces.

"Difficult" Birds

Some gallinaceous birds consume almost exclusively vegetable material. The Koklass, the Blood Pheasant, snowcocks, tragopans and grouse are examples. Feeding these species with game bird pellets or, even worse, with commercial diets for domestic fowl and turkeys, results in obesity, reduced fertility and imbalances in the intestinal microflora. These species should be maintained only where natural-type foods are available year round. These gallinaceous birds should be fed large amounts of fresh vegetables. Pellets should be provided only in small quantities, if at all. Koklass naturally feed on ferns, grasses, leaves, mosses, buds and berries. In captivity they should be provided soft green plants, fruits and berries and no grains. In the summer, grasses and lucerne can be provided. Spinach, romaine lettuce and fresh, frozen vegetables can be substituted in the winter months. Free-ranging Blood Pheasants feed on mosses, lichen, ferns, grass tips and conifer needlebuds. They browse constantly in planted aviaries. Snowcocks eat mostly grasses and leguminous plants. Their chicks feed on these plants immediately after hatching.

Tragopans consume oak trees, bamboo sprouts, grasses, mosses, oaknuts, berries and a few insects. In captivity, tragopans can be fed lucerne, grasses, cucumbers, apples and different kinds of berries. In the spring, summer and autumn, grouse feed on a variety of plants. In the winter, most grouse species are restricted to consuming one or a few plant species. During the winter season, the Spruce Grouse, capercaillies and other grouse species feed almost exclusively on conifer needles, the Black Grouse on birch buds, and ptarmigans on buds from different deciduous trees (birch, alder, willow).

Captive grouse should receive natural foods or at least large amounts of leaves, grass and berries supplemented with a limited quantity of pellets and grain. Capercaillies and ptarmigans require a diet high in crude fiber. In the Sage Grouse, leaves and sprouts of the North American Big Sagebrush are the sole winter food and the main portion of food in the summer.

Some commercial poultry diets contain coccidiostatic agents. Halofuginone is toxic for the Common Pheasant, guineafowl and the Common Partridge. Monensin is toxic for guineafowl. Commercial diets for the Common Turkey contain antiflagellates. The presence of antimicrobial agents can be life-threatening in species that depend on a functional cecal flora and fauna (eg, grouse) for proper digestion.

All gallinaceous birds should have access to grit. The grit container should be emptied and refilled regularly because birds select only stones that are suitable for their body mass. Pellets or complete rations have an adequate supply of calcium and should not be supplemented with lime or crushed shell.

Chicks

Feed should be provided to newly hatched chicks on a large flat plate on which they can move around and practice picking. By five to seven days of age, food can be offered in larger containers. The change from the plate to larger containers should occur by offering feed in both containers at the same time. Small chicks may drown in large water containers. Placing stones or glass marbles in the container will reduce losses.

Chicks of unpretentious species (Common Pheasant, peafowl, guineafowl) are initially fed a starter diet like turkey starter (28% crude protein) and are transferred to a lower protein diet (18-20% crude protein) from the eighth to eighteenth week of age.

Chicks of the vegetarian species are difficult to feed. It is best to provide these birds with foods that are similar to those eaten by their free-ranging conspecifics. A diet composed of turkey starter mixed with mealworms, ant cocoons, chopped hard-cooked eggs, diced romaine lettuce, spinach, dandelion and other green plants is a viable substitute. In several species (some grouse), chicks obtain food by picking at the ground and by cutting off parts of plants with the bill. In these species, it is important that chicks be provided intact plants that are placed in the ground or tied in bundles to facilitate natural food-gathering behavior. Chicks that are to be released into the wild must be introduced to their natural foods to prevent starvation.

The chicks of some gallinaceous birds will not pick downwards in the first days of life. This is because peacock pheasants, Crested Argus, Great Argus and some other gallinaceous hens feed their chicks for several days after hatching.

Reproduction

General Considerations

Gallinaceous birds to be used for breeding purposes should be introduced to each other before the breeding season in surroundings that are novel to all the candidates concerned. The female should be introduced to the enclosure a few hours prior to the male. In some species, it is possible to keep several males together if there are no females present. If females are present, only one male should be housed in an aviary or in one compartment. In monogamous species, only a single pair should be housed together.

Pursuit by the male and mock escape by the female is normal behavior in some species like eared pheasants and francolins. If there is insufficient space for the hen to escape, she may be injured or killed by the cock.

For species in which there are substantial differences in body size between the genders, aviaries can be designed to allow the hens to visit the cock when she wishes. Small holes, just big enough for the hen, are used to connect adjacent enclosures.

Most gallinaceous birds incubate eggs on the ground and should be provided with flat trays containing moss, foliage or hay for nesting material. Tragopans, the Congo Peafowl, the Bronze-tailed Peacock Pheasant, the Crested Argus Pheasant, the Mikado Pheasant, the Salvadori's Pheasant and the cracids nest in trees. A box placed approximately 150 cm from the ground and filled with hay and foliage can be used as an artificial nest.

Most gallinaceous birds are nondeterminant layers, and if the first clutch of eggs is removed, the hen will lay a second and sometimes a third clutch. Hatching is genetically determined and should not be assisted. Because gallinaceous chicks are nidifuguous, the family can stay together only if all the chicks hatch at the same time. Most gallinaceous chicks are independent by three months of age. The exception is the megapode chick, which is independent immediately after hatching.

Foster Breeding

The hens of some gallinaceous birds are unreliable brooders in captivity. Cracid, Common Pheasant and nearly all species of New World quail hens are unamenable brooders in captivity. These hens can be encouraged to produce two or three clutches per year instead of one by using foster parents or an incubator for hatching eggs. Chinese Silk Fowl and Bantams make excellent foster parents. Domestic turkey hens can be used to incubate the eggs of larger gallinaceous birds. Small and fragile eggs should be placed under Golden Pheasant hens, which are cautious brooders and excellent care-providers. Chicks are prone to chilling the first few days post-hatching and must have supplemental body heat from the attending hen.

Gender Determination

Many gallinaceous birds show a marked sexual dimorphism (Table 45.6). Gender can be determined by highly skilled individuals by examining the cloaca in one-day-old chicks or adults. Under certain conditions the hens of some gallinaceous birds behave like, and can have plumage like, the males. Only endoscopic examination of the gonads provides definitive determination of gender in species with similar morphologic characteristics (see Chapter 13).

Artificial Insemination

The semen is collected by massaging the caudal region of the back or the abdomen, followed by stimulation of the cloaca. Fecal contamination of the semen may occur. It is best to collect the semen directly from the spermatic duct with a syringe and a blunted hypodermic needle. The semen may be diluted with Ringer's or Tyrode's solutions by up to a factor of three.

Avian semen has a short half-life and must be used as quickly as possible. The semen is introduced with a syringe and a blunted hypodermic needle into the hen's oviduct. It is best to inseminate the hen just after she has laid an egg. This ensures that the oviduct is open, providing the semen with unrestricted access to the infundibulum.

Restraint

Cocks with spurs can injure handlers, especially when they become increasingly aggressive during the mating season. The beak can also serve as a weapon. Although serious injuries are rare, the face and the eyes of handlers should always be protected from a

Table 45.6   Gender Determination of Selected Species of Gallinaceous Birds Without Marked Sexual Dimorphism

Genus	Plumage	Differences
MEGAPDIIDAE:		
Alectura	Identical	Cocks have neck appendages
CRACIDAE:		
Ortalis	Identical	Voice of cock is deeper
Penelope	Identical	In some species iris colors differ
Nothocrax	Identical	In cocks the tracheal loop is palpable
Pauxi	Identical	In hens, plumage is sometimes a red phase
PHASIANIDAE:		
Numidinae:		
(all genera)	Identical	Cock's call has 3 syllables; hen's has 2
Argusianinae:		
Polyplectron	Similar	Hen's plumage is dull; cocks have spurs
Phasianinae:		
Crossoptilon	Identical	In general, cocks have spurs
Catreus	Similar	Cocks have long, sharp spurs
Ptilopachinae:		
Ptilopachus	Similar	
Perdicinae:		
Tetraogallus	Similar*	In some species, cocks have short spurs
Arborophila	Similar*	In some species, cocks have short spurs
Bambusicola	Similar*	
Frankolinus	Identical	
Pternistis	Identical	In some species, cocks have spurs
Scleroptila	Identical	Cocks have spurs
Ortygornis	Identical	Cocks have spurs
Coturnix	Similar	
Odontophorinae:		
Odontophorus	Similar*	
Tetraoninae:		
Tympanuchus	Similar	
Bonasa	Similar	
Terastes	Similar	
Lagopus	Identical	(only in winter)

*Some species of the genus are identically colored and some are similar.

bird's beak, even in small species. The legs of a gallinaceous bird should be the initial focus for restraint.

Catching gallinaceous birds in an aviary can be done gently with a hooked, long stick. The birds should never be restrained by the feathers alone. The whole body must be secured to prevent a shock molt. Shock molt is most common in tail feathers, but other feathers can be involved. Birds can be nearly "bald" after several failed restraint attempts. In larger species, the base of the wing is fixed with one hand and the legs are controlled with the other hand (see Chapter 44). The abdomen should be supported from below. If assistance is not available, a large bird can be restrained by placing it under one arm and pressing it gently against one's body. Birds can usually be calmed by placing a loose-fitting, lightweight cotton sock over the head to reduce vision.

Disease Considerations

Nutritional Diseases

Vitamin C deficiency does not occur in most birds; however, it has been reported in Willow Ptarmigan chicks, and may occur in other grouse chicks. Clinical signs of vitamin C deficiency are abnormal behavior, enteritis, ruffled plumage, weakness of the wings and legs, bone fractures, retarded growth and death before the age of four weeks. Feeding the chicks natural food stuffs will prevent vitamin C deficiency.

Integument Concerns

Amputation of the comb or the wattles may be indicated following extensive injury, infection or frostbite. Adequate hemostasis is necessary to prevent fatal hemorrhage. Occasional trimming of the keratinous tip of the bill is necessary if the horny layer grows too fast, or is insufficient abrasive materials are available to facilitate normal wear.

Cannibalism may occur in some Galliformes and is characterized by vent-picking, feather-pulling, toe-picking, head-picking and egg-eating. Overcrowding, incorrect feeding, an inappropriate daylight cycle, poor housing conditions (eg, high proportion of toxic gases in the air), genetic predisposition and other factors may all promote cannibalism.

Amputating the comb and wattles and "debeaking" have been used to control cannibalism; however, these control methods should be viewed as cruel and unacceptable procedures.

Trimming of the flight feathers in one wing can be used to prevent birds from escaping from open aviaries, or to reduce the mobility of an aggressive cock during the breeding period. Usually all but the outermost two primaries and the innermost three secondaries are transected, creating an effective and cosmetic wing trim (see Chapter 1). Because the feathers will be replaced during the next molt, trimming must be repeated annually in adults. Other methods, like pinioning or cutting the short tendon of the extensor carpi radialis, make birds permanently unable to fly.

Heterakis sp.

Heterakis isolonche infections have been described in a number of free-ranging and captive Galliformes. This parasite causes typhlitis with clinical signs of infection including diarrhea, weight loss and depression. Mortality rates in captive pheasants may reach 50%. The parasite invades the wall of the cecum and causes lymphocytic infiltration and granuloma formation. In pheasants, the nodules merge, leading to substantial thickening of the cecal wall. The ceca may dilate and increase in size (volume) by up to ten times.

Table 45.7   Checklist of Infectious Diseases in Gallinaceous Birds

Viruses (see Chapter 32)
Poxviridae
  Avian pox
Herpesviridae
  Infectious laryngotracheitis
  Marek's disease
Adenoviridae
  Quail bronchitis
  Inclusion body hepatitis
  Egg drop syndrome = (infectious salpingitis)
  Marble spleen disease
  Hemorrhagic enteritis of turkeys
  Chicken splenomegaly
  Adenovirus infection of the Blue Grouse
Parvoviridae
  Parvovirus infection of chickens
  Parvovirus-like infection of turkeys
Circodnaviridae
  Infectious anemia
Reoviridae
  Viral arthritis
  Other reovirus infections
  Rotavirus infections
Birnaviridae
  Infectious bursal disease
Togaviridae
  Eastern and western encephalitis
  Avian serositis
  Louping-ill
  Israel turkey meningoencephalitis
Coronaviridae
  Coronaviral enteritis of turkeys (bluecomb disease)
  Infectious bronchitis
Rhabdoviridae
  Rabies
Paramyxoviridae
  Newcastle disease
  PMV-2-infection (Yucaipa)
  PMV-3-infection (Wisconsin)
  Turkey rhinotracheitis
  Swollen head syndrome
Orthomyxoviridae
  Avian influenza, fowl plague
Retroviridae
  Leukosis
  Reticuloendotheliosis
  Lymphoproliferative disease of turkeys
Picornaviridae
  Avian encephalomyelitis
  Turkey viral hepatitis
  Infectious nephritis

Bacteria (see Chapter 33)
Staphylococcus spp.
  Staphylococcosis
Streptococcus spp.
  Streptococcosis
Mycobacterium avium
  Tuberculosis
Erysipelothrix rusiopathiae
  Erysipelas
Listeria monocytogenes
  Listeriosis
Clostridium spp.
  Ulcerative and necrotic enteritis (Cl. colinum and Cl. perfringens)
  Botulism (toxin of Cl. botulinum)

Escherichia coli
  Colibacillosis
  Coligranulomatosis
Salmonella spp.
  Salmonellosis
Klebsiella spp.
  Klebsiella infection
Yersinia pseudotuberculosis
  Pseudotuberculosis
Pseudomonas spp.
  Pseudomonas infection
Aeromonas hydrophila
  Aeromonas infection
Bordetella avium
  Bordetellosis (turkey coryza)
Campylobacter spp.
  Avian hepatitis
Borrelia anserina
  Spirochetosis
Treponema spp.
  Infectious typhlitis in chickens
Pasteurella spp.
  Fowl cholera
Actinobacillus salpingitidis
  Actinobacillosis
Haemophilus spp.
  Haemophilus infection
Francisella tularensis
  Tularemia

Mycoplasma (see Chapter 38)
Mycoplasma spp.
Ureaplasma sp.

Chlamydia (see Chapter 34)
Chlamydia psittaci
  Chlamydiosis

Rickettsia (see Chapter 38)
Coxiella burnetii
  Query (Q) fever
Aegyptianella pullorum
  Aegyptianellosis

Mycoses (see Chapter 35)
Aspergillus spp.
  Aspergillosis
Candida albicans
  Candidiasis
Dactylaria gallopavo
  Dactylariosis
Trichophyton spp.
  Favus

Mycotoxicoses (see Chapter 37)
Toxins of Aspergillus spp., Penicillium spp., Fusarium spp. and others

Parasites (see Chapter 36)
Protozoal Parasites:
  Trypanosoma avium
  Spironucleus meleagridis
  Histomonas meleagridis (blackhead disease)
  Trichomonas spp.
  Chilomastix gallinarum
  Entamoeba spp.
  Endolimax spp.
  Eimeria spp.
  Toxoplasma gondii
  Sarcocystis spp.
  Cryptosporidium spp.

Haemoproteus spp.
Leucocytozoon spp.
Plasmodium spp.
Metazoal Parasites
Trematodes
  Prosthogonimus sp.
Cestodes
  Davainea proglottina
  Raillietina spp.
  Amoebotaenia cuneata
  Choanotaenia infundibulum
  Hymenolepis spp.
  Metroliasthes lucida
  Fimbriaria fasciolaris
Nematodes (in digestive tract)
  Capillaria spp.
  Trichostrongylus tenuis
  Heterakis spp.
  Ascaridia spp.
  Gangylonema ingluvicola
  Cheilospirura spp.

Dispharynx nasuta
Tetrameres spp.
Subulura spp.
Nematodes (in respiratory tract)
  Syngamus trachea
Nematodes (in the eye)
  Oxyspirura spp.
Nematodes (in other locations)
  Aproctella stoddardi
  Singhfilaria hayesi
Acanthocephalans
  Mediorhynchus papillosus
Arthropods
  External parasites like lice, fleas, flies, mosquitoes, midges, and ticks occur in most gallinaceous birds. Mites occur above all in intensively reared gallinaceous birds, predacious bugs in some gallinaceous birds.

46

ANSERIFORMES

John H. Olsen

Waterfowl have generally been treated on a flock rather than an individual basis; however, a flock approach to rare birds, pets or small collections is usually not accepted by the client. Waterfowl aviaries are frequently plagued by problems associated with overstocking, poor management practices, and pathogen-contaminated ground or water.

Veterinarians who plan to treat free-ranging or captive Anseriformes in the United States should be aware of pertinent federal and state laws. The Migratory Bird Treaty Act involves the US, Mexico, Canada and Japan, and provides federal protection for all free-ranging birds in the US except for resident exotic species such as the English sparrow, starling, feral pigeon and resident game birds such as pheasant, grouse and quail.

Biology

The Anhimidae are goose-sized birds of fowl-like appearance, with thick, long legs and unwebbed feet. They weigh two to three kilograms. The bill is game bird-like with a downward hook and has none of the filtering fringes (lamellae) common in ducks. Flight feathers are molted gradually so that, like the Magpie Goose, but unlike most waterfowl, they do not pass through an annual flightless period.

The family Anatidae has three subfamilies. Subfamily Anseranatinae contains the Magpie Goose. This bird differs from the rest of the family. The feet are slightly webbed with an unusually long hind toe adapted for semiterrestrial life.

Breeding birds often form trios consisting of a male and two females that lay their eggs in a single nest. All the birds share incubation responsibility. Magpie Geese are the only waterfowl species to provide food to their young. The adults deposit proper foodstuffs in front of their downy chicks.

The subfamily Anserinae includes Whistling Ducks, swans, true geese, Cape Barren Geese and Freckled Ducks. These species undergo a complete annual molt following the breeding season. The flight feathers are shed almost simultaneously so the birds are unable to fly for a period of about three to six weeks. The front toes are fully webbed except in two semiterrestrial species of geese. In all species, the plumage is monomorphic and all species lack iridescent coloration, even on the wings.

Subfamily Anatinae includes Sheldgeese, Shelducks and all the typical ducks. Most of the members of this subfamily molt the body feathers twice each year. Consequently, the breeding (nuptial) and nonbreeding (winter or eclipse) plumage are distinct. In some species the breeding plumage of the male closely resembles that of the female, but more often, the genders have dimorphic plumage. The front surface of the lower tarsus has a linearly arranged (scutellated) scale pattern not seen in the other subfamilies. Iridescent coloration is frequently present in the plumage, particularly among males. The male of sexually dimorphic species is typically larger, more brilliantly patterned and more aggressive. Males of this subfamily do not assist in incubation but, depending on the tribe, participate in brooding the chicks.

Although Anseriformes generally surface feed, they may also graze or feed by diving. Some species are omnivorous while others are strictly herbivorous.

Ducks have anatomic variations in the syrinx that should not be misinterpreted as pathologic lesions. In most ducks, only the male has a left-sided enlargement of the syrinx (syringeal bulla). A syringeal bulla is not present in geese and swans.

Young Anseriformes easily imprint on humans or other species of birds. Pair formation may be difficult in imprinted birds. Homosexual and interspecific pairs are common under captive conditions. Some geese (Cereopsis and Egyptian) may be very aggressive and should not be maintained where they can injure animals or children. Imprinted geese and swans of all species can be dangerous to children.

Physiology

Anseriformes from tropical countries (eg, Whistling Ducks) are prone to frostbite and subsequent gangrene of the toes. These species should be housed indoors during freezing conditions. Otherwise, waterfowl are remarkably tolerant of adverse climatic conditions, especially if open water is available for swimming. They can be maintained successfully in most regions of the world.

In captivity, ducks often live 10-12 years, and geese and swans commonly live for 25 years or more.

Husbandry Practices

Hospitalization

Anseriformes are relatively easy to restrain. Their primary defenses include scratching with sharp toenails, pinching with their bills, striking with their wings or poking at eyes. A dry, warm enclosure with good footing is suitable for brief hospitalization. When confined, waterfowl sometimes stress, so a quiet, dimly lighted enclosure may be preferable. If longer hospitalization is necessary, an enclosure with an accessible pool and padded flooring is necessary to prevent leg and foot problems. Hard surfaces (concrete) may damage the plantar foot surfaces, eventually promoting bumblefoot. Chainlink enclosures should be protected with burlap or other similar materials to prevent birds from abrading their wings, heads or eyes.

Housing

Waterfowl are commonly kept as pairs in small, planted, open pens with a small pool or stream, or in large, open, mixed-species groups with a large pond. Most Anseriformes should have an area for swimming to maintain long-term overall health. Open enclosures allow various free-ranging birds to compete for feed and nesting sites and potentially to introduce infectious diseases. Pests and predators (rats, snakes, otters, raccoons, bobcats, opossums, hawks, owls and eagles) may also complicate waterfowl maintenance in large open exhibits. Burying the fence line will discourage some predators from digging under the fence, and electric fencing will discourage terrestrial predators. Some aviculturists use small aviary mesh to cover pens to reduce access by free-ranging birds, pests and predators.

Covered enclosures allow birds to be full-flighted (most are typically pinioned or wing-clipped to prevent escape from open enclosures). Wing clipping is accomplished by cutting the flight feathers from one wing with a pair of scissors or shears. This procedure impedes flight until the next molt. The feathers should be trimmed at the level of the rachis, not the level of the hollow calamus. This will reduce the chances of water entering the feather shaft, resulting in algae growth and folliculitis. Pinioning is the amputation of the distal portion of the wing, permanently handicapping a bird's flight abilities.

Large ponds should have islands to provide nesting areas and privacy for the birds. Some birds will nest on small floating platforms. Grazing species, such geese, require more land area than do diving ducks. Small ducks can be maintained in small planted pens with an elevated cement water container that holds three to five gallons.

A high water flow rate or filtration is important maintaining clean water and reducing the incidence of disease. Cold water is better for ponds than warm water. Generally, a depth of two feet is adequate for most Anseriformes, although swans and some diving ducks require three to four feet of water. Many waterfowl species require standing water to breed. Anseriformes typically dig or nibble at the pond bank. Lining the banks with concrete blocks, stone or other solid materials will help maintain pond continuity.

The nasal secretions of some marine and semi-marine waterfowl are believed to inhibit the growth mycotic spores. If these species are maintained fresh water, the salt glands producing these secretions may atrophy, affecting the bird's ability to resist infections. These birds may die from hypernatremia if they are returned to salt water.

Nutrition

The types of food consumed, and thus their nutritional components, vary widely between surface-feeding ducks and divers. High protein (28%) gamebird rations are frequently recommended for feeding ducklings; however, it has been found that a ration of 19% protein supplemented with scratch grains on a free-choice basis produced better growth and feed efficiency than higher protein diets (Table 46.4). Diets with 8% animal protein (19% total protein) promoted the best growth. Redhead, Pintail and Canvasback chicks grew best when fed a starting diet containing 2,970 kcal/kg and 19% protein until three weeks of age. After three weeks of age, this pelleted diet was offered free choice with a mixture of cracked corn, wheat and oats or barley (the grain mixture used should depend upon the grains that free-ranging ducks are likely to consume). Amino acid quality of the diet was maintained by the inclusion of 8% fish meal. This diet produced similar results with both dabbling and diving ducks, even though their natural feeding habits differ widely. This did not include species such as the sea ducks and mergansers that feed exclusively on fish.

Rations designed for feeding commercial ducks are not generally recommended for the long-term maintenance of other waterfowl. These diets are designed to produce a carcass to be processed for food and usually contain growth additives and compounds to stimulate feather loss. The fat content in dog foods is much higher than waterfowl can tolerate, particularly when mixed grains are fed as part of the diet.

Many experienced Anseriforme breeders are convinced that all waterfowl need a high-protein diet, and one pelleted ration is fed to all species. This is an inaccurate and dangerous assumption. Many geese are grazers, and most lush grasses seldom exceed 17% protein. Feeding high-protein diets to these birds can cause terminal renal failure. In addition, excessive water consumption is necessary to remove the extra protein, and a relatively short period of water deprivation can be fatal.

Free-ranging ducks and geese consume large quantities of energy-rich foods to establish the fat reserves necessary for migration. The same diet fed to captive birds will predispose them to obesity and fat metabolism problems when they are provided excessive quantities of food.

Geese appeared to have a better ability to utilize dietary fiber than ducks. Captive geese did best when provided alfalfa hay in addition to a pelleted ration. Geese do well when fed the same diets recommended for ducks (Table 46.4). A duck starter diet should be provided for four weeks, followed by the duck grower/finisher diet until maturity. Scratch grains should be added to the grower/finisher diet, approximately 50:50, after eight weeks of age.

When given a choice, ducks prefer pellets to mash. The maximum diameter pellet a duckling can swallow easily dictates acceptable size.

Feeding containers for ducks should be several inches deep and at least one foot square to facilitate their normal forward "shovel-

Table 46.4 Diet for Wild Ducklings

Ingredient	WILD DUCK STARTER RATION	WILD DUCK GROWER RATION
	Pounds per Ton	
Corn meal, No. 2 yellow	933.0	753.0
Oats, heavy, pulverized	200.0	400.0
Wheat standard middlings	300.0	300.0
Soybean oil meal, 50% protein, low fiber	250.0	280.0
Fish meal, 60% protein	160.0	100.0
Fish solubles, dried basis	10.0	10.0
Dried brewer's yeast, 40% protein	20.0	20.0
Whey, dried product, 55% lactose	20.0	20.0
Alfalfa meal, dehydrated, 17% protein (100,000 A/lb)	60.0	80.0
Dicalcium phosphate	10.0	10.0
Calcium carbonate, ground	30.0	20.0
Salt, iodized	5.0	5.0
Manganese sulfate, feed grade	0.5	0.5
Copper sulfate	0.5	0.5
Zinc carbonate	0.25	0.25
DL-methionine (hydroxyanalog)	1.0	1.0
Santoquin		0.25
Vitamin, Unit of Measure	**Amount per Ton**	
Stabilized vitamin A, USP units	10,000,000	12,000,000
Vitamin D_3 ICU	1,500,000	1,500,000
Vitamin E, IU	5,000	5,000
Riboflavin, grams	3	4
Choline chloride, grams	112	250
Niacin, grams	40	40
Calcium pantothenate, pure D-isomer, grams	6	10
Vitamin K (menadione sodium bisulfite), grams	4	4
Vitamin B_{12}, milligrams	6	6
Calculated Analysis (%)		
Protein	20.0	19.0
Fat	6.5	5.0
Fiber	4.0	4.5
Calcium	1.2	1.0
Phosphorus	0.7	0.7

Starter ration to be fed for first three weeks with insoluble grit available at all times. Grower ration to be fed from 21 days of age to maturity with scratch grains free choice. Grit to be available at all times. This diet plus scratch grain free choice can be used as a maintenance ration and for nonlaying breeders.

ing" prehension motion for food collection. Anseriformes should always have access to fresh, uncontaminated water.

Vitamins

Recommended vitamin levels practical for commercial duck rations are in Table 46.5.

Vitamin A: Hypovitaminosis A is associated with poor growth, muscular weakness, retardation of endochondral bone growth and

Table 46.5   Vitamin Requirements for Pekin Ducks

Vitamin	A	B	C
Vitamin A, IU	8000	5000	10,000
Vitamin D_3, IU	1000	500	1000
Vitamin E, IU	25	20	40
Vitamin K, IU	2	1	2
Thiamine, mg	2.0	2.0	2.0
Riboflavin, mg	4.5	4.5	4.5
Niacin, mg	70.0	70.0	50.0
Pantothenic acid, mg	12.0	11.0	15.0
Pyridoxine, mg	3.0	3.0	3.0
Folacin, mg	0.5	0.25	0.5
Biotin, mg	0.15	0.1	0.15
Vitamin B_{12}, mg	0.01	0.005	0.01
Choline, mg	1300.0	1000.0**	1000.0**

* Must be increased to 8 mg/kg if sulfaquinoxaline or other vitamin K antagonist is
 present in the diet.
** growing ducks may be able to synthesize choline.

A = Recommended vitamin allowances for **starting** ducks
B = Recommended vitamin allowances for **growing-finishing** ducks
C = Recommended vitamin allowances for **breeding** ducks

ataxia, paralysis and death. Chronic hypovitaminosis A in ducks
has not been verified but has been suggested as a precipitating
factor in the high incidence of bumblefoot described in
Anseriformes.

Vitamin E: Hypovitaminosis E has not been associated with
encephalomalacia in ducks. Prevention of vitamin E-related muscular dystrophy in ducks is mostly associated with their requirement for dietary selenium. Muscular dystrophy is prevented with
diets containing 1.2 mg vitamin E/kg of food when selenium is
added at a level of 0.1 ppm.

Thiamine (Vitamin B_1): Ducklings begin to lose weight four
days after being placed on thiamine-deficient diets. "Star-gazing"
is a characteristic clinical sign. If deficiencies occur, thiamine
should be added to the drinking water at 100 mg/L.

Riboflavin (Vitamin B_2): Riboflavin deficiencies in ducklings
cause poor growth and high mortality. The "curled toe" syndrome
common in riboflavin-deficient chicks has not been reported in
ducklings. Deficiencies in breeding ducks cause late embryonic
mortality.

Niacin (Nicotinic Acid): Ducklings have a relatively high requirement for niacin, which is required for growth and prevents
severe leg weaknesses. Ducklings receiving a diet deficient in
niacin showed a 100% incidence of bowed legs. Niacin has been
shown to be poorly available from natural feedstuffs, and supplementation with pure niacin may be necessary.

Biotin: The dermatitis associated with biotin deficiency in
chickens has not been described in ducks. A poor growth rate appears to be the only sign of deficiency.

Folic Acid: Deficiencies result in severe anemia as well as reduced growth and poor feathering.

Choline: Ducklings on choline-deficient diets grow poorly, have weak legs, develop perosis and may die.

Ascorbic Acid (Vitamin C): Ducks readily synthesize vitamin C; however, birds receiving supplemental vitamin C have superior erythrocyte and hemoglobin values as well as greater bacteriocidal and lysozyme activity than unsupplemented ducks.

Mineral Requirements

Recommended allowances for minerals in starting ducks, growing Pekin Ducks and breeding Pekin Ducks are found in Table 46.6.

Table 46.6 Mineral Requirements for Pekin Ducks			
Mineral	A	B	C
Calcium, %	0.7	0.6	2.75
Available phosphorus, %	0.5	0.4	0.4
Sodium, %	0.18	0.18	0.18
Chloride, %	0.18	0.14	0.14
Magnesium, ppm	500.0	500.0	500.0
Manganese, ppm	55.0	45.0	35.0
Zinc, ppm	60.0	60.0	60.0
Selenium, ppm	0.2	0.2	0.2

A = Mineral allowance for **starting** Pekin Ducks
B = Mineral allowance for **growing** Pekin Ducks
C = Mineral allowance for **breeding** Pekin Ducks

Reproduction

Breeding Factors

Most ducks become sexually mature at about one year of age. A few exceptions, such as the Bufflehead and Scaup, require longer. Geese often take two years to mature, while swans may take five years to reach sexual maturity. Waterfowl maintained in captivity are prone to hybridize, and related species should not be housed together.

Male Anseriformes have an erectile phallus covered with keratinized papillae. This anatomic feature allows the gender of ducks or geese to be accurately determined at a very early age. Exposure and identification of structures is easier in mature breeding birds. The cloaca is manually everted to visualize the phallus by holding the bird vertically with its head down and abdomen toward the examiner. Gentle, firm pressure with the thumbs on each side of the cloaca will tend to evert the phallus. Two small labia-like structures are found in the female. The phallus can be palpated in its retractile state and needs to be everted only for confirmation; the female requires little effort as a palpable mass cannot be detected.

Swans and geese form a lasting pair bond that is broken only by the death of one of the birds. The surviving bird may have difficulty forming another pair bond, or may not breed again.

Because incubation of the clutch usually begins at the same time, most eggs in a clutch will hatch within a day or two of each other. Once an egg pips, there is usually an interval of 16 to 24 hours before hatching is complete.

Anseriformes have nidifugous young that are covered in down and can eat, swim and dive almost from hatching. The young begin to forage within a day or so of hatching. Normal chicks have sufficient fat and yolk stores to survive for several days without eating.

Embryo and Neonatal Management and Pathology

Inbreeding in domestic birds correlates with a significant increase in infant mortality, which may reach 100% after three to four generations of breeding.

Incubation

Typically, an incubator temperature of 99.3°F and 85% humidity is appropriate for most waterfowl.

Brooder Room Management

Ducklings seem to thrive best if they are provided a thermal gradient and allowed to choose their own temperature. The temperature on the heated side of the enclosure should be about 95-99°F initially and then gradually decreased to about 70°F over a three-week period. It is important that chicks never become chilled. Although they may appear to recover when warmed, many affected chicks develop gastrointestinal problems or liver or kidney failure and die several days later.

With any brooding method, it is important to maintain a clean, dry, warm enclosure with an easily available supply of clean food and water. Drafts should be avoided.

Ducklings are ready for outside pens at two to four weeks of age. It is preferable to use an intermediate facility to acclimate the ducklings to the difference between the very controlled environment of the brooder room and the limited control of outside pens. Providing birds free choice to indoor or outdoor environment is optimal.

Neonatal Problems

The majority of losses during the first two weeks of life are associated with the poorly understood diagnosis of starveout. Starveout is a term coined by poultry pathologists to describe a condition of turkey poults wherein birds never start to eat; they starve after their yolk stores are depleted. Characteristically, deaths occur in waterfowl at 7-14 days of age; the birds have an empty, contracted gastrointestinal tract, a small yellow liver, a distended gall bladder and no fat stores. It has been shown that many species, especially in captive situations, require specific stimuli and encouragement to begin self-feeding, and a lack of these stimuli may contribute to the problem.

Scoters, Harlequins, Oldsquaw ducklings and other specialized species may be particularly difficult to get started eating and must be fed by hand and pampered for considerable lengths of time. Mallard ducklings may be used to stimulate feeding in reluctant eaters. It is easier to raise a brood of young rather than a single bird.

Simulating the natural conditions that a free-ranging hatchling would encounter may stimulate feeding behavior. Newly hatched Mandarin Ducks and Wood Ducks tend to calm down in the brooder and begin to eat after they have been tossed in the air and allowed to drop to the ground. As strange as this may seem, it works because these species are cavity nesters and young often fall 60 feet or more to the ground when they leave the nest. Wood Duck chicks feed best if a cotton floor mop is hung in the brooder.

Ducklings may become wet and chilled in a brooder or when moved to an outdoor area and exposed to heavy rains. A hair dryer can be used to dry the feathers and warm the body. Once the birds are dry, tube feeding with 0.25-3 ml of a prepared formula provides a quick energy source. Steroids, subcutaneous fluids and antibiotics may prevent secondary problems. Large doses of rapidly metabolized steroids (prednisolone sodium succinate 2 mg/60 g chick) should be repeated every 15 minutes (some chicks may require four or five doses) until the chick is warm and stabilized.

Gastrointestinal disorders seem to be particularly common in neonatal birds. A high energy requirement and the need to establish a resident flora in what is a sterile environment at hatching probably account for many of these problems. Impaction of the crop and ventriculus, and less commonly the colon, may be the only lesions seen at necropsy. A precise etiology is rarely identified although inappropriate or excessive food intake is often implicated. Impactions lead to putrefaction of the gastrointestinal contents causing inflammation of the gastrointestinal mucosa and frequently systemic intoxication.

Yolk Sac Disorders: The first is retention of the yolk sac. In general, persistence of the yolk past two weeks of age is abnormal and detrimental. Neonates depend on the yolk sac for the first two to three days of life and if the yolk is not absorbed, the birds will be malnourished. Maternal immunoglobulins, specifically IgG, are absorbed with the yolk. Improper absorption of the yolk could result in the same immunosuppression seen in mammals that do not ingest colostrum.

The yolk sac should be surgically removed if clinical signs, palpation and radiography indicate nonabsorption. Surgery usually is successful if performed before a bird becomes dyspneic. Clinical signs suggesting that surgery is necessary include swollen abdomen, dyspnea, exercise intolerance, inability to stand or walk, inappetence, weight loss or failure to grow. For surgery, birds are anesthetized with isoflurane and placed in dorsal recumbency with the legs pulled caudally. Birds should be given 0.016 ml/g body weight of a 50:50 mixture of 5% dextrose in lactated Ringer's solution and 0.9% sodium chloride to compensate for any blood loss during surgery.

A second syndrome, rupture of the yolk sac, can occur as a sequela to yolk sac retention or yolk sacculitis (the third yolk sac-related syndrome). Rupture can also occur following traumatic events in two- to three-day-old birds with normal yolk sacs. Death results from yolk-related peritonitis and shock. Yolk sacculitis and omphalitis can occur separately or concurrently in a bird and are most frequently associated with gram-negative organisms, especially *Salmonella* sp. and *E. Coli*. Omphalitis is characterized by edema and inflammation of the abdominal wall surrounding the umbilicus. Yolk sacculitis is characterized by enlargement, hyperemia and petechiation of the wall and greenish discoloration and coagulation of the yolk sac. In most cases, omphalitis and yolk sacculitis arise from contamination of the umbilicus. Incubator and brooder sanitation are crucial for prevention of yolk sacculitis.

Miscellaneous Microbial Infections: Bacterial infections in neonates usually cause a multisystemic, fatal septicemia. Bacteriemia occurs so quickly that the entry point for the bacteria cannot be determined. The incidence of bacterial septicemia can be reduced through sound brooder hygiene and by identifying and controlling infections in subclinical parents.

Nutritional Diseases

Angel Wing: This condition is also referred to as healed-over, slipped, crooked, rotating, tilt, sword, spear, reversed, airplane and dropped wing. Angel wing is apparently caused by the weight of the growing flight feathers placing excess stress on the weak muscles of the carpal joint. Gravity encourages the developing wing to hang and finally to twist outward. If untreated, the wing may remain in that position and the ligaments and bones will be permanently deformed. Simply taping the wing on itself (not to the body) in a normal position for three to five days is usually sufficient to correct the problem. Manganese deficiency and hypovitaminosis D_3 have been suggested as etiologies. Genetic factors, environmental influences or management practices have also been implicated. Angel wing seems to occur more commonly in birds fed ad libitum and provided inadequate areas for exercise.

Excessive energy, excessive protein or a deficiency of vitamin E have all been suggested as dietary factors in the occurrence of angel wing. Clearly, a balanced diet formulated for tropical and temperate waterfowl species is required.

Factors that may reduce the incidence of angel wing include exercise (swimming, diving) and plenty of grass and other green foods. Birds originating from low latitudes should not be fed high-energy, high-protein foods. It is clear that waterfowl chicks from different species must be treated differently. Birds originating north of the Arctic Circle should be provided constant light, plenty of water and a constant supply of food that is relatively high in protein. Those originating from equatorial regions should be provided 11 hours of darkness per 24 hours; these birds can consume comparatively less food of a lower quality.

Perosis: Also known as slipped tendon, perosis is characterized by enlargement of the hock, bending deformities of the tibiotarsal and tarsal metatarsal bones and medial luxation of the Achilles tendon.

Open reduction and stabilization of the luxated tendon are successful in some cases. An incision is made through the skin and over the posterolateral aspect of the joint midway between the displaced tendon and lateral condyle of the tibiotarsal bone. The tendon is dissected free of its trochlear and medial adhesions and reduced to its normal position in the trochlear groove. The tendon sheath is sutured to the lateral periosteum and retinaculum with simple interrupted 3-0 absorbable suture. The skin incision is closed with simple interrupted 4-0 nonabsorbable suture. A tongue depressor can be used as a splint for a week. The patient should be using its leg normally by the second postoperative week.

Nutritional Secondary Hyperparathyroidism: Ducklings whose diets are poor in calcium or contain excessive phosphorus may develop fibrous osteodystrophy or osteomalacia. The birds may appear reluctant to move. Abscesses or blisters of the keel often develop in birds that are nonambulatory. Soft bones and enlarged parathyroids are common postmortem findings.

Rickets: Rickets results from a lack of vitamin D. The first clinical signs are lameness, retarded growth and bent or twisted breast bones. Providing a proper diet will reverse the symptoms in two to four weeks unless advanced changes have occurred.

Restraint, Handling and Anesthesia

Heavy-bodied species should not be carried by using the wings or feet alone, although smaller species can be restrained by their wings. Smaller ducks can also be held by grasping the back and wings and using the thumb and fingers to restrain the feet. For larger birds, the base of both wings should be grasped with one hand while the other hand and arm supports the body. These birds should be carried under one arm, with their head facing to the back. The arm is wrapped around the wings and a hand used to support the body and control the legs. A wrap using Velcro adhesive straps or pillowcase-type bag with a hole in the end for the head and neck can be used for restraining waterfowl during certain examinations, blood collection and radiographic procedures.

Field Immobilization and Capture

Several agents have been used to immobilize free-ranging ducks or geese, with sodium amobarbital being the most frequently used. In test studies, an oral dose of 100 mg/kg was found to produce muscle incoordination approximately 20 minutes after ingestion. The test ducks never reached a plane of anesthesia but were immobilized sufficiently to allow easy capture. For field immobilization, one cup of hen scratch was mixed with 900 mg of dissolved amobarbital and allowed to dry in shallow pans (50 pounds of scratch will dry in about four hours with the aid of fans). Animals should not be approached for 60 minutes after feeding to ensure that they are adequately immobilized and will not fly to another location and die. Recovery may take up to eight hours.

The drug has a low therapeutic index and should be used only in a field setting when restraint is critical and all other methods of capture have failed. There was an eight percent mortality rate in one study of ducks. Half of these losses may have been prevented with post-capture gastrolavage or tubing with fresh water to dilute and accelerate passage of the drug.

Anesthesia

Local anesthesia is often sufficient for performing superficial procedures. Lidocaine hydrochloride (2%) is one of the safest local anesthetics for waterfowl; however, general depression can occur with high doses. Reasonable amounts relative to weight are usually safe and effective. Using 1 ml of 2% procaine in ducks and 3 ml in swans was found to provide good local anesthesia with few problems.

Isoflurane anesthesia is convenient for performing minor procedures, positioning for radiographs or major surgery. Mask induction and maintenance for short procedures (< 15 minutes), or mask induction followed by intubation for longer procedures are common. The neck must be extended in intubated, long-necked birds to prevent the trachea from folding over the end of the tube, causing partial or complete airway obstruction.

Induction times for gas anesthetics in waterfowl are frequently prolonged when compared to psittacines, probably due to the substantial subcutaneous fat deposits in the former. Recovery periods are also prolonged. Breathing amplitude (an indicator of tidal volume) has been shown to decrease by 40-50% and the frequency of respiration increases 20-50% when birds are in dorsal recumbency. This causes a 10-60% decrease in minute ventilation, probably due to visceral compression of the air sacs. Positive pressure ventilation can be used to decrease these effects. A peak positive pressure of 15-20 cm of water is adequate.

Cardiac monitoring of anesthetized waterfowl can be done with a doppler flow probe placed under the tongue, against the carotid artery or on the ventral surface of the elbow on the recurrent ulnar artery. An esophageal stethoscope or ECG can also be used. A rectal or esophageal thermometer is useful to monitor body temperature. Time of recovery from anesthesia is directly proportional to the amount of heat loss. The lower the body temperature, the longer the anesthetic recovery period.

Noninfectious Diseases

Bumblefoot

Bumblefoot is believed to be caused by rough, hard surfaces such as concrete pools or pens that cause trauma to the bottom of the birds' feet (see Chapter 16).

Treatment of bumblefoot is difficult and often unrewarding. If a bird is not lame, it may be best to forego treatment that frequently increases the severity of the problem. Suggested therapies that include surgical debulking of the lesion and medical management frequently fail. The bird must be maintained on soft footing during the recovery period. One common treatment is a topically applied combination of dimethylsulfoxide (DMSO) (30 ml), dexamethasone (2 mg) and chloromycetin succinate (200 mg) (or other appropriate antibiotics based on sensitivity). This is applied to the lesion every eight hours. Recovery may take three to six weeks. Another treatment includes daily cleaning of the lesion with iodine scrub followed by the application of camphor spirits (drying agent) and benzoin (toughens the tissues). Supplemental vitamin A and an improved diet may also be helpful (see Chapter 16).

Oil-contaminated Birds

Anseriformes are often affected by oil spills. Mortality of birds affected by oil spills often exceeds 80% but can be reduced to 15% with proper treatment (see Chapter 15).

U.S. Diagnostic Facilities for Resolving Problems in Anseriformes

The federal diagnostic facility is the U.S. Fish and Wildlife Service, National Wildlife Health Center, Madison, Wisconsin. Several states have active wildlife disease programs located at: Fairbanks, Alaska; Sacramento, California; Fort Collins, Colorado; Rose Lake, Michigan; Hampton, New Jersey; Delmar, New York; Fargo, North Dakota; Madison, Wisconsin; and Laramie, Wyoming.

There are three regional wildlife disease programs affiliated with universities. These include the Southeastern Cooperative Wildlife Disease Study, University of Georgia, Athens; Northeastern Center for Wildlife Disease, University of Connecticut, Storrs; and Colorado Wild Animal Disease Center, Colorado State University, Fort Collins. The University of Florida-Gainesville and Virginia Polytechnic Institute and State University-Blacksburg also have active wildlife disease programs. Cornell University has the Duck Research Laboratory located at Box 217, Eastport, New York 11941, telephone (516) 325-0600. The primary focus of the Duck Research Laboratory is on production duck management, nutrition and disease, but it also has involvement with wild fowl. The staff has considerable expertise and diagnostic capability available. The U.S. Department of Agriculture, Veterinary Services Laboratory, Ames, Iowa can also accept diagnostic specimens that have been submitted through appropriate channels.

Amyloidosis

Gross lesions include pallor and enlargement of the liver, spleen or adrenal glands. Less commonly affected organs include the pancreas, kidney, intestine, lung and heart.

The pathogenesis of amyloidosis appears to be complex and is poorly understood. Amyloidosis is found in association with a number of chronic primary diseases and can be induced by some types of immunization. Amyloidosis in domestic ducks has been associated with crowding and social stress. Although there is no treatment for amyloidosis, maintenance of environments with minimal stress and low exposure to infectious diseases should decrease its occurrence.

Capture Myopathy

Capture myopathy has been reported in Lesser Snow Geese and Ross's Geese that were captured with rocket nets and restrained for several hours. The only gross necropsy lesions were pallor of the skeletal muscles and pulmonary and hepatic congestion. The prevalence and importance of this condition in captured free-ranging waterfowl are unknown, but a small number of restrained birds are stiff and reluctant or unable to fly when released (see Chapter 48).

Botulism

Botulism (limberneck, western duck sickness, duck disease, alkali poisoning) occurs from the ingestion of toxins produced by the bacterium *Clostridium botulinum*. It is a paralytic, often fatal disease. The presence of carcasses of invertebrates and vertebrates, rotting vegetation, poor water quality and high temperatures promote growth of *C. botulinum*. High temperature and vertebrate carcasses also promote maggot infestations. Birds that eat maggots may consume the toxin at the same time.

The botulism toxin affects peripheral nerves and results in paralysis of voluntary muscles and an inability to sustain flight. Once paralysis of leg muscles has occurred, ducks may attempt to swim using their wings. By comparison, birds with lead poisoning retain their ability to walk and run. As the disease progresses, paralysis of the neck muscles results in an inability to hold the head erect. Death from drowning is common. Many affected waterfowl (75-90%) can be saved by being provided fluids, a cool environment and antitoxin. Removing toxins and maggots from the stomach by gavage may increase the recovery rate.

Disease prevention requires control of fluctuating water levels during hot summer months and a prompt removal of animal protein to decrease the source of toxin production and maggot infestations. A single waterfowl carcass can produce several thousand toxic maggots. A duck can become intoxicated by eating only two to four maggots. Carcasses should be buried or burned. A commercial type C toxoid is available for mink and has proven to be effective in birds. One-half of the dose recommended for mink can be used in birds.

Lead Poisoning

Clinical signs of lead intoxication include weight loss, weakness and depression, bright green diarrhea, anorexia and variable neurologic disorders such as leg paresis, wing droop and abnormal head tremors.

Blood (2-5 ml) should be collected in lead-free tubes containing sodium citrate. Treatment includes use of chelating agents such as calcium disodium EDTA, DMSA, PA and DTPA (see Chapter 37). Gastric lavage and endoscopy can be used to remove lead shot from the ventriculus. Birds are fasted for 8-12 hours, masked down with isoflurane and intubated. The bird is tilted, head down, at a 45° angle on the table. Large quantities of warm water are pumped into the ventriculus. Water pressure and gravity will force most of the food, grit and lead pellets out of the intestinal tract. Radiographs can be used to confirm that the lead pellets have been removed.

Zinc Poisoning

Zinc toxicity has been reported in captive Anseriformes following the ingestion of pennies minted after 1983 (containing 98% zinc) or metal fence clips (96% zinc). Clinical signs include weight loss, depression, anorexia and posterior paresis. Normal serum levels of zinc are 1.84-4.65 μg/g; normal liver levels are 34.9 μg/g. Abnormal levels seen in an affected group of ducks were 12.6-16.6 μg/g (serum) and 242-548 μg/g (liver). Treatment consists of endoscopic removal of the foreign bodies and chelation therapy (see Chapter 37).

Mycotoxicity

Mold-contaminated foods are frequently unpalatable and avoided by free-ranging waterfowl, while captive birds may be forced to consume the moldy food. Moldy food may contain more than one toxin, and analytical procedures for identification of toxins are not readily available.

Aflatoxin poisoning is caused by the metabolic byproduct of *Aspergillus flavis*, which can be found in feed (especially peanut products and corn). Aflatoxin has been associated with liver cirrhosis in older ducks. Nodular hypoplasia or hepatoma may occur in chronic cases. Young ducks exposed to aflatoxin die at one to two weeks of age, showing signs of inappetence, depressed growth, cyanosis of the feet and legs (caused by subcutaneous hemorrhages), ataxia, convulsions and opisthotonos. Gross lesions include a slightly enlarged, putty-colored liver, pale and slightly swollen kidneys, and petechiae on the kidneys and pancreas. In birds over three weeks of age, the liver is firm and slightly shrunken and has a reticulated pattern; ascites and hydropericardium and petechiation may also be noted.

Immunosuppression with chronic aflatoxicosis may be a problem with waterfowl as it is with some other species.

Fusariotoxicosis is caused by *Fusarium* spp. Their presence on cereal grains is important because of the variety of toxins they produce, including zearalenone (F_2) and tricothecene toxins (including T_2). Zearalenone was found to interfere with sperm production in ganders but not with egg production in geese. Clinical signs of T_2 intoxication include vomition, thirst and depression. Gross lesions were restricted to mucosal necrosis in the esophagus, proventriculus and ventriculus.

Ergotism is caused by toxic alkaloids formed by the fungus *Claviceps purpurea*. Heavy mortality was seen in two- to four-month-old Muscovy Ducks fed wheat containing 1.7% ergot sclerotia. The birds died 48 hours after developing lethargy and diarrhea. Older birds were not affected. Necrosis and gangrene of the extremities, which occur in mammals, have not been reported in waterfowl. Ergotism is unlikely in free-ranging waterfowl that have a choice of food.

Algal Toxins

Algae blooms usually occur in eutrophic waters in warm, sunny weather. Clinical signs may be peracute prostration and death, restlessness, blinking of the eyes, repeated swallowing, salivation and regurgitation. There is no specific treatment, but oral administration of charcoal and mineral oil has been suggested. Access to clean water and food should be provided. There are no specific histologic lesions and there are no tests to detect these toxins. Diagnosis is subjective and based on identifying toxic algae in an affected bird's environment and ruling out other etiologies of similar clinical signs. Algae blooms may be controlled in ponds with copper sulfate, or by increasing water flow to remove nutrients and dilute the algae; however, copper sulfate can also be toxic.

Marine Dinoflagellates

Waterfowl may be poisoned by mollusks living in areas affected by "red tides." Clinical signs include weakness, reluctance to fly, dehydration, nasal and oral discharge, lacrimation, edema of the nictitating membrane, bilateral mydriasis, chalky yellow diarrhea, tachypnea, tachycardia and depressed blood pressure. No specific gross or histologic lesions have been described. Recovery occurred rapidly when affected birds were placed in fresh water.

Chemicals

Fertilizers or pesticides should not be used around birds or where runoff may enter animal enclosures.

Tumors

Spontaneously occurring tumors are infrequently described in waterfowl. The tumors that do occur are histologically similar to those seen in mammals.

Egg-related Peritonitis

Egg-related peritonitis is life-threatening and requires intense and aggressive care.

Infectious Diseases

Aspergillosis

Aspergillosis is commonly seen at necropsy in Anseriformes. Diagnosis and treatment can be difficult (see Chapter 35).

Parasites

Schistosomes in the genera *Trichobilharzia* and *Dendritobilharzia* were considered the cause of high mortality rates (90%) in a group of geese. The principal pathologic changes included thrombosis of the caudal mesenteric vein, fibrinohemorrhagic colitis and hepatomegaly. This parasite is frequently found in waterfowl but is rarely associated with disease. Weight loss and lameness were the principal clinical findings. Parasites were identified in the lumen of the thrombosed vessels.

Proventricular Dilatation

A syndrome similar to that described with neuropathic gastric dilatation in Psittaciformes was documented in two free-ranging Canada Geese. The birds were found in an emaciated state. Postmortem findings included pectoral muscle atrophy and a dilated, thin-walled proventriculus. Nonsuppurative encephalitis with lymphoplasmacytic perivascular cuffing was the principal histologic lesion (see Chapter 32).

Common Surgical Procedures

Anseriformes normally have a high concentration of subcutaneous and intraabdominal fat, making the delineation of anatomic structures (particularly vessels) difficult. Blood that may be present on feathers following a surgical procedure should be carefully removed from goslings, ducklings or cygnets to prevent the parents from traumatizing the area through excessive grooming.

Pinioning

When waterfowl are one to four days of age, they can be quickly and easily pinioned without anesthesia. This procedure causes very little hemorrhage or stress to young chicks. Early pinioning obviates the need for a more complicated procedure at a later date.

continued on page 717

Table 46.9 Bacterial, Fungal; Viral and Parasitic Diseases of Anseriformes* (*see footnote page 715)

Disease/Agent	Host Range	Transmission	Clinical Signs	Treatment/Control
Aspergillosis *Aspergillus fumigatus*	All species varying susceptibility	Airborne spores; moldy litter or feed	Respiratory signs; chronic debility	Prevent exposure; surgical excision of affected tissue
Avian cholera *Pasturella multocida*	Most species highly susceptible; epidemics in wild waterfowl and aviaries, mortality up to 50%	In excrement and respiratory secretions; recovered birds are carriers	Peracute death; acute form - anorexia, dyspnea, diarrhea, mucoid oral discharge; chronic form - dyspnea, diarrhea	Isolate affected birds; burn/bury corpses; autogenous bacterin every three months; A, B, E, F, H*
Avian diphtheria, contagious epithelioma, avian pox, Poxvirus	Undefined, most Anseriformes; seen in Greenwing Teal, Canada and Hawaiian Geese, Mute and Tundra Swans, Mallard Duck	Mosquitoes, direct contact, skin wounds	Wart-like growths on unfeathered skin, dysphagia, dyspnea if lesions in pharynx	Self-limiting, course long; supportive care; control vectors; efficacy/safety fowl pox vaccine undetermined
Avian encephalomyelitis, epidemic tremors Picornavirus	All species; affects chicks 1-2 weeks old	Egg transmission possible	CNS signs in chicks, decreased egg production	No treatment, vaccinate
Avian influenza, fowl plague Orthomyxovirus	Ducks and other Anseriformes; rare; not reported in wild waterfowl	Inhalation, direct contact, excrement	Sinusitis - mild to severe, mucopurulent or caseous	Reduce stress and crowding, supportive care
Chlamydiosis, ornithosis *Chlamydia psittaci*	All species, young mainly; 20-70% mortality in ducklings possible	Excrement; inhalation; asymptomatic carriers	Conjunctivitis, rhinitis, sinusitis, diarrhea, weakness	Chlortetracycline 0.044% in feed 3-6 weeks; doxycycline
Colibacillosis *Escherichia coli*	All species; common	Excrement; ingestion	Septicemia, death, diarrhea, decreased hatchability, omphalitis, salpingitis, bumblefoot	Sanitation, antibiotics based on sensitivity; A, B, G*

Table 46.9 Bacterial, Fungal; Viral and Parasitic Diseases of Anseriformes*

Disease/Agent	Host Range	Transmission	Clinical Signs	Treatment/Control
Duck plague, duck viral enteritis Herpesvirus	Ducks, geese, swans; susceptibility varies; sporadic outbreaks, see in spring; mortality up to 100%	Excrement - ingestion or inhalation, free-ranging waterfowl carriers	Peracute death, hematochezia, depression, photophobia, epiphora	No therapy, live-virus vaccine, prevent access to carriers and outside water
Duck virus hepatitis Picornavirus	Seen in domestics; not reported in free-living waterfowl; ducklings 2-6 weeks old ≤ 90% mortality	Excrement; ingestion or parenteral	Peracute death within hours; sluggishness, paddling of feet, CNS signs	Hyperimmune serum, vaccinate breeders MLV vaccine before laying; vaccinate day old chicks
Eastern and western encephalomyelitis virus Alpha virus/Togavirus	All species; clinical disease rare; not reported in free-living waterfowl	Insect vectors	Asymptomatic or CNS signs; morbidity and mortality highest in chicks	None; vaccine for horses used in ratites and pheasants
Erysipelas *Erysipelothrix insidiosa*	All, 30% mortality in ducklings	Wound infection or ingestion	Depression, diarrhea, inappetance	D.* Bacterin for turkeys may be effective by SC or aerosol (ducklings)
Goose gonorrhea Neisseria-like organism	Geese, captive birds only	Direct cloacal contact; egg transmission	Cloacitis, inflamed/ulcerated phallus; 10% ganders die	
Goose virus hepatitis, goose influenza, goose plague Parvovirus	Common in Europe; not seen in US; domestic goslings < 30 days of age; mortality ≤ 80%	Highly contagious	Coryza, diarrhea, ataxia; survivors stunted, loss of feathers neck and back	Hyperimmune serum; attenuated virus vaccine in Hungary
Leukosis/sarcoma virus	All species; rare		Tumors of the parenchymous organs	

Table 46.9 Bacterial, Fungal; Viral and Parasitic Diseases of Anseriformes*

Disease/Agent	Host Range	Transmission	Clinical Signs	Treatment/Control
Necrotizing enteritis agent unknown, possible flagellate, enteric bacteria, *Clostridium* sp.	Seen in free-living waterfowl, captive geese, mallards; common in breeder ducks, mortality ≤ 40%	Stress predisposes	Depression, subcutaneous and pulmonary hemorrhages, mucoid necrotic enteritis	Neomycin sulfate 0.02% in food for 2-3 weeks; reduce stress
New duck disease, infectious serositis *Cytophaga* sp.	Ducks, geese, swans; sporadic outbreaks in wild; more common domestic flocks; ducklings = acute; older birds = chronic	Probably egg-transmitted	Lethargy, ocular discharge, diarrhea, ataxia, torticollis, often on back paddling legs, acute death	Reduce crowding; bacterin at 2-3 weeks of age; live vaccine experimental; A, C, D, H*
Newcastle disease Paramyxovirus NDV (serotype group 1)	All species; uncommon; few reports clinical disease	Fecal spread likely	Respiratory, conjunctivitis, gastrointestinal, CNS signs	Vaccination for poultry may be effective if legal; depopulate
Pseudotuberculosis *Yersinia* sp.	All species; not uncommon at end of severe winter	Contaminated food supply (rodents and wild birds)	Nonspecific clinical signs	
Reticuloendotheliosis Retroviruses	Unknown; rare; high mortality in 2-week-old domestic ducks	Unknown	Tumors of RE cells and organs	
Salmonellosis *Salmonella* spp.	All; rare in free-ranging; common in captivity, domestic ducklings disease < 2 weeks of age	Excrement; ingestion; carried by rodents, insects, water, wild birds	Depression, sudden death; acute septicemia, enteritis	Sanitation; remove carriers; antibiotics may reduce disease but not stop carriers; B, F, I*
Tuberculosis *Mycobacterium avian*	All; rare in free-ranging; common in captivity	Excrement	Emaciation, diarrhea, debility; often dead, no symptoms	Depopulate infected birds, flame environment; potential treat rare birds

Table 46.9 Bacterial, Fungal; Viral and Parasitic Diseases of Anseriformes*

Disease/Agent	Host Range/Transmission	Clinical Signs	Diagnosis	Treatment/Control
Acuaria *Echinuria uncinata australis*	Unknown	Daphnia is intermediate host	Proventricular ulceration, anorexia, weight loss, anemia, death	Increase water flow to decrease daphnia; J, L, M, N, O*
Air sac mites *Cytodites nudus*	Anseriformes are aberrant hosts		Seen in respiratory passages and air sacs	Difficult
Avioserpens taiwana	Ducks in Taiwan, Indochina and North America; cyclops is intermediate host	Parasite-induced masses, submandibular, thigh, shoulder		Remove masses
Capillariasis *Capillaria contorta*	All; rare	Occasionally, anorexia, dysphagia, diarrhea, necrotizing enteritis	Fecal flotation; barrel-shaped eggs, bipolar plugs; parasites in esophagus, crop, small intestine	J, K, L, N, O*
Cecal worms *Heterakis* sp.	All; rare	Common at postmortem; rarely clinical signs		
Coccidiosis *Eimeria* sp., *Tyzzeria* sp., *Wenyonella* sp.	All; common; mortality ≤ 10% in ducklings; direct transmission	Enteritis, emaciation, anemia, death, renal disease in geese	Fecal flotation; intestinal lesions with merozoites	Amprolium; B, C, Q*
Conjunctival worms *Oxyspirura mansoni*	All; rare	Conjunctivitis, blepharitis, epiphora	Direct visualization; slender, thread-like worms	Manual removal, dilute ivermectin topically
Gape worms of geese *Cyathostoma bronchialis*	Geese; mortality highest in goslings	Carrier adults	Parasite or eggs in tracheal mucus or feces; worms in bronchi and trachea	L, O, P*

Table 46.9 Bacterial, Fungal; Viral and Parasitic Diseases of Anseriformes*

Disease/Agent	Host Range/Transmission	Clinical Signs	Diagnosis	Treatment/Control
Gizzard worms (several nematode species)	Ducks, geese, swans; mortality highest in young; direct life cycle	Unthriftiness, ventricular dysfunction	Eggs in feces; hairlike worms under horny gizzard lining	K, L, N, O*
Heartworms Sarcoma eurycerca	Whistling Swan, Whitefaced Goose; rare	Depression, death, myocardial necrosis	Microfilaria in blood smear; 2-3 adults/host	Unknown
Leeches Hirudinea sp., Theromyzon	Many species; occasional	Anemia, conjunctivitis, asphyxiation, bloody nasal discharge		Drain and disinfect pond
Lice - shaftlice, wetfeather Holomenopen leucocytozoon	Unknown	Moist-appearing feathers; louse feeds on quill; severe irritation		Malathion powder
Lice - chewing Mallophaga spp.	All; common; life cycle 2-3 weeks	Mainly nonpathogenic; feed on feather debris, may cause local irritation	Adults or eggs on feathers	5% carbaryl powder
Ocular trematodes Philophthelmus gralli	Ducks, geese	Conjunctivitis, epiphora	Direct visualization 5 x 1.2 mm	Manual removal
Sarcocystis Sarcocystis ridleyi	Ducks, especially dabblers; more common in adults	Asymptomatic	Small white rice grain masses in muscles	Nonpathogenic
Schistosomiasis Dendritobilhargia pulverulenta	Diving ducks, geese	In arteries, not veins; multi-systemic signs; granulomatous encephalitis	Flukes in aorta and cranial branches	
Simulian black fly	Many species	Anemia, toxicity; transmit leukocytozoon & microfilaria		4% malathion inside buildings

Table 46.9 Bacterial, Fungal; Viral and Parasitic Diseases of Anseriformes*

Disease/Agent	Host Range/Transmission	Clinical Signs	Diagnosis	Treatment/Control
Spirurids *Streptocara* spp.	Ducks; common	Proliferative gastritis, vomiting, weight loss	Parasites in gizzard or under mucus lining gizzard and proventriculus	Unknown
Tapeworms	All; not uncommon; invertebrate or fish = intermediate host	Asymptomatic; catarrhal enteritis, diarrhea, emaciation	Fecal flotation; onchosphere proglottids in feces	R*
Tetrameres	Rare; grasshopper or anthropod is intermediate host.	Poor growth; proventricular dystrophy; anemia	Parasite in mucous glands proventriculus	J, K*
Toxoplasmosis *Toxoplasma gondii*	Geese	Anorexia, anemia, emaciation, diarrhea, CNS signs	Complement fixation; Sabin-Fellman Dye test	C, D*
Trematodes/flukes (numerous species)	Ducks, geese; not uncommon; mollusk is intermediate host	Unthriftiness, enteritis or hepatitis depending on location	Fluke eggs in feces	Difficult; O*

* see Chapters 18, 32, 33, 35 and 36 for further information; treatments: A — sulfaquinoxaline 0.025-0.05% in feed, or penicillin-streptomycin 50,000 U/kg IM; B — sulfadimethoxine-ormetoprim 0.02-0.08% in feed; C — sulfamethazine 0.2-0.25% in drinking water or feed; D — penicillin 50,000 U/kg IM; E — tetracycline 300-400 g/ton feed; F — chlorotetracycline 200-1000 mg/kg PO, 6-10 g/gal drinking water for days; G — lincomycin-spectinomycin IM; H — novobiocin 350 g/ton feed; I — furazolidone 0.022-0.044% in feed; J — piprazine 200-1000 mg/kg PO, 6-10 g/gal drinking water for four days; K — piprazine 45-200 mg/kg PO single dose or 6-10 g in 4 liters of drinking water; L — mebendazole 5-15 mg/kg PO for two days; M — thibendazole 100 mg/kg PO; N — thibendazole 200-500 mg/kg PO; O — levamisole 25-50 mg/kg PO; P — ivermectin 1% (200μg/kg SC); Q — furazolidone in the feed at 0.033% for 14-21 days; R — niclosamide (toxic to geese) 250 mg/kg PO, Droncit, Bunamadine PO.

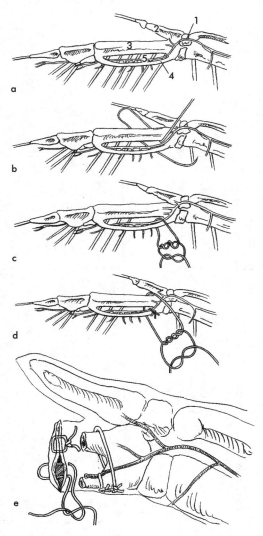

FIG 46.20 Pinioning renders a bird incapable of flight. **a)** Regional anatomy of the carpus: 1) ventral metacarpal artery 2) alula 3) metacarpal III 4) metacarpal IV and interosseous space. **b,c)** Feathers are removed from the carpus and a circumferential incision is made at the midpoint of the metacarpal bones. The skin and muscle are bluntly dissected and pushed proximally using a gauze pad to expose the metacarpal bones. A ligature of absorbable suture is placed around the proximal end of metacarpal IX to ligate the ventral metacarpal artery. **d)** A similar ligature is placed around metacarpal III, also incorporating as much interosseous tissue as possible. The metacarpal bones are excised with bone cutters. **e)** Horizontal mattess sutures are used to close a skin flap over the bone ends. Sufficient skin should be used to cover the bone to prevent pressure necrosis.

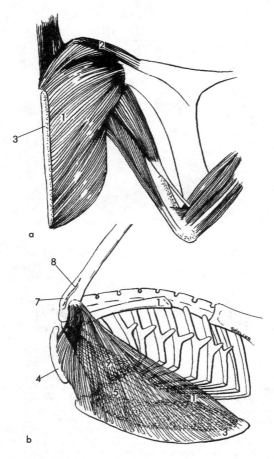

FIG 46.22 Superficial pectoralis tendonectomy for cosmetic deflighting: **a)** The insertion point of the 1) superficial pectoralis muscle and the 2) tensor propotagalis can be excised. **b)** A curvilinear incision (dotted line) is made from a point distal to the pectoral crest extending to a point proximal to the scapulohumeral joint. The wing is then extended fully over the bird's back and should approach the midline of the body. This places maximum tension on the tendon of insertion of the superficial pectoralis muscle. *(continued on next page)*

Toenail clippers, scissors or other cutting device (suture scissors and wire cutting scissors work well) are used for the procedure. The chick is held upside down, preferably with one wing outstretched, and the alula (second digit) is held out from the carpus. The third and fourth metacarpals are then cut as close to the alula and carpus as possible. This will remove all of the primary flight feathers. Although no further treatment is usually necessary, bleeding can be controlled with silver nitrate, Monsel's solution or radiosurgery. The stump can be sprayed with an antibiotic powder.

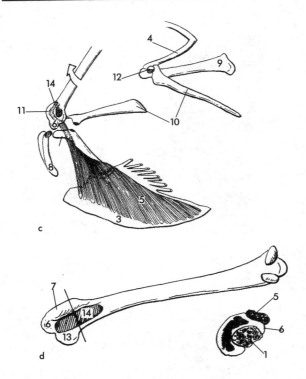

c) The superficial pectoralis muscle is removed at its insertion on the humerus. The insertion of the supracoradoideus muscle on the dorsomedial aspect of the coracoid must be avoided. A two- to three-cm section of the tensor propatagialis is removed. d) Anatomy of the head of the proximal humerus including a cross section showing the relationship of the superficial pectoralis and supracoracoideus muscles. 3) sternum 4) clavicle 5) supracoracoideus muscle 6) head of the humerus 7) dorsal tubercle 8) pectoral crest 9) coracoid 10) scapula 11) attachment of supracoracoideus muscle 12) triosseal canal 13) ventral tubercle and 14) insertion of the superficial pectoralis muscle.

In older birds, pinioning can be performed at the level of the carpus, but is usually performed at the proximal end of metacarpals III and IV. The procedure can be performed using a local anesthetic in a bird that is manually restrained or the bird may be anesthetized with isoflurane (Figure 46.20).

Although bandaging is not usually required, a pressure wrap may be placed over the stump for several days to control mild hemorrhage and protect the incision. Birds should be restricted from the pool for three to seven days to prevent water and bacteria from contaminating the incision. If tissue glue is used to seal the skin, the wound may be sufficiently protected to allow immediate release to water.

Tendonectomy

Suggested alternatives to pinioning include removal of the extensor carpi radialis tendon (tendonectomy) or a wedge resection of the propatagium (patagiectomy). Both techniques are cosmetically and functionally unacceptable.

Another form of tendonectomy involves removing the insertion point of the superficial pectoralis muscle. This will result in a bird that cannot fly but is cosmetically normal.

Beak Repair

Beak injuries that result in an inability to eat, drink and preen will occur in waterfowl. Various attempts at applying prosthetic bills have been described (see Chapter 42).

Air Sac Cannulation

Installation of an air sac cannula as emergency care for airway obstruction is described in Chapter 15. In Psittaciformes, this procedure is usually performed in the abdominal air sac. Successful cannulation of the clavicular air sac has been reported in Pekin Ducks. The clavicular air sac is located just under the skin in the area of the thoracic inlet and can be visualized with minimal dissection.

Castration and Caponizing

Ganders may become very aggressive during the breeding season. As an alternative to removing an aggressive bird, some clients will choose to have the animal castrated to prevent intermale fighting, reduce aggression toward people and prevent additional offspring. The procedure is performed on an anesthetized bird placed in lateral recumbency. The wings are extended and taped above the body. Geese are very muscular, so full caudal extension of the up leg is necessary to expose the surgery site. The area of the last two ribs cranial to the femur is plucked and prepped for surgery.

The lungs extend almost to the last intercostal space, so care is necessary when making a one-half-inch vertical incision between the last two ribs. Retractors are necessary to keep the ribs separated. Blunt dissection through the air sac reveals the testicle. Two curved hemostats are clamped between the testicle and body wall and left in place for two minutes. The outer hemostat is then pulled up and away from the other hemostat, tearing the testicle free. Minimal bleeding can be expected. Alternatively, two hemostatic clips may be applied between the testicle and body wall, taking care not to occlude the aorta or vena cava. The opposite testicle is removed in a similar manner. Several affected birds have been reported to maintain their original personality, but their bellicose nature associated with previous breeding seasons did not develop. This procedure can be most safely performed in young birds.

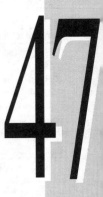

RAMPHASTIDAE

Hans Cornelissen
Branson W. Ritchie

These birds are indigenous to South America, ranging from southern Mexico to northern Argentina. Of the 43 species of toucans, toucanets and aracaris, only a few are frequently seen in captivity, including the Toco, Keel-billed, Red-billed and Channel-billed Toucans, and the Green Aracari (rare).

The *Ramphastos* spp. most commonly encountered as companion birds are the Toco and Keel-billed Toucans. If hand-raised, these birds are tame, easily handled and highly inquisitive. These large, active birds require plenty of space for exercise and produce a voluminous, moist excrement, which may account for the low numbers of these birds that are maintained as pets.

Gender Determination

Sexual dimorphism occurs in some Ramphastidae, while others are monomorphic and gender must be determined by endoscopy (Table 47.2). Spot-billed Toucans have individually distinct beak patterns that can be photographed and used for identification.

In general, male Ramphastids have a larger beak than females. To determine the beak's length, the lower margin of the upper mandible is measured from the edge of the facial skin outward toward the tip. In Toco Toucans, the beak of the male is generally greater than 16 cm in length, while in the female the measurement is less than 15.5 cm.

Behavior

Toucans can be loud and aggressive, particularly if untamed. Tame birds that are not given sufficient attention may also become very aggressive toward their keepers. Ramphastids are best restrained by initially removing them from the enclosure with a net or large towel. The bird can then be controlled by holding the beak in one hand and using a towel loosely wrapped around the body to control the wings and feet. Toucans should never be handled by the head and neck alone, as is commonly done with psittacine birds.

The active, curious nature of these birds often leads them to pick up and consume nonedible

Table 47.2	Gender Dimorphism	
Genera	Male	Female
Selenidera sp.	Black head feathers	Brown head feathers
S. culik	Black neck and underparts	Chestnut neck, grey underparts
Pteroglossus viridis	Black head feathers	Brown head feathers
P. inscriptus	Black head feathers	Brown head feathers

foreign bodies found in the enclosure (eg, rocks, pieces of wood, screws, string, coins). Resulting impactions can cause perforation or stasis of the gastrointestinal tract, which may lead to death. These birds are capable of being extremely destructive and can injure their beaks when biting on solid objects.

Toucans are active, inquisitive birds that are best housed as pairs in large flights with numerous, variably sized perches. These birds are carnivorous, and if housed in mixed-species aviaries may consume smaller aviary inhabitants.

Husbandry

An adequate maintenance diet for toucans would consist of fresh fruits (eg, melons, papaya, berries, tomatoes) supplemented with a low-iron, formulated diet. Paprika may be added to the diet to maintain the bright coloration of the beak. During the breeding season, the diet should be supplemented with crickets (up to 800 per day when a pair is raising chicks), small mice and crushed hard-boiled eggs. Fresh water for drinking and bathing should always be available. Toucans like to bathe and should be provided with large, easy-to-clean water containers.

The diet recommended for toucans is low in iron, which may reduce the chances of iron storage disease. The recommended level of iron for poultry is 40-60 ppm and the suggested diets for toucans approximate these levels. Many dog foods contain high levels of iron (up to 1500 ppm) and these high-iron foods should be avoided in a diet designed for Ramphastids. Grapes and raisins are also high in iron and should be avoided. Vitamin C enhances the absorption of iron, and citrus fruits should be offered on a limited basis.

These birds may normally pass some undigested food. Birds that are losing weight and consistently excreting undigested food should be evaluated.

Reproductive Characteristics

Toucans are best bred in large, planted flight enclosures with plenty of privacy. The walls of the enclosure should be covered with a cloth or plastic barrier to protect young chicks from collision injuries while they are learning to fly or, more appropriately, stop.

Courtship behavior is characterized by the males feeding the females, and both adults share incubation and rearing responsibilities. Sexual maturity generally occurs by three years of age.

Toco Toucans usually lay three to four eggs per clutch with an 18-day incubation period. Red-breasted Toucans usually have two to three eggs with a 16- to 17-day incubation period.

Toucan chicks may leave the nest within 45 days of hatch and are generally weaned from two to four months of age. Cannibalism of young chicks by the parents is common if the diet is not supplemented with crickets, mice or mealworms.

Toucan chicks have been successfully hand-raised from the egg. Initially, the diet consisted of small diced pieces of grape, banana, and pinkie mice soaked in water and offered by forceps. By three days of age, soaked monkey biscuit was added to the diet. The neonates were fed every two hours for the first twelve hours and then every three hours for 16 days, when the feeding frequency was reduced to four times per day. The eyes were open at three to four weeks of age. It is important to remember that these birds do not have a crop and should be fed smaller quantities and more frequently than psittacine neonates. Weaning may occur from two to four months of age. A neonate should be expected to gain weight daily and any weight loss is an indication of a problem. The weight should double each week.

Toucans can be anesthetized using isoflurane delivered through a modified face mask. Blood collection techniques are similar to those described for other avian species. Normal blood parameters are listed in the Appendix.

Diseases

Liver Disease

Toucans are frequently diagnosed with iron storage disease, liver cirrhosis and chronic acute hepatitis. They are among the species of birds most susceptible to iron storage disease. It remains unclear whether hemochromatosis in toucans is caused by hereditary factors, excess dietary iron or a defect in iron metabolism.

Toucans with hemochromatosis may die acutely with no premonitory signs or can develop clinical signs, including emaciation, dyspnea and abdominal enlargement (ascites). Affected birds typically have an enlarged, yellow liver with ascites. [*Editor's note: Liver biopsy may be the only reliable method of diagnosing the disease antemortem.*]

A low iron diet (< 150 mg/kg) and weekly phlebotomies to remove a blood volume equivalent to one percent of body weight have been suggested as methods to prevent hemochromatosis in Ramphastids with high serum iron levels.

Infectious Diseases

The normal aerobic and microaerophilic microflora of clinically normal toucans include *Escherichia coli, Staphylococcus* spp. and *Streptococcus* serotype D. These organisms were detected in the cloaca of 90% of 53 asymptomatic toucans representing five different species. *Klebsiella pneumonia* was recovered from 50% of the clinically normal Red-billed and Plated-billed Mountain Toucans examined in one study. Birds from aviaries with good hygiene had fewer gram-negative bacteria than birds from less well maintained facilities. However, the fact that pathogenic gram-negative bacteria were commonly recovered from normal birds suggests that toucans are able to withstand colonization of the gastrointestinal tract by these bacteria better than are psittacine birds.

Avian pseudotuberculosis (*Yersinia pseudotuberculosis*) has been documented as a cause of acute death following a brief period of lethargy in toucans. Infections are most frequently associated with a rapid bacteremia and peracute death. Postmortem findings include pneumonia, hepatomegaly and splenomegaly. The enlarged liver and spleen are generally covered with numerous raised, white-to-yellow-orange foci. Chronic debilitating infections have also been defined with *Y. pseudotuberculosis*. In these cases, bacteremia results in formation of granulomas in numerous parenchymatous organs.

Small rodents, such as mice and rats, which normally are part of the toucan diet, are known to carry *Y. pseudotuberculosis* and may serve as a reservoir for infection. The aviary should be rodent-proof, and only laboratory-raised mice and rats should be offered as food items.

An experimental *Y. pseudotuberculosis* vaccine appears to be clinically effective in reducing the prevalence of infections.

Parasites

Three species of *Plasmodium* (*P. huffi*, *P. nucleophilum tucani* and *P. rouxi*) have been documented in toucans. High levels of *P. huffi* usually result in death.

Fluke eggs and numerous giardia were found in the feces of a Red-bellied Toucan with loose droppings that contained undigested food. Metronidazole resolved the giardia infection in four days but had no effect on the flukes. Treatment with praziquantel (10 mg/kg) IM daily for three days followed by the same dose orally daily for 11 days was effective in stopping the passage of fluke eggs.

Giardia is frequently identified in fecal samples collected from asymptomatic toucans. Currently, no clinical disease has been associated with these infections.

Ascarids, coccidia and capillaria are other parasites frequently encountered in toucans. These infections are treated in a manner similar to those described for psittacine birds (see Chapter 36).

Metabolic Diseases

Idiopathic diabetes mellitus is frequently diagnosed in toucans. Weight loss, glucosuria (1 mg/dL), hyperglycemia (700 mg/dL often occur), polyuria and polydipsia are frequent clinical findings. The frequency with which this disease occurs suggests that the etiology is related to management or diet rather than genetic defects. Pancreatic islet cell tumors and hypothyroidism have also been suggested as causes for diabetes mellitus in toucans.

Protamine zinc insulin (0.1-0.5 units q12h) has been suggested as a possible treatment. However, maintaining proper blood glucose in toucans with insulin is difficult. Long-term therapy is generally associated with pancreatic atrophy, which causes pancreatic exocrine insufficiency, eventually leading to death.

A toucan being fed a fruit and dog food kibble diet was found to have diabetes mellitus with a blood glucose level of 1587 mg/dL. Changing the diet to a 100% formulated diet supplemented with prozyme reduced the blood glucose level to 365 mg/dL, suggesting this bird's diabetes was dietary related.

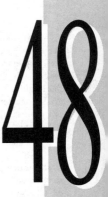

RATITES

James Stewart

There is no scientific classification "ratite," but the term is used to collectively describe the ostrich (from Africa), rhea (from South America), emu (from Australia), cassowary (from Australia and the New Guinea archipelago) and the kiwi (from New Zealand). Once considered to be a single category of related primitive birds, the ratites are now considered to be derived from unrelated groups of flighted birds that have adapted to a highly specialized terrestrial lifestyle.

Ostrich

The ostrich is the largest living bird, reaching over 200 kg in weight and 2.7 m in height. Four subspecies are currently recognized.

Struthio camelus camelus (North African ostrich) ranges from Morocco to Ethiopia and Uganda. A male *S. c. camelus* has a red coloration of the skin of the neck and thighs and a bald crown of the head. The hens of all races are indistinguishable. The eggs can be differentiated among subspecies, and those of the nominate species are characterized by fine stellate pores.

S. c. massaicus (East African or Masai ostrich) inhabits Kenya and Tanzania. The male has a red neck and thigh and the crown of the head is feathered.

S. c. molybdophanes (Somali ostrich) is found in Ethiopia and Somalia. The male has a blue-gray neck and thighs and the crown of the head is bald.

S. c. australis (South African ostrich) ranges throughout southern Africa. The neck and thighs of the male are gray and the head is feathered. The large pores in the shells of this subspecies leave the egg with a pitted appearance.

A hybridized ostrich that is a combination of *S. c. australis, S. c. massaicus* and *S. c. syriacus* is referred to as a "domestic" or "African black" ostrich. The careful breeding of this bird since the 1870s has resulted in a smaller, calmer bird that has higher quality feathers than its free-ranging relatives.

Rhea

Weighing 25 kg and standing 1.5 m in height, the rhea is the largest bird of the western hemisphere. Two distinct species are recognized. The Common Rhea ranges throughout the central continent, and as many as five subspecies have been described. Darwin's Rhea, including three subspecies, is a smaller bird residing in the eastern foothills of the Andes.

Cassowary

Cassowaries are stout, heavy-bodied birds reaching 85 kg in weight and 1.5 m in height. They are distinguished by a large bony casque on the forehead that is used to deflect brush as they dart through their dense rain forest habitat. Three species are found in New Guinea; one also ranges in northern Australia. Cassowaries are solitary, the males are highly aggressive and these birds adapt poorly to most captive settings.

Emu

Emus are closely related to cassowaries and share the same type of feather. The shaft and aftershaft are equally well developed, giving each feather the appearance of being doubled. The single existing species is found throughout Australia, while the Tasmanian and Kangaroo Island emus became extinct only in the past century. Adult emus may weigh 55 kg and stand 1.7 m in height.

Other Ratites

Included among the ratites is the kiwi, and frequently the tinamous. Both groups are specialized ground-dwelling birds that bear little resemblance and no relationship to the larger species.

Clinically Relevant Anatomy and Physiology

Musculoskeletal System

The ventral midline area of the abdominal wall consists only of the aponeuroses of the abdominal muscles. A surgical incision made along the midline penetrates the skin, subcutaneous fat (minimal) and a dense fibrous abdominal tunic. The next layer is retroperitoneal fat, which may be two to eight centimeters thick, especially in the emu. When a laparotomy is performed, the bulk of this adipose tissue should be peeled away prior to closing the body wall.

Respiratory System

Unlike other birds, the sternum is fixed and bears the weight of the resting ratite. Respiration occurs by lateral excursions of the chest wall, which must be considered during anesthesia and recovery.

Emus have a longitudinal cleft in the trachea 10-15 cm cranial to the thoracic inlet that opens into a resonation chamber for vocalization.

The presence of this expandable pouch may complicate inhalation anesthesia in mature emus. If positive pressure ventilation is used to inflate the air sacs and ventilate the lungs, air may be directed into and thus inflate the pouch. Inflation of the pouch can be prevented by wrapping the lower neck with a self-adhesive bandage, taking care not to place excessive pressure on the major vessels of the neck.

Digestive System

Ratites have no crop, and the large proventriculus serves the feed storage function. Material deposited into the esophagus during tube-feeding is routinely regurgitated, creating a risk for aspiration. Consequently, gavage feeding requires that a tube extend into the proventriculus.

The distal extremity of the ostrich proventriculus passes dorsal to the ventriculus and empties into this organ through a large opening on its caudal aspect. Ventricular foreign bodies can be easily removed through an incision made into the proventriculus.

Though the proventriculus and ventriculus can normally contain small stones, gastric impaction from the consumption of foreign bodies is a common problem in ratites, particularly in juvenile birds.

Reproductive System

Ratites of both genders possess a genital prominence that extends from the ventral aspect of the cloaca. This prominence may be visualized or palpated to determine the gender of any aged individual. Gender determination is easiest in chicks between one and three months of age. A lubricated gloved finger is used to expose the cranioventral aspect of the cloaca.

The male ostrich chick has a phallus that is conical in cross section, contains a palpable core of fibroelastic tissue and is characterized by the presence of a seminal groove. By comparison, the clitoris in the hen is laterally compressed, soft and lacks the seminal groove. The clitoris of the adult female remains approximately one to two centimeters in length. By six months of age the phallus of the male is approximately three to five centimeters in length and is readily detected on the ventral wall of the cloaca by palpation. The phallus of the adult male ostrich is "J"-shaped and when everted curves to the left. The phallus of the emu and rhea is considerably smaller, and the males are usually distinguished from females by the spiral conformation of the phallus.

Anatomic Considerations for Sample Collection and Supportive Care

Blood samples can be collected by routine venipuncture techniques used in most other avian species. Venipuncture can be performed using the jugular, brachial and medial metatarsal veins. The right jugular vein is larger than the left as in other avian species and is a convenient site for venipuncture or placement of intravenous catheters. The brachial vein is inaccessible in the reduced wings of the cassowary and emu, but is well developed in the large wings of the ostrich and can be easily accessed. The medial metatarsal vein is readily accessible in sedated or immobilized adult ratites and in unsedated chicks. The medial metatarsal vein generally is not used in standing adults due to the potential for being kicked. Reference hematologic and biochemical values for the ostrich, emu and cassowary are listed in the Appendix.

Intravenous catheters can be placed in any of the vessels used for venipuncture. The medial metatarsal vein is a common preference for intravenous catheterization of chicks. Catheterization of the brachial vein (18 ga) is preferred in adults. A 14 ga catheter can be placed in the jugular vein of an adult ostrich. Catheters should be secured in place using tissue adhesive followed by a light bandage.

Samples for cytology and for culture and sensitivity can be collected from the oviduct of adult hens (see Chapter 29). Abdominocentesis can be performed on birds with clinical signs suggestive of intestinal torsions, penetrating foreign objects, egg yolk peritonitis or retained eggs. A teat cannula is the safest device for use for abdominocentesis in ratites (see Chapter 10).

Oral medications are relatively simple to administer by orogastric tube to chicks or tractable adults. Occasional feedings can be provided by placing an equine stomach tube directly into the proventriculus; however, to perform gastric lavage or supply sustained enteral nutrition, an equine stomach tube is passed through an esophagostomy incision and is sutured into place. The tube is most easily placed by introducing it orally into the esophagus, making an incision over the cranial end of the tube and retracting it back through the incision. Blended canine maintenance kibble administered q8h has been suggested as an effective enteral nutrition product.

Subcutaneous medications can be given in the knee web cranial to the thigh.

The pectoral musculature of ratites is greatly reduced, and the large thigh muscles are frequently selected as a site for intramuscular injections. It has been suggested that this site may be inappropriate for the administration of nephrotoxic or renally excreted drugs because of the renal portal system. However, in one study involving the clearance of aminoglycoside, there was no difference in plasma levels when the drug was given in the posterior or anterior portions of the body. This finding suggests that the renal portal system may not be of importance when considering drug administration in ratites. The epaxial musculature along either side of the spine serves as an alternative site to the thigh muscles for IM injections.

Adult Bird Management

Identification

It is suggested that all ratites be permanently identified. The importance of properly identifying birds is dramatically illustrated by a case in which an ostrich was identified on a health certificate as an "African black" and was insured for twenty thousand dollars. The bird died, and at necropsy the veterinarian identified the bird as a "blue-necked" ostrich, and the animal was cremated. The insurance company declared that the dead bird was not insured.

The implantation of a microchip provides one fail-safe method of identification. Sterilized microchips can be implanted immediately after hatching in the left side of the pipping muscle approximately two to three centimeters below the ear. These chips help in the recovery of stolen birds, satisfy most insurance company requirements for identification and provide unmistakable identification for record keeping purposes.

Nutrition

In South Africa, range-raised ostriches are fed on alfalfa pastures supplemented with maize. Captive ratites seem to maintain a good state of health and reproduction when fed a diet that contains 16-20% protein, 10% fat and 10% fiber. Diets with 18% protein produced the best weight gains in one small nutritional study that compared only the effects of varying levels of protein. The calcium to phosphorus ratio should be about two to one.

The adequacy of the breeder diet is reflected in the eggs produced. Generally speaking, hens deficient in carbohydrates, proteins and fats produce fewer, smaller eggs. Vitamin and trace mineral deficiencies can result in nutrient-deficient eggs. The effects may be graded with the level of the deficiency. Characteristic lesions may be noted at various stages of incubation or several days post-hatch.

Thiamine deficiencies are thought to cause star-gazing, and riboflavin deficiencies may be a cause of curled toe deformities in ratite embryos. Pantothenic acid and biotin have been associated with curling of the feathers and hyperkeratosis of the skin, particularly around the mouth, beak, feet and neck.

In a group of ostrich chicks fed crushed corn, hypovitaminosis E was suspected to have been the cause of muscle degeneration. Vitamin E and selenium deficiencies also may occur in birds fed locally produced foods from regions with low levels of selenium in the soil.

Angular limb deformities are probably multifactorial, with decreased exercise, genetics and diets of high fat and protein all being involved.

Restraint and Transportation

Clients and veterinarians should be aware of the dangers associated with handling ratites and should be well versed in restraint techniques. Male ostriches are particularly aggressive during the breeding season and must be handled with caution. Any handling procedure is best performed in an area with solid walls in which the lights can be dimmed. Many basic procedures can be performed in these confined areas without the need for excessive physical restraint.

The natural defense of ratites is the kick, enhanced by the well developed toenails. Ostriches kick straight forward at chest level to the bird, followed by a downward sweep of the foot. Emus and cassowaries may kick either forward or backward and may incorporate wide lateral swings into the range of motion. All ratites jump with great agility, and when restrained, cassowaries roll onto their backs with their legs flailing.

When physical restraint is necessary, it is best to make slow, methodical movements. Working with untrained birds is an exercise in patience. It is important when handling chicks to use gentle restraint because rough handling can cause fractures, tendon damage and severe bruising. Whenever possible, larger chicks are usually herded rather than carried, but they may also be guided by placing one hand across the sternum and the other below the pelvis.

Most adult ostriches will become tractable when the head is covered with a dark, tight-fitting cloth hood, such as a sweatshirt sleeve. The sleeve is placed over the arm, the bird is grasped by the beak and the sleeve is then inverted over the head of the ostrich. The natural curiosity of a captive ostrich is usually sufficient to tempt the bird close enough to the handler to grasp the beak. A long smooth shepherd's hook can also be used to grasp the ostrich around the neck and lower the head, but the handler must be prudent of potential injuries to himself or the bird.

Ostriches may also be restrained without a hood if one person holds the head and neck horizontal to the ground while a second person provides upward and forward pressure to the pelvis. Grasping ostriches by the wings is a common cause of fractures and paralysis. Emus can be crowded into a corner and restrained by standing straddled over the bird's hips while holding the bird across the sternum with the hands.

Mechanical Restraint

Enclosures designed with catch pens, alley systems and stanchions facilitate the restraint of ratites. Facilities designed for cattle and horses usually include fencing inappropriate for use with ostriches. One side of the standard horse trailer is suitable to accomplish most procedures on an adult ostrich. A stanchion is used in the commercial feather industry to restrain ostriches for the clipping and plucking of feathers and is excellent for veterinary procedures. The stanchion consists of two thigh-high side-bars in the formation of a "V," with a strap to be placed over the shoulders and a bar to be positioned behind the legs and below the pelvis, thus restricting the bird's motion in all directions.

Chemical Restraint

The author's preference for smaller birds (under 20 kg) is face mask induction with four per cent isoflurane, followed by intubation and maintenance at two to three percent levels. Injectable agents are adequate for short procedures such as wound repair or casting in large birds. The author's agent of choice is tiletamine-zolazepam administered intravenously at 2-8 mg/kg depending upon the desired duration of anesthesia. Induction time is less than 15 seconds, and cardiac and respiratory functions are well maintained. The duration of anesthesia for a single dose is approximately 20-40 minutes, and supplemental doses may be administered as needed.

Alternatively, ketamine hydrochloride may be administered IV at 2-5 mg/kg when used in conjunction with either xylazine at 0.2-0.3 mg/kg or diazepam at 0.2-0.3 mg/kg. Ketamine alone gives unacceptable results.

For surgical anesthesia, large ratites are generally induced with low doses of tiletamine-zolazepam by intravenous administration and maintained on either 2-4% halothane or 2-4% isoflurane. Mature ostriches can be intubated using 14-18 mm cuffed endotracheal tubes. Intermittent positive pressure ventilation can be performed with a peak pressure of 15-20 cm of H_2O. The tidal volume of ratites is considered to be 10-15 ml/kg. Birds may become apneic immediately after or commonly at 15-20 minutes into anesthesia. These birds should be provided IPPV at 6-30 breaths per minute until $paCO_2$ levels have stabilized.

Bradycardia, apnea, hypercapnia, hypocapnia and movement are complications of anesthesia in ratites. Glycopyrrolate (0.011 mg/kg) was effective in reversing bradycardia (<30 bpm) in one bird. Heart rates in young ostriches at rest are normally 100-150 bpm and in the adults, 80 bpm. The respiratory rate in a group of anesthetized ostriches was 25-40 bpm and the heart rate was 65-70 bpm.

Ratites can easily injure themselves during the ataxic phase of anesthetic recovery, particularly following injectable agents. Extubation should occur in recovery when the bird is swallowing. Large, shaded areas, padded with mats or straw and clear of objects or walls within reach of the flailing legs can be used for recovery. Alternatively, a bird may be packed in a crate that is heavily padded with straw to restrict extension and flailing of the legs. Because ratites respire with lateral excursions of the chest, the sternal position for recovery is preferred. Small ratites can be recovered by wrapping them in a towel and using manual restraint. Adults should remain hooded with minimal disturbances. When the bird sits sternally with the head held upright, the hood should then be removed.

Transportation

The individual compartment of a standard horse trailer is well suited for the routine transport of one adult ostrich. The compartment should be modified to have solid smooth walls to the floor, and adequate traction can be provided by covering the floor with wet wood shavings or sand. Hauling birds at night tends to keep them calm and reduces the possibility of overheating. Food and water should be offered two to three times per day, but should be removed from the compartment while traveling.

Ostrich Management

Ostriches are gregarious in nature, with one male breeding several hens. The breeding group in intensive operations consists of one male and one to three females.

A paddock with 5,000 square feet would be considered minimum for a pair of adult ostriches. Fencing should be approximately two meters tall, clearly visible to a running bird and designed so that the feet or neck cannot become entangled within the fence. The bottom of the fence can be raised 40 cm from the ground to prevent the bird's legs and feet from becoming entangled. Stranded wire fence (barbed or smooth) should never be used for ratites.

Breeding Behavior

In general, ostriches reach puberty around two years of age, but are not at full reproductive maturity until four years of age. Birds in the northern US have a laying season from May to September, while birds in the southern US may produce all year.

Ostrich hens are indeterminate layers and if the eggs are removed, a hen may lay an egg every other day throughout the breeding season. Forty is the average for hens in captivity; however, some birds may produce 70-100 eggs per year.

Both sexes may have periods of reproductive quiescence within the breeding season, each lasting three or four weeks. During this time the female stops laying and the male "goes out of color" (ie, the bright red coloration of the face and tarsal scutes fades).

Emu

Breeding Behavior

Emus are managed in a manner similar to ostriches, but with proportionately smaller facilities. Emus are short-day breeders, with a breeding season that lasts from October to March in the United States.

Medical Disorders and Therapies

Many of the infectious diseases are shared by psittacines, waterfowl and other common companion and aviary birds. Sound management dictates that ratites should not be reared in close proximity to other types of birds.

Waste management, sanitation and human movement patterns within the flock are essential in preventing the transmission of infectious agents from paddock to paddock or from farm to farm. Ratite clinicians must be acutely aware of the role they can play in the transmission of disease through improper hygienic practices. New birds should be quarantined in an area separated from the remainder of the group for at least one month. During this period, the birds should receive a thorough physical examination and should be treated for parasites.

Reproductive Abnormalities

A diagnosis of reproductive tract disease is based upon the reproductive history, physical examination (including cloacal palpation and eversion of the phallus), and diagnostic tests including hematology and serum biochemistry, oviduct cultures, abdominocentesis, radiology and ultrasonography.

Prolapse of the phallus has been described in male ostriches. A partial prolapse may occur in reproductively active males with no adverse effects. The precise etiology is unknown, but debilitation toward the end of the breeding season and extreme weather fluctuations have been suggested as causes. Full prolapse requires replacement of the phallus into the cloaca, with or without a purse-string suture, and administration of nonsteroidal anti-inflammatory agents. If the phallus is traumatized, daily washes with a disinfectant solution and administration of systemic antibiotics may be indicated. The prognosis is good if the damage is not too extreme.

Intersex appears to be common in the ostrich. The black pigment of the male's feathers is due to a lack of estrogen. A mature

Table 48.2   Infectious Diseases Reported in Ratites

	Ostrich	Rhea	Emu	Cassowary
VIRAL				
Coronavirus	x			
Alphavirus			x	
Avipoxvirus	x	x	x	x
Influenzavirus type A	x			
Paramyxovirus type 1	x	x	x	x
BACTERIAL				
Bacillus anthracis	x			
Bordetella avium	x	x		
Clostridium botulinum	x			
Campylobacter jejuni	x	x		
E. coli	x	x	x	x
Edwardsiella tarda	x			
Pasteurella multocida	x			
Haemophilus paragallinarum	x	x		
Clostridium perfringens type C	x	x	x	
Clostridium colinum	x			
Salmonella spp.	x	x	x	x
Treponema sp.		x		
MYCOBACTERIAL				
Mycobacterium avium	x	x	x	
MYCOPLASMAL				
Mycoplasma sp.	x			
Mycoplasma synoviae	x			
Mycoplasma gallisepticum	x			
Mycoplasma meleagridis	x			
CHLAMYDIAL				
Chlamydia psittaci	x		x	
MYCOTIC				
Aspergillus fumigatus	x	x	x	
Aspergillus flavus	x		x	
Aspergillus niger	x			
Candida albicans	x	x	x	
Rhizopus oryzae	x			

black bird that sexes cloacally as a hen will not reproduce and may have inactive ovaries, testes or both. Many young hens may be very dark brown or even have a few black feathers, but become gray with maturity.

Prolapse of the vagina can occur without egg laying and may be seen in hens less than one year of age. These prolapses are thought to be caused by unseasonably cold temperatures. Replacement and application of a retention suture are usually corrective.

Peritoneal hernias occur in the caudal abdominal cavity, allowing the intestines and uterus to prolapse into the pericloacal region. Affected hens appear to have a large pericloacal swelling. Ultrasound is diagnostic. Surgical repair is required.

E. coli, Pseudomonas spp., *Acinetobacter* spp. and other gram-negative bacteria are common causes of oviduct infections in ostriches. Affected hens generally present with a history of erratic egg production, cessation of egg production or malformed or odoriferous eggs. The hen may have a discharge below the cloaca and may have a peculiar odor. Affected hens often have white blood counts ranging from 20,000-100,000 (pronounced heterophilia in acute cases or lymphocytosis in chronic cases); however, the severity of the infection varies with the etiologic agent. In mild cases, only the uterus or shell gland (metritis) may be affected, and in these hens clinical signs range from the formation of abnormal shells to the cessation of breeding.

Therapy for metritis should include appropriate antimicrobial therapy, multiple vitamin and calcium injections. Surgical (laparotomy) or nonsurgical (vaginal) flushing of the oviduct can be used to remove accumulated debris.

Egg binding may occur in ratite hens and is thought to be caused by genetic factors, malnutrition, cold weather or lack of exercise. Many affected hens are asymptomatic, while others may present with a history of tenesmus or with a vaginal prolapse. An impacted egg may be palpable in the caudal abdomen. Radiology or ultrasound may be required for diagnosis. Medical treatment consists of increasing the bird's ambient temperature along with the injection of multivitamins, calcium and oxytocin (prostaglandin may be superior, see Chapter 29). Impacted eggs should be removed surgically.

Gastrointestinal Abnormalities

Ingestion of foreign bodies is a common problem in ratites. These birds are likely to swallow anything that fits into their mouths, and their keen eyesight and curiosity all but ensure that they will find many unusual items in their pen. Stones, sand, hardware and long-stemmed grasses are common offenders. Ingestion of foreign bodies can be reduced by making certain that pastures and paddocks are covered with grass and do not contain abundant or clearly visible rocks or sand.

The most common clinical presentation includes lethargy accompanied by small, firm, fecal balls and a distended abdomen. Occasionally, affected birds may appear lame or be unwilling to rise due to weakness or pain. A cloacal prolapse may occur in chicks with proventricular impaction. Eighty-five percent of impactions occur in birds under six or seven months of age, with 10-12% occurring in birds six to twelve months of age and 3-5% occurring in adults.

An impacted proventriculus can frequently be palpated on the left side of the abdomen by identifying the caudal and dorsal extremities of this organ. Impactions with rocks or sand can best be detected by palpating caudal to the sternum. Impactions caused by grasses and leaves may be more difficult to palpate. Radiography can be used to document the presence of foreign bodies and an enlarged stomach. Ultrasound and gastroscopy may be other effective diagnostic techniques.

Psyllium administered by stomach tube may be effective in resolving mild cases of gastric distension, but true impactions can be resolved only by surgical removal of the foreign material. The proventriculus may be approached via either a midline or left paramedian incision that extends caudally from the caudal margin of the ventriculus. A 15 cm skin incision is made caudal to the end of the sternum just to the left of midline, and the peritoneum is incised to expose the proventriculus. Allis tissue forceps or stay sutures can be used to manipulate the proventriculus. The proventriculus is temporarily sutured to the abdominal wall to minimize contamination of the coelomic cavity with ingesta. The proventriculus is then incised and the contents are removed. Closure is in two layers with a simple continuous primary closure that is oversown with a continuous inverting suture pattern.

Birds can be offered alfalfa pellets and corn as soon as they are fully recovered from anesthesia.

Many ingested objects will penetrate the wall of the ventriculus or proventriculus causing peritonitis. The diagnostic procedures are the same as those used for gastric impaction. A proventriculotomy to remove the foreign body and surgical removal of necrotic peritoneum is indicated. Other common digestive disorders include cloacal prolapse and intussusception. Cloacal prolapse may be associated with diarrhea, or more frequently, with tenesmus due to constipation. Treatment of the prolapse is similar to methods used in other birds, but the initiating cause must be addressed to prevent recurrence. Intussusception is caused by hypermotility and gastrointestinal tract irritation and is often the result of an abrupt dietary change, especially when the new diet is higher in fiber.

Fractures

Tibiotarsal fractures in small birds under 15 kg are best repaired with a through-and-through, six-pin, modified external fixation device (see Chapter 42). Plates may be used in larger birds if bone quality is normal. Fractures of the phalanges, fractures of the distal metaphysis of the tarsometatarsus and luxations of the metatarsal-phalangeal or interphalangeal joints can be stabilized with fiberglass casts, to which most ratites readily adapt.

Wing fractures in ostriches frequently occur secondary to improper restraint. These may be resolved by placing the wing in a normal anatomic position and taping it to the body for six weeks; however, intramedullary pinning usually produces more satisfactory results. A small diameter pin may enter the distal caudal surface of the humeral shaft and be advanced through the fracture site into the proximal fragment. The wing is then taped to the body for a period of six weeks to provide rotational stability to the fracture site.

Ruptured Aorta

Ostriches are prone to spontaneous rupture of the aorta.

Degenerative Myopathy

A large percentage of the young ostriches, rheas and emus submitted for necropsy have evidence of degenerative myopathy. In birds, several etiologies for degenerative myopathy have been reported, including capture myopathy, selenium or vitamin E deficiency, furazolidone and ionophore toxicity. Clinical signs of degenerative myopathy that have been described in ratites include depression, reluctance to rise or move, and a rapid progression to death (two to five days).

Furazolidone is a nitrofuran antibiotic commonly used in the poultry industry. Ionophore coccidiostats, such as monensin, lasalocid and salinomycin, are frequently added to chick starter feeds. These compounds may be contributing factors in the development of degenerative myopathy, and ratite producers should avoid the use of turkey or chick starter feeds that contain furazolidone and ionophores.

Some authors believe that capture myopathy, which has been described in ratites with some frequency, is simply the acute manifestation of a chronic subclinical deficiency of selenium or vitamin E. Degenerative myopathy appears to be primarily a disease of young ratites and higher levels of vitamin E may be required for growth.

Therapy and Prevention

Treatment with vitamin E followed by immediate correction of the diet is the recommended therapy and is generally effective in early cases. It is probably safer to supplement a bird with vitamin E rather than selenium. The latter has a low therapeutic index and can readily reach a toxic level.

Neoplasms

Neoplasias have been reported in all ratites with none of particular prevalence. Lymphoid tumors have been described in ratites, and their similarity to tumors caused by leukosis virus in poultry warrants further investigation.

Viral Disease

Newcastle disease was the only disease of viral etiology reported in the ostrich prior to 1987. Recent international interest in ostrich production, particularly in the United States and Israel, has prompted further viral investigations. Numerous viruses have been detected in ratites by virus isolation or electron microscopy, but the clinical relevance of most of these findings is uncertain. Newcastle disease virus, coronavirus, reovirus, influenzavirus and togavirus have been associated with specific diseases.

Coronavial particles were reported in the small intestines of an 18-day-old ostrich chick that died following a one-week history of anorexia, lethargy, weakness and diarrhea.

Avian influenza was associated with high levels of mortality among ostriches in South Africa. Clinical signs in affected birds included respiratory signs, conjunctivitis, green discoloration of the urine and death.

Fowlpox infections are well documented in ostriches. This disease presents primarily as the dry form, although diphtheritic lesions may also occur. Vesicles that turn to encrustations form along the eyelids, ear openings, beak, neck and legs. Morbidity may be high but mortality is low. A commercial fowlpox vaccine administered at 10-14 days of age appears to provide some protection.

Eastern equine encephalomyelitis virus has been associated with high mortality (14 of 23 birds in one outbreak) among flocks of emus in the southeastern United States. Clinical signs include profuse hemorrhagic diarrhea, depression, ataxia and death. Terminally, affected birds may become recumbent and develop hemorrhagic hyperemesis. Paired serum samples can be used to document an increase in antibodies indicating an active infection. Some infected birds will respond to supportive care.

An inactivated equine vaccine is apparently effective in preventing the disease in emus. The initial vaccination is given at three months of age followed by boosters at six-month intervals. Written consent from the client and clearance from the insurance carrier should be obtained before the extralabel use of this vaccine is initiated.

Bacterial Disease

Clostridial enteritis is a common disorder in ratites of all ages and is often associated with the excessive consumption of wet soil. Botulism, clinically characterized by paralysis and death, has historically been a significant industry problem in adult ostriches in South Africa.

Tuberculosis is a common finding in adult ostriches. Affected birds develop a chronic wasting syndrome with visceral tubercles that can be detected by exploratory laparotomy. Salmonella outbreaks have been described in three- to six-week-old birds presented with acute weight loss, lethargy and bilaterally symmetrical distal limb edema. *Staphylococcus* sp. is frequently associated with omphalitis and septic arthritis.

Ostriches are the only birds susceptible to anthrax, and the symptoms and diagnostic methods are identical to those for mammalian hoofstock. Commercial anthrax vaccines are safe and effective in ostriches, following standard recommendations for hoofstock. The client and insurance company should provide written consent before the extralabel use of this vaccine.

Mycotic Disease

In South Africa, aspergillosis causes the condemnation of up to ten per cent of inspected ostrich carcasses. Granulomatous nodules are most frequently distributed through the parenchyma of the lung, and only occasionally in the air sacs (see Chapter 22). Infections in older birds are enhanced by the inhalation of dust from dry feeds and soil. Outbreaks in chicks are associated with prolonged antibiotic therapy or inadequate hatcher and brooder hygiene.

Candidiasis of the proventriculus, esophagus and mouth may occur in ostrich chicks. Infections are most common in birds maintained in damp environments or secondary to proventricular impaction or the long-term use of antibiotics. Chlorhexidine, ketoconazole or nystatin have been discussed as effective therapies. Candidiasis may be prevented with good hygiene and a dry environment.

Mycoplasma and Chlamydia

Serologic tests designed for poultry occasionally yield positive results. Mycoplasma have been identified on culture as well, but there is no firm evidence to implicate these microbes as the cause of clinical disease in ratites.

A pigeon-like isolate of chlamydia has been diagnosed in rheas and ostriches. Treatment of chlamydial infections in ratites with chlortetracycline (CTC) at the rate of 400 g per ton of feed for 45 days may be expected to be effective (see Chapter 34).

Parasites

Protozoa

Intestinal protozoa including *Cryptosporidium, Toxoplasma, Histomonas, Giardia* and *Trichomonas* spp. have been discussed as causes of severe and transient diarrhea in ratites (see Chapter 36). Coccidiosis is a common finding in emu chicks, but is not confirmed as a clinically important problem in ostriches.

Cestodes

The tapeworm *Houttuynia struthionis* is abundant on South African ostrich farms and has been seen sporadically in the United States. Chicks are particularly susceptible, becoming unthrifty with high mortality rates. The intermediate host is unknown, but infestations can be controlled with regular use of fenbendazole at 15 mg/kg orally.

Nematodes

The wireworm *Libyostrongylus douglassi* is an economically important parasite of ostriches. The adult worms and third and fourth stage larvae reside in the glandular crypts of the proventriculus. The resultant inflammation obstructs gastric secretions and inhibits digestion. Diagnosis is made by identification of the trichostrongyloid-type egg in the feces. The eggs can be confused with those of the harmless cecal worm, *Codiostomum struthionis*. Levamisole hydrochloride dosed at 30 mg/kg is routinely administered monthly to chicks and four times per year to adults. Fenbendazole (15 mg/kg) and ivermectin (0.2 mg/kg) are also considered to be effective.

Tracheal worms *Syngamus trachea* have been associated with hemorrhagic tracheitis in emus. The ostrich guinea worm, *Dicheilonema spicularum,* is a large filarial worm found in the subperitoneal connective tissue.

Filariid nematodes *Chandlerella quiscali* were removed from the spinal cord and lateral ventricles of the brain of emus with clinical signs that included torticollis, ataxia and abnormal gait followed by recumbency and death. Only two- to five-month-old emus were affected. Grackles are the normal host for *C. quiscali*, which is transmitted by *Culicoides* sp.

Prevention of this cerebrospinal nematode may be possible by control of the vector, elimination of the environmental conditions conducive to transmission of the parasite and prevention of larval migration. *Baylisascaris* sp. has also been shown to cause neurologic signs in ratites (see Chapter 36).

Arthropods

Ostriches are subject to infestation by a variety of external parasites, both host-specific and indiscriminate. The ostrich louse, *Struthiolipeurus struthionis*, is commonly found on ostriches worldwide. Infestation is easily diagnosed by identification of the nits glued to the barbs along the shaft of feathers, particularly under the wing. Ticks from a variety of mammalian, avian and reptile hosts have been reported to infest ostriches.

External parasites may be treated with monthly applications in five percent carbaryl or two to four percent malathion in either powder or liquid form. Benzene hexachloride is highly toxic to ostriches and should be avoided. Quill mites are responsive to monthly treatments with ivermectin at standard doses.

Respiratory Problems

Upper respiratory tract infections may be caused by bacteria, mycoplasma, fungi (*Aspergillus* spp.) or possibly viruses. Treatment is based on the etiology. Affected birds should be isolated immediately and flockmates should be carefully observed.

Ocular Problems

Cataracts are frequently seen in ostriches. They are more common in older birds, but may occur also in chicks only a few months of age. Bilateral cataracts must be removed, and surgery has been successful.

Lacerations, abrasions or ulcerations to the eye may cause epiphora or blepharospasms. Subpalpebral flukes may cause chronic epiphora in birds raised in moist areas.

Eye infections generally cause the production of a purulent discharge and will usually be bilateral. Cytology and cultures are necessary to determine the etiologic agent. Ocular discharges are common with upper respiratory infections. A blocked nasolacrimal duct is recognized clinically by epiphora and swelling within the lower lid. The lacrimal duct can be cannulated and flushed to determine if a blockage has occurred and to correct the problem.

Feather Loss (With or Without Skin Involvement)

Bacterial folliculitis has been described in ratites and is most commonly caused by *Staphylococcus* spp.

Feather picking can be caused by overcrowding, excessive exposure to light at night and a lack of available food. Feather picking is common in adult ostriches maintained in small, barren paddocks and may be a reflection of malnutrition or environmental stresses.

Neural Diseases

Toxins that can cause neurologic lesions in ratites may include plants, oil, grease and insecticides. Endotoxins produced by bacteria can lead to severe ataxia. Infectious causes of neurologic problems include viruses, bacteria, fungi or parasites. Paramyxovirus, EEE virus and Newcastle disease virus have all been associated with neurologic signs in ratites. Overheating may cause ataxia or seizures. The normal body temperature of ratites is approximately 103°F. Birds, particularly chicks, that are panting with extended wings are overheated. Treatment should include cold water baths. Hypoglycemia can cause ataxia and tremors in anorectic neonates. Oral or IV dextrose as well as tube feeding with high-carbohydrate diets three to four times daily is usually curative.

Hatchery Management

The Egg

Hatchability exceeding 90% of fertile eggs should be expected with well managed commercial ostrich operations. The maintenance of accurate records, including the analysis of unhatched eggs, is an absolute necessity for the elucidation of incubation and hatchery problems.

Shell quality is influenced by nutrition, disease and genetics, as well as by the conditions of the nest site and the egg handling methods.

Egg washing is a controversial issue in ratite production. It is better to provide the breeding pair with a clean, dry area in which to lay eggs rather than attempting to clean or disinfect dirty moist eggs.

Incubation

The minimum ventilation requirement for the incubation of ostrich eggs is calculated at 50 cubic feet of fresh air per hour per 100 eggs.

Ratite eggs should be incubated in the vertical position with the air cell end upward. Following poultry protocol, the egg rotation angle should be 45° from vertical, shifting a minimum of six times per day.

The weight loss of eggs is fairly linear throughout incubation, and weighing an egg weekly can be used to monitor an embryo's development and guide adjustments in humidity.

It is important to determine when mortality occurred in a dead embryo. Losing ten per cent of fertile eggs during incubation is considered normal, with peaks of loss at 3-4 days (organogenesis) and 40 days (respiration change) of incubation. Embryonic death at other times may be caused by incorrect incubation parameters, nutritional deficiencies in the egg, infectious agents, genetic abnormalities, improper egg storage or toxins.

Fluctuating incubation temperatures result in unthrifty chicks. High temperatures result in an early hatch, small dry chicks, increased embryonic mortality and malformations. Low temperatures result in soft, large, weak chicks with a delayed hatch. Excessive humidity (inadequate moisture loss from the egg) may cause a delayed hatch, small air cells, wet edematous chicks and mild degeneration of the leg muscles. Humidity that is too low (excess moisture loss from the egg) results in large air cells, increased malpositions due to sticky chicks (dry albumen), albumen plugs in the non-air cell end of the egg and weak, dehydrated chicks with poor survivability.

Hatching

Ratite eggs are transferred to a hatcher with the same temperature and humidity settings as the incubator three to five days prior to the anticipated date of hatch.

The social facilitation of pipping and hatching is strongly developed in ratite chicks, and light, sound and motion help stimulate a hatch.

Chick Management

Ratite chicks are precocial, hatching with a full coat of natal feathers, open eyes and the ability to stand within hours. They should be removed from the hatcher at one to two days of age and placed in brooder pens with other neonates that do not vary more than three weeks in age. Chicks should be expected to lose weight for three to five days following hatch and then to begin a steady increase in weight gain.

Young chicks should have access to supplemental heat that can be provided by infrared lamps, heated floors or space heaters. Chicks should be maintained at decreasing temperatures with age (90°F one to two weeks, 85°F to 12 weeks). Indoor flooring should be inedible, provide good traction and be easily cleaned. The general consideration for air circulation is 0.012 cubic feet per minute/per pound of bird for each degree F. For example, if the temperature is 70° and ten birds weighing 50 lbs each are in the space (500 lbs total), then the air exchange requirement is 0.012 x 500 x 70 or 420 cubic feet per minute.

As soon after hatching as ambient temperatures permit, chicks should be moved to outdoor grazing areas with fencing that is low to the ground and with holes no larger than 2.5 cm. Chicks should be considered cold-intolerant and provided supplemental heat in cold weather until they are six months of age. Chicks should be housed with birds of similar age to prevent injuries. Young chicks require constant attention to keep them tame and to quickly detect any developmental problems.

To reduce the chances of foreign body ingestion, chicks should be carefully monitored during their initial introduction to a pasture. Using a grassy area that has been well groomed (cut to three inches) and placing chicks with slightly older birds to serve as feeding models are the best techniques to introduce chicks to pasture. Initial introduction periods should be 10-15 minutes in length with daily doubling of the time in the paddocks.

Chick Problems

"Wet" is the term applied to chicks that have not lost sufficient weight during incubation and are consequently edematous at hatching. Most birds will lose the excess water several days after hatch.

"Sticky" Chicks

This condition occurs when the inner shell membrane is excessively dry, causing the chick to stick to the membrane. Assisted hatching is mandatory in these chicks or they will not survive.

External Yolk Sac

If the umbilicus does not close properly, the yolk will protrude from the abdomen to varying degrees. In mild cases, the yolk can be placed in the abdomen, the umbilicus covered with antibiotic ointment and gauze, and the abdomen wrapped with self-adherent bandage. Systemic antibiotic therapy should be initiated immediately. If a large quantity of the yolk sac is externalized or the umbilicus has sealed, the yolk sac should be surgically removed. The prognosis for chicks with externalized yolk sac is poor.

Retained Yolk Sac

Chicks that fail to absorb the yolk sac are generally weak, depressed and may peck erratically at the air with or without their eyes closed. A distended abdomen in a depressed chick less than two weeks old is a characteristic finding.

Retained or infected yolk sacs may represent 15-40% of a chick's total body weight and should be surgically removed in conjunction with the administration of broadspectrum antibiotics. *E. coli* is frequently cultured from retained yolk sacs. To remove the yolk sac, the chick is placed in dorsal recumbency and the abdomen is prepared for surgery. The skin is incised circumferentially around the umbilicus and the incision is extended transversely at the three and nine o'clock positions to the lateral distance required to allow easy removal of the intact yolk sac. The body wall is then incised in a corresponding pattern being careful to not damage the underlying yolk sac. The yolk sac is exteriorized by placing gentle traction on the umbilical stump. The yolk stalk is clamped, clipped or ligated just distal to the intestine to allow the stalk to be transected and the yolk sac to be removed. The body wall is closed with a monofilament, absorbable material in a simple continuous pattern. Broadspectrum antibiotic therapy is indicated pending culture results. Trimethoprim-based antibiotics can be administered until the results of yolk sac culture and sensitivities are available. Some chicks begin to eat and gain weight within a day or two of surgery while others require nutritional support by tube-feeding for several days before they resume normal growth.

Stress

Young chicks require a stable social group that might include a parental figure in the form of a natural parent, older counselor chick or a human substitute. Complete social isolation of young chicks is tantamount to death.

Management systems in which chicks are transferred through a series of pens are disturbing to the birds. Relocating or mixing chicks from different groups may alter the social structure causing some chicks to be harassed or rejected by dominant birds.

Musculoskeletal Disorders of Chicks

Rolled toe in ostrich chicks is a problem frequently seen in backyard operations the first few days after hatching. In ostriches, rolled toe syndrome seems to be caused by genetic abnormalities, incubation problems or inappropriate substrates during the first week of life while the phalanges are mineralizing. A firm flat surface such as packed dirt or concrete induces proper toe formation. Rolled toe deformities may be corrected with a variety of simple splints.

Rotational and angular deformities of the legs are a common problem in the rearing of all ratite chicks and should be viewed primarily as a management problem. Leg deformities are more common in birds that are pushed to grow too fast (high-protein, high-fat diets) combined with reduced exercise, and are maintained in areas with poor footing (sand, straw, Astroturf). Weight gains should be linear, and several days of excess weight gain may induce bone deformities. Chicks are best raised on moderate protein diets (20%) in large pastures with plenty of room for exercise.

Treatment of afflicted individuals can be attempted with a variety of external splints and slings or by derotational osteotomy and fracture repair, but the prognosis is exceptionally poor. Rerotation following surgery commonly occurs.

Spraddle Leg

Spraddle leg is caused by a deformity in the coxofemoral joint that prevents the legs from being adducted. This condition, usually associated with edematous chicks, is manifested by the legs being directed laterally resulting in the inability to stand. Hobbling the legs with a self-adherent bandage or placing the chick in a restrictive box that forces the legs together is usually effective if initiated immediately after the problem is noted. The problem can be prevented by ensuring proper weight loss of the egg during incubation.

Ruptured or Slipped Achilles Tendon

Rupture or slippage of the Achilles tendon may occur secondary to valgus or varus deformities of the leg. Manganese deficiency has been suggested as a possible predisposing factor. Management practices must be scrutinized if multiple cases occur in a flock. Feed analysis, feeding frequency, exercise programs, concurrent rotations or angular deformities are areas to evaluate. Surgical repair can be attempted (see Chapter 46).

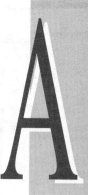

Conversion Factors: SI Units / Gravimetric Units

Analyte	To convert From	To	Multiply by	To convert From	To	Multiply by
Albumin	g/dL	g/L	10.0	g/L	g/dL	0.1
Ammonia	µg/dL	µmol/L	0.5871	µmol/L	µg/dL	1.7
Bilirubin	mg/dL	µmol/L	17.1	µmol/L	mg/dl	0.059
Calcium	mg/dL	mmol/L	0.25	mmol/L	mg/dL	4.0
Chloride	mEq/L	mmol/L	1.0	mmol/L	mEq/L	1.0
Chloride	mg/dL	mmol/L	0.272	mmol/L	mg/dL	3.5
Cholesterol	mg/dL	mmol/L	0.02586	mmol/L	mg/dL	38.7
Corticosterone	µg/dL	nmol/L	28.9	nmol/L	µg/dL	0.0346
Cortisol	µg/dL	nmol/L	27.59	nmol/L	µg/dL	0.0362
Creatinine	mg/dL	µmol/L	88.4	µmol/L	mg/dL	0.0113
Globulin	mg/dL	g/L	10.0	g/L	mg/dL	0.1
Glucose	mg/dL	mmol/L	0.05551	mmol/L	mg/dL	18.0
Insulin	µU/ml	pmol/L	7.175	pmol/L	µU/ml	0.1296
Iron	µg/dL	µmol/L	0.1791	µmol/L	µg/dL	5.58
Lead	µg/dL	µmol/L	0.04826	µmol/L	µg/dL	20.72

Conversion Factors: SI Units / Gravimetric Units

Analyte	To convert			To convert		
	From	To	Multiply by	From	To	Multiply by
Magnesium	mEq/L	mmol/L	0.5	mmol/L	mEq/L	2.0
Magnesium	mg/dL	mmol/L	0.4114	mmol/L	mg/dL	2.43
Phosphate (inorganic)	mg/dL	mmol/L	0.3229	mmol/L	mg/dL	3.097
Potassium	mEq/L	mmol/L	1.0	mmol/L	mEq/L	1.0
Pressure	mmHg	Pa (pascal)	0.1333	Pa (pascal)	mmHg	7.5
Progesterone	ng/dL	nmol/L	0.032	nmol/L	ng/dL	31.25
Protein	g/dL	g/L	10.0	g/L	g/dL	1.0
Sodium	mEq/L	mmol/L	1.0	mmol/L	mEq/L	1.0
Thyroxine	μg/dL	nmol/L	12.87	nmol/L	μg/dL	0.0777
Triglycerides	mg/dL	mmol/L	0.01129	mmol/L	mg/dL	88.5
Urea	mg/dL	mmol/L	0.167	mmol/L	mg/dL	6.0
Urea nitrogen (BUN)	mg/dL	mmol/L	0.7140	mmol/L	mg/dL	1.4
Urea nitrogen (BUN)	mg/dL	mmol urea/L	0.3670	mmol urea/L	mg/dL	2.72
Uric acid	mg/dL	mmol/L	59.48	mmol/L	mg/dL	0.0168

Biochemistry and Hematology Reference Ranges for Selected Psittacine Species*

Determination	African Grey	Amazon	Lovebird	Budgerigar	Parakeet	Cockatiel	Cockatoo
Alkaline phosphatase (U/L)	20-160	15-150	10-90	10-80	20-120	20-250	15-255
ALT (U/L)	5-12	5-11	-	-	-	5-11	5-11
AST (U/L)	100-365	130-350	110-345	145-350	145-395	95-345	145-355
Amylase (U/L)	210-530	205-510	-	-	-	-	-
BUN (mg/dL)	3.0-5.4	3.1-5.3	-	-	-	2.9-5.0	3.0-5.1
Calcium (mg/dL)	8.5-13	8.5-14	8.5-14	6.5-11	6.5-13	8.0-13	8.0-13
Cholesterol (mg/dL)	160-425	180-305	95-335	145-275	150-400	140-360	145-355
Creatinine (mg/dL)	0.1-0.4	0.1-0.4	0.1-0.4	0.1-0.4	0.1-0.4	0.1-0.4	0.1-0.4
CO$_2$, total (mmol/L)	13-26	13-26	14-25	14-25	14-24	13-25	14-25
CPK (U/L)	165-412	55-345	52-245	90-300	50-400	30-245	95-305
GGT (U/L)	1.0-10	1.0-12	2.5-18	1.0-10	1.0-12	1.0-30	1.0-45
GLDH (U/L)	0-9.9	0-9.9	0-9.9	0-9.9	0-9.9	0-9.9	0-9.9
Glucose (mg/dL)	190-350	190-345	195-405	190-390	205-345	200-445	185-355
LDH (U/L)	145-465	155-425	105-355	145-435	145-445	120-455	220-550
Lipase (U/L)	35-350	35-225	-	-	-	30-280	25-275
Phosphorus (mg/dL)	3.2-5.4	3.1-5.5	3.2-4.9	3.0-5.2	3.0-5.3	3.2-4.8	2.5-5.5
Potassium (mmol/L)	2.9-4.6	3.0-4.5	2.1-4.8	2.2-3.9	2.3-4.2	2.4-4.6	2.5-4.5
Sodium (mmol/L)	157-165	125-155	132-168	139-165	138-166	130-153	130-155

Biochemistry and Hematology Reference Ranges for Selected Psittacine Species*

Determination	African Grey	Amazon	Lovebird	Budgerigar	Parakeet	Cockatiel	Cockatoo
Total bilirubin (mg/dL)	0-0.1	0-0.1	0-0.1	0-0.1	0-0.1	0-0.1	0-0.1
Total protein (g/dL)	3.0-4.6	3.0-5.0	2.4-4.6	2.5-4.5	2.3-4.7	2.4-4.1	3.0-5.0
Triglycerides (mg/dL)	45-145	49-190	45-200	105-265	55-250	45-200	45-205
Uric acid (mg/dL)	4.5-9.5	2.3-10	3.5-11	4.5-14	4.5-12	3.5-10.5	3.5-10.5
Bile acids (μmol/L)	20-85	20-98	25-95	20-65	25-78	25-85	20-70
T_4 (μg/dL)	0.3-2.1	0.1-1.1	0.2-4.3	0.5-2.1	0.6-2.3	0.7-2.4	0.7-4.1
Pre-albumin (g/dL)	0.03-1.35	0.35-1.05	-	-	-	0.8-1.6	0.24-1.18
Albumin (g/dL)	1.57-3.23	1.9-3.52	-	-	-	0.7-1.8	1.8-3.1
Alpha-1 (g/dL)	0.02-0.27	0.05-0.32	-	-	-	0.05-0.40	0.05-0.18
Alpha-2 (g/dL)	0.12-0.31	0.07-0.32	-	-	-	0.05-0.44	0.04-0.36
Beta (g/dL)	0.15-0.56	0.12-0.72	-	-	-	0.21-0.58	0.22-0.82
Gamma (g/dL)	0.11-0.71	0.17-0.76	-	-	-	0.11-0.43	0.21-0.65
A/G ratio	1.6-4.3	1.9-5.9	-	-	-	1.5-4.3	2.0-4.5
WBC (x 10³)	5.0-11	6.0-11	3.0-8.5	3.0-8.5	4.5-9.5	5.0-10	5.0-11
RBC (x 10⁶)	2.4-3.9	2.4-4.0	2.3-3.9	2.4-4.0	2.2-3.9	2.2-3.9	2.2-4.0
HCT (%)	38-48	37-50	38-50	38-48	36-48	36-49	38-48
Hb (g/dL)	1.0-16	1.0-17.5	3.0-18	2.0-16	2.0-16	1.0-16	1.5-16

Biochemistry and Hematology Reference Ranges for Selected Psittacine Species*

Determination	African Grey	Amazon	Lovebird	Budgerigar	Parakeet	Cockatiel	Cockatoo
MCV (fl)	90-180	85-200	90-190	90-200	85-195	90-200	85-200
MCH (pg)	28-52	28-55	27-59	25-60	25-60	28-55	28-60
MCHC (g/dL)	23-33	22-32	22-32	23-30	24-31	22-33	21-34
Hets (%)	55-75	55-80	50-75	50-75	50-75	55-80	55-80
Eos (%)	0-2	0-1	0-1	0-2	0-2	0-2	0-2
Baso (%)	0-1	0-1	0-1	0-1	0-1	0-2	0-1
Mono (%)	0-3	0-3	0-2	0-2	0-2	0-2	0-1
Lymphs (%)	25-45	20-45	25-50	25-45	25-45	20-45	20-45

*University of Miami Avian and Wildlife Laboratory
Methods - Routine chemistry: Lithium heparinized plasma, 24 hrs after sample acquisition analyzed on Kodak Ektachem and Dupont Analyst machinery; Total protein by refractometer; Protein fractions by electrophoresis; Bile acids and T_4 by RIA; Hematology: Absolute numbers determined by Unopette method/hemacytometer; Spun HCT; Hemoglobinometer for Hb determination

Biochemistry and Hematology Reference Ranges for Selected Psittacine Species*

Determination	Conure	Macaw	Eclectus	Senegal	Pionus	Quaker	Jardine's
Alkaline phosphatase (U/L)	80-250	20-230	150-250	-	-	-	-
ALT (U/L)	5-13	5-12	5-11	-	-	-	-
AST (U/L)	125-345	100-300	120-370	100-350	150-365	150-285	150-275
Amylase (U/L)	100-450	150-550	200-645	-	-	-	-
BUN (mg/dL)	2.8-5.4	3.0-5.6	3.0-5.5	-	-	-	-
Calcium (mg/dL)	7.0-15	8.5-13	7.0-13	6.5-13	7.0-13.5	7.0-12	7.0-13
Cholesterol (mg/dL)	120-400	100-390	130-350	-	130-295	-	-
Creatinine (mg/dL)	0.1-0.4	0.1-0.5	0.1-0.4	0.1-0.4	0.1-0.4	-	-
CO_2 total (mmol/L)	14-25	14-25	14-24	-	-	-	-
CPK (U/L)	35-355	100-300	220-345	100-330	-	-	-
GGT ((U/L)	1.0-15	1.0-30	1.0-20	1.0-15	-	-	-
GLDH (U/L)	0-9.9	0-9.9	0-9.9	-	-	-	-
Glucose (mg/dL)	200-345	145-345	145-245	140-250	125-300	200-350	200-325
LDH (U/L)	120-390	70-350	200-425	-	-	-	-
Lipase (U/L)	30-290	30-250	35-275	-	-	-	-
Phosphorus (mg/dL)	2.0-10	2.0-12	2.9-6.5	-	2.9-6.6	-	-
Potassium (mmol/L)	3.4-5	2.0-5	3.5-4.3	-	3.5-4.6	-	-
Sodium (mmol/L)	135-149	140-165	130-145	-	145-155	-	-

Biochemistry and Hematology Reference Ranges for Selected Psittacine Species*

Determination	Conure	Macaw	Eclectus	Senegal	Pionus	Quaker	Jardine's
Total bilirubin (mg/dL)	0-0.1	0-0.1	0-0.1	-	-	-	-
Total protein (g/dL)	3.0-4.2	2.1-4.5	4.0-4.4	3.0-4.2	3.2-4.6	3.0-3.8	2.8-4.0
Triglycerides (mg/dL)	50-300	60-135	70-410	-	-	-	-
Uric acid (mg/dL)	2.5-11	2.5-11	2.5-11	2.3-10	3.5-10	3.5-11.5	2.5-12
Bile acids (µmol/L)	20-45	20-75	10-65	20-85	-	-	-
T$_4$ (µg/dL)	0.5-2	0.5-2.3	0.5-2.5	-	-	-	-
Pre-albumin (g/dL)	0.18-0.98	0.05-0.7	0.4-1.04	-	-	-	-
Albumin (g/dL)	1.9-2.6	1.24-3.11	2.3-2.6	-	-	-	-
Alpha-1 (g/dL)	0.04-0.23	0.04-0.25	0.09-0.33	-	-	-	-
Alpha-2 (g/dL)	0.08-0.26	0.04-0.31	0.11-0.27	-	-	-	-
Beta (g/dL)	0.07-0.47	0.14-0.62	0.17-0.43	-	-	-	-
Gamma (g/dL)	0.12-0.61	0.10-0.62	0.18-0.55	-	-	-	-
A/G ratio	2.2-4.3	1.6-4.3	2.62-4.05	-	-	-	-
WBC (x 10^3)	4.0-11	6.0-12	4.0-10	4.0-11	4.0-11.5	4.0-10	4.0-10
RBC (x 10^6)	2.5-4.0	2.4-4.0	2.4-3.9	2.4-4.0	2.4-4.0	2.3-4.0	2.4-4.0
HCT (%)	36-49	35-48	35-47	36-48	35-47	35-46	35-48
Hb (g/dL)	12.0-16	11.0-16	11.5-16	11.0-16	11.0-16	11.0-15	11.0-16

Biochemistry and Hematology Reference Ranges for Selected Psittacine Species*

Determination	Conure	Macaw	Eclectus	Senegal	Pionus	Quaker	Jardine's
MCV (fl)	90-190	90-185	95-220	90-200	85-210	90-200	90-190
MCH (pg)	28-55	27-53	27-55	27-55	26-54	26-55	26-56
MCHC (g/dL)	23-31	23-32	22-33	23-32	24-31	22-32	21-33
Hets (%)	55-75	58-78	55-70	55-75	50-75	55-80	55-75
Eos (%)	0-2	0-1	0-1	0-1	0-2	0-1	0-1
Baso (%)	0-1	0-1	0-2	0-1	0-1	0-2	0-1
Mono (%)	0-2	0-3	0-2	0-2	0-2	0-3	0-2
Lymphs (%)	25-45	20-45	30-45	25-45	25-45	20-45	25-45

University of Miami Avian and Wildlife Laboratory

Serum Biochemical Values for Juvenile Eclectus Parrots

Parameter	30-day Mean (SD)	90-day Mean (SD)	All Mean (SD)
NA (mEq/L)	141 (2)	154 (3)	148 (6)
K (mEq/L)	2.9 (1.0)	2.7 (0.6)	2.8 (0.7)
CL (mEq/L)	105 (3)	115 (3)	111 (5)
CA (mg/dL)	9.5 (0.5)	9.1 (0.4)	9.3 (0.4)
PHOS (mg/dL)	7.9 (0.8)	5.7 (0.9)	6.8 (1.2)
UREA (mg/dL)	1.5 (2.3)	2.0 (3.1)	1.7 (2.4)
CREAT (mg/dL)	0.3 (0.1)	0.4 (0.1)	0.4 (0.1)
UA (mg/dL)	0.8 (0.9)	3.9 (1.5)	2.0 (1.6)
CHOL (mg/dL)	181 (43)	300 (69)	268 (80)
GLUCOSE (mg/dL)	249 (16)	265 (19)	258 (18)
LDH (IU/L)	235 (145)	268 (70)	228 (101)
AST (IU/L)	85 (21)	216 (47)	140 (58)
ALT (IU/L)	4 (3)	7 (3)	4 (3)
ALP (IU/L)	421 (85)	565 (217)	489 (159)
GGT (IU/L)	5 (2)	2 (1)	4 (2)
CK (IU/L)	555 (164)	643 (262)	616 (472)
TP (g/dL)	2.6 (0.4)	2.9 (0.4)	2.9 (0.5)
ALB (g/dL)	1.2 (0.2)	1.3 (0.2)	1.3 (0.3)
GLOB (g/dL)	1.3 (0.3)	1.6 (0.3)	1.5 (0.3)
A:G (ratio)	0.9 (0.1)	0.8 (0.1)	0.9 (0.2)
ALB (Elect) (g/dL)	1.8 (0.5)	2.1 (0.4)	2.2 (0.4)
GLOB (Elect) (g/dL)	0.7 (0.2)	0.7 (0.2)	0.8 (0.2)

Hematology Values for Juvenile Eclectus Parrots

Parameter	30-day Mean (SD)	90-day Mean (SD)	All Mean (SD)
RBC (x 10^6 /µl)	1.95 (0.28)	3.22 (0.51)	2.69 (0.67)
HB (g/dL)	8.83 (1.15)	15.42 (2.38)	12.46 (3.01)
HCT (%)	33.7 (4.4)	53.8 (3.0)	43.8 (8.4)
MCV (fl)	174 (25)	169 (27)	166 (26)
MCH (pg)	43.9	49.1 (9.9)	45.5 (10.7)
MCHC (g/dL)	26.1 (2.5)	28.7 (4.1)	27.7 (5.0)
WBC (cells/µl)	18500 (6900)	10900 (3700)	13700 (6300)
WBC Est (cells/µl)	17000 (6000)	10500 (4000)	13500 (6000)
BANDS (%)	0.2 (1.1)	0.4 (0.9)	0.5 (1.5)
HET (%)	62.8 (7.7)	52.1 (10.2)	53.9 (11.4)
LYMPH (%)	30.4 (6.3)	40.8 (10.4)	39.5 (11.5)
MONO (%)	5.5 (3.0)	5.2 (2.7)	5.0 (2.7)
EOS (%)	0.0 (0.0)	0.1 (0.4)	0.1 (0.3)
BASO (%)	1.2 (1.0)	1.5 (1.0)	1.1 (1.0)
BAND # (cells/µl)	34 (188)	48 (111)	70 (221)
HET # (cells/µl)	11800 (5400)	5900 (2800)	7700 (4800)
LYMPH # (cells/µl)	5500 (2100)	4200 (1200)	5100 (2000)
MONO # (cells/µl)	930 (520)	532 (331)	639 (428)
EOS # (cells/µl)	0	9 (43)	8 (44)
BASO # (cells/µl)	209 (199)	175 (158)	152 (169)
HET: LYMPH (ratio)	2.2 (0.8)	1.4 (0.6)	1.6 (0.8)
PP (Refrac) (g/dL)	2.8 (0.6)	3.9 (0.6)	3.5 (0.8)

Hematology Values for Juvenile Cockatoos

Parameter	30-day Mean (SD)	90-day Mean (SD)	All Mean (SD)
RBC # (x10^6/μl)	196.(0.22)^a	2.84 (0.49)^b	2.53 (0.63)
HB (g/dL)	8.12 (0.83)^a	14.04 (1.23)^c	11.43 (2.90)
HCT (%)	30.1 (2.8)^a	47.6 (4.1)^c	39.7 (9.0)
MCV (fl)	155 (17)^a	172 (28)^b	160 (23)
MCH (pg)	38.9 (11.7)^a	49.0 (12.9)^b	43.8 (10.8)
MCHC (g/dL)	24.6 (7.9)^a	28.5 (6.2)^{bc}	27.2 (6.1)
WBC# (cells/μl)	13700 (7400)^a	10000(2800)^b	12900(6300)
WBC Est (cells/μl)	13200 (6700)^a	10400 (2800)^b	13100 (5900)
BAND (%)	1.3 (2.3)^{ab}	1.3 (2.3)^{ab}	1.3 (2.3)
HET (%)	54.8 (9.7)^a	49.0 (8.1)^b	50.8 (11.7)
LYMPH (%)	36.4 (8.1)^a	43.6 (8.4)^b	41.2 (11.9)
MONO (%)	6.9 (3.4)^a	4.9 (3.4)^{bc}	5.8 (3.4)
EOS (%)	0 (0)	0 (0.2)	0 (0)
BASO (%)	0.6 (0.9)^{ac}	1.2 (1.1)^b	0.9 (1.1)
BAND # (cells/μl)	150 (275)^a	130 (290)^a	160 (325)
HET # (cells/μl)	7800 (5000)^a	4400 (2200)^b	6500 (4500)
LYMPH # (cells/μl)	4900 (2600)^a	3900 (2000)^a	4900 (2500)
MONO # (cells/μl)	880 (530)^a	440 (450)^a	690 (525)
EOS # (cells/μl)	0 (0)	0 (0)	0 (0)
BASO # (cells/μl)	67 (130)^a	115 (130)^a	100 (140)
HET: LYMPH (ratio)	1.6 (0.6)^a	1.2 (0.4)^b	1.4 (0.8)
PP Est (Refrac) (g/dL)	2.3 (0.5)^a	4.0 (0.8)^b	3.2 (0.9)

a,b,c = Values for parameters are statistically different (P<0.05) when letters are different.

Serum Biochemical Values for Juvenile Cockatoos

Parameter	30-day Mean (SD)	90-day Mean (SD)	All Mean (SD)
NA (mEq/L)	139 (3)[a]	150 (3)[c]	145 (6)
K (mEq/L)	4.0 (0.8)[a]	3.1 (0.4)[b]	3.6 (0.7)
CL (mEq/L)	105 (4)[a]	115 (4)[c]	110 (6)
CA (mg/dL)	9.2 (0.6)[a]	9.5 (1.0)[ab]	9.6 (0.7)
PHOS (mg/dL)	7.0 (0.6)[a]	5.1 (1.0)[c]	6.1 (1.1)
UREA (mg/dL)	1.6 (1.9)[a]	2.6 (2.5)[b]	2.0 (2.2)
CREAT (mg/dL)	0.31 (0.06)[a]	0.42 (0.07)[ab]	0.4 (0.1)
UA (mg/dL)	1.2 (0.9)[a]	5.1 (1.8)[c]	2.9 (2.3)
CHOL (mg/dL)	165 (32)[a]	350 (122)[b]	251 (105)
GLU (mg/dL)	247 (20)[a]	249 (29)[ab]	253 (24)
LDH (U/L)	393 (348)[a]	367 (218)[a]	371 (285)
AST (U/L)	98 (54)[a]	195 (73)[c]	143 (79)
ALT (U/L)	2 (2)[a]	3 (3)[ab]	2 (3)
ALP (U/L)	593 (202)[a]	478 (167)[c]	579 (239)
GGT (U/L)	2.35 (1.75)[a]	2.79 (1.54)[ac]	2.55 (1.67)
CK (U/L)	595 (205)[a]	368 (156)[b]	510 (235)
TP (g/dL)	2.2 (0.4)[a]	3.1 (0.6)[b]	2.8 (0.7)
ALB (g/dL)	0.8 (0.2)[a]	1.2 (0.3)[b]	1.1 (0.3)
GLOB (g/dL)	1.3 (0.4)[a]	1.9 (0.4)[b]	1.7 (0.5)
A:G (ratio)	0.6 (0.2)[ab]	0.6 (0.1)[b]	0.6 (0.2)
PRE ALB (g/dL)	0.4 (0.1)[a]	0.5 (0.2)[b]	0.5 (0.2)
ALB (Elect) (g/dL)	1.1 (0.3)[a]	1.7 (0.5)[bc]	1.5 (0.5)
ALPHA GLOB (g/dL)	0.2 (0.1)[a]	0.3 (0.2)[c]	0.2 (0.1)
BETA GLOB (g/dL)	0.3 (0.2)[a]	0.3 (0.1)[a]	0.3 (0.1)
GAMMA GLOB (g/dL)	0.2 (0.1)[a]	0.3 (0.1)[b]	0.3 (0.1)

a,b,c = Values for parameters are statistically different (P) when letters are different.

Hematology Values for Juvenile Macaws

Parameter	30-day Mean (SD)	90-day Mean (SD)	All Mean (SD)
RBC# (x 10⁶/μl)	1.9 (0.3)ᵃ	3.7 (0.5)ᶜ	2.9 (0.8)
HB (g/dL)	7.7 (0.9)ᵃ	15.4 (1.0)ᶜ	12.3 (3.3)
HCT (%)	30.9 (3.3)ᵃ	49.5 (2.5)ᶜ	41.7 (8.4)
MCV (fl)	165.5 (25.4)ᵃ	137 (19.2)ᶜ	149 (24.7)
MCH (pg)	41.7 (6.1)ᵃ	42.8 (5.8)ᵃ	42.3 (6.2)
MCHC (g/dL)	25.1 (1.9)ᵃ	31.1 (1.3)ᵇ	28.7 (2.9)
WBC (cells/μl)	19300 (8300)ᵃᵇ	17700 (4900)ᵇ	19200 (6900)
WBC Est (cells/μl)	17700 (5100)ᵃᵇ	18300 (4500)ᵃᵇ	18600 (5880)
BANDS (%)	0.8 (1.6)ᵃ	0.3 (1.2)ᵃ	0.6 (1.7)
HET (%)	58.9 (11.1)ᵃ	53.9 (9.4)ᵃᵇ	55.3 (10)
LYMPH (%)	33.8 (9.7)ᵃ	41.6 (9.6)ᵇᶜ	39.0 (10)
MONO (%)	5.9 (3.3)ᵃ	3.6 (2.0)ᵇ	4.4 (2.9)
EOS (%)	0 (0)ᵃ	0.1 (0.2)ᵃ	0 (0.2)
BASO (%)	0.7 (0.9)ᵃ	0.6 (1.2)ᵃᵇ	0.5 (1.0)
BANDS # (cells/μl)	134 (344)ᵃ	59 (230)ᵃ	110 (313)
HET # (cells/μl)	10200 (7600)ᵃᵇ	9400 (4000)ᵇᶜ	10100 (5800)
LYMPH # (cells/μl)	5500 (3100)ᵃ	7000 (2500)ᵇ	6800 (3200)
MONO # (cells/μl)	910 (643)ᵃ	627 (418)ᵇ	750 (545)
EOS # (cells/μl)	0 (0)ᵃ	9.3 (51)ᵃ	4.6 (35)
BASO # (cells/μl)	115 (190)ᵃ	75 (165)ᵃᵇ	91 (175)
HET: LYMPH (ratio)	2.0 (1.0)ᵃᵇ	1.4 (0.6)ᵇᶜ	1.6 (0.8)
PP (refrac) (g/dL)	1.8 (0.40)ᵃ	3.5 (0.4)ᶜ	2.9 (0.8)

a,b,c = Values for parameters are statistically different (P<0.05) when letters are different.

Serum Biochemical Values for Juvenile Macaws

Parameter	30-day Mean (SD)	90-day Mean (SD)	All Mean (SD)
NA (mEq/L)	137 (1.4)a	151.1 (2.5)c	145 (6.2)
K (mEq/L)	3.3 (0.5)a	2.7 (1.0)b	2.9 (0.8)
CL (mEq/L)	101 (4)a	112 (3)c	106 (5.5)
CA (mg/dL)	9.5 (0.5)a	10 (0.5)b	9.9 (0.5)
PHOS (mg/dL)	7.3 (0.6)a	5.6 (0.6)c	6.5 (1.0)
UREA (mg/dL)	1.0 (1.7)a	3.4 (2.2)c	2.4 (2.3)
CREAT (mg/dL)	0.4 (0.1)a	0.4 (0.1)a	0.4 (0.1)
UA (mg/dL)	0.6 (0.4)a	3.9 (1.2)c	2.3 (2.1)
CHOL (mg/dL)	119 (37.2)a	231 (48.9)c	165 (62.0)
GLU (mg/dL)	264 (32)a	290 (27)b	281 (30)
LDH (U/L)	131 (75)a	114 (55)a	138 (84)
AST (U/L)	84(17)a	127 (36)b	104 (31)
ALT (U/L)	3 (2)a	4 (2)a	3 (2)
ALP (U/L)	1072 (346)a	786 (276)b	970 (397)
GGT (U/L)	2.0 (1.0)a	1.2 (1.2)b	1.8 (1.2)
CK (U/L)	596 (330)ab	442 (280)b	550 (312)
TP (g/dL)	1.7 (0.3)a	3.0 (0.3)c	2.6 (0.6)
ALB (g/dL)	0.7 (0.2)a	1.4 (0.2)c	1.2 (0.3)
GLOB (g/dL)	0.8 (0.4)a	1.5 (0.4)c	1.3 (0.6)
A:G (ratio)	0.7 (0.4)a	0.9 (0.1)b	0.8 (0.3)
PRE ALB (g/dL)	0.2 (0.1)a	0.5 (0.1)c	0.3 (0.1)
ALB (Elect) (g/dL)	1.0 (0.3)a	1.8 (0.3)c	1.5 (0.4)
ALPHA GLOB (g/dL)	0.2 (0.1)a	0.3 (0.1)a	0.3 (0.1)
BETA GLOB (g/dL)	0.3 (0.1)a	0.4 (0.1)a	0.3 (0.2)
GAMMA GLOB (g/dL)	0.2 (0.1)a	0.3 (0.2)a	0.3 (0.1)

a,b,c = Values for parameters are statistically different (P<0.05) when letters are different.

Normal Hematologic and Biochemical Values in Toucans

Parameter	Value
RBC (10^3/mm^3)	2.5-4.5
WBC (10^3/mm^3)	4.0-10.0
PCV (%)	45-60
Buffy Coat (%)	0-1
Hets (%)	35-65
Lymphs (%)	25-50
Basos (%)	0-5
Eosins (%)	0-4
Thromb	present
Calcium (mg/dL)	10-15
Glucose (mg/dL)	220-350
LDH (U/L)	200-400
AST (U/L)	130-330
TP (g/L)	30-50
UA (mg/dL)	4-14
Iron (μg/dL)	<350
TIBC (μg/dL)	<550

Blood Chemistry in Canary Finches

Parameter	Mean Value	SD	$P_{2.5}$-$P_{97.5}$
Ca (mg/dL)	7.99	1.84	5.1-13.4
P (mg/dL)	3.28	1.21	1.6-5.6
Na (mmol/L)	139.2	8.18	125-154
Cl (mmol/L)	108.88	8.85	93-123
K (mmol/L)	3.58	0.69	2.7-4.8
Gluc (mg/dL)	345.88	30.27	291-391
Trig (mg/dL)	184.78	55.46	120-312
Crea (mg/dL)	0.48	0.25	0.1-1
NH3 (mmol/L)	221.18	110.42	87-467
ALT (U/L)	11.58	7.92	2-30
AST (U/L)	98.93	34.73	45-170
LDH (U/L)	1582.63	325.72	1580-1816[male] 1300-1632[female]
AP (U/L)	265.05	79.62	146-397
Chol (mg/dL)	165.45	44.52	110-286
Amyl (U/L)	481.78	141.84	277-787
CK (U/L)	302.1	106.94	177-556
TP (g/dL)	2.84	0.75	2.0-4.4
Uric (mg/dL)	8.93	3.31	4.3-14.8

Kodak Ektachem®-25°C.

Plasma Chemistry Reference Values for Racing Pigeons

Parameter	$P_{2.5}$-$P_{97.5}$
Sodium (mmol/L)	141-149
Potassium (mmol/L)	3.9-4.7
Calcium (mmol/L)	1.9-2.6
Magnesium (mmol/L)	1.1-1.8
Inorganic phosphorus (mmol/L)	0.57-1.33
Chloride (mmol/L)	101-113
Plasma iron (μmol/L)	11-33
Iron binding capacity (mmol/L)	30-45
Osmolality (mOsm/kg)	297-317
Glucose (mmol/L)	12.9-20.5
Creatinine (μmol/L)	23-36
Urea (mmol/L)	0.4-0.7
Uric acid (μmol/L)	150-765
Urea:Uric acid (ratio)	1.8 ± 1.8 (mean ± sd)
CPK (U/L)	110-480
AP (U/L)	160-780
AST (U/L)	45-123
ALT (U/L)	19-48
GLDH (U/L)	0-1
LDH (U/L)	30-205
Bile acids (μmol/L)	22-60
GGT (U/L)	0-2.9
Total protein (g/L)	21-33
Albumin:Globulin (ratio)	1.5-3.6
Prealbumin (g/L)	1-4
Alpha globulin (g/L)	2-3
Beta globulin (g/L)	3-6
Gamma globulin (g/L)	1-3

Thyroxine before and 16 h after stimulation with 2 U/kg TSH, 6-35/100-300 nmol/L Corticosterone before and 90 min after stimulation with 250 mg/kg ACTH, 0.2-1.24/2.22-11.2 μg/dL
Recommendations of the German Society for Clinical Chemistry, Enzymes 30°C.

Blood Cells of Domestic Pigeons

Type Cell	Number
Erythrocytes (x 10^{12}/L)	3.1-4.5
Leukocytes (x 10^9/L)	13.0-22.3 morning<evening
Heterophils (x 10^9/L)	4.3-6.2
Eosinophils (x 10^9/L)	0.1-0.3
Basophils (x 10^9/L)	0.1-0.5
Lymphocytes (x 10^9/L)	10.9-12.2
Monocytes (x 10^9/L)	0.4-1.1
Thrombocytes (x 10^9/L)	7.0-27.0
Hemoglobin (mmol/L)	8.1-9.9
Hematocrit (vol %)	42.5

Hematology of Selected Gallinaceous Birds, Differential

Species	Heterophils (%)	Lymphocytes (%)	Monocytes (%)	Basophils (%)	Eosinophils (%)
Domestic Fowl	19.8-32.6	45.0-75.0	8.1-16.5	1.7-4.3	1.5-2.7
Domestic Turkey	43.4	50.6	1.9	3.2	0.9
Pheasant	48.0	34.0	8.0	10.0	1.0
Guineafowl	43.5	36.2	8.4	4.5	7.4
Common Quail	33.8-50.0	40.0-46.0	1.0-2.0	0.8-3.0	1.0-4.0
Japanese Quail	20.8-52.0	40.0-73.6	1.0-2.7	0.2-3.0	1.0-4.3

Note: In both, Currasows and Guans, hemolysis occurs in EDTA tubes. It is not know whether or not this in vitro hemolysis exists in other gallinaceous birds.

Hematology of Selected Gallinaceous Birds, Blood Parameters

Species	RBC (10⁶/ml)	PCV (%)	Hb (g%)	MCV (μm³)	WBC (10³/ml)
Domestic Fowl	2.2-3.3	24-43	8.9-13.5	120-137	19.8-32.6
Domestic Turkey	2.3-2.8	36-41	10.3-15.2	129	23.5-26.8
Pheasant	2.2-3.6	28-42	8.0-18.9	104-150	
Guineafowl	1.7-2.8	39-48	11.4-14.9		15.5
Peafowl	2.1	33-41	12.0		
Common Partridge	1.8-3.3	28-34	7.4-11.8	117-155	
Rock Partridge	2.6	37	11.1		
Bobwhite Quail	3.4-5.4	38	11.6-15.8		
Common Quail	3.8-5.4	40-53	12.9-15.8		16.2-24.0
Japanese Quail	3.3-4.1	37-46	10.7-15.8		19.7-25.0
Chachalaca	2.7	35-45			

RBC = Red blood cells, PCV = Packed cell volume, hematocrit, Hb = Hemoglobin, MCV = Mean cell volume (erythrocytes), WBC = White blood cells

Blood Chemistry of Selected Gallinaceous Birds

Species	Total Protein (g%)	Albumin (g%)	Globulin (g%)	Creatine (mg %)	Uric Acid (mg %)	Glucose (mg %)	Cholesterol (mg %)	Ca (mg %)	P (mg %)	Na (mEq/L)	K (mEq/L)
Domestic Fowl	3.3-5.5	1.3-2.8	1.5-4.1	0.9-1.8	2.5-8.1	227-300	86-211	13.2-23.7	6.2-7.9	131-171	3.0-7.3
Domestic Turkey	4.9-7.6	3.0-5.9	1.7-1.9	0.8-0.9	3.4-5.2	275-425	81-129	11.7-38.7	5.4-7.1	149-155	6.0-6.4
Pheasant	6.9	5.2	1.7		2.3-3.7	335-397			164-172		
Guineafowl	3.5-4.4				2.9-5.1					149-157	
Common Quail	3.4-3.6									180	1.4
Bobwhite Quail								14.1-15.4			
Japanese Quail		1.2-1.9									
Peafowl					1.8-3.7	273-357				154-162	
Rock Partridge					2.5-4.2	270-312				145-163	
Chachalaca					3.7-7.9	235-345				158-164	

Serum Chemistry and Enzyme Values, Nonreproductive Adult Mallards

Assay	Male		Female	
	Mean	SD	Mean	SD
TPR (g/dL)	3.8	0.7	4.2	0.5
ALB (g/dL)	1.5	0.4	1.7	0.2
GLU (mg/dL)	185.0	47.0	215.0	34.0
AMY (U/L)	2631.0	630.0	2766.0	684.0
CHE (U/L)	794.0	249.0	812.0	197.0
ALT (U/L)	26.3	8.0	29.9	9.9
AST (U/L)	16.2	4.3	15.8	4.7
GGT (U/L)	7.7	4.2	8.0	4.8
ALP (U/L)	26.3	8.0	44.2	22.7
LDH (U/L)	199.0	83.0	147.0	80.0
CA (mg/dL)	9.4	1.9	9.8	1.1
MG (mEq/L)	1.8	0.4	1.8	0.3
PHOS (mg/dL)	2.9	1.0	3.0	1.0
UA (mg/dL)	4.0	1.3	4.5	1.8
CRN (mg/dL)	0.25	0.08	0.28	0.07
BITO (mg/dL)	0.16	0.05	0.16	0.04
BIDI (mg/dL)	0.07	0.01	0.07	0.01

Serum Chemistry and Enzyme Values for Adult Female Mallards of Differing Reproductive States

Assay	Pre-egg Laying		Egg Laying		Incubating		Molt	
	Mean	SD	Mean	SD	Mean	SD	Mean	SD
TPR (g/dL)	5.6	2.9	6.3	1.2	4.4	0.6	4.5	1.2
ALB (g/dL)	2.0	0.3	2.3	0.2	1.6	0.2	1.7	0.2
GLU (mg/dL)	238.0	21.0	258.0	51.0	211.0	53.0	199.0	30.0
AMY (U/L)	3058.0	527.0	3821.0	741.0	2700.0	626.0	2346.0	1012.0
CHE (U/L)	1337.0	280.0	1563.0	592.0	1002.0	266.0	894.0	219.0
ALT (U/L)	31.0	10.3	34.2	19.4	30.6	13.1	41.1	17.1
AST (U/L)	18.0	3.4	23.7	6.7	22.1	7.4	22.6	12.6
GGT (U/L)	19.8	19.8	199.6	283.0	7.5	4.7	20.8	36.9
ALP (U/L)	63.6	56.8	124.9	56.7	34.3	15.8	36.0	18.1
LDH (U/L)	165.0	50.0	177.0	57.0	215.0	107.0	268.0	2.2
CA (mg/dL)	14.0	4.1	21.9	5.6	10.3	2.0	10.6	4.2
MG (mEq/L)	2.3	0.5	3.6	0.8	1.6	0.3	1.6	0.5
PHOS (mg/dL)	4.6	1.7	8.1	2.4	3.7	1.0	4.1	2.2
UA (mg/dL)	5.2	1.1	9.1	5.1	5.5	1.7	4.9	1.7
CRN (mg/dL)	0.34	0.06	0.33	0.15	0.42	0.15	0.33	0.08
BITO (mg/dL)	0.23	0.08	0.43	0.28	0.20	0.11	0.21	0.05
BIDI (mg/dL)	0.07	0.04	0.15	0.22	0.06	0.04	0.06	0.01

Serum Chemistry and Enzyme Values for Adult Male Mallards of Differing Reproductive States

Assay	Pre-egg Laying		Egg Laying		Incubating		Molt	
	Mean	SD	Mean	SD	Mean	SD	Mean	SD
TPR (g/dL)	4.6	0.6	4.5	0.8	4.2	0.5	3.9	0.8
ALB (g/dL)	1.8	0.2	1.6	0.2	1.7	0.3	1.5	0.3
GLU (mg/dL)	234.0	33.0	233.0	32.0	199.0	26.0	185.0	29.0
AMY (U/L)	3123.0	583.0	2869.0	614.0	3203.0	785.0	2991.0	748.0
CHE (U/L)	1326.0	344.0	1380.0	399.0	984.0	470.0	983.0	452.0
ALT (U/L)	34.6	9.4	35.8	13.1	27.6	12.1	28.4	19.2
AST (U/L)	17.3	4.0	20.5	8.0	20.8	15.7	18.1	8.1
GGT (U/L)	8.5	7.6	10.6	12.6	9.3	6.0	16.5	36.0
ALP (U/L)	40.2	25.3	44.1	44.8	38.4	48.0	35.3	44.2
LDH (U/L)	168.0	66.0	219.0	107.0	263.0	203.0	202.0	152.0
CA (mg/dL)	10.9	1.0	11.0	1.9	9.9	1.0	9.3	2.2
MG (mEq/L)	2.0	0.2	2.0	0.4	1.8	0.4	1.8	0.9
PHOS (mg/dL)	3.7	0.9	3.6	0.9	2.8	0.5	3.1	1.4
UA (mg/dL)	5.2	1.2	5.2	1.5	5.7	1.9	4.7	2.3
CRN (mg/dL)	0.35	0.08	0.36	0.10	0.34	0.12	0.30	0.12
BITO (mg/dL)	0.22	0.09	0.20	0.09	0.18	0.04	0.20	0.08
BIDI (mg/dL)	0.07	0.02	0.06	0.01	0.07	0.02	0.08	0.05

Serum Chemistry and Enzyme Values for Juvenile Mallards

Assay	Age 5 days		Age 18 days		Age 42 days		Age 48 days	
	Mean	SD	Mean	SD	Mean	SD	Mean	SD
TPR (g/dL)	3.4	0.6	4.3	1.3	4.0	0.8	3.2	1.0
ALB (g/dL)	1.4	0.2	1.5	0.3	1.6	0.4	1.4	0.4
GLU (mg/dL)	239.0	54.0	215.0	93.0	189.0	27.0	186.0	45.0
AMY (U/L)	3230.0	760.0	3984.0	1297.0	3005.0	302.0	2395.0	699.0
CHE (U/L)	1423.0	696.0	984.0	559.0	827.0	253.0	818.0	248.0
ALT (U/L)	21.3	9.1	30.5	10.5	26.1	7.0	23.9	7.1
AST (U/L)	22.3	7.4	88.5	54.1	9.4	5.1	17.4	5.7
GGT (U/L)	1.2	2.8	4.6	3.6	5.3	5.7	6.1	3.6
ALP (U/L)	411.0	89.0	386.0	194.0	217.0	32.0	185.0	47.0
LD-L (U/L)	425.0	153.0	629.0	251.0	169.0	70.0	233.0	83.0
CA (mg/dL)	13.0	10.3	9.6	1.7	10.9	1.6	8.4	1.8
MG (mEq/L)	2.8	0.8	1.8	0.7	2.0	0.2	1.6	0.5
PHOS (mg/dL)	7.9	2.8	7.6	1.3	6.2	1.3	5.0	1.7
UA (mg/dL)	12.2	5.4	10.9	3.8	4.0	0.7	4.0	1.8
CRN (mg/dL)	0.47	0.42	0.55	0.65	0.28	0.10	0.21	0.11
BITO (mg/dL)	0.40	0.11	0.43	0.31	0.20	0.0	0.17	0.05
BIDI (mg/dL)	0.08	0.02	0.10	0.04	0.06	0.0	0.06	0.02

Hematological and Biochemical Values for Ratites

Parameter	Ostrich Mean	Ostrich SD	Emu Mean	Emu SD	Cassowary Mean	Cassowary SD
WBC (x 10³/μl)	5.5	1.9			18.0	4.5
Heterophils (%)	62.6	7.6			77.7	25.8
Lymphocytes (%)	34.1	7.0			19.7	10.4
Monocytes (%)	2.8	1.3			2.4	2.4
Eosinophils (%)	0.3	0.5				
Basophils (%)	0.2	0.5				
PCV (%)	32.0	3.0			50.8	3.7
RBC (x 10⁶/μl)	1.7	0.4			2.1	0.3
Hb (g/dL)	12.2	2.0			14.5	0.5
MCV (fl)	174.0	42.0			245.0	41.0
MCHC (g/dL)	33.0	5.0			28.5	1.6
MCH (pg)	61.0	16.0			70.0	11.5
Total protein (g/dL)	3.7	0.7	4.2	0.5	6.1	0.5
Osmolality (mOsm/kg)	286.0	49.0				
Glucose (mg/dL)	250.0	70.0	158.0	22.0	208.0	47.4
Triglycerides (mg/dL)	90.0	45.0	325.0	591.0	180.0	72.0

Hematological and Biochemical Values for Ratites (continued)

Parameter	Ostrich		Emu		Cassowary	
	Mean	SD	Mean	SD	Mean	SD
Cholesterol (mg/dL)	97.0	45.0	104.0	31.0	80.0	16.0
BUN (mg/dL)	2.4	0.6	2.5	0.9	9.3	0.6
Uric acid (mg/dL)	8.2	2.7	4.7	2.0	6.0	0.6
Calcium (mg/dL)	9.2	2.4	10.5	1.3	11.4	0.2
Phosphorus (mg/dL)	4.8	1.2	5.4	1.0	5.0	0.1
Sodium (mEq/L)	147.0	34.0			149.0	2.1
Potassium (mEq/L)	3.0	0.8			4.1	1.0
Chloride (mEq/L)	100.0	16.0			108.0	0.0
Magnesium (mEq/L)	2.2	0.8			2.3	0.3
ALP (U/L)	575.0	248.0			84.0	44.0
ALT (U/L)	2.0	1.7	15.4	4.3	80.0	21.0
AST (U/L)	131.0	31.0	104.0	24.0	698.0	532.0
GGT (U/L)	1.5	2.9	4.4	3.4		
LDH (U/L)	1565.0	660.0	240.0	91.0	1060.0	516.0
CK (U/L)	688.0	208.0	264.0	170.0		

Class Aves: A List of Orders, Common and Scientific Names

APTERYGIFORMES
Kiwi *Apteryx* sp.

STRUTHIONIFORMES
Cassowary *Casuarius* spp.
Emu *Dromiceius novaehollandiae*
Greater Rhea *Rhea americana*
Lesser Rhea *Pterocnemia pennata*
Ostrich *Struthio camelus*

TINAMINIFORMES
Tinamou *Eudromia* spp.
Bustard (Houbara) *Chlamydotis undulata*

GRUIFORMES
Blue Crane *Tetrapteryx paradisea*
Brolga *Grus rubicunda*
Crowned Crane *Balearica pavonina*
Demoiselle Crane *Anthropoides virgo*
Hooded Crane *Grus monacha*
Manchurian Crane *Grus japonensis*
Sandhill Crane *Grus canadensis*
Sarus Crane *Grus antigone*
White-naped Crane *Grus vipio*

RALLIFORMES
Coot (European) *Fulica atra*

CHARADRIIFORMES
Sanderling (eroliinae) *Crocetha ulba*
Turnstone *Arenaria interpres*

LARIFORMES
Black-headed Gull *Chroicocephalus ridibundus*
Herring Gull *Larus argentatus*
Kittiwake (Black -legged) *Rissa tridactyla*

ALCIFORMES
Black Guillemot *Cepphus grylle*

SPHENISCIFORMES
Fairy Blue (Little) Penguins *Eudyptula minor*
Humboldt penguin *Spheniscus humboldti*
Jackass Penguin *Spheniscus demersus*

PELECANIFORMES
Brandt's Cormorant *Phalacrocorax penicillatus*
White Pelican *Pelecanus onocrotalus*

COLUMBIFORMES
Pigeons
Crowned (Blue) Pigeon *Goura cristata*
Nicobar Pigeon *Caloenas nicobarica*
Pheasant Pigeon *Otidiphabs noblis*
Rock-Pigeon (Racing, King) *Columba livia*
Tooth-billed Pigeon D*idunculus strigirostris*
Wood-Pigeon *Palumbus palumbus*
Doves
African Collared Dove *Streptopelia roseogrisea*
Emerald Dove *Chalcophabs indica*

Galapagos Dove *Nesopelia galapagoensis*
Luzon Bleeding-heart *Galliculomba luzonica*
Mourning Dove *Zenaida macroura*
Namaqua Dove *Oena capensis*
Plain-breasted Ground Dove *Columbigallina minuta*
Turtle-Dove *Streptopelia turtur*

PSITTACIFORMES
Lovebirds
Black-cheeked Lovebird *Agapornis nigrigenis*
Black-collared Lovebird *Agapornis swindernianus*
Black-winged Lovebird *Agapornis taranta*
Fischer's Lovebird *Agapornis fischeri*
Grey-headed Lovebird *Agapornis canus*
Lilian's (Nyassa) Lovebird *Agapornis lilianae*
Masked Lovebird *Agapornis personatus*
Red-faced Lovebird *Agapornis pullarius*
Rosy-faced Lovebird *Agapornis roseicollis*
Macaws
Blue and Yellow (Gold) Macaw *Ara ararauna*
Buffon's Macaw *Ara ambigua*
Green-winged Macaw *Ara chloroptera*
Hyacinth Macaw *Anodrohynchus hyacinthinus*
Illiger's Macaw *Ara maracana*
Military Macaw *Ara militaris*
Red-shouldered Macaw *Diopsittaca noblis*
Scarlet Macaw *Ara macao*
Yellow-collared Macaw *Ara auricollis*
Conures
Australian Conure *Enicognathus ferrugineus*
Blue-crowned Conure *Thectocercus acuticaudatus*
Brown-throated Conure *Eupsittula pertinax*
Cactus Conure *Eupsittula cactorum*
Dusky-headed Conure *Eupsittula weddellii*
Finsch's Conure *Psittacara finschi*
Golden Conure *Guaruba guarouba*
Green-cheeked Conure *Pyrrhura molinae*
Green Conure *Psittacara holochlora*
Maroon-bellied Conure *Pyrrhura frontalis*
Mitred Conure *Psittacara mitrata*
Nanday Conure *Nandayus nenday*
Painted Conure *Pyrrhura picta*
Patagonian Conure *Cyanoliseus patagonus*
Peach-fronted Conure *Eupsittula aurea*
Pearly Conure *Pyrrhura perlata*

Slender-billed Conure *Enicognathus leptorhynchus*
Sun Conure *Aratinga solstitialis*
White-eyed Conure *Psittacara leucophthalma*

Parakeets
Alexandrine Parakeet *Psittacula eupatria*
Blossom-headed Parakeet *Psittacula roseata*
Blyth's Parakeet *Psittacula caniceps*
Derbyan Parakeet *Psittacula derbiana*
Grey-cheeked Parakeet *Brotogeris pyrrhoptera*
Monk (Quaker) Parakeet *Myiopsitta monachus*
Moustached Parakeet *Psittacula alexandria*
Orange-chinned Parakeet *Brotogeris jugularis*
Red-fronted (Kakariki) Parakeet *Cyanoramphus novaezelandiae*
Rose-ringed Parakeet *Psittacula krameri*
Yellow-fronted (Kakariki) Parakeet *Cyanoramphus auriceps*
Black-headed Caique *Pionites melanocephalus*
White-bellied Caique *Pionites leucogaster*

Parrots
African Grey Parrot *Psittacus erithacus*
Amboina King Parrot *Alisterus amboinensis*
Australian King Parrot *Alisterus scapularis*
Barraband's Parrot *Gypopsitta barrabandi*
Black Parrot *Coracopsis nigra*
Blue-bonnet *Psephotus haematogaster*
Blue-winged Parrot *Neophema chrysostoma*
Bourke's Parrot *Neopsephotus bourkii*
Budgerigar *Melopsittacus undulatus*
Eastern Rosella *Platycercus eximius*
Eclectus Parrot *Eclectus roratus*
Elegant Parrot *Neophema elegans*
Golden-shouldered Parrot *Psephotus chrysopterygius*
Great-billed Parrot *Tanygnathus megalorhynchos*
Green Rosella *Platycercus caledonicus*
Green-winged King Parrot *Alisterus chloropterus*
Ground Parrot *Pezoporus wallicus*
Hawk-headed Parrot *Deroptyus accipitrinus*
Kakapo *Strigops habroptilus*
Mulga Parrot *Psephotus varius*
Night Parrot *Geopsittacus occidentalis*
Northern Rosella *Platycercus venustus*
Orange-bellied Parrot *Neophema chrysogaster*
Paradise Parrot *Psephotus pulcherrimus*
Pennant's Rosella *Platycercus elegans*
Pileated Parrot *Pionopsitta pileata*

Princess Parrot *Spacthopterus alexandrae*
Red-capped Parrot *Purpureicephalus spurius*
Red-rumped Parrot *Psephotus haematonotus*
Red-winged Parrot *Aprosmictus erythropterus*
Regent Parrot *Spathopterus anthopeplus*
Ringneck Parrot *Barnardius zonarius*
Scarlet-chested Parrot *Neophema splendida*
Short-tailed Parrot *Graydidascalus brachyurus*
Superb Parrot *Polytelis swainsonii*
Thick-billed Parrot *Rhynchopsitta pachyrhyncha*
Timor Red-winged Parrot *Aprosmictus jonquillaceus*
Turquoise-Parrot *Neophema pulchella*
Vasa Parrot *Coracopsis vasa*
Western Rosella *Platycercus icterotis*

Amazon parrots
Blue-fronted Amazon *Amazona aestiva*
Cuban Amazon *Amazona leucocephala*
Festive Amazon *Amazona festiva*
Green-cheeked Amazon *Amazona viridigenalis*
Hispaniolan Amazon *Amazona ventralis*
Lilac-crowned Amazon *Amazona finschi*
Mealy Amazon *Amazona farinosa*
Orange-winged Amazon *Amazona amazonica*
Puerto Rican Amazon *Amazona vittata*
Red-spectacled Amazon *Amazona pretrei*
Red-lored Amazon *Amazona autumnalis*
Tucuman Amazon *Amazona tucumana*
Vinaceous Amazon *Amazona vinacea*
White-fronted Amazon *Amazona albifrons*
Yellow-lored Amazon *Amazona xantholora*
Yellow-crowned Amazon *Amazona ochrocephala*
Yellow-billed (Jamaican) Amazon *Amazona collaria*
Yellow-shouldered Amazon *Amazona barbadensis*
Yellow-faced Amazon *Amazona xanthops*

Fig parrots
Desmarest's Fig Parrot *Psittaculirostris desmarestii*
Double-eyed Fig Parrot *Opopsitta diophthalma*
Edward's Fig Parrot *Psittaculirostris edwardsii*
Salvadori's Fig Parrot *Psittaculirostris salvadorii*

Pionus parrots
Blue-headed Parrot *Pionus menstuus*

Bronze-winged Parrot *Pionus chalcopterus*
Dusky Parrot *Pionus fuscus*
Plum-crowned Parrot *Pionus tumultuosus*
Red-billed Parrot *Pionus sordidus*
Scaly-headed Parrot *Pionus maximiliani*
White-capped Parrot *Pionus senilis*
White-headed Parrot *Pionus seniloides*

Poicephalus parrots

Brown-headed Parrot *Poicephalus cryptoxanthus*
Cape Parrot *Poicephalus robustus*
Jardine's Parrot *Poicephalus guilielmi*
Meyer's Parrot *Poicephalus meyeri*
Niamnian Parrot *Poicephalus crassus*
Red-bellied Parrot *Poicephalus rufiventris*
Ruppell's Parrot *Poicephalus rueppellii*
Senegal Parrot *Poicephalus senegalus*
Yellow-faced Parrot *Poicephalus flavifrons*

Lories

Black-capped Lory *Lorius lory*
Black Lory *Chalcopsitta atra*
Blue-streaked Lory *Eos reticulata*
Cardinal Lory *Chalcopsitta cardinalis*
Chattering Lory *Lorius garrulus*
Dusky Lory *Pseudeos fuscata*
Duyvenbode's Lory *Chalcopsitta duivenbodei*
Ornate Lory *Trichoglossus ornatus*
Purple-bellied Lory *Lorius hypoinochrous*
Purple-naped Lory *Lorius domicella*
Rainbow Lory *Trichoglossus haematodus*
Red Lory *Eos bornea*
Violet-necked Lory *Eos squamata*
Yellow-streaked Lory *Chalcopsitta sintillata*

Lorikeets

Goldie's Lorikeet *Psitteuteles goldiei*
Little Lorikeet *Glossopsitta pusilla*
Scaly-breasted Lorikeet *Trichoglossus chlorolepidotus*
Varied Lorikeet *Psitteuteles versicolor*

Cockatoos

Black Cockatoo *Calyptorhynchus funereus*
Blue-eyed Cockatoo *Cacatua ophthalmica*
Ducorps's Cockatoo *Cacatua ducorps*
Galah *Eolophus roseicapillus*
Gang-gang Cockatoo *Callocephalon fimbriatum*
Glossy Cockatoo *Calyptorhynchus lathami*
Goffin's Cockatoo *Cacatua goffini*
Lesser Sulphur-crested Cockatoo *Cacatua sulphurea*
Little (Slender-bill) Corella *Cacatua sanguinea*

Long-billed Corella *Cacatua tenuirostris*
Mitchell's Cockatoo *Cacatua leadbeateri*
Palm Cockatoo *Probosciger aterrimus*
Red-vented Cockatoo *Cacatua haematuropygia*
Red-tailed Cockatoo *Calyptorhynchus magnificus*
Salmon-crested Moluccan Cockatoo *Cacatua moluccensis*
Sulphur-crested Cockatoo *Cacatua galerita*
White Umbrella Cockatoo *Cacatua alba*
Cockatiel *Nymphicus hollandicus*
Kaka *Nestor meridionalis*
Kea *Nestor notabilis*

ANSERIFORMES

Subfamily Anseranatinae
Tribe Anseranatini

Cuban (Black-billed) Whistling (tree) Duck *Dendrocygna arborea*
Eyton's (Plumed) (Grass) Whistling Duck *Dendrocygna eytoni*
Fulvous Whistling Duck *Dendrocygna bicolor*
Javan (Lesser) Whistling Duck *Dendrocygna javanica*
Magpie Goose *Anseranas semipalmata*
Northern Black-bellied (Red-billed) Whistling Duck *Dendrocygna autumnalis*
Spotted Whistling Duck *Dendrocygna guttata*
Wandering (East Indian) Whistling Duck *Dendrocygna arcuata*
White-Backed (African) Whistling Duck *Thalassornis leuconotus*
White-faced Whistling Duck *Dendrocygna viduata*

Tribe Anserini
(Swans and True Geese)

Bar-headed Goose *Eulabeia indica*
Barnacle Goose *Branta leucopis*
Bewick's Swan *Olor bewickii*
Black-necked Swan *Sthenelides melancoryphus*
Black Swan *Chenopis atrata*
Brent (Russian) (Dark-Bellied) Brant *bernicla*
Canada (Atlantic) Goose *Branta canadensis*
Coscoroba Swan *Coscoroba coscoroba*
Emperor Goose *Philacte canagica*
Freckled (Monkey) Duck *Stictonetta naevosa*
Graylag (Domestic) Goose (Western) *Anser anser*
Lesser White-fronted Goose *Anser erythropus*
Mute Swan *Cygnus olor*
Nene (Hawaiian) Goose *Branta sandvicensis*
Pink-footed Goose *Anser brachyrhynchus*
Red-breasted Goose *Rufibrenta ruficollis*
Ross's Goose *Chen rossii*

Snow (Lesser) (Blue) Goose *Chen caerulescens*

Swan Goose *Anser cynoides*

Trumpeter Swan *Olor buccinator*

Western (Yellow-billed) Bean Goose *Anser fabalis*

Whistling Swan *Olor columbianus*

White-fronted (European) Goose *Anser albifrons*

Whooper Swan *Olor cygnus*

Sub-Family Antinae
Tribe Tadornini
(Shelducks and Sheldgeese)

Abyssinian Blue-winged Goose *Cyanochen cyanopterus*

Andean Goose *Chloephaga melanoptera*

Ashy-headed Goose *Chloephaga poliocephala*

Australian Shelduck *Casarca tadornoides*

Cape Barren (Cereopsis) Goose *Cereopsis novaehollandiae*

Common (European) Shelduck *Tadorna tadorna*

Crested Shelduck *Pseudotadorna cristata*

Egyptian Goose *Alopochen aegyptiacus*

Kelp (Patagonian) (Lesser) Goose *Chloephaga hybrida*

Magellan (Lesser) (Upland) Goose *Chloephaga picta*

Orinoco Goose *Neochen jubatus*

Paradise (New Zealand) Shelduck *Casarca variegata*

Radjah Shelduck (Moluccan) (Black-Backed) *Radjah radjah*

Ruddy-headed Goose *Chloephaga rubidiceps*

Ruddy Shelduck *Casarca ferrugina*

South African (Cape) Shelduck *Casarca cana*

Spur-winged (Gambian) Goose *Plectropterus gambensis*

Tribe Cairinini
(Perching Ducks)

African (South) Black Duck *Melananas sparsa*

African Pygmy Goose *Nettapus auritus*

American (Baldpate) Wigeon *Mareca americana*

Australian Shoveler *Spatula rhynochotis*

Australian Wood Duck (Maned Goose) *Chenonetta jubata*

Bahama (Lesser) (Northern White-Cheeked) Pintail *Paecilonetta bahamensis*

Baikal Teal *Nettion formosum*

Blue-winged (Prairie) Teal *Spatula discors*

Brazilian (Lesser) Teal *Amazonetta brasiliensis*

Brown (Chillian) Pintail *Dafila georgica*

Brown (New Zealand) Teal *Nettion aucklandicum*

Cape (South African) Shoveler *Spatula capensis*

Cape Teal *Nettion capense*

Chestnut Teal *Nettion castaneum*

Chiloe Wigeon *Mareca sibilatrix*

Cinnamon (Northern) Teal *Spatula cyanoptera*

Common (European Green-Winged) Teal *Nettion crecca*

Common (Northern) Shoveler *Spatula clypeata*

Common (Northern) Pintail *Dafila acuta*

Cotton (Indian) Pygmy Goose (Cotton Teal) *Nettapus coromandelianus*

European (Eurasian) Wigeon *Mareca penelope*

Falcated Duck *Eunetta falcata*

Gadwall (Gray Duck) *Chaulelasmus streperus*

Garganey *Querquedula querquedula*

Green Pygmy Goose *Nettapus pulchellus*

Grey Teal (East Indian) *Nettion gibberifrons*

Hartlaub's Duck *Pteronetta hartlaubii*

Hottentot Teal *Punanetta hottentota*

Knob-billed (Old World Comb) Duck *Sarkidiornis melanotos*

Madagascan (Bernier's) Teal *Nettion bernieri*

Mandarin Duck *Dendronessa galericulata*

Muscovy Duck *Cairina moschata*

Red (Argentine) Shoveler *Spatula platalea*

Red-billed Pintail *Paecilonetta erythrorhyncha*

Ringed Teal *Callonetta leucophrys*

Silver (Northern) (Versicolor) Teal *Punanetta versicolor*

South American (Chilean Speckled) Teal *Nettion flavirostre*

White-winged Wood Duck *Asarcornis scutulatus*

Wood Duck (North American) (Carolina Duck) *Aix sponsa*

Tribe Anatini (Dabbling Ducks)

American (North) Black Duck *Anas fulvigula*

Blue (Mountain) Duck *Hymenolaimus malacorhynchos*

Bronze-winged (Spectacled) Duck *Speculanas specularis*

Crested (Patagonian) Duck *Lophonetta specularioides*

Falkland Flightless Steamer-Duck *Tachyeres brachypterus*

Flying Steamer Duck *Tachyeres patachonicus*

Grey Duck (New Zealand) *Anas superciliosa*

Hawaiian Duck (Koloa) *Anas wyvilliana*

Laysan Teal *Anas laysanensis*

Magellanic Flightless Steamer-Duck *Tachyeres pteneres*

Mallard (Northern) (Domestic) Duck *Anas platyrhynchos*

Marbled Teal *Marmaronetta angustirostris*

Meller's Duck *Anas melleri*

Philippine Duck *Anas luzonica*

Pink-eared (Zebra) Duck *Malacorhynchus membranaceus*

Salvadori's Duck *Salvadorina waigiuensis*
Spot-billed (Indian) Duck *Anas poecilorhyncha*
Torrent (Chilean) Duck *Merganetta armata*
Yellow-billed (South African) Duck *Anas undulata*

Tribe Aythya (Pochards)

Australasian (White-Eye) (Hardhead) Pochard *Aythya australis*
Baer's Pochard (Siberian White-Eye) *Aythya baeri*
Canvasback *Aythya valisineria*
Common (Ferruginous) (White-Eyed) Pochard *Aythya nyroca*
European (Eurasian) Pochard *Aythya ferina*
Greater (European) Scaup *Aythya marila*
Lesser Scaup *Aythya affinis*
Madagascan (White-Eye) Pochard *Aythya innotata*
New Zealand Scaup (Black Teal) *Aythya novaeseelandiae*
Pink-headed Duck *Rhodonessa caryophyllace*
Red-Crested Pochard *Netta rufina*
Redhead Duck *Aythya americana*
Ring-necked Duck *Aythya collaris*
Rosy-bill (Rosybilled) Pochard *Metopiana peposaca*
Southern (South American) Pochard *Phaeoaythia erythrophtalma*
Tufted Duck *Aythya fuligula*

Tribe Somteria (Eiders)

Common (European) Eider *Somateria mollissima*
King Eider *Somateria spectabilis*
Spectacled (Fischer's) Eider *Somateria fischeri*
Steller's Eider *Polysticta stelleri*
Tribe Merginia (Sea Ducks)
Auckland Island Merganser *Mergus australis*
Barrow's Goldeneye *Glaucionetta islandica*
Black (European) Scoter *Melanitta nigra*
Brazilian Merganser *Mergus octosetaceus*
Bufflehead *Bucephala albeola*
Common (European) Goldeneye *Glaucionetta clangula*
Goosander (Curasian) *Mergus merganser*
Harlequin (Atlantic) Duck *Histrionicus histrionicus*
Hooded Merganser *Lophodytes cucullatus*
Labrador Duck *Camptorhynchus labradorius*
Long-tailed (Oldsquaw) Duck *Clangula hyemalis*
Red-breasted (Common) Merganser *Mergus serrator*
Scaley-sided (Chinese) Merganser *Mergus squamatus*
Smew *Mergellus albellus*
Surf Scoter *Melanitta perspicillata*
White-winged (European) (Velvet) Scoter *Melanitti fusca*

Tribe Oxyurini (Stiff-Tailed Ducks)

Black-headed Duck *Heteronetta atricapilla*
Blue-billed (Australian) Duck *Oxyura australis*
Lake (Argentine) (Ruddy) (Blue-billed) Duck *Oxyura vittata*
Maccoa Duck *Oxyura maccoa*
Masked Duck *Oxyura dominica*
Musk Duck *Biziura lobata*
Ruddy Duck (North American) *Oxyura jamaicensis*
White headed Duck *Oxyura leucocephala*

RAPTORS

American Kestrel (Sparrow Hawk) *Tinnunculus sparverius*
Bald Eagle *Haliaeetus leucocephalus*
Barn Owl *Tyto alba*
Common (European) (Rock) Kestrel *Tinnunculus tinnunculus*
Common Buzzard *Buteo buteo*
Eagle Owl *Bubo bubo*
Eastern Turkey Vulture *Cathartes aura*
European Sparrow Hawk *Accipiter nisus*
Forest Eagle Owl *Bubo nipalensis*
Golden Eagle *Aquila chrysaetos*
Goshawk *Accipiter gentilis*
Great Horned Owl *Bubo virginianus*
Grey Eagle Buzzard *Geranoaetus melanoleucus*
Griffon Vulture *Gyps fulvus*
Little Owl *Athene noctua*
Long-eared Owl *Asio otus*
Merlin (Pigeon) Hawk *Aesalon columbarius*
Peregrine Falcon *Hierofalco peregrinus*
Prairie Falcon *Hierofalco mexicanus*
Red Kite *Milvus milvus*
Red-necked Falcon *Chiquera chiquera*
Rough-legged Buzzard *Buteo lagopus*
Saker Falcon *Hierofalco cherrug*
Screech Owl *Megascops asio*
Short-eared Owl *Asio flammeus*
Snowy Owl *Nyctea scandiaca*
South American Black-collared Hawk (Fishing Buzzard) *Busarellus nigricollis*
Striped Owl *Asio clamator*
Tengmalm's Owl *Aegolius funereus*
Ural Owl *Strix uralensis*

CICONIIFORMES

Black Stork *Ciconia nigra*
Cattle Egret *Bubulcus ibis*
Greater Adjutant Stork *Leptoptilos dubius*
Grey Heron *Ardea cinerea*
Hermit Ibis *Geronticus eremita*
Marabou Stork *Leptoptilos crumeniferus*
Night Heron (Black-Crowned) *Nycticorax nicticorax*
Striated Heron *Butorides striatus*
White Stork *Ciconia ciconia*
Yellow-crowned Night Heron *Nyctanassa violacea*

GALLIFORMES
Brush-Turkey *Alectura lathami*

Numidinae
Crested Guineafowl *Guttera pucherani*
Domestic Guineafowl *Numida meleagris forma domestica*
Helmeted Guineafowl *Numida meleagris*
Plumed Guineafowl *Guttera plumifera*
Vulturine Guineafowl *Acryllium vulturinum*

Pavoninae
Congo Peafowl *Afropavo congensis*
Green Peafowl *Pavo muticus*
Indian Peafowl *Pavo cristatus*

Meleagridinae
Common Turkey *Meleagris gallopavo*
Domestic Turkey *Meleagris gallopavo forma domestica*
Oscillated Turkey *Meleagris ocellata*

Argusianinae
Bronze-tailed Peacock-Pheasant *Polyplectron chalcurom*
Crested Argus *Rheinardia ocellata*
Great Argus *Argusianus argus*
Grey Peacock-Pheasant *Polyplectron bicalcaratum*
Palawan Peacock-Pheasant *Polyplectron emphanum*
Phasianinae Bar-tailed Pheasant *Calophasis humiae*
Blue-eared Pheasant *Crossoptilon auritum*
Brown-eared Pheasant *Crossoptilon mantchuricum*
Bulwer's Wattled Pheasant *Lophura Bulweri*
Cheer Pheasant *Catreus wallichii*
Common (Ring-necked) Pheasant *Phasianus colchicus*
Copper Pheasant *Graphephasianus soemmeringii*
Elliot's Pheasant *Calophasis ellioti*
Golden Pheasant *Chrysolophus pictus*
Lady Amherst's Pheasant *Chrysolophus amherstiae*
Mikado Pheasant *Calophasis mikado*
Reeve's Pheasant *Syrmaticus reevesii*
Salvadori's Pheasant *Lophura inornata*
Siamese Fireback *Lophura diardi*
Silver Pheasant *Lophura nycthemera*
Swinhoe's Pheasant *Lophura swinhoii*

Lophophorinae
Himalayan Monal *Lophophorus impejanus*

Pucrasiinae
Koklass *Pucrasia macrolopha*

Ithagininae
Blood Pheasant *Ithaginis cruentus*

Gallinae
Domestic Fowl *Gallus gallus forma domestica*
Red Junglefowl *Gallus gallus*

Tragopaninae
Satyr Tragopan *Tragopan satyra*

Ptilopachinae
Stone Partridge *Ptilopachus petrosus*

Perdicinae
Black Francolin *Francolinus francolinus*
Chinese Bamboo Partridge *Bambusicola thoracica*
Chukar Partridge *Alectoris chukar*
Common Partridge *Perdix perdix*
Common Quail *Coturnix coturnix*
Himalayan Snowcock *Tetraogallus himalayensis*
Japanese Quail *Coturnix japonica*
Jungle Bush Quail *Perdicula asiatica*
Painted Quail *Coturnix chinensis*
Redlegged Partridge *Alectoris rufa*
Rock Partridge *Alectoris graeca*
Roulroul (Crested Wood Partridge) *Rollulus roulroul*

Odontophorinae
Bobwhite Quail *Colinus virginianus*
California Quail *Callipepla californica*
Gambel's Quail *Callipepla gambelii*
Scaled Quail *Callipepla squamata*

Tetraoninae
Black Grouse *Lyrurus tetrix*
Blue Grouse *Dendragapus obscurus*
Common Capercaillie *Tetrao urogallus*
Hazelhen (Common) *Tetrastes bonasia*
Prairie Chicken *Tympanuchus cupido*
Red Grouse *Lagopus lagopus scoticus*
Ruffed Grouse *Bonasa umbellus*
Sage Grouse *Centrocercus urophasianus*
Sharp-tailed Grouse *Tympanuchus phasianellus*
Spruce Grouse *Falcipennis canadensis*
Willow Ptarmigan (Grouse) *Lagopus lagopus*

Cracidae
Black-billed Turaco *Tauraco schuetti*
Common Piping Guan *Aburria pipile*
Great Curassow *Crax rubra*
Guinea Turaco *Tauraco persa*
Helmeted (Northern) Curassow *Pauxi pauxi*
Lady Ross's Turaco *Musophaga rossae*
Purple-crested Turaco *Tauraco porphyreolophus*
Razor-billed Curassow *Mitu mitu*
Wattled Curassow *Crax globulosa*
White-crested Turaco *Tauraco leucolophus*

UPUPIFORMES
Hoopoe *Upupa epops*

CAPRIMULGIFORMES
Indian Edible-nest Swiftlet *Collocalia unicolor*
Quetzal *Pharomachrus mocinno*
Tawny Frogmouth *Podargus strigoides*

PASSERIFORMES
African Silverbill *Euodice cantans*

American Bare-eyed Thrush
Planesticus nudigenis
American Goldfinch *Spinus tristis*
American Tree-Sparrow *Spizella
arborea*
Antbirds and gnateaters
Formicariidae
Apostle-bird *Struthidea cinerea*
Ashey (Brown-eared) Bulbul
Hemixos flavala
Australian Magpie *Gymnorhina
tibicen*
Avadavat (Strawberry-Finch, Red
Munia) *Amandava amandava*
Barn Swallow *Hirundo rustica*
Bearded Manakin *Manacus manacus*
Bengalese (Society) Finch *Lonchura
domestic*
Birds of Paradise *Paradisaeidae*
Black (Pied) (Pied Bell-Magpie)
Currawong *Strepera graculina*
Black-eared Wheatear *Oenanthe
hispanica*
Black-faced Cuckoo-Shrike *Coracina
novaehollandiae*
Black-faced Babbler *Turdoides
melanops*
Black-throated Grass-(Parson-)
Finch *Poephila cincta*
Blackbird (Common) *Merula merula*
Bluejay *Cyanocitta cristata*
Blue Tit *Cyanistes caeruleus*
Blue Waxbill (Angola Cordon-bleu)
Uraeginthus angolensis
Broad-tailed (Long-tailed) Paradise
Whydah *Steganura interjecta*
Brown-headed Cowbird *Molothrus
ater*
Brown Tree-Creeper *Climacteris
picumnus*
Bushlark (Horsfield's, Cinnamon)
Mirafra javanica
Canary *Serinus canaria*
Cape May Warbler *Dendroica tigrina*
Cardinal (Creasted) *Paroaria
coronata*
Catbird *Dumetella carolinensis*
Cedar Waxwing *Bombycilla
cedrorum*
Chaffinch *Fringilla coelebs*
Chatham Islands Robin (-Flycatcher)
Miro traversi
Common Bullfinch *Pyrrhula
pyrrhula*
Common Cardinal *Cardinalis
cardinalis*
Common Raven *Corvus corax*
Cowbird *Molothrus aeneus*
Crested Lark *Galerida cristata*
Crested Oropendola *Psaracolius
decumanus*
Crimson Finch *Neochmia phaeton*
Cuban (Grassquit) Finch *Tiaris
canora*
Cutthroat Finch *Amadina fasciata*
Diamond Firetail (Diamond
Sparrow) *Stagonopleura guttata*
Double-barred Finch *Stizoptera
bichenovii*
Eastern Bluebird *Sialia sialis*
European Goldfinch *Carduelis
carduelis*
European Robin *Erithacus rubecula*

Fox Sparrow *Passerella iliaca*
Glossy (Superb) Starling
Lamprospreo superbus
Golden-collared Manakin *Manacus
mvitellinus*
Golden-headed Manakin *Pipra
erythrocephal*
Goldfinch *Carduelis carduelis*
Gouldian Finch *Chloebia gouldiae*
Great Tit *Parus major*
Green Avadavat *Stictospiza formosa*
Green Catbird *Ailuroedus
crassirostris*
Greenfinch *Chloris chloris*
Grey-headed Wheatear *Oenanthe
moesta*
Hawaiian Crow *Corvus tropicus*
Hawfinch *Coccothraustes
coccothraustes*
Hooded Siskin *Spinus magellanicus*
House Sparrow *Passer domesticus*
Jackdaw *Coleus monedula*
Java Sparrow (Rice Bird) *Padda
oryzivora*
Large-billed Seed Finch (Suriname
Finch, Twa twa's) *Oryzoborus
crassirostris*
Long-tailed (Shaft-tailed) Grass-
Finch *Poephila acuticauda*
Magpie *Pica pica*
Melba Finch (Grey-naped Pytilia)
Pytilia melba
Mockingbird *Mimus polyglottos*
Mynah (Hill) birds *Gracula religiosa*
Nutmeg Mannikin (Spice-Finch)
(Spotted Munia) (Rice-bird)
Lonchura punctulata
Orange-cheeked Waxbill *Estrilda
melpoda*
Painted Firetail *Emblema picta*
Pekin Robin *Leiothrix lutea*
Pied wagtail *Motacilla alba*
Pin-tailed Parrot-Finch *Erythrura
prasina*
Purple Grackle *Quiscalus quiscula*
Red (hooded) Siskin *Spinus
cucullatus*
Red-breasted Flycatcher
Erythrosterna parva
Red-capped Manakin *Pipra mentalis*
Red-cheeked (Cordon-blue) Blue
Waxbill *Uraeginthus bengalus*
Red-headed Barbet *Eubucco
bourcierii*
Red Wattlebird *Anthochaera
carunculata*
Red-winged Pytilia (American
Aurora finch, Crimson-winged
Waxbill) *Pytilia phoenicotera*
Rock Robin *Petroica archboldi*
Rook (European) *Corvus frugilegus*
Rothschild's (Bali) Myna *Leucospar
rothschildi*
Rufous-sided Towhee *Pipilo
erythrophthalmus*
Rufous-tailed Weaver *Histurgops
ruficauda*
Siberian Rubythroat *Calliope
calliope*
Silvereye *Zosterops lateralis*
Siskin (Euroasian) *Spinus spinus*
Sky-lark *Alauda arvensis*

Spotted Pardalote *Pardalotus punctatus*
Starling (Common) *Sturnus vulgaris*
Superb Lyrebird *Menura novaehollandiae*
Swainson's (Olive-backed) Thrush *Catharus ustulatus*
Tree Sparrow (Eurasian) *Passer montanus*
Ultramarine Grosbeak *Cyanoloxia cyanea*
Vesper Sparrow *Pooecetes gramineus*
Violaceous Euphonia *Euphonia violacea*
Waxwing (Bohemian) *Bombycilla garrulus*

Weebill *Smicrornis brevirostris*
Welcome Swallow *Hirundo neoxena*
White-rumpted Canary *Ochrospiza leucopygia*
White-throated Sparrow *Zonotrichia albicollis*
Wood Thrush *Hylocichla mustelina*
Yellow-backed (Orange-winged) Pytilia (Red-faced Waxbill) *Pytilia afra*
Yellow-tufted (Helmeted) Honeyeater *Lichenostomus melanops*
Zebra Finch *Taeniopygia guttata*

INDEX

NOTES

NOTES

NOTES

NOTES

NOTES

NOTES

NOTES

NOTES